Fundamentals
of Diagnostic
Mycology

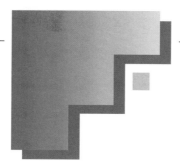

Fundamentals of Diagnostic Mycology

Fran Fisher, M.Ed., M.T.(ASCP)

formerly,
Associate Professor
Department of Medical Laboratory Sciences
University of Florida
Gainesville, Florida

Norma B. Cook, M.A., M.T.(ASCP)

Professor Emeritus, formerly Clinical Education
Coordinator
Clinical Laboratory Sciences Program
Health Sciences Department
Western Carolina University
Cullowhee, North Carolina

W.B. SAUNDERS COMPANY
A Division of Harcourt Brace & Company
Philadelphia / London / Toronto / Montreal / Sydney / Tokyo

W.B. SAUNDERS COMPANY
A Division of Harcourt Brace & Company

The Curtis Center
Independence Square West
Philadelphia, Pennsylvania 19106

Library of Congress Cataloging-in-Publication Data

Fisher, Frances W.
  Fundamentals of diagnostic mycology / Fran Fisher, Norma B. Cook.

  p.   cm.

  ISBN 0–7216–5006–6

  1. Medical mycology.   I. Cook, Norma B.   II. Title.
    [DNLM: 1. Mycoses—diagnosis.   WC 450 F533f 1998]

  QR248.F55   1998   616.9′69—dc21

  DNLM/DLC   97-29245

FUNDAMENTALS OF DIAGNOSTIC MYCOLOGY   0–7216–5006–6

To Leanor D. Haley,
Student and Consummate Teacher of Mycology,
Who Inadvertently Set Our Feet on the Path to This Book
Through Courses She Taught Us Years Ago
At the Centers for Disease Control and Prevention
in Atlanta, Georgia

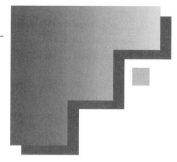

Foreword

At first glance, this is a text written by experienced educators. Each chapter contains tools that will make teaching mycology easier and more organized. From pronunciation guidelines for difficult terms and names to concise objectives, evaluation questions, and answer keys, this book adds immeasurably to the mycology guides currently available. One particularly handy feature is the extensive student laboratory schedule that takes into consideration growth rates, safety factors, and student knowledge gained in the associated chapter. The writers are realists and have adapted the schedules to different time constraints. The well-designed laboratory work sheets will help instill observation skills in your mycology students. From a teaching point of view, it would be difficult to find a mycology textbook that includes so many educator-friendly features as this one.

The usefulness of this text extends beyond academia. As a person who has worked at the "bench" for years, I see within its pages the distilled experience and expertise of its writers. The authors have provided concise yet detailed verbal descriptions of the important medical fungi that read like mini-biographies. These descriptions include up-to-date immunologic and probe testing where applicable as well as lists of organisms with which the fungus might be confused. Accompanying sketches depict ideal as well as less-than-perfect presentations of each organism. The inclusion of a normocytic red blood cell in each sketch makes relative sizes easier to determine. Photographs of the more commonly encountered organisms round out this detailed and practical presentation, which should prove useful to the most seasoned mycologists.

For many years, I have had the pleasure of knowing the authors. Both have graciously served in the American Society for Clinical Laboratory Science and its state organizations in many capacities. They have given so much time and talent to furthering our profession. This book is a just tribute. Within its pages, this text holds a lifetime of information, technical skill, and wisdom in mycology. Students, educators, and microbiologists are most fortunate that these authors decided to share their experiences in such a meaningful and productive way.

Shirley L. Adams, B.S., M.S., CLS(NCA),
CLDir(NCA), SM(AAM),
MT(ASCP)SM

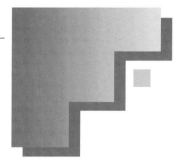

Preface

This book stems from a casual conversation between two newly met colleagues who discovered a mutual interest in clinical mycology combined with shared excitement about teaching clinical mycology and regrets about the lack of a text that combined the features we felt were important. The conversation ended with "Maybe we should write that book" and, several years later, we have. One goal was to write a text for students in the medical laboratory sciences at all levels and for practitioners in the clinical laboratory that presented sufficient basic information about symptoms and infections without the ghastly pictures of "worst case" sufferers that cause the reader to close the book in disgust. We also wanted to present the important facts about fungi most often isolated in clinical laboratories in their usual manifestations, without diversionary treks into the exotic and unusual, in an organized and consistent manner. Our combined 50+ years of teaching have shown us that the contents of any book are without value unless students open it, so we wanted to use a style that was interesting and easy to read. We also sought to include a coherent system for teaching laboratory skills in clinical mycology. Finally, we wanted the reader to acquire a system for identifying an unknown fungus—beyond the simple memorization of facts to pass (necessary) examinations. We believe this book attains these goals.

Fundamentals of Diagnostic Mycology is a self-contained introductory course, complete with detailed laboratory exercises and workable schedules for courses in three different time frames. Each chapter begins with objectives that alert the reader to the important points to follow and ends with related questions, to "Assess What You Have Learned." Answers to the questions are provided in Appendix A. No laboratory exercises are included in Chapter One, providing a breathing space for the student to learn basic concepts and vocabulary, but laboratory exercises tied to the objectives and to the schedules provided are included in each of the remaining chapters. Chapters One and Two should be studied first. Chapters Three through Eight open with a general discussion of the fungi to be studied, including new vocabulary, the types of infections, identifying features, and methods for isolation and identification of the organisms. The theme is to "learn the similarities of the group, then focus on a few distinctive features of each organism," rather than to memorize a daunting list of all the characteristics of each fungus. After the first two chapters are completed, Chapters Three through Eight can be studied in any order; taking them out of order will require adjustments for the laboratories, which present basic skills in the initial sessions and build on these through the course.

The book is illustrated with almost 300 drawings and photomicrographs, most of which were supplied by the authors. Norma learned the skill of photography, and Fran honed her artistic skills by providing detailed sketches for the final creation of the artwork. The *unique feature* of the line drawings is the "GEBEs" (**G**ood **E**xamples of **B**ad **E**xamples), depicting fungi as they are likely to appear in microscopic preparations, which accompany the drawings and photomicrographs of the ideal appearance of the organism. Key features that suggest the identity of a fungus or a group of similar fungi are emphasized in the legend accompanying the GEBE and in the text. Another *unique feature* of the drawings is the inclusion of a red blood cell, rather than the usual metric ruler, to set the scale for the mycotic structures; we believe laboratorians will find it easier to use the red blood cell as a basis for comparison. Composite figures pull similar fungi together in one figure so that their similarities and differences can be compared easily.

Throughout the book important terms are emphasized in the objectives and as they are introduced in the text. Appendix B is the glossary for the book, with definitions as expected, and with pronunciations for all terms and names of fungi. The *unique feature* is the pronunciations, which are written as they sound in English rather than with the esoteric symbols and markings used in standard dictionaries, which many people find difficult to translate into sounds. Pronunciations *"auf English"* are also found in the introduction for each fungus because we believe that talking about the fungi contributes to learning about them, and that students hesitate to use words when they are unsure of the pronunciation.

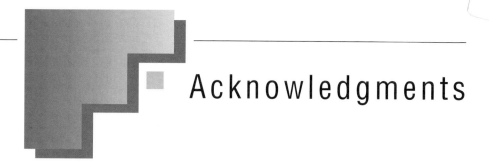

Acknowledgments

Honest authors acknowledge all those who inspired them to start, and encouraged them to finish, and so we do this, beginning with the students who made us learn more of the facts and more of the reasons for things by their questions, and who drove us—in the interest of continued sanity for all—to develop less demanding, more effective ways of serving mycology to them. Joeline and John Davidson, Ron Ferrigno, Maurice and Diana Plemons, Dr. Lawrence Selby, and Dan Southern helped ensure that Norma's photographs became reality. Shirley Adams, Cathy Horton, and Erma Konitsy critiqued the text effectively, but gently. Mary Stevenson Britt did her best to assure the continuing health and sanity of the authors; Donna S. Wanat contributed to the usefulness of the pronunciations in the glossary. We thank all of them now, publicly, as we have thanked them before, with all of the other family and friends who encouraged us when we hit a snag, listened when we whined, and nagged us when we needed it. The last special "thank you" is for Gordon and Stephen Cook, and Russ Bayne, who fed us often and well, and who drove us out to play whenever they could.

Fran Fisher
Norma B. Cook

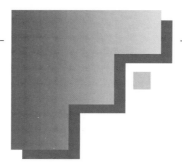

Contents

Color plates follow page xvi.

Color Plates

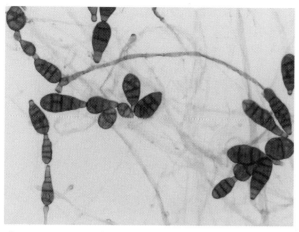

1. *Alternaria* species are difficult to miss because of the dark pigment in the septa, hyphae, and reproductive structures. The conidia are characteristically club shaped, with a few that are ovoid to almost round. They have broad bases and tapered tips with horizontal and transverse septa and are smooth or echinulate. They are borne in chains on septate branched or unbranched conidiophores that become knobby as the conidia are produced.

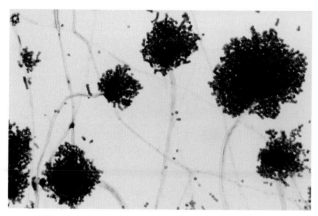

3. *Aspergillus niger* has long, smooth, and usually colorless conidiophores. They may be dark where they enlarge to form globose-shaped vesicles. Two sets of flask-shaped, biserate phialides completely cover the vesicle and give rise to numerous chains of large, globose, echinulate black conidia.

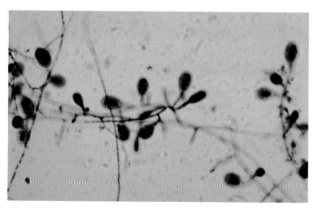

5. *Chrysosporium* species have hyaline, septate hyphae. The ovoid or club-shaped conidia may vary somewhat in size and shape, and they may seem almost too heavy for the delicate lateral micronematous conidiophores that support them. Conidia may also be borne directly on hyphal pedicles. A remnant of the cell wall often remains attached to the conidia when they are released by the fracture of their supporting cell.

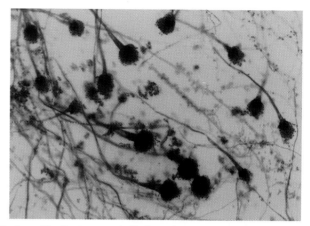

2. *Aspergillus fumigatus* typically has relatively long, smooth conidiophores that gradually enlarge to form swollen club-shaped vesicles. A single row of flask-shaped phialides covers the upper one half to one third of the vesicle and gives rise to compact chains of smooth to echinulate, globose conidia.

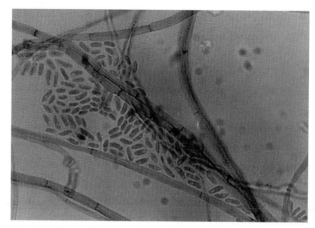

4. *Aureobasidium pullulans* is typically a mixture of two types of hyphae. Microscopic preparations contain large thick-walled dematiaceous hyphae that break up into arthroconidia when mature and thin-walled hyaline hyphae. Cylindrical, hyaline conidia aggregate as they are formed from denticles and other points on conidiogenous cells.

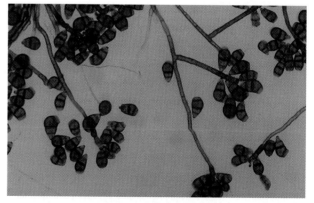

6. *Curvularia* species produce dark curved, multicellular conidia resembling crescent rolls. Conidia develop in a sympodial pattern around dark geniculate conidiophores. Typically mature conidia contain four cells separated by transverse septa. One of the central cells is darker and larger than the others, creating the swollen appearance.

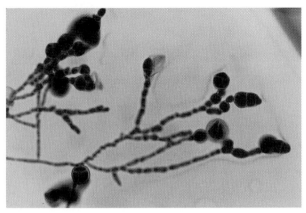

7. *Epicoccum* species have septate yellow-to-orange hyphae that become brown with age. Conidiophores are short and thick, lumpy, and beaded with many branches. In older cultures the conidiophores are clustered together to form sporodochia. The conidia are initially hyaline, round to clavate, smooth, and nonseptate. When mature the larger conidia are dark brown to black, echinulate, round to club shaped, and multicellular with muriform septa.

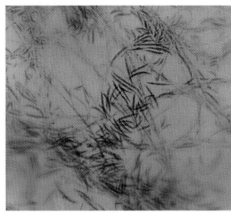

8. *Fusarium* species have delicate septate hyphae. Two kinds of conidia are formed. The microconidia are hyaline, one or (more rarely) two celled, and oval to cylindrical. The macroconidia are hyaline, multiseptate, sickle or cylindrical shaped, and borne singularly and in whorls on branched or unbranched phialides or directly from the hyphae. They have pointed ends and distinct foot cells. Most conidia are free in preparations because their attachments are so tenuous.

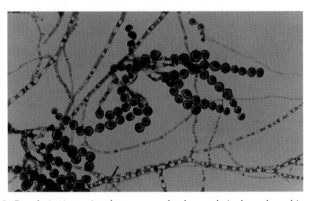

9. *Scopulariopsis* species show septate hyphae and single or branching micronematous conidiophores. The conidiophores support flask-shaped annellides either singly or in groups, or they may form a penicillus. Large globose to lemon-shaped, echinulate, one-celled conidia are formed in long chains. The truncate base of one conidium is attached to the rounded end of the one below it. The denser center of the conidia often stains more intensely than the periphery so that the conidia appear to have thick walls.

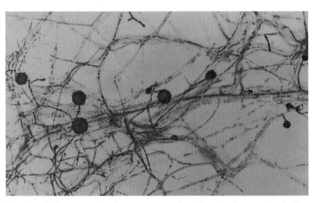

10. *Sepedonium* species have septate, hyaline hyphae and single or branched micronematous conidiophores of various lengths. Conidia are unicellular, globose to ovoid. Typically, conidia in varying stages of growth are present. As conidia mature they develop thick walls that sometimes form tuberculate extensions resembling the mould form of *Histoplasma*.

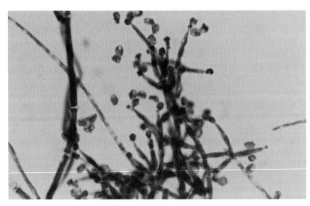

11. *Trichoderma* species form delicate septate hyphae. Conidiophores are erect, single, or branched at wide angles to the hyphae and to one another. Single-celled, smooth, or echinulate conidia are borne on vase-shaped hyaline phialides that are formed at wide angles to the conidiophore. This photograph of a young culture shows the oval conidia developing at the tips of phialides. However, in mature cultures conidia remain clustered in spherical groups.

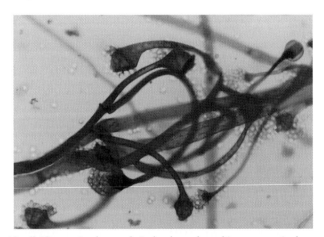

12. *Absidia* species have relatively short, branching sporangiophores that arise in groups of two or more from internodes along the wide aseptate hyphae. Pyriform sporangia are filled with round to oval single-celled sporangiospores. When sporangial walls dissolve, details of the cone-shaped columella, an apothesis, and a collarette can be seen more clearly. Rhizoids may be present, but unlike *Rhizopus* species, sporangiophores arise internodally on arched stolons between the nodes where rhizoids develop.

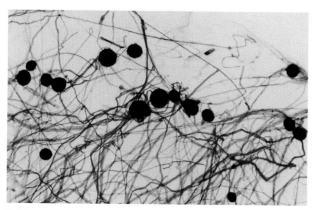

13. *Mucor* species have long, straight sporangiophores that may be single or branched. Sporangia are round and contain smooth, ovoid or elliptical sporangiospores. When sporangial walls dissolve, round hyaline sporangiospores are released, revealing a columella of various shapes with a collarette at its base. Chlamydospores may be present in the wide aseptate hyphae, but rhizoids and stolons are absent.

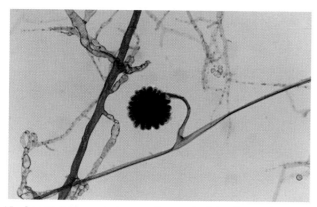

15. *Syncephalastrum* species are characterized by the production of tubular merosporangia that arise from and surround globose to ovoid vesicles. The vesicles are supported by sporangiophores that often branch and are curved. The sporangiospores that fill the merosporangia, like marbles filling a test tube, are one celled and ovoid to round. Rudimentary rhizoids may develop (not shown). The hyphae are sparsely septate.

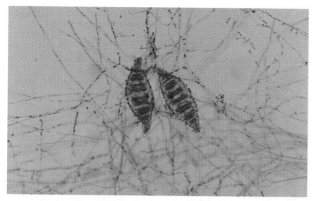

17. *Microsporum canis* produces many large, spindle-shaped macroconidia with pointed ends. They have thick, rough outer walls and contain 6 to 15 cells divided by thin- to medium-width septa. The apex of the macroconidium is often knobby and asymmetrical. Microconidia (not present in this preparation) are unicellular and clavate or pyriform with thin, smooth walls.

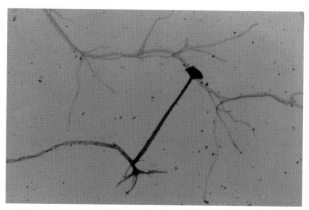

14. *Rhizopus* species characteristically have long, straight, unbranched nodal sporangiophores that arise from arching stolons opposite prominent rhizoids. Intact sporangia are large and round (not shown). The sporangiophores arise singly or in groups of two or more. The columella, as seen here, forms a half circle with a flattened base. Sporangiospores vary with the species but are frequently round to ovoid, smooth to echinulate, and hyaline to dark brown. There are no collarettes. The hyphae are aseptate or sparsely aseptate.

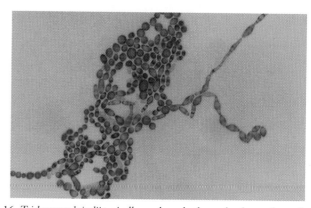

16. *Trichosporon beigelii* typically produces both true hyphae and pseudohyphae. The hyphae are hyaline and septate, and as they mature they break up into arthroconidia. At first the arthroconidia are rectangular, but they become rounded as the hyphae fragment. The disassociated arthroconidia resemble a string of oval beads. Blastoconidia that develop from the hyphae are unicellular and, like the arthroconidia, are found in a variety of shapes and sizes.

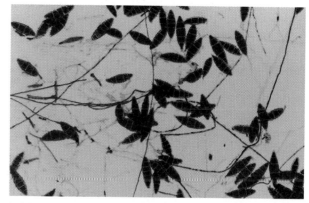

18. *Microsporum gypseum* has septate, hyaline hyphae and produces numerous large echinulate, ellipsoid to spindle-shaped macroconidia. They have relatively thin outer and septal cell walls and contain up to six cells. When present the microconidia are clavate and are produced sessilely on the hyaline hyphae.

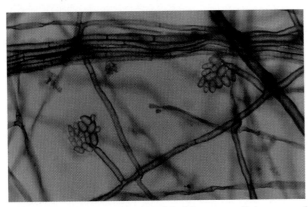

19. *Exophiala jeanselmei* produces black budding yeast cells in young cultures that, with time or after several transfers, give rise to short, dematiaceous, septate aerial hyphae. Micronematous conidiophores support cylindrical or flask-shaped annellides. They are tapered at their apices and elongate as annelations are formed with the production of each new annelloconidium. The annelloconidia are unicellular, hyaline to light brown, and elliptical, and they accumulate in clusters at the tips of annellides.

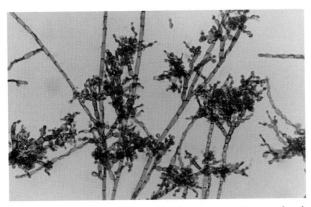

21. *Fonsecaea compacta* closely resembles *Fonsecaea pedrosi*, except that the branching conidiophores and chains of conidia are more compact and are not as easily dissociated; the conidia are more ovoid and somewhat smaller. *Cladosporium*, *Rhinocladiella*, and *Phialophora* types of anamorphic conidiation all may be present. Several mycologists believe that *F. compacta* is a variant of *F. pedrosoi*.

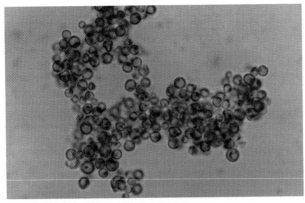

23. *Cryptococcus neoformans* is photographed in a lactophenol–cotton blue stain wet mount. *C. neoformans* is a globose, unicellular budding yeast surrounded by polysaccharide capsules; they may form short chains. They do not produce true hyphae or pseudohyphae. In this very densely packed field, dark-walled budding yeasts appear as large ovoid forms of various sizes that do not demonstrate visible capsules; if present, the capsules are very thin.

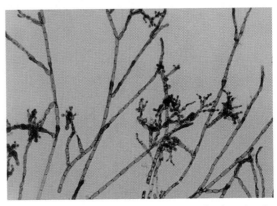

20. *Fonsecaea pedrosoi* has dematiaceous, septate hyphae that branch. This photograph of a young culture demonstrates the early development of *Cladosporium* and *Rhinocladiella* types of conidiation. The conidiophores in *Cladosporium*-type conidiation typically branch and bear short chains of dark oval to elliptical conidia in a finger-like arrangement. Scars are produced on conidia at points of attachment or branching and are called *shield cells*. In *Rhinocladiella*-type conidiation, brown unicellular oval conidia are produced around the top and along the sides of swollen, club-shaped conidiophores. Single scars are produced on conidia and on conidiophores at the point of attachment. *Phialophora*-type conidiation with flask-shaped phialides is not seen in this field; it is the least common type found.

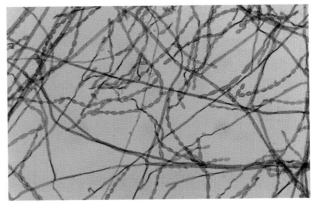

22. *Xylohypha bantiana* produces septate, dematiaceous hyphae. Branched and unbranched chains of oval, unicellular, brown conidia develop in *Cladosporium*-type sporulation. Conidia are borne directly on the sides and tips of hyphae or on micronematous septate conidiophores. The long chains may contain 25 or more conidia that angle away from the hyphae.

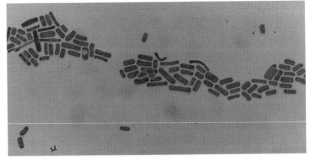

24. *Geotrichum candidum* produces true hyphae. One-celled rectangular arthroconidia are formed by fragmentation of the double-septate hyaline hyphae. The arthroconidia of various sizes are found in chains and may have rounded or square ends after they are released by fission of the septa. They do not form blastoconidia but may germinate from one corner.

CHAPTER 1

The Basics

Upon completion of this chapter the reader should be able to:

Instructional Objectives

1. Define the following terms: mycology, mycosis (mycoses), fungus (fungi), mycelium (mycelia), hypha (hyphae), septate, aseptate, conidium (conidia), spore, holomorph, teleomorph, anamorph, synanamorph, thallus (thalli), mould, yeast.

2. Describe the tissues involved in each of the following infections: superficial mycoses, cutaneous mycoses, subcutaneous mycoses, systemic mycoses.

3. List at least two reasons for the increasing importance of the "opportunistic fungi."

4. State the standard ending for each of the levels of formal taxonomy.

5. Explain why one fungus may hold a position in more than one taxonomic class.

6. Distinguish among the four classes of fungi that infect humans.

7 Explain the differences among vegetative, aerial, and reproductive hyphae.

INTRODUCTION

Mycology, the study of fungi, is easier in many respects than the study of bacteria. Both colony morphology and microscopic structures of fungi are larger than those of bacteria. The field of study is smaller. Rippon recognizes about 200 of the approximately 100,000 known species of fungi as "pathogens" of humans; fewer than 60 species are consistently associated with human infections. By contrast, the family Enterobacteriaceae alone was reported in 1992 to have more than 28 validly published genera divided into more than 112 species. Biochemical studies and differential tests often are not needed to identify fungi. The study of the body, or shape, of the organism—its morphology—usually provides enough information, especially when the patient's history is known.

These facts do not mean that learning clinical mycology (the study of fungi infecting humans) is easy—it is just easier than learning bacteriology. A new vocabulary must be learned—the terms for structures and the names of the organisms—but another blessing is that as a rule the names of fungi change less rapidly than the names of bacteria. Techniques vary, reflecting a reliance on morphology instead of biochemical tests to identify fungi. Equipment varies, a concession to differences in the texture of the colonies and the kinds of techniques used. The time frame for identification also varies, in recognition of the slower growth rate of most fungi. Bacteria can usually be identified in 48 hours; most fungi require at least 5 days just to produce an identifiable colony.

Patterns of mycotic (fungal) diseases differ from those of bacterial infections. Few fungi are transmitted directly from person to person. Epidemics are rare and can usually be traced to exposure to a common source. Mycoses (mycotic infections) occur in someone with lowered resistance or a defective immune system, the compromised host, far more often than in a person who is not compromised. Indeed, Rippon asserts that anyone who develops a fungal infection—unless he or she is exposed to an overwhelming dose—has a defect in the immune system.

Mycology, like bacteriology, is part of clinical microbiology. Its increasing importance is reflected in the increasing numbers of positive cultures. The increase is probably artificial in part, related to improved techniques for isolation and identification and a better system of reporting mycotic infections, but a real increase has also occurred. A critical element in the real increase is the changing practice of medicine to prolong life in more seriously ill patients, which creates a large susceptible population.

Whether the study of fungi is more or less difficult than the study of bacteria is actually a rhetorical question. The competent microbiologist must be able to isolate and identify fungi or know someone who can. Competence does not always mean knowing how to do everything. It sometimes means knowing your limitations and asking for help.

PRESENTATION OF FUNGI

We believe that one of the barriers to the study of fungi is, simply, that the names are difficult to pronounce. If the name is merely a jumble of letters, students find it difficult to remember and use the names, and they hesitate to risk embarrassment by asking questions or using the names. Consequently, a phonetic pronunciation of the name of the fungus is given when an organism is presented, and an appendix provides an alphabetized list with pronunciations of all the fungi in the book. The pronunciations are not based on any standardized dictionary or international system for pronunciations; nor are they necessarily used by all mycologists. We have created the list in the expectation that the pronunciations will be useful. We do not always agree with each other about pronunciations, and we have had several lively discussions about some of them before reaching a compromise. Nonetheless, the pronunciations that are presented are an attempt to make the student's task easier by providing a consistent style for use by those who have no prior knowledge of the field. Inevitably, individuality creeps in, and variations in pronunciation will continue to exist.

A standard format is used in each chapter to present the organisms. Features that are associated with most of the organisms in the chapter are presented in the Introduction, including patterns of infection, characteristics of the colonies and the microscopic structures, and so forth. Following the Introduction, individual fungi are presented. Each chapter concludes with a section called "Assess What You Have Learned"; an answer key is provided in Appendix A. Every chapter but this one also includes specific directions for laboratory exercises. Appendix C provides schedules for laboratory courses of three different lengths. The format for presentation of the organisms, with general comments on each section, follows.

■ **Teleomorph.** Some of the fungi that infect humans have more than one sexual or perfect form of the organism, the *teleomorph,* and others have no teleomorph. The reasons for this and a more complete discussion of teleomorphs are given later in this chapter. The asexual or imperfect form of the organism related to the teleomorph is the *anamorph.*

■ **Reservoir.** The reservoirs are the places where the fungus is found in nature—soil, water, vegetation, or some combination of these. This section also identifies the areas of the world in which the fungus is most likely to be found as an agent of infection.

■ **Unique Risk Factors.** For all fungi, either general debilitation or an incompetent immune system is a risk factor. These are not cited again and again. Unique risk factors, such as a hobby or travel to a particular area, are presented when relevant.

■ **Human Infection.** General patterns of infection for organisms in the chapter are noted in the Introduction. Details of infections with a particular fungus are discussed in the presentation of the organism.

■ **Specimen Sources.** This is a simple list of the sites *most likely* to be cultured. The fact that a specimen source is omitted from this list *does not mean* that the fungus cannot be isolated from that specimen, only that it is uncommon.

■ **Specimen Collection and Handling.** Specimen collection is presented in Chapter 2. When all of the organisms in a chapter can be treated identically, specimen collection and handling are presented in the Introduction. Important reminders, and factors related to a specific fungus, are stated in the discussion of the organism.

Direct examination presents special methods for preparing specimens or special stains that should be used when a particular fungus or group of fungi is suspected. The details of microscopic morphology in specimens are given as part of the discussion of the microscopic morphology of colonies.

■ **Special Precautions.** With every organism, you are reminded that specimens and cultures should be handled within a biologic safety cabinet (an area that is enclosed to prevent the spread of microorganisms to the laboratory environment) with a fan that "pulls" any particles into a filter before the air is returned to general circulation. Certainly this is not universal practice, but it should be. Some laboratorians believe that, since many of the fungi are widely present in the environment, they present little hazard and use of a biologic safety cabinet is unnecessary. Although it is true that the fungus may not be a threat to the practitioner, the presence of the organism in the environment means that contamination of specimens is quite possible. When cultures (rather than specimens) are being manipulated, use of a biologic safety cabinet greatly reduces the chance of contaminating the laboratory with the fungus. Finally, until the fungus grows out in culture, no one can know whether it is harmless for those with competent immune systems or a dangerous pathogen.

■ **Culture Media.** This section is remarkably similar for all the fungi. The chapter introductions include a general discussion of media, and much the same information is provided in abbreviated form for specific organisms. The important variations are in the selective media to be used, if any, and the media for subcultures.

Temperature considerations are also similar for most organisms. The fact that the same information is given consistently about media and temperature should suggest learning the generalities, then focusing on the information that differs, rather than attempting to learn every detail for every organism.

■ **Differential Tests.** Differential tests are not used when identification can be made satisfactorily on the basis of colony and microscopic morphologies. When differential tests are important, they are listed, along with the characteristic results.

■ **Macroscopic (Colony) Morphology.** The basic rules for describing colony morphology are given in Chapter 2 and are applied throughout the remainder of the book. The chapter presents characteristic features that are useful in identifying fungi. Like Koneman and Roberts, we use colony morphology as a practical guide to the group to which the fungus belongs, but the fungi are presented alphabetically rather than by group. The morphology of the colony is often the important first clue to the identity of the fungus; don't neglect a good description, for it makes the rest of the identification process much easier. At best the colony description narrows the list of organisms that could be causing the infection. Unfortunately the morphology of some fungi is so varied that the colony may not indicate clearly what the organism is—but it does provide information about what it is not. The age of the colony, the preferred temperature of growth, the average rate of growth, and the medium used are key facts that allow interpretation of the colony morphology.

■ **Microscopic Morphology.** An attempt has been made to walk a tightrope between providing enough information to make this text useful as a reference and drowning you in details. One feature that is expected to be helpful is the inclusion of a normocytic ("normal cell") red blood cell with an average diameter of 7 μm in every drawing to help readers compare the structures they are seeing with a familiar object of standard size.

The discussion of all organisms but two is accompanied by at least one line drawing demonstrating a good example of the microscopic structures of the fungus and the way those structures fit together. In most cases a second drawing is also provided, showing a good example of a bad example (GEBE) of the fungus. The GEBEs are a sort of reality check, recognizing that we rarely see the perfect example but that most slide preparations contain enough clues to allow at least tentative identification of the fungus.

Direct Examination refers to the appearance of the fungus in specimens. The information is placed immediately following the description of the fungus in culture rather than adjacent to specimen collection, because many fungi look somewhat different in the specimen than they do in culture. Placing the two microscopic descriptions side by side makes it easier to compare them.

Helpful Features for Identification are cited as a summary for each fungus as a quick reference to help determine whether the characteristics of the unknown organism fit the description (and for a quick review before a test). In addition, tables are included in the chapters to summarize important features of each fungus and to compare similar organisms.

Organisms from Which the Fungus Must Be Differentiated are listed. Wise readers will focus on the features that are key characteristics of a fungus rather than cluttering up their minds with every detail.

VOCABULARY AND TERMINOLOGY

How It Is Presented and Used

Kwon-Chung and Bennett describe *fungi* as "a group of nonmotile eukaryotic organisms that have definite cell walls, are devoid of chlorophyll, and reproduce by means of spores" (p. 4, 1992); they also reproduce by means of conidia. The cell walls contain chitin or cellulose, or both. Fungi are heterotrophs ("hetero," different; "troph," nourishment), using many different organic compounds as sources of their required nutrients. Nutrients are absorbed from the substrate rather than digested. Parasites are organisms that grow on or in another host organism and derive benefit from the host. As parasites, fungi are capable of growing on both living and dead organic materials. The fact that fungi are eukaryotes (organisms with a true nucleus surrounded by a membrane) separates them from bacteria. Mammalian cells, including those of humans, are also eukaryotic, which helps explain the problems in developing treatments for mycotic infections. The absence of chlorophyll distinguishes fungi from algae and most higher plants.

In this text we have departed from the traditional approach to vocabulary in which the authors pour out a torrent of new terms in the first chapter. Our intention is to initially present the minimum number of terms needed to begin the study of fungi. Subsequently, as new organisms and structures are introduced, the terminology will follow. In each chapter new terms are emphasized, and those that are essential for understanding are defined. A glossary of terms used in the text is provided as an appendix. In it the pronunciation is given for terms that are important and that seem unpronounceable.

Most fungi are composed of filamentous (tubular) structures called **hyphae** (sing. **hypha**), which grow by elongation at the tips or by branching (Fig. 1.1). Hyphae may be **septate** or **aseptate;** septa are the cross walls in the hyphae. Masses of hyphae form the **mycelium** (pl. **mycelia),** which comprises the colony of the fungus; the colony mass is also called a **thallus.** Mycelia are di-

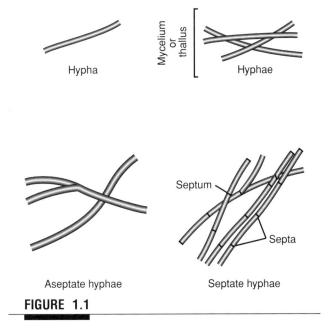

FIGURE 1.1

A hypha *(upper left)* is a single filamentous strand. Fungi of medical importance are more likely to have septate hyphae *(lower right)* than aseptate hyphae *(lower left).* Multiple strands *(upper right)* are hyphae; multiple masses of hyphae constitute a mycelium or thallus, and multiple groups of mycelium are mycelia or thalli. The relative width of the hyphae and the presence of septa are important characteristics for identifying fungi.

vided into three types (Fig. 1.2). The *vegetative* mycelia grow in or on the medium; their role is in the absorption of nutrients from the medium. *Aerial* hyphae grow above the surface of the agar, forming most of the visible portion of colonies. *Fertile* or *reproductive* mycelia are the mycelia from which the reproductive structures arise. The three types are found in one colony and generally cannot be distinguished unless we can determine what function is being performed. The size and shape of the

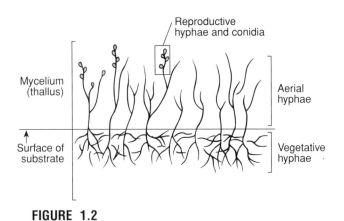

FIGURE 1.2

The vegetative hyphae (vegetative mycelium) anchors the fungus to the substrate. The portion of the fungus growing above the surface is the aerial hyphae (aerial mycelium). The portions of the aerial hyphae that develop conidia or spores are the reproductive hyphae (reproductive mycelium). The three types of hyphae constitute the thallus.

hyphae, and specialized structures that are present, are important in identification of fungi.

Fungi that form hyphae, as most do, are *moulds.*[1] A smaller number of fungi are *yeasts,* composed predominantly of unicellular forms. The thermally dimorphic fungi develop mould-form colonies at room temperature and another form at human body temperature. *Conidium,* in the general sense in which the term is used here, refers to any reproductive structure. Conidium is used more precisely later for reproductive structures produced by an asexual mode; the reproductive structures produced sexually by fungi, and the asexual propagules of the Zygomycetes, are *spores.*

MYCOTIC INFECTIONS

A General Discussion

A normal host is protected from mycotic infection by a combination of circumstances. Fungi generally grow as well or better at temperatures of 25° to 30°C than they do at the normal human body temperature of 37.5°C. They require more oxygen than is available in most human tissues. In addition, the normal host is protected from fungi by the same physical, chemical, and cellular defenses that normally prevent bacterial infections. "Humoral" defenses are those involving fluid-borne products of the immune system such as antibodies. Humoral defenses are not active in most mycoses, a fact that causes problems with the development of serologic methods for the detection and identification of fungi.

The type of tissue(s) attacked by each of the fungi infecting humans is remarkably stable; that is, those that attack the hair or skin usually confine their attention to those tissues and do not move into other areas of the body. Of course exceptions occur, which makes the life of a mycologist (anyone who studies fungi) more interesting. A few fungi consistently attack a wide variety of tissues, whereas most others must have a particular opportunity to do so. The increasing use of invasive treatments and of medications that affect the immune system, as well as the increasing incidence of human immunodeficiency virus (HIV) infection and acquired immunodeficiency syndrome (AIDS), has resulted in a concomitant increase in unusual mycotic infections—cases where the etiologic agent (causative organism) has never before been reported in that tissue, or in any tissue. Nonetheless, most mycotic infections are caused by a relatively small number of fungi that have a track record for infecting humans and, moreover, for attacking a limited number of kinds of tissue.

We can usually surmise the group of organisms likely to be responsible when the source of the specimen is known. Therefore, a *mycosis (pl. mycoses)* is identified by the tissue attacked, and the group of infecting fungi is given a related name (Table 1.1). For example, when fungi attack the muscle and bone, the infection is called a subcutaneous mycosis and the fungi are subcutaneous mycotic agents or subcutaneous fungi.

Five broad categories are used to group the mycoses: opportunistic, superficial, cutaneous, subcutaneous, and systemic. The category in which a fungus is placed is primarily related to the tissue attacked and the severity of the damage or—if you prefer—to how far the fungus penetrates into the body and how much it is able to disseminate. The types of mycoses are introduced here in general terms and discussed in greater depth in the related chapters of this text.

The *opportunistic fungi,* as a group, are "wild cards," infecting a great variety of tissues in compromised hosts when the opportunity appears. They have been isolated from subcutaneous and systemic infections as well as from lesions of the skin. Infections occur in patients who are immunocompromised, that is, whose immune system is not functioning normally. The opportunistic fungi are found in the environment in all areas of the world; they are probably also found in your refrigerator. They have

TABLE 1.1 Types of Mycotic Infections

Type of Mycosis	Tissues Involved	Representative Fungi
Superficial	Outer "dead" layers of skin and hair	*Exophiala, Malassezia, Piedraia, Trichosporon*
Cutaneous	Keratinized portions of hair, skin, and nails	*Epidermophyton, Microsporum, Trichophyton*
Subcutaneous	Muscle, bone, and connective tissue	*Cladosporium, Exophiala, Fonsecaea, Pseudallescheria, Phialophora, Sporothrix, Wangiella, Xylohypha*
Systemic	Any tissue— especially of the pulmonary, lymphatic, and circulatory systems	*Blastomyces, Coccidioides, Histoplasma, Paracoccidioides*
Opportunistic	Any organ or tissue	*Aspergillus, Candida, Mucor, Rhizopus*

The five types of mycotic infections are compared in terms of the tissues most likely to be affected. Examples of fungi that can cause each mycosis are also given.

---

[1]McGinnis considers "mould" as the proper spelling for the colony type that develops when fungi develop hyphae. His terminology has been adopted throughout this text.

the same structural form under all conditions of growth; that is, they are monomorphs ("one body"). Opportunistic fungi are discussed in Chapter 3.

Superficial mycoses are infections of the outer "dead" layers of the skin and hair. Because they don't penetrate into living tissue, they don't stimulate the host's defenses. Little if any discomfort is associated with superficial mycoses. Usually the patient seeks treatment because the infection is unsightly. The four fungi that are most often associated with superficial infections are discussed in Chapter 4.

Cutaneous mycoses are also infections of the skin and hair, as well as of the nails, penetrating to a deeper level of these tissues than the superficial agents. Although cutaneous fungi do not penetrate into living tissue, their physical presence and the metabolites they produce are irritating. The defenses of the host, rather than the fungi, are responsible for the inflammation and the attendant discomfort. Three genera of fungi are primarily responsible for cutaneous mycoses. Since the superficial and cutaneous fungi all attack the hair and skin, some authors have placed them together in a single group of cutaneous agents. Cutaneous mycoses are discussed in Chapter 5.

As we've already noted, fungi that attack the muscle, bone, and connective tissues are designated subcutaneous, and the infections are *subcutaneous mycoses*. Infections typically are the result of a traumatic inoculation that introduces the fungus into the body. A prick from a thorn, a scratch, a cut—any minor or not so minor injury to the skin is a traumatic inoculation. Subcutaneous mycoses tend to remain localized at the site of the injury. Subcutaneous mycoses and the fungi that cause them are presented in Chapter 6.

Systemic mycoses have the potential to affect any tissues of the body. The four fungi that are the traditional agents of systemic mycoses are considered true pathogens; that is, they can initiate infection in people with normal immune systems if the infecting dose is large enough. Because most infections result from inhalation of the fungus, they begin in the lung. The systemic pathogens are endemic (native) to specific geographic areas; they are unlikely to initiate infections elsewhere. People who live outside of the endemic areas must go to these areas to become infected—not that this is proposed as a good idea. One additional important characteristic shared by the systemic pathogens is that they are thermal dimorphs; that is, they have "two bodies," depending on the temperature at which they are growing. Thermal dimorphs have one structural form at room temperature and another form at body temperature. Other fungi, especially some yeasts, also cause systemic infections. Yeasts are discussed in Chapter 7, and the systemic mycoses are presented in Chapter 8.

Classification according to the type of tissue attacked is very useful for the clinical laboratory. If the source of a specimen is known, good decisions can be made about which media to use for primary inoculation of the specimen. We devote a chapter to each of the five categories of fungi that consistently cause human disease. Disease states are discussed briefly in each of the chapters; the primary focus is on the presentation of characteristics that allow identification to at least the genus level of most of the fungi isolated in the laboratory.

CLASSIFICATION OF MEDICALLY IMPORTANT FUNGI

The classification of fungi and the taxonomy of the organisms are entangled with many discussions, much controversy, and innumerable changes. Campbell cites from Kendrick (*The Whole Fungus: The Sexual-Asexual Synthesis* [1979]):

> We are still far from agreement about the ultimate shape of our taxonomic scheme (and about the nomenclature with which to express it). . . . The facts still do not of themselves or by themselves create a system for us. . . . There must still . . . be room for the intuition born of experience, and the often rather divergent ideas expressed in this book show that the boredom born of unanimity and uniformity has not yet set in among mycologists.

This statement is as true now as it was when it was published. Taxonomic classification depends on pigmentation, growth temperatures, the pattern of conidiogeny and/or sporogeny, the appearance of microscopic structures, and other factors. Use of the scanning electron microscope and research into DNA composition and molecular biology—especially antigenic structure—have dictated many changes in fungal nomenclature and taxonomy. More can be expected. Use of these parameters sometimes increases confusion for the clinical mycologist who must rely on characteristics that can be seen with the naked eye and conventional microscopes.

Fungi reproduce asexually or sexually. Some reproduce by both means. Asexual reproduction is called "imperfect"; this is the anamorphic state of the fungus. Most fungi that cause infections in humans reproduce only asexually in the clinical laboratory. Sexual reproduction is the "perfect," or teleomorphic, state. In some species the teleomorphic state is known, but in many cases it is not known. Teleomorphs for fungi continue to be identified. Most mycologists believe that all fungi have perfect states and that these will be detected when the correct combination of nutritional and environmental conditions is identified. Fungi that reproduce sexually have a teleomorph and at least one anamorph. If the teleomorph(s) has more than one anamorph—and many do—the anamorphs are called **synanamorphs,** just as brothers and sisters are called siblings. Strangely enough, one anamorph may also be associated with more than one teleomorph. The complete fungus, the teleomorphs and

TABLE 1.2   Relationship Among Anamorphs, Teleomorphs, and Holomorphs

Holomorphs	
	1st Anamorph + 2nd Anamorph + 3rd Anamorph + 4th Anamorph + . . . = Synanamorphs
	Teleomorphs

The relationship between the perfect, teleomorphic, form and the imperfect, anamorphic, form is shown. Note that the teleomorph and the anamorph together comprise the holomorph. Notice also that related anamorphs are all synanamorphs of one another.

the related anamorphs, is the **holomorph.** Table 1.2 shows the relationship among these three forms.

If the teleomorph is not known the fungus belongs to a group called "Fungi Imperfecti," or Deuteromycetes. When both sexual and asexual states of a fun-

gus are known, the perfect form is usually placed in the taxonomically correct Class and Order, whereas the imperfect form remains with the Fungi Imperfecti. This apparent schizophrenia is accepted because (1) the anamorphic form has a history that must be pre-

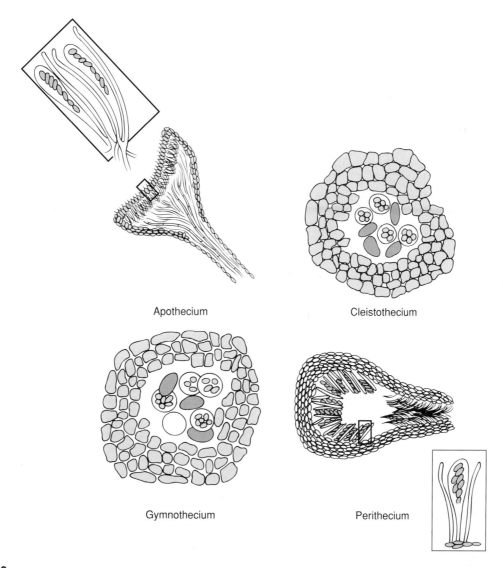

FIGURE 1.3

Four of the five types of ascocarps are shown: apothecium, cleistothecium, gymnothecium, and perithecium. They differ in whether they have an opening and in the ease with which ascospores are released as well as in their size and shape. Asci (sacs) within the ascocarp contain the ascospores. The *inset* shows details of the structures of two ascocarps: the apothecium and the perithecium.

served, and (2) the anamorph is the form isolated from patients.

Fungi are distinctive at both the cellular and molecular levels. They possess an organized nucleus surrounded by a membrane. Meiosis is the process of nuclear reduction and division that results in the formation of haploid nuclei without division of the cytoplasm. These haploid nuclei have half the number of chromosomes found in mature cells. Mitosis is the division of the nuclear chromosomes between two daughter cells (the cells produced from a mature "mother" cell by blastogenesis [discussed later]). Sexual reproduction involves the union of nuclei or gametes through meiosis. Meiosis and mitosis are explained in any basic biology text and are not discussed further.

Meiosis, sometimes followed by mitotic division, occurs in the sexual formation of ascospores within an ascus in the Class Ascomycetes. Some Ascomycetes exhibit free ascospores, and others produce asci within a fruiting body called an ascocarp (Fig. 1.3). If the ascocarp is entirely enclosed, with no opening, it is called a *cleistothecium*. Asci are released when the cleistothecium ruptures at maturity. A *perithecium* is a flask-shaped fruiting body with an opening through which the ascospores can escape. *Gymnothecia* are the third type of ascocarp. These resemble cleistothecia except that the outer walls of the ascocarp are loosely organized so that the asci are randomly released through openings in the walls. A fourth type of ascocarp is the cup-shaped *apothecium*; asci are formed on the inside of the cup. The fifth ascocarp is the *ascostroma*, in which asci are produced in locules (compressions or cavities) in hard masses of supporting hyphae called a *stroma* ("mattress").

Basidiospores are produced by both meiosis and mitosis on short denticles (pegs) on the outer surface of a club-shaped cell called a *basidium*. Fungi that reproduce sexually with basidiospores are members of the Class Basidiomycetes.

In the Class Zygomycetes a round, thick-walled zygospore is formed from fusion of the tips of two compatible hyphae in a zygosporangium. Zygospore production may be heterothallic or homothallic. In heterothallic zygosporogeny two compatible thalli mate. In homothallic zygosporogeny the fungus is self-fertilizing; only one thallus is involved. Fungi that reproduce sexually also have one or more asexual means of reproduction. Ascomycetes and Basidiomycetes reproduce asexually by forming conidia. Zygomycetes reproduce asexually by producing sporangiospores within a saclike structure called a *sporangium*. The reproductive processes are karyogamy (fusion of two nuclei) and mitosis, followed by cleavage of the protoplasm and nuclear material and formation of free cells. Table 1.3 compares the three Classes of perfect fungi to the Fungi Imperfecti. Sexual reproductive structures are shown in Figure 1.4.

Fungi Imperfecti (Deuteromycetes) reproduce only by asexual means, by mitosis. Asexual reproduction involves only nuclear and cytoplasmic reproduction. Most mycologists identify asexual reproductive structures as conidia. The exception that is generally recognized is the sporangiospore produced by the Zygomycetes. Sporangiospores *are* asexual spores produced in a sac, the sporangium, by mitosis.

The unicellular conidia of yeasts are produced by a "blowing-out" or "budding" process called *blastogenesis*. The blastoconidia formed are typically released by fission (splitting); they divide into two approximately equal parts. Moulds with fertile mycelia give rise to a number of reproductive conidia in a process called *conidiogeny*. Conidiogeny is asexual "genesis," that is, the production of specialized reproductive structures. The cells that produce the conidia are called *conidiogenous cells*. Conidia are produced by moulds and yeasts. In some instances the conidiogenous cell *is* the *conidiophore* ("phore," to carry or bear). At other times a conidiophore only supports the

TABLE 1.3 Comparison of Fungi Classes

Sexual Reproduction	Class	Asexual Reproduction	Hyphae
Perfect Fungi			
Ascospores	Ascomycetes	Conidia	Septate
Basidiospores	Basidiomycetes	Conidia	Septate
Zygospores	Zygomycetes	Sporangiospores	Aseptate
Fungi Imperfecti			
None	Deuteromycetes	Conidia	Septate

The similarities and differences among four classes of fungi are shown in terms of methods of sexual and asexual reproduction, and hyphal structure. Three of the four classes reproduce sexually; Deuteromycetes does not. Three of the four classes form conidia by both thallic and blastic conidiogeny; Zygomycetes does not form conidia.

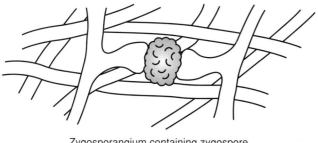

Zygosporangium containing zygospore

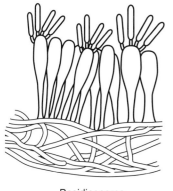

Basidiospores

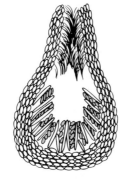

Ascospores

FIGURE 1.4

Three types of sexual reproductive structures are shown: zygospore, basidiospore, and ascospore. A single zygosporangium containing zygospore *(top)* is produced by the mating of two compatible hyphal branches. Multiple basidiospores form on denticles at the tips of the club-shaped basidia *(lower left)* within a basidium. Ascospores *(lower right)* form within asci inside the protective ascocarp; a perithecium is shown.

reproduce by forming one or more of these conidia in addition to producing more specific structures by thallic conidiogeny.

Taxonomy of Fungi. A currently used taxonomy begins with the "layers" of the Kingdom Myceteae and Division Amastigo**mycota** that are common to the medically important fungi. At this point the tree breaks out into multiple subdivisions: classes, orders, genera, and species. We present only those classes, orders, and genera that contain medically important fungi included in this text (Table 1.4). Pay particular attention to the endings of the names (printed in bold type) for classes and orders. The same suffix is always used for a given level; learning the ending is much easier than learning all the other names and where they fit into the taxonomic tree. Another reason to fix attention on the ending is that, in some cases, only the ending changes. For example, Monili**ales** is the Order and Monili**aceae** is the Family. This family tree is included in Table 1.4 to show the relationships among these organisms and to provide a reference during study of the remainder of this text—this is *not* something to be memorized. As each organism is presented, the Class *or* the Family to which it belongs is stated as a reminder of the associations among the organisms.

The genera *Actinomyces*, *Nocardia*, and *Streptomyces* belong to the Kingdom Monera, where they are classified

conidiogenous cell. Conidiogenous cells differ in appearance, in how they produce conidia, and in the changes that occur during conidiogeny. Several different kinds of asexual conidia are produced; they are distinguished by their size, shape, and manner of production. Details are provided as various kinds of asexual conidia are encountered in the study of different organisms.

Conidia are formed in two ways (Fig. 1.5). *Blastic conidiogeny* involves budding or blowing out. In blastic conidiogeny the new conidium begins to enlarge and then is differentiated from the parent cell by the development of a septum in the hypha or cell. Arthroconidia, blastoconidia, and chlamydoconidia are produced blastically. The second mode is *thallic conidiogeny*, pertaining to the mass of hyphae. The young conidium does not develop until after the formation of a septum in the parent cell. Conidia produced by thallic conidiogeny are easily recognized because of the distinctive shapes and arrangement of components. Blastic conidiation is more primitive, sort of the ABCs of conidiation (*a*rthroconidia, *b*lastoconidia, *c*hlamydoconidia—get it?). Many moulds

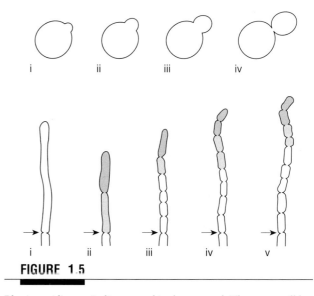

FIGURE 1.5

Blastic conidiogeny is diagrammed in the *top* panel. The young cell begins to enlarge before the septum forms to wall it off from the parent. You see the bud beginning to emerge (i) and increasing in size (ii, iii) before the wall begins to form between the parent and the daughter cell (iv). The alternative, in thallic conidiogeny, is shown in the *bottom* series of drawings. Here the septum forms first (i). After the first septum has developed in the parent cell to create a new cell, the *new* cell becomes a parent in turn (ii). And so on (iii), and so on (iv), and so on (v).

TABLE 1.4 Family Tree of Medically Important Fungi

Kingdom: Myceteae (Fungi)
Division: Amastigo**mycota**

  Class: Zygo**mycetes**
    Order: Mucor**ales**
      Genera: *Absidia*
            Mucor
            Rhizomucor
            Rhizopus
            Syncephalastrum

  Class: Asco**mycetes**
    Order: Endomycet**ales**
      Genera: *Endomyces**
            Hansenula
            Saccharomyces

  Class: Loculoasco**mycetes**
    Order: Myriang**ales**
      Genus: *Piedraia*

  Class: Plecto**mycetes**
    Order: Microasc**ales**
      Genus: *Pseudallescheria*

  Class: Basidio**mycetes**
    Order: Ustilagen**ales**
      Genus: *Filobasidiella*†

  Class: Blasto**mycetes**
    Family: Cryptococc**aceae**
      Genera: *Candida*
            Cryptococcus
            Malassezia
            Phaeoannellomyces
            Phaeococcomyces
            Rhodotorula
            Torulopsis
            Trichosporon

  Class: Hypho**mycetes**
    Family: Monili**aceae**
      Genera: *Acremonium*
            Aspergillus
            Blastomyces
            Chrysosporium
            Coccidioides
            Epidermophyton
            Geotrichum
            Gliocladium
            Histoplasma
            Microsporum
            Paecilomyces
            Paracoccidioides
            Penicillium
            Scopulariopsis
            Sepedonium
            Sporothrix
            Trichoderma
            Trichophyton

    Family: Dematia**aceae**
      Genera: *Alternaria*
            Aureobasidium
            Bipolaris
            Cladosporium
            Curvularia
            Drechslera
            Exophiala
            Fonsecaea
            Helminthosporium
            Nigrospora
            Phialophora
            Wangiella
            Xylohypha

    Family: Tuberculari**aceae**
      Genera: *Epicoccum*
            Fusarium

*Teleomorph of *Geotrichum.*
†Teleomorph of *Cryptococcus.*
This family tree includes fungi that cause infections in humans and that are included in this text; it is not an exhaustive taxonomic list for all fungi or even for all fungi infecting humans. Consider this list as a reference to the relationships among these fungi as you proceed with your studying, and pay careful attention to the endings of the names (shown in bold type) because these show how the fungi relate to one another.

in the Order Actinomycet**ales.** They are fungus-like bacteria that have been tossed back and forth from kingdom to kingdom. The Actinomycet**ales** were traditionally studied with fungi because they are found as the agents of mycetoma (a subcutaneous infection sometimes caused by fungi) and are therefore isolated from the same specimens. Also, certain physical characteristics, such as a slow rate of growth, made them seem more like fungi than bacteria. *Actinomyces, Nocardia,* and *Streptomyces* are now classified with bacteria as gram-positive filamentous rods because of metabolic and cellular characteristics such as susceptibility to antibiotics, procaryotic cell structure, and cell wall composition. We have not included the Actinomycetales in this text because we believe they should be included in the study of bacteria.

LABORATORY EXERCISES

Laboratory exercises have not been designed to accompany this first chapter because we believe it important for you to ease into those exercises after becoming somewhat familiar with the methods described in Chapter 2 and with the vocabulary. Each subsequent chapter does contain suggested exercises, step-by-step plans that show one way to approach the laboratory study of these organisms. Most exercises are necessarily done over two to four sessions separated by days or weeks to allow time for the organisms to grow in culture. In some cases the tasks simply cannot be done in one 3-hour session. Multiple exercises are scheduled for most class meetings.

Schedules for mycology courses of 10 days', 8 weeks', and 16 weeks' duration are included in Appendix C. Each proposed schedule has space for you to enter the scheduled date of the laboratory. The exercises are listed in the first column. The shaded boxes in each row show when a session for the exercise is to be done; numbers in the boxes show which session is planned for a specific day.

The detailed plans contain a list of demonstrations and demonstration materials, the sessions for each exercise, and a list of tasks in which the authors have attempted to weave the strands of the sessions together into a smooth fabric. The printed plans must, of course, be modified for individual situations in consideration of the time, and stock cultures of fungi, available.

Prepare for labs by at least reading the "session" for each exercise scheduled and the task outline for that class. Read the introduction in Appendix C before the first laboratory meeting. Attend to the safety precautions that are repeated again and again. Draw the fungi! And have fun.

ASSESS WHAT YOU HAVE LEARNED

Responses to the questions below are located in Appendix A.

1. Organisms in the Kingdom Myceteae are differentiated from microorganisms in other kingdoms by certain characteristic features. Name at least three of these characteristics.
2. Mycotic infections predominantly occur through two routes. What are they?
3. Name three factors that contribute to mycotic infections or that predispose the host to acquire a mycotic infection.
4. State the standard endings for the following taxonomic groups. Don't be fooled—remember that not all taxonomic groups have a standard ending.

   a. Division
   b. Class
   c. Order
   d. Family
   e. Genus
   f. Species

5. Name the five broad categories used to group "mycoses" and the specific tissues affected in each type of mycosis.

For questions 6 through 12, **MATCH** the definition **(lettered)** with the term **(numbered).** NOTE: Some responses may not be used.

6. aseptate
7. conidiogenous cell
8. etiologic agent
9. hyphae
10. mycelium
11. mycosis
12. spore

   a. cell from which conidia are produced
   b. fungal infection
   c. fungus causing the infection
   d. mass of hyphae
   e. reproductive structures produced asexually
   f. reproductive structures produced sexually
   g. tubular structures comprising mould-form growth of fungi
   h. with cross walls
   i. without cross walls

13. Name the three types of hyphae. Describe and define each type.
14. Describe the relationship among anamorphs, teleomorphs, synanamorphs, and holomorphs. What taxonomic Class(es) of fungi is (are) associated with each of the -morphs?
15. What is the difference between a truly pathogenic fungus and an opportunistic fungus?
16. Explain how a fungus may hold a position in more than one taxonomic Class and why this occurs.
17. BONUS: What blood cell is included in drawings in the text as a basis for comparing the size of mycotic cells and structures? What is its diameter?

Morphology and Methods

Instructional Objectives

1. Define the following terms: antimicrobial, antimycotic, antibiotic, selective medium, saprobe, dematiaceous, moniliaceous, hyaline, rapid grower, intermediate grower, slow grower, obverse, texture, glabrous, velvety, yeastlike, cottony, granular, topography, rugose, crateriform, cerebriform, verrucose, anergic.

2. Match the mycosis with the kind of specimen that should be collected.

3. Explain in general terms how specimens to be cultured for dermatophytes and for other fungi should be transported.

4. List (and learn to abstain from) behaviors that are banned from the mycology laboratory for reasons of safety.

5. Describe procedures that keep the laboratory clean and prevent cross-contamination of cultures, specimens, and people.

6. Explain how to clean up after a "lab accident."

7. State the advantages and disadvantages of using test tubes and Petri dishes for fungal cultures.

8. Explain why direct examination should always be done of specimens to be cultured for fungi (if sufficient material is available).

9. Describe, in general terms, appropriate methods for processing tissues; mucoid, thick, or cloudy specimens; and clear fluids.

10. Outline the general steps in making a wet prep.

11. Explain when and why each of the following procedures should be done:
    a. wet mount (wet prep)
    b. India ink prep
    c. Scotch tape prep
    d. calcofluor white stain
    e. lactophenol cotton blue prep
    f. slide culture
    g. subculture

12. Explain why antimicrobials are added to media for fungal cultures and why such media should always be paired with nonselective media.

13. List the features of gross colony morphology that should always be described, and explain why this is an essential element of identifying fungal cultures.

14. State four conditions that have retarded the development of immunologic methods for identification of fungi and diagnosis of mycoses.

15. Briefly describe each of the immunologic methods used for the study of fungi.

■

SPECIMENS

Specimen Selection. The type of specimen that is selected for culture is obviously dictated by the site of the infection. Table 2.1 shows the preferred specimen for common infections; media recommended for culture and the most frequent fungal isolates for each kind of specimen are also shown. Details of specimen selection, collection, and processing vary among hospitals and laboratories; in recognition of this we have elected to omit the details of specimen handling. Such a discussion would necessarily be general; the important protocols are the ones included in the laboratory in which you work or study. If necessary, more comprehensive microbiology texts such as the *Manual of Clinical Microbiology*, published by the American Society for Microbiology, should be consulted. The subtle aspect of specimen selection is the important one—taking it with as little contamination as possible from the area most likely to yield a positive culture. Selecting the specimen, collecting it at the appropriate stage of the infection, and obtaining an adequate quantity all are critical to the quality of the specimen. The quality of the specimen is the key element in ensuring that the agent of the infection is isolated and identified. "Garbage in, garbage out" does not apply solely to using computers.

To culture *dermatophyte infections of the skin*, the edge of the lesion—not the center—should be scraped for culture after the skin surrounding the lesion has been thoroughly scrubbed with alcohol sponges to disinfect it. In *nail infections* the tip of the nail is disinfected before the surface is scraped; the debris at the rim is discarded, but deeper material should be collected for culture. In *hair infections* collection of large masses of hair, or even entire hairs, is unnecessary. Instead, the base of infected hairs should be collected by clipping or plucking the hairs.

Exudate (drainage from the site) is the most important specimen from *abscesses and other subcutaneous infections*. If tissue clipped from the edge or base of the infection is to be cultured, it should be transported and cultured separately.

In *systemic infections* and suspected cryptococcoses, multiple specimens may be cultured. Sputa and other res-

TABLE 2.1 Specimen Selection

The quality of the specimen is the key element in ensuring that the agent of the infection will be isolated and identified.

Type (Site) of Infection	Specimen(s) to Collect	Recommended Media	Probable Agents	Notes
Central nervous system	Cerebrospinal fluid	BHI and SABHI, with and without blood	*Cryptococcus*	Filter or centrifuge the cerebrospinal fluid; use the filtrate or sediment to inoculate culture media
Eye	Corneal scrapings, discharge from the eye	SDA with and without antimicrobials	*Fusarium* and other opportunistic pathogens	
Fungemia	Blood, bone marrow	BHIA or BHIB in biphasic bottles or specialized containers for lysis-centrifugation or automated methods	*Aspergillus, Candida, Histoplasma, Torulopsis*	
Hair	Intact hairs, especially the base of the hair shaft	SDA with antimicrobials, DTM	Dermatophytes Cutaneous fungi	Use KOH or KOH with stain to clear the specimen before examining it
Mucocutaneous tissues of mouth and nose	Scrapings of affected areas	SDA and SABHI, with and without antimicrobials and with and without blood	*Blastomyces Paracoccidioides*	
Nails	Scrapings of the surface and the underside of the nail	SDA with antimicrobials, DTM	Dermatophytes *Candida*	Use KOH or KOH with stain to clear the specimen before examining it
Respiratory system	Sputa, bronchial washings, transtracheal aspirate, biopsied tissue	SDA with and without antimicrobials, SABHI with and without antimicrobials	Systemic fungi Yeast	
Skin	Scrapings from rim of lesions	SDA with antimicrobials, DTM	Dermatophytes Cutaneous fungi	Use KOH or KOH with stain *if necessary* to clear the specimen before examining it
Subcutaneous lesions	Aspirates, tissue from wall and base of lesion	SDA with and without antimicrobials, SABHI with and without antimicrobials	Subcutaneous fungi	Look for "granules" in aspirates and drainage from lesions
Urinary tract infections	Urine	SDA with and without antimicrobials, SABHI with and without antimicrobials	*Candida Torulopsis* Systemic fungi	Filter or centrifuge the urine; use the filtrate or sediment to inoculate culture media
Vaginal infections	Vaginal discharge	SDA	Yeast	

A *general* guide to specimen selection is presented here for quick reference. Consult your procedure manual or a reference text for a more detailed discussion before actually attempting specimen collection and before advising anyone else about proper specimen collection.

SDA, modified Sabouraud's dextrose agar; BHI, brain-heart infusion agar (A) or broth (B); SABHI, combination of SDA and BHI; KOH, potassium hydroxide; DTM, dermatophyte test medium.

piratory secretions are obvious specimens since the systemic mycoses almost always begin with a pulmonary infection. The sputum should be a "deep-cough" or induced specimen to ensure as much as possible that the agent of the infection will be found. Urine should also be collected, and the sediment should be cultured; a speci-

men collected in the early morning is preferred. Cerebrospinal fluid and blood cultures may also be requested.

Histoplasma capsulatum is found in the blood in some stages of disease and in some kinds of infections. Because the fungus is an intracellular pathogen, smears and cultures should be collected from the *buffy coat* (the layer of leukocytes and platelets found at the interface between the plasma and the red blood cell mass when blood is centrifuged or allowed to settle). The buffy coat is most likely to yield positive results.

Specimen Collection. In most settings laboratory personnel are unlikely to be expected to collect any specimens except blood cultures, hair, skin, or nails. Nonetheless, nurses and physicians reasonably expect laboratory personnel to know *how* specimens should be collected. An obvious critical element of specimen collection is disinfection of the area surrounding the infection so that the smallest possible amount of normal flora is included in the specimen. The general process is to remove any crusts or debris from the lesion, then scrub the surrounding skin thoroughly with soap and water followed by a disinfectant scrub before the specimen is obtained. Nails are treated in the same fashion; hair cannot really be disinfected, although exposed skin surrounding the culture site can be scrubbed.

Laboratory personnel are also occasionally asked to be present when bone marrow, cerebrospinal fluid, tissue biopsies, or aspirates from subcutaneous mycoses are collected so that the specimen can literally be plated immediately. The possible variations in these processes due to the site being cultured, the suspected organisms, and the systems used in individual laboratories make it impossible to give detailed procedures here. Every laboratory should consider the possibility that such a request will be made and develop a general protocol because the request, when it comes, is almost always for immediate action. Prepare ahead of time by determining the supplies that should be included in a kit that can be taken to the patient's bedside, media that may be required, and, perhaps most important, what steps can be taken to provide the maximum assurance that cultures are inoculated without contamination. Smears should also be prepared for microscopic examination. Finally, remember that you are likely to be the resident authority as to what can and cannot be done to ensure reliable results from the smears and cultures.

With one exception, specimens are placed in sterile dry containers and transported as rapidly as possible to the laboratory. The exception is a specimen of hair, skin, or nail to be cultured for dermatophytes. These can be placed between two clean glass slides, wrapped in paper, and fastened securely together with a rubber band. Alternatively, the material to be cultured can be placed on a piece of bibulous paper or stationery that is then folded into a packet in such a way as to keep the specimen from spilling out and placed in an envelope for transport. Any urgency in transporting these specimens is occasioned by the need to get the culture started; the organisms survive several days to several weeks within the specimen in the transport container as long as it remains dry.

Specimen Processing. This is discussed briefly in relation to the fungus when it is important. We have elected to omit detailed protocols for collection and processing. Instead, consult the procedure manual for your laboratory or a more comprehensive microbiology text.

SAFETY PROCEDURES

Precautions to Provide a Safe Working Environment

The standard laboratory precautions taken in a hospital microbiology laboratory apply when work is being done with fungi. Accidental exposure to fungi in the laboratory may occur by inhalation of airborne conidia or ingestion of the conidia when pipetting by mouth is done or because handwashing procedures were not followed. Fungi can also be introduced through broken or cracked skin; lesions should always be covered with a bandage even when surgical gloves are worn. Smoking, eating, drinking, applying makeup, and storing food are all *verboten!* Mouth pipetting is also prohibited, of course. People who wear contact lenses should not remove or clean the lenses in the laboratory; ideally contacts should not be worn in the laboratory or should be worn with safety glasses. All people working in the mycology laboratory should receive training in safety precautions and a written manual of safety procedures. Universal precautions, instituted to prevent infections with hepatitis B virus and human immunodeficiency virus, should be used in the study of fungi in both medical laboratories and school laboratories. *Handwashing* is a universal precaution that cannot be overemphasized.

Laboratory professionals must assume responsibility for the safety of everyone who enters the mycology laboratory, including housekeeping and maintenance personnel, physicians, house staff, and clerical workers.

Examine all moulds in a certified biologic safety cabinet or laminar flow hood of Class II or III to help prevent infections and avoid laboratory contamination. Yeast cultures can be treated like bacterial cultures, but care should always be taken to prevent aerosols and to dispose of contaminated needles, blades, or glassware properly.

The work area should be cleansed with a good disinfectant daily (or after use) when inoculation of primary cultures, subculturing, and identification procedures are completed to prevent contamination of the laboratory, laboratory personnel, and other cultures. A good disinfectant is one that is inexpensive, nonstaining, effective against a wide spectrum of microorganisms, and harmless to the people using it. Following disinfection the area should be washed with soap and water. Fresh clean disinfectant should be an arm's length away when cultures or specimens are being handled so that spatters and minor spills can be dealt with immediately. If contaminated specimen containers are received, they should be rejected when a new specimen can be obtained. When this is not possible, the container should be wiped with disinfectant before it is otherwise handled.

Containers should be provided for towels and other materials used for cleaning. Some institutions provide lab coats that are changed every day. After use, coats that are obviously contaminated should be placed in properly labeled containers and autoclaved before being laundered. All coats should, of course, be laundered frequently. They should be autoclaved with gas (ethylene oxide) or steam (30 minutes at 15 psi [121°C]). An alternative that is becoming increasingly common is to use disposable lab coats or gowns like those used in the operating room.

Disposable pipettes, syringes, and glass slides should be placed carefully in biohazard bags or containers of disinfectant after they are used. Nondisposable pipettes and syringes should be placed in containers of disinfectant labeled "BIOHAZARD" to be decontaminated before they are washed. Recommended disinfectants are 70% to 95% alcohol, 5% phenol, or 5% hypochlorite (Wescodyne, Amphyll, or Alcide, respectively) prepared according to the manufacturer's directions.

Contaminated needles and scalpels should be placed in a puncture-proof container and properly decontaminated. Glassware and tubes or Petri dishes containing contaminated specimens and culture materials should be carefully placed in biohazard bags—to avoid creating aerosols—and autoclaved. Uncontaminated broken glassware is deposited in strong cardboard boxes and labeled "BROKEN GLASSWARE."

Centrifuges should contain carriers that can be sealed tightly when fungi or material that may contain fungi are centrifuged; these should be opened only in a biologic safety hood after aerosols created by centrifugation have had time to settle.

Glassware and "trash" should be autoclaved for 1 hour at 15 psi (121°C). The process should be monitored with biologic indicators. Intact containers that are being decontaminated before they are washed should be capped loosely to allow free passage of steam into the containers. The mouths of biohazard bags should be pulled together loosely and fastened once with a rubber band so that, again, steam can penetrate into the bags to effect sterilization.

Precautions in Responding to Accidents. No one except the person cleaning up the breakage or spill— a laboratory worker, not housekeeping personnel, please!—should be allowed into the area of the accident until it has been decontaminated. To clean up after an accident wear rubber gloves and a surgical mask. The area around the contamination should be flooded with disinfectant for 1 hour. Don't pour disinfectant directly on the broken glass or spilled material. That can cause aerosols of conidia or spores; pouring at least spreads the contamination around. Spilled liquids and agar and the broken glass should be covered with paper towels that have been soaked in disinfectant.

After an hour, use an autoclavable or disposable brush and pan to pick up any broken glass. Place it in leakproof pans with other disposable materials to be autoclaved. Contaminated clothing should be removed and placed in a tray to be autoclaved. Materials from the spill and those used to clean it up should be placed in leakproof containers (labeled "BIOHAZARD") to be autoclaved. Thoroughly disinfect and scrub any equipment or furniture that cannot be removed and sterilized. Most institutions require an incident report to be made to the appropriate office. A record should be kept in the laboratory, including any injuries that occurred and the personnel involved, the source of the specimen and culture, the identity of the organism when this is known, and actions taken.

If a tube breaks the centrifuge should be turned off *immediately.* After 20 minutes, when the aerosols have settled, the centrifuge can be opened. The containers should be autoclaved unopened, but the caps should be loosened so that steam can enter the containers. The accident is cleaned up with the same procedure used for any other area of the laboratory. Autoclave and discard the cleaning materials.

MATERIALS AND METHODS

Fungus cultures can be done in either Petri dishes or test tubes; each has advantages and disadvantages (Table 2.2). If tubes are used, they should be larger than those used for bacteria (at least 25 × 125 mm) and preferably have cotton plugs rather than screw caps. The larger size is required because colonies of fungi are larger and require more "head room" to develop. Cotton plugs are recommended because fungi require oxygen, which is admitted more freely by the cotton than by a screw cap. The tradeoff is that in tubes that are plugged with cotton the medium dries out more rapidly, so commercial suppliers do not sell media with cotton closures. If the laboratory is not going to substitute sterile cotton plugs for the screw caps—and few are—the caps should be seated loosely after the agar is inoculated to allow as much oxygenation as possible. Caps should also be checked every 2 to 3 days and loosened if they have mysteriously become tight again.[1]

Petri dishes provide a larger surface area for the fungal cultures and an ample supply of oxygen, but they have two disadvantages. First, the agar tends to dry out when cultures have to be incubated for more than 5 or 6 days, as many fungal cultures do. Second, the lids of Petri dishes are readily displaced if they are dropped, jostled, or otherwise handled roughly, which can release thou-

---

[1]The "mysterious" tightening is caused by formation of gaseous waste products as the fungus metabolizes the medium.

TABLE 2.2 Comparative Advantages of Petri Dishes Versus Test Tubes

Characteristic*	Petri dish	Test tube
Surface area	*Large (approximately 7500 mm² for a 100-mm plate)	Small (approximately 1500 mm² for a 25 × 125-mm tube)
Oxygen supply	*Good	Poor
Rate of drying	Relatively fast	*Relatively slow
Security of closure	Poor—lid is easily displaced	*Good
Probability of disseminating the fungus	Relatively large	*Relatively small
Detection of mixed cultures	*Relatively easy	Relatively hard

*Positive characteristic of the container is indicated by the asterisks.
Knowledge of the comparative advantages of Petri dishes and test tubes allows a laboratorian to make an informed choice as to the appropriate container for various uses. Each mycologist must decide what characteristic(s) is most important, and where he or she is willing to compromise, when faced with a specific application.

sands of conidia or spores into the laboratory environment. To prevent drying, humidify the incubator with an open container of water. To prevent lost lids, tape the lid of the dish on or use a special closure (available from Remel as ShrinkSeal Bands, catalog # 52-2600), which is moistened before it is applied so that the lid is effectively shrink-wrapped to the bottom. A third choice is to substitute a 9 × 50-mm plate with a lid that snaps on (available from Falcon as Tight Seal Petri dishes, catalog # 1006) for the conventional 10 to 15 × 100-mm dish. Michael Rinaldi, who is from the University of Texas Health Science Center in San Antonio, recommends these because they have a better surface-to-medium ratio, "almost never dry out," and require less space for storage and incubation. They also have an added safety feature because two hands are needed to open them.

Subculture of a fungus (inoculation of a fresh tube or plate of medium from a growing colony) may be required for several reasons. For some fungi the temperature range at which it will grow is important in identification, or it may be necessary to determine if the organism is dimorphic. Different media may be needed to enhance pigment production in the isolate or to encourage reproduction so that the structures used to differentiate fungi can be examined. Finally, subculture may be necessary to pre-

vent bacterial overgrowth by removing the slower-growing fungus from the original mixed culture and planting it on selective media.

Mould cultures cannot be manipulated as easily as cultures of bacteria or yeast because of the characteristic fuzzy growth that tends to wrap around the needle being used and stick tenaciously instead of slipping easily onto the new culture medium or the slide. One trick mycologists use is a different kind of needle, a *teasing needle*, which is thicker and stronger than the conventional loop used for bacteria (Fig. 2.1); teasing needles resemble the dissecting needles used in high school biology labs. Another trick that is useful when subcultures are done is to remove a bit of the agar along with the mycelium and seat this agar plug in a small slit or a roughened area in the new medium. In doing such transfers it is important to ensure that the base of the culture, not the top, is in contact with the new medium.

An electric incinerator rather than a gas Bunsen burner with an open flame should be used for mycology because of the tendency of the mycotic elements to adhere to the needle. When the needle is heated the conidia (spores) and hyphae tend to sizzle and spatter; some of the "spattered" elements may be viable, contaminating the laboratory environment and personnel. The alternative, if incinerators are not available, is to use beakers containing a layer of sand that is overlaid with disinfectant.[2] The needle is rubbed up and down in the sand to remove clinging bits of fungus before the needle is flamed with the Bunsen burner; the disinfectant controls the mycotic elements until the beaker can be autoclaved.

[2]SAFETY TIP: If an electric incinerator is not available to sterilize needles, half-fill a 250-ml beaker with sand, then pour in enough disinfectant to cover the sand and the debris that will accumulate. Rubbing the contaminated needle in the sand scrubs the clinging mycelium off the needle; the disinfectant inactivates the mycotic elements. *The needle must still be sterilized in a flame;* using the sand simply keeps the mycotic elements from spattering all over the countertop (and you). Autoclave the beaker and its contents.

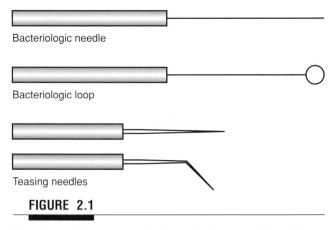

Bacteriologic needle

Bacteriologic loop

Teasing needles

FIGURE 2.1

The wire used for teasing needles (two variations shown) is much heavier and stiffer than that used for bacteriologic needles and loops.

Most moulds can be identified by careful examination of the gross (colony) and microscopic morphology of the isolate, especially if the patient's symptoms and history—including travel and hobbies—are considered. Biochemical tests are not often used for moulds other than to determine if the organism grows better in the presence of certain nutrients than it does without them. Other methods assess the ability of the organism to ferment or assimilate carbohydrates or to decompose certain proteins or amino acids. Some of the cutaneous and subcutaneous fungi do require biochemical tests; yeast frequently cannot be identified by morphology alone, and further biochemical testing is necessary. The methods are introduced in the chapters in which the fungi are discussed and are provided in Appendix D.

MICROSCOPIC EXAMINATION OF FUNGI

Examination of Specimens

A direct microscopic examination should be done of all specimens received for culture for fungi. The methods are not highly sensitive, but the physician and patient deserve a rapid preliminary report of what was seen in the specimen. Sometimes mycotic elements are seen in direct smears and allow diagnosis when the culture is negative. Negative preparations do not rule out a mycotic infection; the smear may have been made from the wrong area of the specimen, or few conidia may be present. Moreover, false-positive results can occur when specimens are contaminated with a fungus during the collection of the specimen or the preparation of the culture and smear.

Nonetheless specimens should be examined directly for fungi for at least two reasons. First, if yeast forms or mycelial elements are seen, the diagnosis of a mycosis is supported, especially if the patient's symptoms are consistent with a mycotic infection. Second, the appearance of the fungus in the specimen may provide clues to its identity before it has had time to grow. This is important for early treatment of the patient, and it helps tailor the selection of media for primary culture. Although it takes little material for direct examination, sometimes there *is* little material; in such instances inoculation of cultures *always* takes precedence over the slide preparations (unless, of course, the patient's physician says different).

The methods used for microscopic preparations for fungi differ in several respects from those used for bacteria. Although mycelial elements and yeasts are certainly visible in gram-stained smears done routinely to look for bacteria, Gram's stains are ordinarily not done to detect fungi. Because the fungal cells are larger than bacteria, dried stained smears of the specimen are usually unnecessary. Instead *wet preparations* (simple coverslipped suspensions of the microorganism in fluid), commonly called *wet mounts* or *wet preps*, are done. Several mounting fluids may be used. All methods are provided, step by step, in Appendix D. A portion of the specimen (or culture) is suspended in 1 or 2 drops of water or physiologic saline, allowed to settle, and examined. A coverslip is always used to reduce the chance of contaminating the observer or the microscope and to improve the optical properties of the specimen. In seating the coverslip on the preparation, be careful to lower it slowly into place to reduce the number of air bubbles in the preparation. Wet preps are examined with the high-power lens; a brightfield microscope, using reduced light[3] to improve the contrast between the specimen and the mounting fluid, or a phase-contrast microscope is used. Do not use oil immersion on wet preps; it is unnecessary and can be messy and dangerous with viable organisms.

Some specimens need special attention before the wet prep is done. Specimens must be handled with good aseptic technique so that they are not contaminated. Clear liquids, such as urine or cerebrospinal fluid, should be concentrated by centrifugation or filtration before they are examined. The supernatant can be saved for other tests. Look for flecks of blood or mucus in cloudy liquids or purulent aspirates because these are most likely to contain fungi; these portions should be included in the slide preparation. Biopsy specimens, other tissues, and nail samples must (preferably) be minced first (cut into tiny bits with a scalpel) or ground gently with a small amount of sterile sand. Mincing is preferred because grinding the specimen sometimes also grinds up the fungal elements if they are large and fragile. Sputa, respiratory secretions, and gastric aspirates usually are relatively thick and mucoid. They should be digested and concentrated with a mucolytic agent such as an aqueous solution of the enzyme N-acetyl-L-cysteine (without added sodium hydroxide), just as they are digested to be cultured for mycobacteria. After the sediment is resuspended in sterile water, a drop is examined in a wet prep.

The most widely accepted wet mount is a potassium hydroxide (KOH) preparation, so named because the suspending fluid is a 10% to 15%$^{W/V}$ solution of KOH instead of water or saline; the concentration of KOH varies with specimen type. Glycerol can be added to the KOH to keep the solution from crystallizing. The KOH readily dissolves most cellular debris without affecting the chitinous cell walls of the fungus. Eventually the fungus will also be dissolved, so KOH preps cannot be kept permanently. Add a drop of KOH solution to a small amount of specimen on the slide—1 drop of a well-mixed liquid specimen is enough. Mix gently and cover with a coverslip. The preparation is examined after the cellular materials have had time to settle. Sometimes the speci-

---

[3]Reduce the light by closing the iris diaphragm, NOT by lowering the condenser!

men-KOH mixture must stand at room temperature for 5 to 10 minutes before the debris is cleared enough for the fungal elements to be visible. An alternative to allowing the mixture to stand is to heat it gently—and perhaps repeatedly—to hasten dissolution of the debris. Do NOT boil it. Most often the fungi appear as yeast forms or fragments of hyphae against the colorless background, but conidia or spores and other fungal structures may also be seen.

The visibility of the mycotic elements is improved by an easy variation on the KOH preparation; mix KOH with blue-black ink or methylene blue stain (2 parts KOH:1 part ink or stain) before adding it to the specimen.[4] *Dimethyl sulfoxide* (DMSO), a penetrating agent, can also be added to the KOH to speed up the digestion of the debris by enhancing penetration of the KOH. DMSO should not be used for hair or thin scales of skin because the specimen may dissolve along with the debris.

Calcofluor white was originally used for fabric and paper to make the whites look "whiter." This colorless dye binds to chitin and cellulose and fluoresces when exposed to ultraviolet light. A mixture of equal parts of 10%$^{W/V}$ KOH and 0.1%$^{W/V}$ calcofluor white creates a solution that will simultaneously clear the debris and stain the fungal elements. A wet prep is done in the usual fashion, and the preparation is examined with a fluorescent microscope. Fungal elements fluoresce "apple green" or white, depending on the combination of filters used in the microscope; usually a dim reddish background is seen. The calcofluor white stain is best for detecting viable fungal elements in clinical specimens.

India ink preparations are wet preps that use India ink (Pellikan brand) as the mounting fluid; nigrosin, an alternative stain, is not recommended because it is less convenient unless large quantities are used by the laboratory. They are primarily used for detecting the encapsulated yeast *Cryptococcus neoformans*. India ink is a *negative stain*, creating a dark background against which the yeast appear to be surrounded by so-called halos—the clear polysaccharide capsules that resist the stain. One way to make an India ink prep is simply to substitute the ink (or a 1:1 dilution of ink in water) for the water used for a simple wet mount; otherwise the procedure is unchanged. An alternative is to place a drop of the specimen on a clean microscope slide and coverslip it. Then place a drop of India ink at the edge of the coverslip. The ink gradually mixes with the specimen, providing a good gradient of intensifying shades of India ink as the background. All of the area under the coverslip should be examined with a brightfield microscope and 10 to 20× magnification. As before, reduce the light.[5] When bright round refractile areas are seen, switch to the high-power lens to look for

the characteristic halo formed by the capsule of *Cryptococcus*. Mononuclear leukocytes can be confused with the *Cryptococcus*. Look closely for the structural detail that is present in leukocytes and absent in the yeast cells. Because of its low sensitivity (it is less reliable than flipping a coin), the India ink prep cannot be relied on as the only screening method but it can be useful. It is more appropriately used as one of the steps in identifying a yeast after isolation.

Stains are sometimes used for direct examination of specimens for fungi, especially tissue specimens that have been fixed and sectioned in the histology laboratory. Fixation involves treating the tissue with a series of solutions to prevent shrinkages or distortion and preserve it for further study. Then the tissue is cut into sections or slices mere micrometers wide so that it can be stained to emphasize details of the structures. *Wright's stain, Giemsa stain,* or *Wright-Giemsa stain* is routinely used in the hematology laboratory for the study of blood films. In mycology one of these is often used to search for the yeast form of *Histoplasma capsulatum*, one of the systemic pathogens, within cells in blood smears or bone marrow preparations. The stain should be used in conjunction with other staining methods.

Five additional special stains can be used to identify fungi in tissue; they are more likely to be used in histology than in mycology. *Hematoxylin and eosin (H&E) stain* is routinely used in the histology laboratory for staining tissue sections; fungal elements are pink to pinkish blue. H&E demonstrates the tissue response of the host and stains some fungi well, but others are not stained or are stained poorly; it should be used with other staining methods. The *periodic acid–Schiff (PAS) stain* uses periodic acid to affect the cell wall of the fungus so that it can take up the carbolfuchsin stain; usually the counterstain is a solution of light green stain. The mycotic elements appear red or purple against a green background; picric acid may also be used as a counterstain, creating a less desirable orange background. The *methenamine silver (MS) stain* is recommended as the best stain for detecting fungal elements in tissue sections. Fungi are black, with paler lavender-gray areas in the center of the cell. Bacteria and *Pneumocystis carinii* are also stained; they can be differentiated from fungi with attention to details such as size, shape, and the internal structures present. *Meyer's mucicarmine (MM) stain* is considered excellent for demonstrating *C. neoformans* in tissue sections. The mucin in *Cryptococcus* stains rose to red; nuclear material stains black and other tissue elements are yellow. Fluorescent antibody staining methods are also available for specific fungi; they are discussed with immunologic methods and in relation to specific organisms. Techniques for these staining methods are not included in Appendix D because the methods of specimen preparation and staining are not usually used in the mycology laboratory and are well beyond the introductory scope of this book.

---

[4]Ink is handy to use but diffuses more slowly than methylene blue stain.

[5]Reduce the light by closing the iris diaphragm, NOT by lowering the condenser!

Examination of Cultures

Microscopic examination of colonies of fungi is critically important, because this is the key to identification of the organisms. Many fungi are identified solely on the basis of gross and microscopic morphologies. Yeast colonies resemble bacterial colonies; they usually can be examined satisfactorily with a simple wet prep. Place a drop of water on the slide, and suspend a *tiny* portion of the colony in it—*just* enough to make the water *begin* to look cloudy. Add a coverslip, wait for the cells to settle, and examine the slide with a brightfield microscope using 10 to 20× magnification and reduced light. Bacteria resemble grains of sand under this magnification, while yeast cells are much larger (approximately 5 to 6 μm, about the size of a normal red blood cell) and more refractile. Again, blue-black ink or methylene blue stain can be mixed with the water to create a colored background, but this is not necessary.

Mould colonies require different techniques. The trick is to make a preparation from the filamentous mass of mycelium without getting it so hopelessly disrupted that no details can be seen and without knocking all the conidia or spores loose from their supporting structures. Most technologists prefer *lactophenol–cotton blue* (LPCB) as the mounting fluid. Phenol in the solution kills the fungus and lactic acid fixes it so that it doesn't shrivel up. The dye is

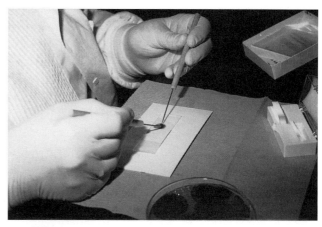

FIGURE 2.2

To make a "tease mount" use two teasing needles to separate the strands of hyphae suspended in mounting fluid. Wear gloves. Use a slow, gentle movement to avoid disrupting the conidia (spores) any more than necessary. Work over a paper towel or mat soaked with a disinfectant.

cotton blue (Poirrier's blue). All of the hyaline elements stain a deep blue against a lighter blue background; *dematiaceous* (brown-to-black) elements are also stained, but the characteristic dark color is obvious. An alternative to the LPCB prep is to suspend the cotton blue in *polyvinyl*

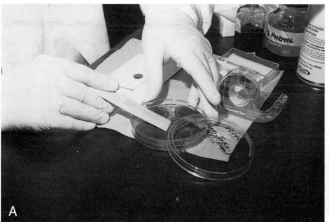

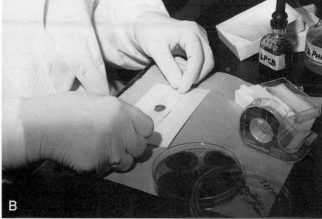

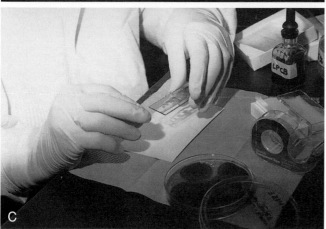

FIGURE 2.3

For a Scotch tape prep *(A)*, wrap a piece of Scotch tape around a tongue blade so that the sticky side is exposed. Touch the surface of the colony lightly with the tape. *B,* Lay the tape, sticky side down, on a drop of mounting fluid on a slide. *C,* Finally, wrap the ends of the tape over the ends of the slide, preferably without "scooting" the tape around in the mounting fluid and disrupting the conidia.

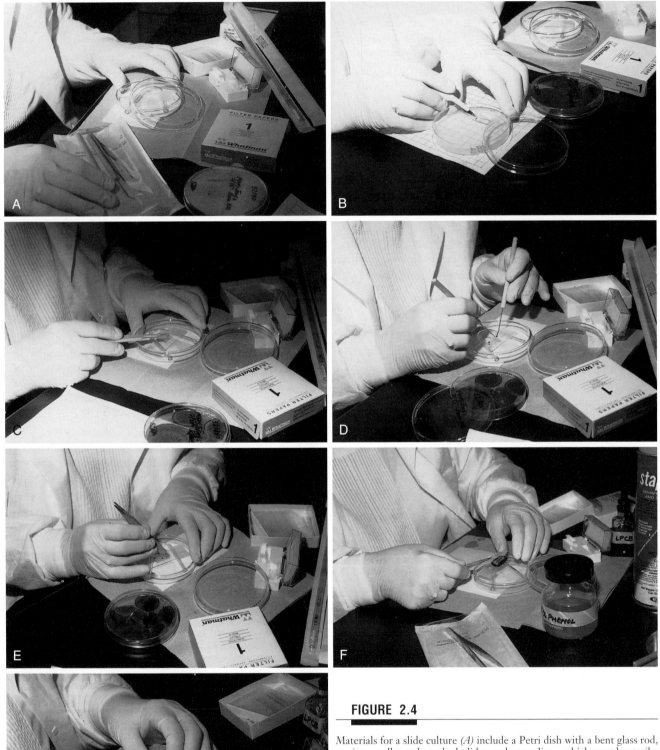

FIGURE 2.4

Materials for a slide culture (*A*) include a Petri dish with a bent glass rod, teasing needles and a scalpel, slides, and coverslips—which must be sterile. *B*, First, cut a rectangular block of agar from a fresh plate of potato dextrose or modified Sabouraud's agar. Then place a sterile slide across the bent rod in the Petri dish (*C*) and transfer the agar block onto the slide. *D*, Touch a sterile needle to the colony being studied and "tickle" the sides of the block with the teasing needle bearing the fungus. *E*, Aseptically lay a coverslip over the inoculated agar to create a "sandwich" and *gently* tap the coverslip so that it won't fall off during incubation. When the culture has grown, gently twist the coverslip to separate it from the agar block (*F*) and lower it onto a drop of mounting fluid (*G*).

alcohol[6] (PVA) to create a *polyvinyl alcohol–cotton blue* (PVA-CB) mounting fluid that also yields blue mycotic structures against a blue background and that hardens to create a permanent slide of the preparation.

Two procedures that are frequently used for examination of cultures are tease mounts and Scotch tape preps. Both should be done within a biologic safety cabinet to prevent infections in personnel and contamination of the laboratory. The *tease mount*, with either mounting fluid, requires as much patience as skill. After placing 1 or 2 drops of the mounting fluid on the slide, *gently* remove a small portion of the colony from the agar and place it in the mounting fluid. Then use two teasing needles to gently "tease" the strands of the mycelium apart (Fig. 2.2). This is a challenge to both ingenuity and patience, but if you are too hasty or rough, you will end up with a muddled mass and have to begin again. Patience is the key. After teasing is completed, coverslip the preparation and examine it microscopically.

Because of the problems with making a tease mount that is usable, many technologists prefer making a *Scotch tape prep*. For the Scotch tape prep wrap a piece of clear cellophane tape (not the "invisible" kind) around a tongue blade so the sticky side is out. Touch the colony with the sticky tape, then lay the tape, sticky side down, on a drop of mounting fluid on a slide (Fig. 2.3). The tape serves as the coverslip. Step-by-step procedures for tease mounts and Scotch tape preps are provided in Appendix D.

Another technique, the *slide culture*, is needed when you can't get enough information for identification from an LPCB or Scotch tape prep. Slide cultures are also useful to make permanent mounts for a study collection or for teaching. *A slide culture should NEVER be attempted if one of the systemic pathogens is suspected.* This specialized procedure should be done within a biologic safety cabinet. A variety of media can be used; potato dextrose agar (PDA) or potato flake agar (PFA) is recommended if you wish to study the reproductive structures of the fungi, because production of these are enhanced by PDA and PFA. The general process is to cut a block of agar from a Petri dish, aseptically transfer it to a sterile glass slide, inoculate the sides of the block, then cover the block with a sterile coverslip (Fig. 2.4). An agar "sandwich" is created, with the slide and coverslip serving as the bread. Slide cultures dry out extremely fast, so they must be incubated in a moist chamber. A Petri dish can be used, with a piece of wet filter paper that helps hold the moisture and keeps the water from sloshing up on the agar. Sterile glass rods, bent in a V shape, can also be used to hold the slide out of the water in the chamber. When the culture has grown enough for reproductive structures to be seen, two permanent mounts can be prepared. "Har-

vest" the culture by carefully removing the coverslip and mounting it on a slide with LPCB or PVA-LPCB. Then discard the agar block from the original slide into a biohazard container. Add a drop of mounting fluid to the growth remaining on the slide. Coverslip it and examine it microscopically. The stepwise procedure can be found in Appendix D. Slide cultures should be inoculated and harvested within a biologic safety cabinet.

CULTURAL METHODS FOR FUNGI

In deciding what kind of container (Petri dish or culture tube) to use for incubation of fungal cultures, mycologists face a dilemma (see Table 2.2). The need to provide adequate oxygen for the cultures and keep them moist is incompatible with the need to protect personnel from infection and prevent contamination of the work area with the conidia that are produced. We recommend using large (25 × 125-mm) glass test tubes with cotton plugs for primary culture media and Petri dishes for the media for subcultures *when you have determined that you are NOT working with one of the systemic pathogens.* Petri dishes can be sealed with tape, or with the ShrinkSeal. Media should be as fresh as possible. The optimum is to make it the day it is used, but this is impractical for most clinical laboratories. Leanor Haley suggested that laboratories that use small amounts of media for examining the morphology of yeast in corn meal agar can purchase or prepare it in tubes, then melt the agar and pour it into Petri dishes as the medium is needed. This process is also recommended for other situations in which small amounts of media are used.

Media for Primary Culture. Ideally, four media should be used for *primary cultures*, the tubes or plates inoculated directly from the patient's specimen. A combination of media is always desirable because it broadens the chances of quickly isolating the etiologic agent of the infection. Emmon's modification of Sabouraud's dextrose agar (SDA) is a general-purpose isolation medium containing 2% dextrose and 2% agar; it has a neutral pH (7.0). We prefer it because it provides the basic nutrition that will support the growth of almost any fungus, and it is the medium most often used for studying fungi. This means that isolates should resemble the pictures and descriptions in texts better than if another medium is used.

When a specimen is likely to contain normal bacterial flora—sputum, for example—antimicrobial agents may be added to the basic SDA. *Antimicrobial* agents are directed at "all" microbes. *Antibiotics* are antimicrobial agents used against bacteria, and *antimycotics* are agents that kill or inhibit fungi. The antibiotics that are most often used are chloramphenicol and gentamicin; penicillin and streptomycin are also used. Cycloheximide (also known as Acti-Dione) is the antimycotic agent most of-

---

[6]PVA is classified as a carcinogenic substance. It should be handled carefully. Work with it within a biologic safety cabinet and avoid getting it on your skin.

ten incorporated into media for the culture of fungi. Cycloheximide inhibits the *saprobic fungi* (fungi that do not harm the host, although they eat dead organic material); most of the fungi infecting humans are resistant to cycloheximide. A **selective medium** is a medium engineered to select for the fungi of interest while inhibiting other microorganisms. Whenever a selective medium such as SDA with chloramphenicol and cycloheximide (SDA + C&C), or SDA with chloramphenicol is used, *it is imperative to pair it with a nonselective medium!*

Brain-heart infusion agar (BHIA) is also suggested for cultivation of fungi; this enriched medium, to which blood can be added, is useful for the more fastidious fungi. SABHI medium, a combination of SDA and BHI, is preferred by some mycologists who believe that it has the best features of each. Antimicrobial agents can be added to both BHI and SABHI. A more specialized medium, inhibitory mold agar (IMA) with chloramphenicol but without cycloheximide, is recommended when the physician suspects the infection is caused by a fungus sensitive to cycloheximide. The combination of nutrients and mineral salts increases the chance of isolating the etiologic agent. Sheep blood agar plates are useful, especially for the isolation of yeast or the yeast phase of the dimorphic fungi. Standard trypticase soy agar with sheep blood can be used, or sheep blood can be added to BHIA.

Media for Subcultures. PDA is the classic medium for subculture when you wish to encourage the fungus to produce reproductive structures and other typical features that help identify the organism; slide cultures are often made using PDA. It is also widely used to enhance pigment production. Rinaldi recommends preparing fresh PFA from instant mashed potatoes to create a medium that is even more effective in enhancing reproduction and pigmentation. Other media used for identification of specific groups of fungi are mentioned throughout the book in discussing the fungi to which they relate. Detailed descriptions of these media, and methods for preparation, can be found in Appendix D. These media are available commercially from a number of laboratory supply houses, either prepared or as the powdered base.

Overcoming Mycelia Sterilia. *Mycelia sterilia*, that is, sterile isolates or sterile hyphae, occurs more commonly with some genera of fungi than with others; a sterile culture produces large amounts of white cottony mycelium and absolutely no reproductive structures. To identify the culture the culture must be induced to produce conidia, spores, or fruiting bodies.

No single medium or set of environmental conditions stimulates production of reproductive structures by all fungi, so a battery of conditions should be used. The basic premise is that unsatisfactory growth conditions kindle conidiogeny or sporogeny. Sterile cultures are transferred to nutritionally poor media such as dilute hay infusion agar, soil extract agar, or 2% water agar (in which tap water may be substituted for distilled water). Other substrates such as moist filter paper, wooden sticks partially immersed in water, leaves, bean pods, or carrot wedges may also stimulate development of reproductive structures.

If a combination of nutritionally poor media and exposure to ultraviolet radiation does not enhance conidiogeny or sporogeny, the isolate is likely to remain sterile, and nameless, in the clinical laboratory.

Incubation of Cultures. Most fungi are moulds when they grow at room temperature (25° to 30°C) and at human body temperature (35° to 37°C). A few genera form yeast colonies whether they are growing at 25° to 30°C or 35° to 37°C. At least five of the fungi that infect humans are thermally dimorphic, that is, they are moulds at 25° to 30°C and another form at human body temperature. Customarily all primary cultures for fungi are incubated at 25° to 30°C; Kwon-Chung and Bennett report better primary isolation of the opportunistic fungi and the dimorphic pathogens at 30°C. If dimorphic pathogens are suspected by the physician, an additional set of media can be inoculated for primary culture and incubated at the higher temperature, but this is not recommended. More often all media are incubated at 25° to 30°C initially and, when a potential dimorphic organism is isolated, an attempt is made to convert it to the tissue (yeast) phase by subculturing it and incubating the new set of cultures at 37°C.

The pathogenic fungi are aerobic organisms. A good supply of oxygen is mandatory if they are to be isolated in primary culture. Generally the moulds produce conidia or spores most actively when they are incubated aerobically. Primary cultures of yeast should also be incubated aerobically, but they are better adapted than the moulds to growth in reduced oxygen levels. In fact, to induce yeast to produce reproductive structures, one method is to make subcultures beneath the agar or coverslip.

IMPORTANT FEATURES OF COLONIES

Conditions of Growth. Each type of colony in a culture should be described. The first step in examining a colony is to record the medium on which it is growing, the age of the culture, and the temperature at which it was incubated. All of these are germane to the identification of the fungus. Age of the culture when the colony is *mature*, that is, produces identifiable conidia or spores, helps categorize the isolate. Age interacts with the medium and the number of conidia in the specimen to affect pigmentation, colony size, and the kinds of microscopic structures present, as well as features such as the texture and topography of the colony.

The type of medium is important because, logically, fungi grow better on highly nutritious media than on poor media, but they conidiate better on nutritionally poor agar. The kind of medium used is also important because fungi grow at different rates on different media, and the rate of growth is a clue to the identity of the fungus. Of course, the mass of conidia and spores in the specimen also affects the number of colonies and the rate of growth. The monomorphic yeasts routinely mature in less than 5 days, usually in 48 to 72 hours.

Moulds are considered to be **rapid growers** if the colony matures in less than 5 days. Most moulds that produce mature colonies in less than 5 days are **saprobes,** organisms that use dead organic material for nutrition and do not harm the normal host (Table 2.3). **Intermediate growers** produce colonies in 6 to 10 days. Many opportunistic fungi are in this group. Organisms that consistently cause infection, particularly the dermatophytes, also belong to this intermediate category. **Slow growers,** as expected, need 11 or more days—sometimes up to 8 weeks—to produce identifiable colonies. Most of the fungi infecting humans, especially the systemic and subcutaneous fungi, are slow growers. For the beginner it is helpful to compare an unknown organism with known cultures of varying ages to assign the growth rate.

Perhaps the most important reason to know the temperature of growth is to get an early clue about the presence of one of the dimorphic fungi. It is also important because some fungi, especially the saprobes, won't grow at temperatures above 30°C. A few fungi are *thermotolerant*, that is, they grow at temperatures above 37°C.

Pigment. After the "where" and "when" aspects of the culture have been described, look at the pigment displayed by the colony. For most fungi the pigment is the same on the front and the reverse of the colony. A few moulds, notably the dermatophytes, have a reverse pigment that differs from the **obverse** (surface) pigment. In these cases, record both colors. You should also note whether the pigment is confined to the colony or has diffused into the medium.

Many of the fungi are dematiaceous, that is, produce colonies with dark olive-green to dark brown-to-black pigment on the surface *and on the reverse* of the colony. Microscopic structures such as hyphae, conidiophores, and conidia are also darkly pigmented whether or not they have been stained. Fungi that are not dematiaceous are **hyaline** or **moniliaceous** (clear) and colorless or pastel.

Texture. After recording the pigment, give attention to the texture. **Texture** is best defined as the way the colony looks as if it would feel if you were bold enough to touch it (but please don't). Texture is dictated by the length of the aerial mycelium and the number of conidia or spores present. This is not a cut-and-dried, either-or feature. The texture of a colony may be intermediate between two definitions. Other colonies seem to have more than one texture, although usually one texture predominates. Be strong, and decide on one term to describe texture. The descriptive terms most often used for texture are glabrous, velvety, yeastlike, cottony, and granular (Fig. 2.5).

Glabrous colonies appear *leathery* or waxy. They have little if any aerial mycelium, and the colony almost seems to merge with the agar. A **velvety** colony resembles plush or velvet fabric, or *suede*. Fungi with velvety (suede) textures have short aerial hyphae of approximately equal length, and few conidia or spores are visible to the naked eye. **Yeastlike** colonies closely resemble colonies of coagulase-negative staphylococci; they are sometimes described as "bacteria like." The difference between colonies of staphylococci and colonies of yeast is that yeast colonies appear drier and duller; no aerial mycelium is produced, but some yeast develop a delicate fringe around the colony on blood agar plates after 24 hours or longer. **Cottony** (synonyms are *woolly, floccose*)[7] colonies develop when the fungus produces large quantities of long aerial hyphae; the hyphae usually become tangled. A few of these colonies may totally fill the tube or Petri dish. Colonies that are **granular** (powdery)[8] are formed by fungi that conidiate or sporulate heavily. Most granular colonies have even hyphae and abundant conidia. However, even a cottony colony that produces large numbers of conidia or spores is granular.

Topography. The **topography** of a colony is the way the colony surface is arranged—its peaks and valleys—just as a topographic map describes the "lay of the land" for a hiker. Infinite variation in topography is possible, and

TABLE 2.3 Growth Rates

Group	Growth Rate (days)	Representative Fungi
Rapid growers	<5	Saprobes Opportunistic fungi Yeasts
Intermediate growers	6–10	Opportunistic fungi Dermatophytes Subcutaneous fungi
Slow growers	>11	Systemic fungi Subcutaneous fungi

The growth rate of a colony is one of the general characteristics that is important for preliminary differentiation of fungi.

[7]Technically, woolly colonies are denser and more matted than cottony or floccose colonies.
[8]Colonies that are granular have a coarser texture than powdery colonies because the granules, i.e., conidia or spores, are larger.

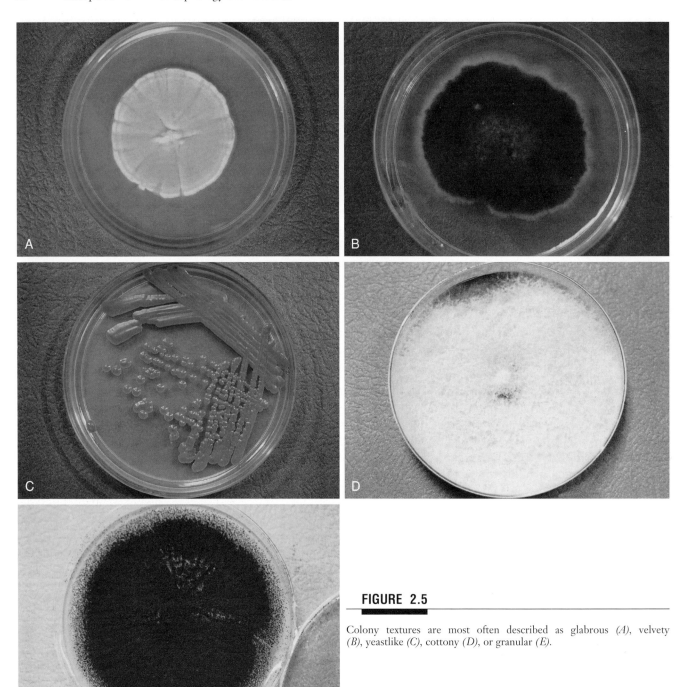

FIGURE 2.5

Colony textures are most often described as glabrous *(A)*, velvety *(B)*, yeastlike *(C)*, cottony *(D)*, or granular *(E)*.

this variation can be matched with lengthy, tedious descriptions. A rational approach dictates limiting the terms to be used to those that occur most often: flat, folded, rugose, crateriform, cerebriform, and verrucose (Fig. 2.6).

Flat colonies predominate in mycology; the form is efficient and requires no extra effort or enzymes from the fungus. *Rugose* colonies have radial grooves that radiate from the center of the culture toward the rim like the spokes in a bicycle wheel. *Folded* colonies have random folds rather than grooves. The folds may be long or short, parallel or at right angles, or in some combination of these patterns. To remember *crateriform* colonies, think of a volcano or the way mashed potatoes are pushed down to hold the gravy. In crateriform colonies a central depression is surrounded by a raised edge. This is probably the least common of the common forms of topography. *Verrucose* colonies have many warts or rough knobs on the surface. Finally, *cerebriform* colonies look like a brain. Some fungi form colonies that are raised, with elaborate folds and convolutions—a distinctive look.

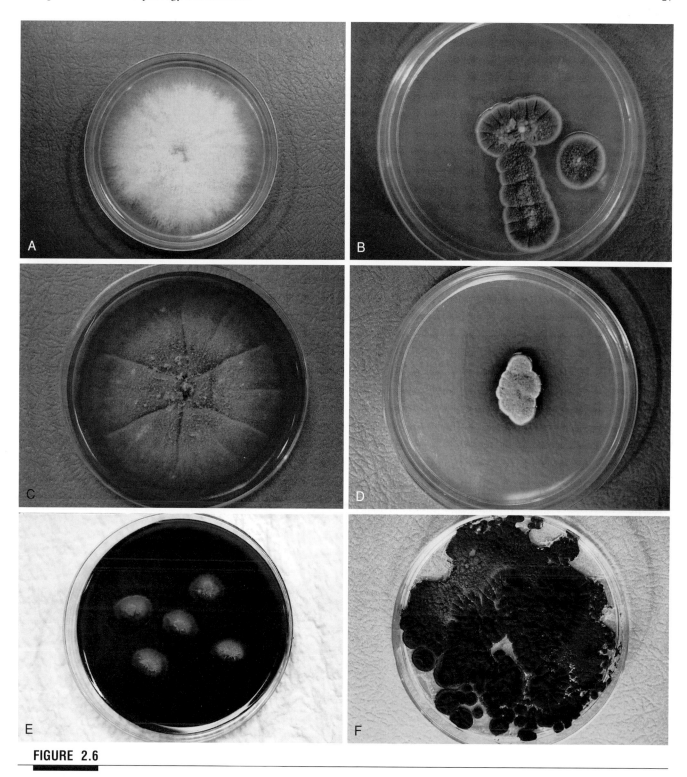

FIGURE 2.6

Topography of fungi describes the surface of the colonies. The topographies most often seen are flat *(A)*, folded *(B)*, rugose *(C)*, crateriform *(D)*, cerebriform *(E)*, or verrucose *(F)*.

Describing colony morphology is a task worth doing well. In doing it, remember the goal—to identify the culture, not to create a prize-winning description. As much as possible confine the description to the terms used here. If you can't do that, at least incorporate these terms so that someone else will know what is meant.

IMMUNOLOGIC METHODS

Even when specimens are properly collected, and the cultures and smears are done flawlessly, they may not demonstrate the agent of the infection. Development of immunologic methods is considered important primarily because most of the fungi responsible for systemic infections grow slowly. In the past, unfortunately, many fungi were identified long after the patient's funeral. The antimycotic agents used to treat infections (except topical agents for skin infections) typically have side effects because they are directed at the eukaryotic fungal cell, and human cells are also eukaryotic. Treatment often combines excision of the infected tissue with administration of antimycotic drugs.

Immunology is probably the fastest growing subspecialty within mycology. Interest in detection of mycoses by their antigens and the antibodies they elicit has existed for a long time but, until recently, technology was too unsophisticated to allow adequate separation and purification of fungal antigens. One problem is that fungi generally are not good antigens. Another is that in many mycoses the fungi are sequestered in one area of the body and do not have intimate contact with the patient's immune system. Unlike bacteria, most fungi do not have weapons that help them penetrate healthy tissues. A third problem, in terms of developing diagnostic tests, is that cellular immunity rather than humoral immunity has the important role in protecting the host against fungi. Finally, cross-reactions occur between antigenically related fungi and sometimes between fungi that are not known to be related. Nonspecific substances in patient sera, such as C-reactive protein, cause false-positive results in certain tests.

Despite the problems, new technology has created the opportunity to develop immunologic methods that can be used to screen sera for antibodies, examine specimens for fungal antigens, and identify atypical and non-conidiating cultures with greater accuracy than ever before. The methods vary with the specific fungus, as much because of the interests of the researchers as the antigenic differences among the fungi.

The optimum procedure is to use a *battery* (array) of antisera for the multiple fungi that are known to cause the type of infection under investigation. For example, in pulmonary or systemic infections all of the agents to which the patient could have been exposed would be sought. Testing for multiple fungi allows detection of cross-reactions. Generally the antibody titer to the infectious agent is higher than the antibody titer for the cross-reacting antigen. *Serial testing* involves testing a series of serum samples drawn from the patient at 2- to 3-week intervals; it permits assessment of the course of the disease. Rising titers generally indicate a poor prognosis, while declining titers suggest recovery from the infection. Serial testing is always recommended if initial tests are negative but the infection persists with symptoms indicative of a mycosis. Using more than one method for antibody detection also increases the likelihood that antifungal antibodies will be detected if they are present. The type of immunoglobulin produced varies with the stage of disease, and different immunoglobulins are detected by different immunologic methods. Table 2.4 reviews important characteristics of the human immunoglobulins.

Patients who are severely immunosuppressed due to therapy for another disease (such as treatment for cancer) or because of the nature of the primary disease (such as acquired immunodeficiency syndrome) may be ***anergic,*** that is, unable to mount an immune response to foreign

TABLE 2.4 Characteristics of Human Immunoglobulins

Immunoglobulin Class	IgM	IgG	IgA	IgE	IgD
Time Produced	First	Second	Third	Last	—
Detected by Complement Fixation Methods	Yes (classic pathway)	Yes (classic pathway)	Yes (alternate pathway)	No	—
Average Molecular Weight	900,000	150,000	350,000	190,000	150,000
Diffusible in Agar Gel	No	Yes	Yes	—	—
Normal Serum Concentration (mg/dl)	85–205	1000–1500	200–350	0.01–0.07	3
Present in Secretions	No	No	Yes	No	No
Precipitation	++	+++	+	No	No
Agglutination	+++	++	+	No	No
Skin Tests	No	No	No	Yes	No
Other	Indicates new infection	—	Suggests chronic infection	Immediate hypersensitivity	—

Knowledge of the properties of human immunoglobulins is important both in interpreting test results and for selecting the appropriate method of detecting the antibody at different stages of infection.

antigens. In such cases efforts can be directed at detecting the fungal antigen in tissues and other specimens. The procedures are generally the same as those used for antibody detection. The difference lies in using antiserum as the reagent to detect the antigen instead of using preparations of antigen to detect patient antibodies.

Finally, cultures of some fungi can be identified by immunologic methods. This may be necessary because the fungus is not producing the structures typically used for its identification or to speed up the identification process in serious infections. Exoantigens are antigens external to the fungus, because they diffused naturally or were extracted. Exoantigen and immunofluorescence tests are the most widely used procedures for identification of cultures. Details of serodiagnostic tests that are currently available are discussed in conjunction with specific fungi.

PRESERVATION OF CULTURES

Cultures are preserved for future reference or teaching; they also can be used as controls. Cultures of significant pathogens should always be saved, especially if they have unique identifications or are rarely reported for the specimen from which they were isolated. Finally, preservation of cultures allows you to recover a culture collection when the working cultures become infested with mites.

Methods of Culture Preservation. Three widely used methods are available to the clinical laboratory: storing in water, freezing, and adding a mineral oil overlay. *Lyophilization* (freeze drying) also effectively preserves most fungi, but the special equipment required is not generally available in clinical laboratories.

Storage in water requires a fresh culture. The conidia and spores are washed off in sterile water and placed in sterile labeled vials. Yeast cultures can be transferred directly to sterile water in small sterile vials that are sealed and stored at room temperature. Subculture involves aseptically transferring a portion to plating media. The detailed procedure is given in Appendix D.

Freezing simply requires labeling the tubes in which the fungus is growing, tightening the caps of the glass tubes, and placing them in a rack in the freezer at $-70°C$. Dangerous pathogens, that is, the systemic fungi, should be placed in crush-proof metal shipping containers, with a label on the outer container, before they are put in the freezer. To subculture remove the tube from the freezer, unscrew the cap, and remove a small piece of growth from the frozen agar and plant it on PDA. Return the stock culture to the freezer before it thaws out.

Mineral oil overlays to preserve fungal cultures simply means layering sterile oil over the entire slant in the test tube, capping the tube tightly, and storing it at room temperature. We do not recommend mineral oil overlays primarily because we have found the process to be less satisfactory than either of the other two methods. Our other reasons are that the process is messy, the cultures are ugly, and subculture produces a nasty, oily mess of mycelium with which to contend.

Combating Mite Infestations. Contamination of culture collections with mites that feed on fungi is a disaster. The mites travel from culture to culture carrying fungi and bacteria on their multiple tiny legs, quickly munching their way through any fungal cultures in the area. Mites enter the laboratory on food, hair, and skin; on clinical specimens; and in cultures imported from a mite-infested laboratory.

The options are to (1) shut down the laboratory; (2) leave on vacation; or (3) discard and autoclave all remaining cultures, then clean the entire area with disinfectant. If cultures must be saved, cotton plugs with drops of naphthalene will kill the pests overnight; the treated culture should then be refrigerated until needed. An alternative is to transfer the mite-infested fungus to a tube of medium containing hexachlorocyclohexane to kill the mites.

If refrigerators or incubators are infected, use naphthalene or paradichlorobenzene to disinfect them. Wipe the surfaces with 70% alcohol, then place the disinfectant in an open Petri dish and leave it for a week. Follow the institution's rules for dealing with hazardous materials to discard the chemicals.

Cultures can be protected from mites by storing them on a freestanding table or bench with legs. Place each table leg in a Petri dish filled with petroleum jelly.

QUALITY CONTROL METHODS

Quality control—the combination of procedures for ensuring that media, methods, equipment, and personnel are performing optimally—is a vital and inescapable component of any laboratory wishing to produce reliable results in an efficient, cost-effective manner. At a minimum any laboratory that is identifying cultures from clinical specimens should maintain stock cultures of viable organisms that can be used for periodic checks of methods. Specific needs vary among hospitals and laboratories according to the scope of the laboratory and the preferences of those who work there. We simply assume that all laboratorians of good conscience accept the basic premise that quality control must be done and refer the reader to the laboratory's procedure manual and comprehensive microbiology books.

SUGGESTED EXERCISES FOR CHAPTER 2

(M o r p h o l o g y   a n d   M e t h o d s)

Exercise 1 (1st Session)

Purpose. To demonstrate the prevalence of airborne fungal contaminants in the laboratory environment—even before the first lab session begins! NOTE that the same procedure could be done in a lecture room, dorm room, family home, restaurant, and so forth.

Initial Process. Select a plate of Sabouraud's dextrose agar from the supply table. Choose an area of the laboratory to culture—the window ledge, a table top, the floor, and so forth. Label the bottom of the Petri dish with your name or initials, today's date, and the specific site cultured.

Place the plate of medium in the selected site in an upright position. Remove the lid and *leave the lid off for the duration of the lab session.*

At the end of today's laboratory session, replace the lid and put the culture in the 25–30°C incubator.

Exercise 1 (2nd Session)

Remove your environmental culture (Exercise 1) from the incubator. Note the number of different kinds of fungal colonies present and describe the gross morphology of two of them.

Make tease mounts and Scotch tape preps of the colonies you described, using the procedures in Appendix D. Make drawings of both fungi, recording the results on separate LABORATORY WORK SHEETS.

Save the culture and the WORK SHEETS. As you learn more mycology you may eventually be able to identify the organisms.

Exercise 2 (Single Session)

Purpose. To acquire more experience in making a tease mount (wet prep), to learn the advantages and disadvantages of the technique and to develop knowledge of the microscopic structures of the saprophytic fungi.

Suggested Fungus Cultures

Alternaria
Aspergillus
Cladosporium
Penicillium

Initial Process. Obtain one of the fungus cultures prepared for Exercise 2 from the supply table. Label it with your name or initials and today's date, and mark it "Exercise 2." The same culture will be used for Exercises 2 through 4 so that the results of the three methods can be compared fairly.

Record the gross (macroscopic) characteristics of the colony on the LABORATORY WORK SHEET, following the example that has been provided for you in Figure C.1 in Appendix C.

Follow the instructions for tease mounts (wet preps) found in Appendix D. Work within a biologic safety cabinet. Be patient and handle the fungus gently so that your first preparation will be a success. Label the slide with your initials and the name of the organism.

Examine the wet prep microscopically, using low power first to scan fields until you find an area of the preparation that appears to have an even distribution of fungal structures and where the mass of hyphae is not too dense. Remember that the task is to see "all" the important structures *and* to see how they are connected to one another.

When you have found a good area of the preparation, switch the objective to high power. Examine several fields. Then complete the section of the LABORATORY WORK SHEET for the tease mount, *including drawings* of the structures and how they are connected to one another. Lay the preparation aside so that you can reexamine it later, if necessary, and so that you can swap your preparations with those done by another student for additional experience (if time permits). Discard the preparations at the end of the day.

Exercise 3 (Single Session)

Purpose. To practice making a Scotch tape prep, to compare Scotch tape preps to tease mounts and slide cultures, and to develop knowledge of the microscopic structures of the saprophytic fungi.

Initial Process. Use the same fungus culture that you used for Exercise 2. Check the characteristics of the colony on the LABORATORY WORK SHEET to ensure that you didn't make an error in recording them *and* to fix them more firmly in your mind.

The instructions for a Scotch tape prep are given in Appendix D. Work in a biologic safety cabinet. Do be careful—the tape has a nasty habit of sticking to your gloves. Label the slide with your initials and the name of the organism.

Examine the Scotch tape prep microscopically, using low power first to scan fields until you find a "good" area of the preparation—one that is not crowded or dense. The task is still to see the important structures *as well as* how they are connected to one another.

Switch to the high-power objective when you have found a good area of the prep and examine several fields. Then complete the LABORATORY WORK SHEET for the Scotch tape prep, *including drawings* of the structures.

Put the Scotch tape prep with the tease mount so you can reexamine it later, if necessary, and so that you can swap your preparations with those someone else made to study if time permits during this session. Discard the tease mounts and Scotch tape preps into a biohazard container at the end of the session.

Exercise 4 (1st Session)

Purpose. To learn how to set up a slide culture, to see how slide cultures compare to the results obtained with the other two techniques, and to increase your knowledge of the microscopic structures of the saprophytic fungi.

Initial Process. Get a slide culture "setup" from the supply table; use the fungus culture for Exercise 2 one more time. Check the gross characteristics of the colony on the LABORATORY WORK SHEET again, even if it does seem like a waste of time—the morphology may have changed since the last time you looked!

Use the instructions for slide cultures in Appendix D. You should be concerned about spreading the conidia or spores of the fungus in the laboratory

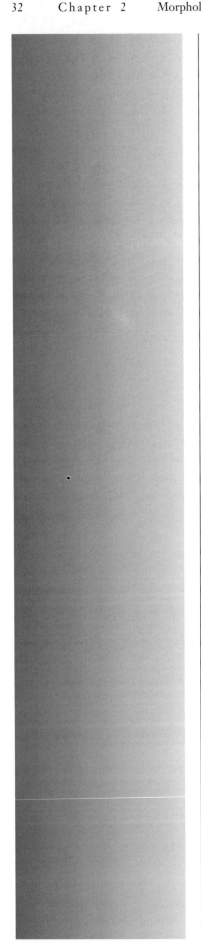

whenever you work with a culture; use the biologic safety cabinet. With a slide culture you must also use good aseptic technique so that the final product isn't a mixture of the fungus and bacteria or, worse, of two fungi.

When the slide culture is done, be sure that the Petri dish is labeled correctly with your name or initials, the name of the organism, and today's date, and place the completed slide culture in the 25–30°C incubator. Record the work you have done to this point on the LABORATORY WORK SHEET. The drawings will be completed during the second session for Exercise 4.

Before the next laboratory session you should check the slide culture every 2 to 3 days and add sterile water if the filter paper appears dry. Put the water on the filter paper *only*—*not* on the slide, *not* on the coverslip, *not* on the agar block.

Exercise 4 (2nd Session)

Retrieve your slide culture from the 25–30°C incubator and examine it. Use a microscope to check the intact culture (on the microscope slide) to determine whether it is mature enough to be harvested. Be **very** careful not to touch the coverslip with the microscope objective—you will not be happy if you knock the conidia off the hyphae and have to set the slide culture up again. This examination process is described in Appendix D.

If sufficient growth is present,[9] "harvest" the slide culture. The process has been demonstrated by your instructor, and the technique is given in Appendix D.

Label both slides with the name of the organism, the medium on which it was grown, and the age of the culture when it was harvested. This information will be important when the slide is reviewed later in preparation for a practical examination or when another of your classmates examines it. Place the preparations in a slide "flat" and allow the preparations to dry before you begin the microscopic examination. Slide flats are the heavy cardboard folders with indentations to hold 10 to 20 slides that are used by pathologists and hematologists. Initially the coverslip is floating on the mounting fluid and is easily dislodged.

Time will be allowed in the next laboratory session to complete this exercise; examining the preparations before they have dried will ruin the slides (and your disposition). After the preparations have dried several days (or during the next laboratory session) you can seal the edges of the coverslips. Then they can safely be examined, and oil immersion can be used without damaging the preparation.

Complete the LABORATORY WORK SHEETS by *drawing each fungus* and labeling the structures.

Exercise 4 (3rd Session)

If you have not already done so, make permanent mounts of the slide cultures of the saprobic fungi by sealing the edges of the coverslips. Be sure that each preparation is labeled properly (which means including the name of the organism, the age of the culture when it was harvested, and medium on which it grew). Put the slides aside so that the seal can dry before they are examined and added to your slide collection.

---

[9]In this context "sufficient" means that conidia and other microscopic structures have developed enough to give you the evidence needed to identify the culture. Synonyms for "sufficient growth" are "mature culture," "ready," "ripe," and "adequate growth."

ASSESS WHAT YOU HAVE LEARNED

Responses to the questions below are located in Appendix A.

1. List at least three general requirements that should be met if specimens collected for fungal culture are to be of good quality.
2. Describe specific procedures for the collection of hair, skin, and nails to be cultured for fungi.
3. What are accepted standards for specimen containers and for the delivery of specimens for fungal cultures to the laboratory?
4. Name four specimens that can be collected to recover the etiologic agents of systemic fungal infections or cryptococcoses. How should each of these specimens be prepared for culture?
5. List five procedures that help keep the laboratory clean and prevent cross-contamination of cultures, specimens, and personnel.
6. Compare Petri dishes to test tubes for culturing fungi.
7. State two reasons for subculturing fungi from the primary plates.
8. Most mould cultures can be identified by observing their _____ and _____ morphology.
9. What elements of the patient history can be valuable aids in identifying the etiologic agent of a fungal infection? (Name four.)
10. Two reasons for always doing a direct microscopic examination of a specimen submitted for fungus culture are:

For questions 11 through 16, **MATCH** the textures and topographies **(numbered)** with the appropriate definition or description **(lettered)**. NOTE that some responses will not be used.
11. cerebriform
12. cottony
13. crateriform
14. granular
15. velvety
16. verrucose

    a. featuring many warts and rough knobs
    b. large number of conidia/spores
    c. long, thin, tangled aerial hyphae
    d. radial grooves from the center of the colony
    e. resembling the surface of the brain
    f. short aerial hyphae of approximately equal length
    g. volcano-like

17. Outline the steps in making and studying a simple wet prep.
18. Name the mounting fluid most frequently used in clinical mycology. State the names and functions of the three main ingredients.
19. Explain when each of the following procedures should be done: KOH prep, India ink prep, tease mount/LPCB prep, Scotch tape prep, slide culture.
20. List four media that are recommended for the primary culture of specimens from which fungi are to be isolated.
21. Why should antimicrobial agents be added to media for fungus culture? What agents are most often used?
22. Name two media recommended for subculture of isolates to enhance the development of pigment and/or conidia.

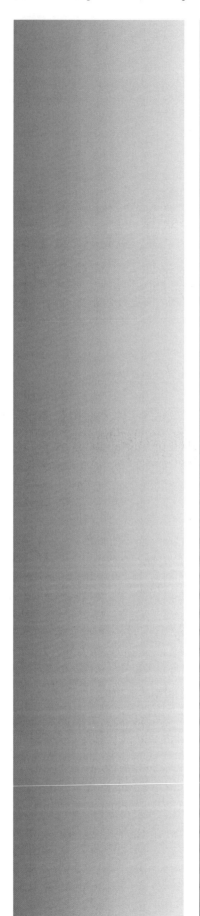

23. What conditions of growth and features of the gross (colony) morphology of a fungus should always be recorded?
24. Define dematiaceous, moniliaceous, hyaline, anergy.
25. List four types of immunologic tests used for detection and identification of antibodies to fungi and two types used for detection and identification of fungal antigens.

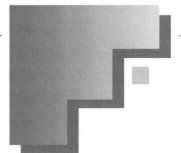

Some Opportunistic Fungi

Upon completion of this chapter the reader should be able to:

Instructional Objectives

1. Define "opportunistic pathogen." Explain why these fungi are increasingly important in the medical community.

2. Define the following terms: apex, apophysis, collarette, columella, contaminant, geniculate, glabrous, hilum, merosporangium, muriform, penicillus, pyriform, rhizoid, vesicle.

3. Compare the following pairs of words: acropetal and basipetal, determinate and indeterminate, nodal and internodal, synchronous and nonsynchronous, uniseriate and biseriate. Explain how they are similar and how they differ.

4. Explain how to judge whether the fungus isolated (presumptively) is the etiologic agent of the infection.

5. Differentiate among the three groups of opportunistic fungi by colony morphology and the presence (or absence) of hyphal septa.

6. List the four types of aspergillosis, and briefly describe how each of them is initiated and the tissues and organs involved.

7. Describe the zygomycoses in terms of the route of inoculation and the tissues and organs involved.

8. Distinguish between hyalohyphomycosis and phaeohyphomycosis.

9. Recognize or describe the distinguishing characteristics of the gross morphology of *Acremonium, Aspergillus, Chrysosporium, Epicoccum, Fusarium, Gliocladium, Paecilomyces, Penicillium, Scopulariopsis, Sepedonium, Trichoderma*, the dematiaceous opportunists, and the Zygomycetes (*Absidia, Mucor, Rhizomucor, Rhizopus,* and *Syncephalastrum*).

10. Recognize or describe the distinguishing characteristics of the microscopic morphology of *Acremonium, Aspergillus, Aureobasidium, Bipolaris, Chrysosporium, Curvularia, Drechslera, Epicoccum, Fusarium, Gliocladium, Helminthosporium, Nigrospora, Paecilomyces, Penicillium, Scopulariopsis, Sepedonium, Trichoderma,* and the Zygomycetes (*Absidia, Mucor, Rhizomucor, Rhizopus,* and *Syncephalastrum*).

11. Use colony morphology and patterns of conidiation (and symptoms of the infection, when relevant) to identify each of the opportunistic pathogens described in the chapter.

∎

INTRODUCTION

"Opportunistic fungi" must be studied because they *can* cause infections, and because they are the fungi most frequently isolated in the clinical hospital laboratory. This chapter presents characteristic features that are useful in identifying these organisms. Like Koneman, and Rippon, we use colony morphology as a practical guide to the group to which the fungus belongs, but the fungi are presented alphabetically rather than by group—with one exception. The fungi that belong to the Zygomycetes are presented as a group at the end of the chapter because of their many similarities. Colony morphology alone is rarely enough for identification of a fungus; sometimes the variation in colony morphology is so great that it only adds to the confusion. On the other hand, microscopic morphology is frequently sufficient to identify the organisms to genus, if not to species. Occasionally biochemical tests must also be done, especially for the dermatophytes and yeast.

Infections in Humans. The fungi in this chapter are called opportunists because they usually infect people who are significantly injured or debilitated in some fashion—diabetics, for example. The improved ability of medical science to keep people with severe injuries or serious disease alive has contributed to an increase in the number and kind of opportunistic mycotic infections.

These fungi—in fact, most fungi (even those labeled pathogens)—are found to be more common in soil or water or on plants than as agents of disease. People sometimes pick them up in passing through an area where the fungi are present and carry them around without becoming infected. The fungi are considered **contaminants** of the individual or *commensals.* Contaminants are present without causing infection; they are transients. Commensals are organisms that live on or in another organism, the *host*—the person, plant, or animal entertaining the commensal—without injuring or benefitting the host. The fungi identified as *opportunistic pathogens* cause infection only when the injured or weakened condition of the host creates an opportunity. Opportunistic fungi generally share the properties of producing mature colonies in less than a week and of rarely infecting patients who are otherwise healthy.

Aspergillus, especially *Aspergillus fumigatus,* is one of the few genera of opportunistic pathogens consistently associated with disease. *Aspergillosis* is the general term for the infection caused by any species of *Aspergillus.* The four leading types of aspergillosis are colonization, allergy, disseminated infection, and toxicity. Pulmonary colonization and allergic reactions to the conidia are induced by the inhalation of large numbers of conidia; they are usually primary conditions, that is, the first infection, injury, or disease. X-rays of the airspaces of the lung may show *aspergillomas* (fungus balls); aspergillomas are colonies of *Aspergillus.* Dissemination of the infection from the lungs to other organs is by the *hematogenous* (blood-borne) route when hyphae penetrate blood vessel walls and enter the bloodstream. Damaged areas of tissue called *infarcts*, caused by lack of blood and oxygen to the area, may occur in distal organs, that is, organs located at a distance from the site where the fungus has established itself. Reactions to toxins contained within cells of *A. fumigatus*, endotoxins, develop when food that is contaminated with the organism is eaten or when large numbers of conidia are inhaled. Cutaneous aspergillosis occurs most frequently in immunosuppressed patients who have had some injury to the skin or subcutaneous tissue. It may also develop in intravenous drug users who use contaminated needles.

The Zygomycetes are the other opportunistic pathogens consistently associated with human disease. *Zygomycosis (mucormycosis)* is any infection caused by one of the Zygomycetes. It is most often initiated by the inhalation of sporangiospores by susceptible people; allergic reactions or infections of the lungs or paranasal sinuses may result. Zygomycotic infections of the cornea, ear, cutaneous, and subcutaneous tissues may follow traumatic inoculation of sporangiospores, and gastrointestinal infections can result from eating contaminated food. In established infections the zygomycetes[1] may penetrate blood vessels in the area, allowing the fungus to spread to other sites. The Zygomycetes (especially *Mucor* and *Absidia*) may also move through the blood as emboli, plugs, or masses of foreign material that affect other tissues, especially the brain. In sinus infections the fungi can move along the nerve trunks to involve the central nervous system. Zygomycosis is a particularly threatening infection because the fungi grow so rapidly that enormous tissue damage can result even if the infection is successfully treated; infections in the sinuses or brain may be fatal. Fortunately, this rapidly progressing or *fulminating* form of acute zygomycosis is relatively uncommon.

Hyalohyphomycosis is a mycotic infection caused by a hyaline mould. The term is largely reserved for infections caused by opportunistic fungi that occasionally cause infection, in contrast with the hyaline *Aspergillus* species, which have a track record for causing infections designated as aspergillosis. The counterpart of hyalohyphomycosis is *phaeohyphomycosis*, the term for mycotic infections caused by dematiaceous moulds that are not consistently associated with infections. Symptoms of hyalohyphomycosis, and phaeohyphomycosis, are similar, whatever fungus is responsible. Identification of the causative agent is important because treatment varies for different agents of both these mycoses.

[1]No, this isn't an error in proofreading. When a family or genus name is used like this, without capitalization or italics, it is being used as a general term to represent a group of organisms—a nickname, if you will—just as you talk about "staph" and "strep" without referring to a particular species.

Determining the Role of the Fungus in the Host. Because the opportunistic fungi are found widely in the environment, reliable diagnosis requires more than simple identification of the organism (Table 3.1). The questions are, "Is the organism an opportunist that is causing an infection? Or is it a contaminant or a normal commensal?" The first step in proving the fungus is *pathogenic*, that is, causing the pathologic condition, is to show that the symptoms are consistent with a mycotic infection. In addition, structures of the fungus should be seen in material obtained from the infected site. The fungus should be isolated in cultures of the infected area—preferably in multiple specimens from the infection. The morphology of the fungus should be consistent with the symptoms the patient demonstrates. Finally, to complete the diagnosis of a mycotic infection and recognize the fungus as a pathogen, it must be identified correctly. Confidence in the diagnosis is highest when mycelial elements are seen in preparations of tissue or other specimens during direct examination and when the organism is isolated from multiple cultures of the infection.

Reproductive Structures. The opportunistic fungi, and most others, reproduce only by asexual methods in routine cultures. The conidia are produced from conidiophores, structures that bear (Greek phoros, "bearing") the conidia. Conidiogeny may occur directly on the conidiophore, which serves as the conidiogenous cell, or conidia may be produced from a specialized conidiogenous cell located between the conidium and the conidiophore. Phialides and annellides are examples of conidiogenous cells. With both phialides and annellides the first conidium is *holoblastic*[2] and each successive conidium is *enteroblastic*.[3] *Phialides* are *determinate* conidiogenous cells, meaning the phialide stops elongating when the first conidium is produced (Fig. 3.1). *Annellides* are *indeterminate* conidiogenous cells that continue to grow

[2]Involving all the cell wall layers of the conidiogenous cell.
[3]Involving only the inner cell wall of the conidiogenous cell.

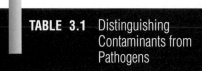

TABLE 3.1 Distinguishing Contaminants from Pathogens

1. Are the symptoms of the infection consistent with the symptoms caused by a fungus?
2. Were fungal elements seen in tissue or other material obtained from the infection?
3. Did a fungus grow in a culture of the infection?
4. Was more than one culture positive for the same fungus?
5. Is the fungus isolated capable of causing the symptoms of the infection being investigated?

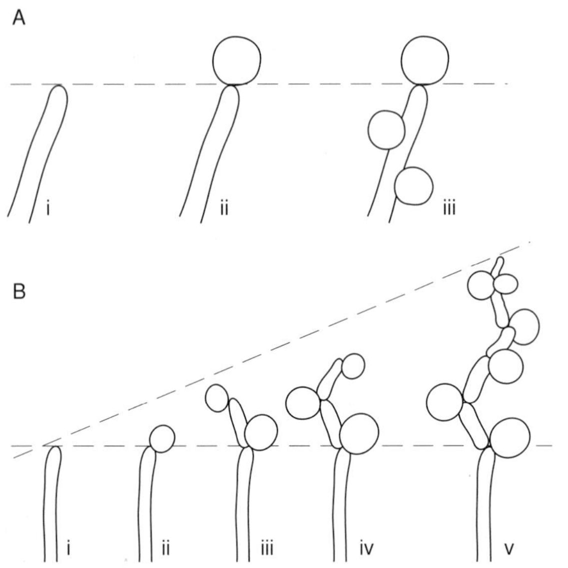

A

B

FIGURE 3.1

As the dashed line shows, determinate conidiophores *(A)* stop growing when they begin to produce conidia. The dashed line shows the tip of the conidiophore in its position without any conidia (i), after the first conidium formed (ii), and after additional conidia formed below the first one (iii). In contrast, *in*determinate conidiophores *(B)* continue to elongate after conidiogeny has started. In *B*, the horizontal dashed line shows the tip of the conidiophore without conidia (i) and when the first conidium was generated (ii); the slanted dashed line shows how the conidiophore has continued to grow as successive conidia were formed (iii, iv, v).

longer as conidia are produced. A ring of the cell wall forms a scar, an *annellation*, at the tip of the annellide as each *annelloconidium* is released. *Poroconidia* are holoblastic conidia produced through pores (openings) in the cell wall of the conidiogenous cell or conidiophore.

In fairness, the kind of conidium or conidiogenous cell usually cannot be determined simply by observation with a brightfield microscope. This terminology is not introduced to make the study of mycology seem enormously complex. Rather, it is included for those readers who would otherwise be puzzled by the different terms used for structures that appear similar.

Characteristic Features of Groups of Opportunistic Fungi. The contaminant/opportunistic fungus can be assigned to one of three groups by the morphology as a convenient first step in identification, in the same way that bacteria are conveniently grouped by whether they are gram positive or gram negative, cocci or rods. The basis for the grouping is the pigment of the colony and the presence or absence of septa in the hyphae.

The dematiaceous opportunistic fungi, both the contaminant/opportunistic types and those that consistently cause infection, are typically **glabrous** or velvety. The pigment is, of course, dark brown or black on the surface and the reverse of the colony (Fig. 3.2). The microscopic structures (Fig. 3.3) of dematiaceous fungi are also dark,

in comparison with the hyaline or moniliaceous fungi. Organisms in the Dematiaceous Group are easily differentiated to genus, and sometimes to species, by the size, shape, and arrangement of the reproductive structures. For some genera the differences in microscopic structures are so subtle that species are not easily identified by neophytes. The organisms seen in the clinical laboratory reproduce only by asexual methods. The dematiaceous contaminants presented in this unit are *Aureobasidium, Alternaria, Bipolaris, Curvularia, Drechslera, Epicoccum, Helminthosporium,* and *Nigrospora.*

A second group of contaminants/opportunistic fungi is distinguished by a single microscopic feature or, more accurately, by the absence of that feature. Fungi that have few or no septa in the hyphae (see Fig. 1.1) belong to a single taxonomic group, the Zygomycetes. Like the dematiaceous fungi, these organisms are easily differentiated to genus, and perhaps to species, by the size, shape, and arrangement of microscopic structures.

The zygomycetes have similar colony morphologies, but not to the extent seen with the Dematiaceous Group. The zygomycetes produce colonies that are cottony, with rather nondescript white, gray, or brownish surface pigment and equally nondescript reverse color. These organisms usually develop rapidly, producing detectable colonies in 1 or 2 days.

The zygomycetes all have essentially the same microscopic structures; the differences lie in the shapes and arrangements of them. They are perfect fungi, meaning that they can reproduce by both sexual and asexual modes. Sexual reproduction is by means of zygospores (see Fig. 1.4). The primary asexual reproductive structure for all the fungi in this group is the sporangiospore. As already noted, zygomycetes have few or no septa in their hyphae. The are also distinguished to genus by the shape and arrangement of the microscopic structures; in the zygomycetes these features are markedly different from those of the other fungi that infect humans. Details are presented later in this chapter, in the discussion of specific organisms. The Zygomycetes to be studied in this chapter include *Absidia, Mucor, Rhizomucor, Rhizopus,* and *Syncephalastrum.*

The third major group of opportunistic pathogens or contaminants consists of fungi that have septa in the hyphae, produce pastel or white colonies, and have microscopic structures that are not darkly pigmented. This Hyaline Group contains more fungi than either of the other two groups. It can be subdivided by the shape and complexity of the conidiophores (Fig. 3.4). Some fungi produce *simple (micronematous)* conidiophores; they cannot be distinguished from the vegetative hyphae unless conidia are attached. Others produce branching structures or distinctively shaped *complex (macronematous)* conidiophores; they are readily differentiated from the vegetative hyphae. The Hyaline Group is further separated into genera, and often to species, by the size, shape, and complexity of the conidia and the way they are pro-

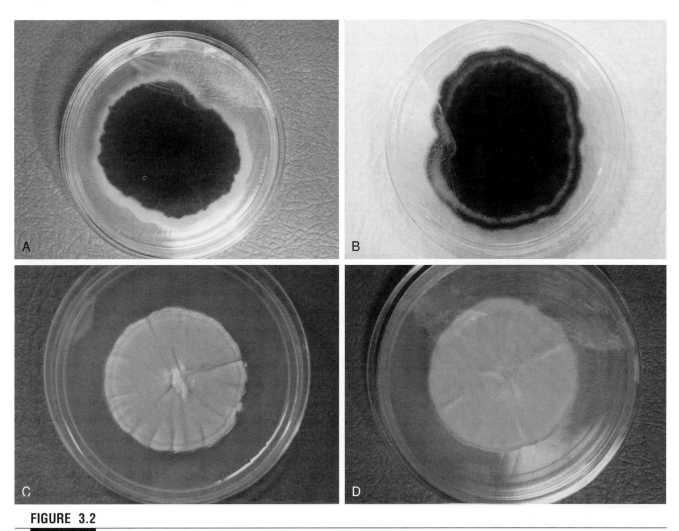

FIGURE 3.2

Both the obverse *(A)* and reverse *(B)* pigments of dematiaceous fungi are dark brown to black, in contrast with moniliaceous organisms, which have a light surface pigment *(C)* and usually also have a light or pastel reverse pigment *(D)* (although the surface pigment of moniliaceous organisms may be dark).

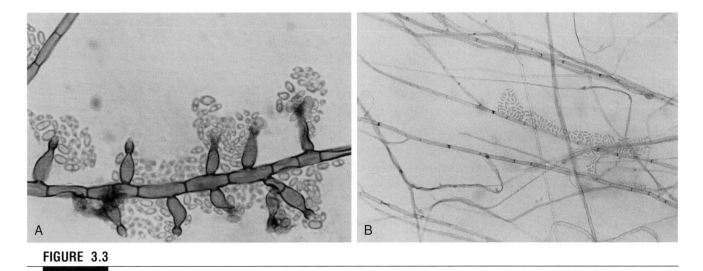

FIGURE 3.3

The microscopic structures of dematiaceous fungi such as *Phialophora verrucosa (A)* are dark brown, dark green, or black in unstained preparations, while the hyphae, conidiophores, and/or conidia of moniliaceous fungi *(B)* are hyaline and colorless.

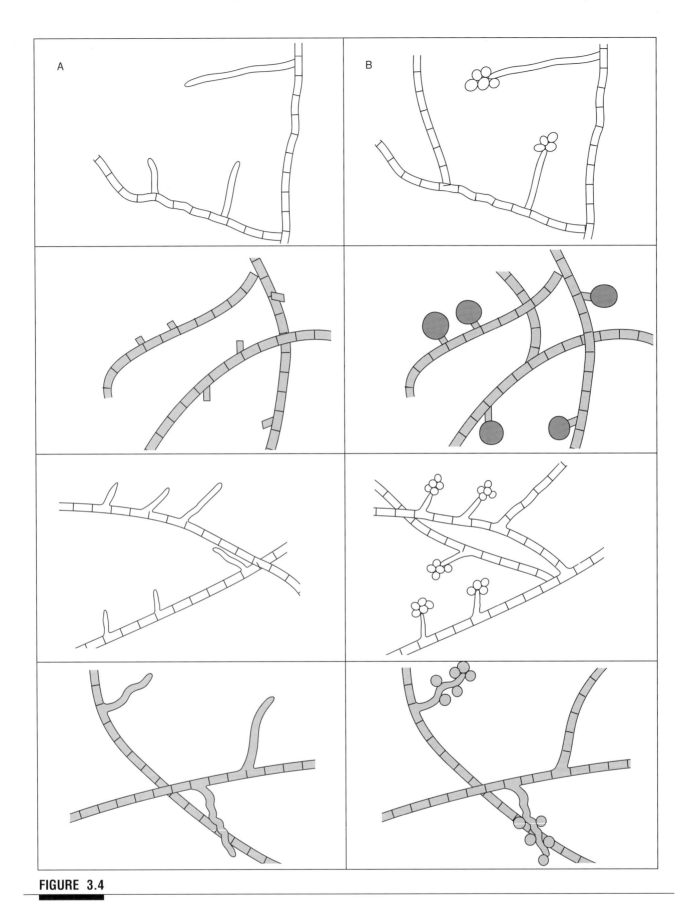

FIGURE 3.4

In panels *A* to *D*, simple (*micro*nematous) conidiophores are compared with complex (*macro*nematous) conidiophores. *A* and *B* show simple conidiophores, which resemble sticks or pegs. When no conidia are attached, as shown in *A*, simple conidiophores cannot be distinguished from hyphae and the fungus cannot be identified. When conidia are attached (*B*), the process of identification can begin. *C* and *D* show that complex conidiophores are very different from hyphae because of their distinct shapes or branching patterns. Even when no conidia are attached (*C*) you can see which structures are conidiophores and begin to think of possible identities of the organisms as—from top to bottom—*Gliocladium*-like, *Penicillium* species, possible *Nigrospora*, and a potential *Phialophora*-type. The presence of conidia (*D*) certainly helps with identification, but even without them the conidiophores provide useful clues.

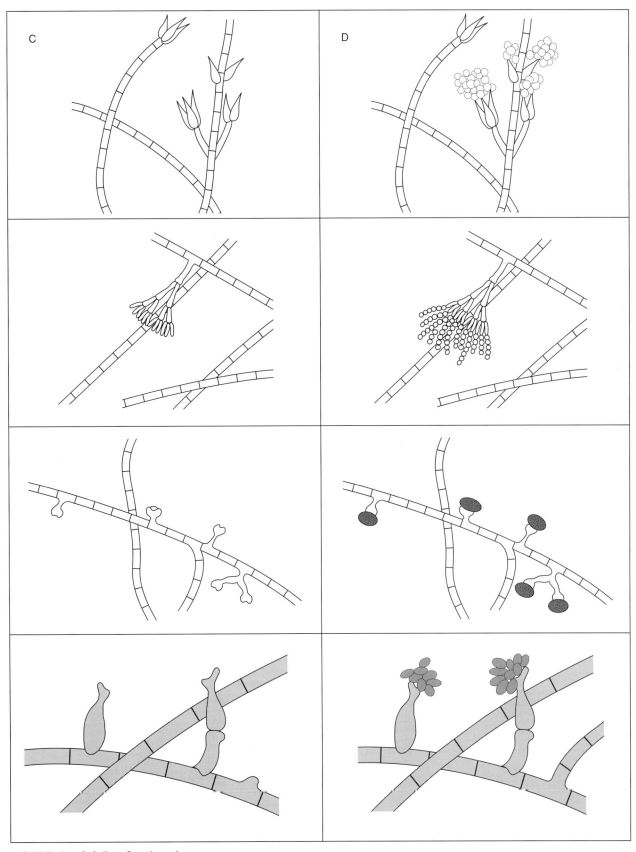

FIGURE 3.4 C & D   *Continued*

duced and by the presence of special structures. The Hyaline group of opportunistic pathogens to be studied includes *Acremonium, Aspergillus, Chrysosporium, Fusarium, Gliocladium, Paecilomyces, Penicillium, Scopulariopsis, Sepedonium,* and *Trichoderma.*

LABORATORY METHODS FOR SOME OPPORTUNISTIC FUNGI

Collection and handling of specimens, inoculation of primary cultures, and microscopic examination are generally the same for all of the contaminants/opportunistic pathogens. The features applicable to all of these organisms are introduced here; the occasional exception is presented when the organism concerned is discussed.

Distinguishing Contaminants from Pathogens. One important fact to remember is that any of the fungi described in this chapter are normally found in the environment on plants and animals as contaminants, but they are also capable of causing disease when the opportunity presents itself. The mycologist's job is to work with the physician and to learn enough about the patient to help make an informed judgment about whether the isolated fungus is or is not the etiologic agent of disease (see Table 3.1). The number of mycotic elements seen in a direct preparation of a fresh specimen and the amount of growth in the culture help enormously in making this decision. Other important elements are the (probable) immunocompetence of the host, whether or not the specimen source is normally sterile, and the presence of the fungus in multiple specimens from the same or related sites.

Specimen Sources. Any kind of specimen may be received for culture. The most likely specimens are sputa and other respiratory secretions, urine, cerebrospinal fluid, blood, corneal scrapings, aspirates from abscesses, and biopsies of infected tissue.

Specimen Collection and Handling. Specimens that are cultured for opportunistic pathogens are generally handled just like any other fungus culture. They should be placed in sterile containers and transported to the laboratory as rapidly as possible. Several of the fungi are sensitive to refrigeration; these are identified when they are discussed.

Immunology. Little is known about the immunologic structure of most of the opportunistic pathogens, except *A. fumigatus* and the Zygomycetes. The others have not been important enough, medically speaking, to have been studied thoroughly.

Special Precautions. Since these fungi are opportunists rather than true pathogens, special precautions are not necessary to prevent laboratory-acquired infections. A wise worker will, however, work with these fungus cultures—any fungus cultures—in a biologic safety cabinet to avoid contaminating the work area with conidia that may be released when cultures are opened.

Culture Media. Opportunistic fungi are not nutritionally fastidious; they can be isolated on any standard mycology medium as well as on old bread and orange peels. The commonly used medium is Emmon's modification of Sabouraud's dextrose agar (SDA) without antimicrobials, but brain-heart infusion agar (BHIA) and SABHI (a combination of SDA and BHIA) without antimicrobials also serve. Media with antibacterial agents may be used to prevent overgrowth by bacteria, but media (SDA, SABHI, or BHIA) with the antimycotic agent cycloheximide (Acti-Dione) should not be used because most of the opportunistic fungi are sensitive to cycloheximide. Rely on the adage "when in doubt, leave it out." One of the major themes of this text is that selective media should ALWAYS be paired with media without antimicrobial agents.

Occasionally additional media are recommended to enhance development of a particular feature for identification; these are introduced in the discussion of the organisms. The most common recommendation is that the initial colony be subcultured to potato dextrose agar (PDA) or potato flake agar (PFA) to encourage *conidiation* (production of conidia) and pigmentation. Harsher measures, such as those discussed in Chapter 2 to deal with Mycelia Sterilia, may be required.

Teleomorphs are not included with the contaminants and opportunistic fungi, although they are known for many of these organisms. Study of these fungi is still in an embryonic state because their involvement in human infection was not recognized. As a result of increasing frequency of isolation of the opportunistic organisms, they are studied more intensely. Some of the generic names can be expected to change, and changes in the nomenclature of the teleomorphs will undoubtedly follow.

Contaminant/Opportunistic Pathogen

ZYGOMYCETES

ABSIDIA SPECIES

Absidia is discussed with the other four Zygomycetes at the end of this chapter.

Contaminant/Opportunistic Pathogen

MONILIACEAE

ACREMONIUM SPECIES[4] (Ack-ruh-moan'-ee-um)

■ **Reservoirs.** *Acremonium* species are found in soil and sewage and on vegetation and in foodstuffs. They are spread by an airborne route.

■ **Unique Risk Factors.** None.

■ **Human Infection.** Infections with *Acremonium* were rare, but increasing numbers are being reported. The fungus has been associated with various types of hyalohyphomycosis, primarily *mycetoma* (a fungal "tumor" or mass), and mycotic *keratosis* (a "condition"—in this case an infection—of the cornea). It has also been involved in systemic infections such as endocarditis, osteomyelitis, arthritis, and pulmonary infection as well as infections of the skin, nails, and hard palate. *Acremonium* species have been reported to colonize contact lenses.

■ **Specimen Sources.** Corneal scrapings, aspirates from lesions, respiratory secretions and pleural fluid,

[4]Formerly *Cephalosporium* species.

blood, biopsies of tissue and skin, nail clippings, cerebrospinal fluid, and gastric secretions are most likely to be submitted for culture.

■ **Special Precautions.** None are needed. Specimens should be handled within a biologic safety cabinet.

■ **Culture Media.** Modified SDA without cycloheximide.

Temperature Considerations. *Acremonium* species grow at 25° to 37°C. The optimum temperature is 30°C.

■ **Macroscopic (Colony) Morphology.** On modified SDA at 25°C, after 4 to 5 days, colonies of *Acremonium* are smooth and waxy or velvety. Later they may be cottony. The color varies enormously, from white to gray to rose, with a beige, light yellow, or light pink reverse. One species, *Acremonium falciforme*, produces colonies that are gray-violet with a violet-purple reverse pigment.

■ **Microscopic Morphology** (Figs. 3.5 through 3.7). The hyphae of *Acremonium* are delicate, thin, hyaline, and septate; they may form intertwining ropes. The slender conidiophores are phialides. They form directly on the hyphae in an upright arrangement, usually at right angles to the hyphae. Conidiophores are hyaline, solitary, and unbranched, tapering from the (3 μm) base to the

[handwritten: clear]

[handwritten: Segmented]

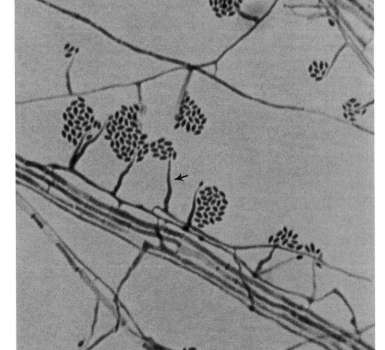

FIGURE 3.5

Acremonium species characteristically have slender, intertwined hyphae such as those seen in the lower left quadrant of this field. Phialides are upright and taper at the tip *(arrow)*, with irregular clusters of elliptical conidia at the tips of the conidiophores. (From Rippon JW: Medical Mycology: The Pathogenic Fungi and the Pathogenic Actinomycetes, 3rd ed. Philadelphia, WB Saunders, 1988, p 763.)

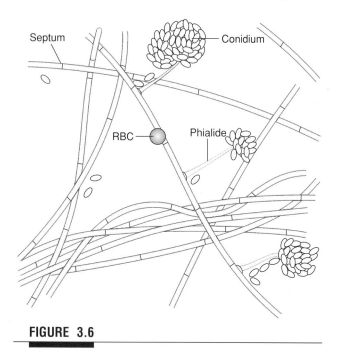

FIGURE 3.6

The hyphae of *Acremonium* are often interwoven into ropelike strands; septa are present. The clusters of elliptical phialoconidia are the most obvious feature of *Acremonium*. Phialides that form right angles with the hyphae and that taper from the base to the tip also suggest *Acremonium*. The red blood cell (RBC) is approximately 7 μm in diameter. It is included in all drawings to provide a perspective on the size of the fungal elements.

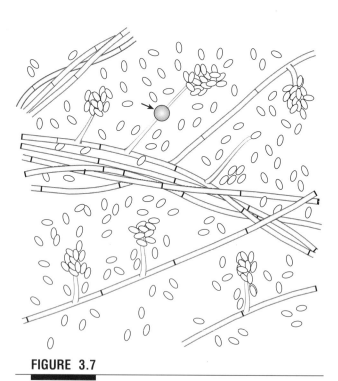

FIGURE 3.7

Even in bad preparations the presence of elliptical conidia and upright conidiophores that taper from the base to the tip suggests that the fungus is *Acremonium*, especially if some of the conidia are in clusters. Interwoven ropelike hyphae further suggest the identity of the fungus. Colony morphology helps to distinguish *Acremonium* from similar organisms. The red blood cell (arrow) of approximately 7 μm is included to indicate the relative sizes of the mycotic elements.

apices (tips) where *phialoconidia*, asexual reproductive structures formed from phialides, are produced. Conidia are usually *elliptical* (egg shaped) but are crescent shaped in some species. They are approximately 3 × 6 μm and typically are unicellular (single celled) and hyaline, with smooth walls. Phialoconidia are produced individually. A mucoid substance holds them together to create spherical clusters ("slimy balls") around the tip of the determinate conidiogenous cell, the *phialide*. When the medium is dry, short chains of conidia may develop.

In *direct examination* of specimens *Acremonium* species are seen as fragments of hyaline septate hyphae. Small (<1.5 to 2 μm in diameter) white-to-yellow granules are produced rarely. A dense mass of slender hyaline hyphae with occasional **vesicles** (swellings) and numerous swollen cells is seen in the granules, which are soft, lobulated, and *vermiform* (wormlike).

■ **Helpful Features for Identification of *Acremonium* Species**

> Unicellular hyaline phialoconidia on long, tapering, upright phialophores
> Clusters of conidia at the tips of the phialides

■ **Organisms from Which *Acremonium* Must Be Differentiated** (Table 3.2 and Fig. 3.8)

> *Fusarium*
> *Verticillium*
> *Gliocladium*
> *Trichoderma*
> *Sporothrix schenckii*
> *Cylindrocarpon*

Contaminant/Opportunistic Pathogen

DEMATIACEAE

ALTERNARIA SPECIES (All-tur-nair'-ee-uh)

■ **Reservoirs.** *Alternaria* species are found worldwide as a soil saprophyte and as a plant pathogen.

■ **Unique Risk Factors.** None.

■ **Human Infection.** *Alternaria* species have been reported to cause phaeohyphomycosis, sinusitis, asthma, osteomyelitis, eye and ear infections, and cutaneous infections. Sinusitis and asthma due to *Alternaria* occur more frequently than the other conditions.

■ **Specimen Sources.** Aspirates, respiratory secretions, tissue biopsies, and scrapings of infected areas are most likely to be submitted for culture.

TABLE 3.2 *Acremonium* and Fungi that Resemble *Acremonium*

Fungus	Size of Conidia (μm)	Shape of Conidia	Arrangement of Conidia	Width of Hyphae (μm)	Length of Conidiophore (μm)	Shape of Conidiophore	Arrangement of Conidiophores	Colony Morphology	Growth Rate	Other Helpful Features
Acremonium	3 × 6	Elliptical phialoconidia	Slimy balls at tip of conidiophore	3	30–35	Tapers smoothly from base to tip	Solitary, at roughly right angles to hyphae	Cottony texture; pastel surface pigment	Rapid	No macroconidia
*Cylindrocarpon**		Curved cylinder with rounded ends	Solitary	4	50	Branched; may resemble penicillus	Solitary	Floccose; white to purple	Rapid	Macroconidium lacks foot cell and pointed tip
Fusarium	3 × 6 and 5 × 50	Cylindrical microconidia, fusiform macroconidia	Solitary micro, whorls of macroconidia	4	50–100	Tapering phialides	Solitary, occasional whorls	Cottony pastel (typically pink or purple)	Rapid	Colony pigment is water soluble
Gliocladium	6–7	Spherical	Clusters	4–5	70	Penicillus	Alternate on hyphae	Floccose or granular pastel	Rapid	Popcorn balls on tripods
Trichoderma	2 × 3	Elliptical	Spherical clusters	2–3	12–30	Sticklike, with septa and branching	Branching at wide angles, with phialides	Moniliaceous	Rapid	Fat vaselike phialides with round clusters of oval conidia
Sporothrix	2 × 4	Pyriform	Rosettes and sleeves	1–2	Short	Tapers from base to middle, then swells into small vesicle	Solitary, at right angle to hypha	Dematiaceous	Intermediate	Dimorphic
Verticillium†		Oval or tear shaped	Clusters or balls		Short	Simple or branched, tapering from base to tip	Erect; simple or branched	Velvety or cottony, with pastel or white color	Rapid	Single conidia or irregular balls at tips of conidiophores

*This is the only place *Cylindrocarpon* is found in this text.
†*Verticillium* is found here and in Figure 3.8 but is presented nowhere else in this text.

45

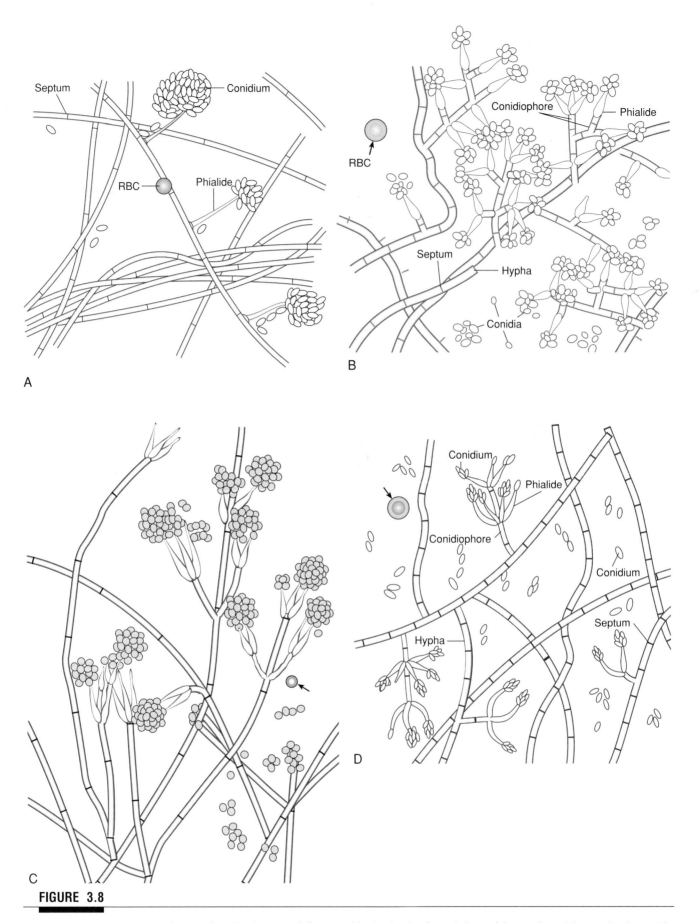

A

B

C

D

FIGURE 3.8

Fungi with clusters of conidia at the tips of conidiophores are differentiated by the details of morphology of the conidia and the conidiophores. The hyaline species presented in this text are presented together in this composite. *Acremonium (A)* has conidiophores that taper from the base to the tip and stand at right angles to the hyphae; conidia are elliptical. In *Gliocladium (C)* the conidiophores are erect, but each separates into multiple metulae and phialides; conidia are round. The conidiophore of *Trichoderma (B)* is macronematous, with multiple branches and vase-shaped phialides; conidia are oval. *Verticillium (D)* produces conidiophores that are somewhat vaselike but without the multiple branches of *Trichoderma;* conidia are distinctly elliptical, in small packets. Colony morphology and growth rate are also useful characteristics for differentiating these fungi. The 7-μm red blood cell (arrow) shows the relative sizes of the mycotic elements.

■ **Special Precautions.** None are needed, but cultures should be handled within a biologic safety cabinet.

■ **Culture Media.** Modified SDA.

Temperature Considerations. Alternaria species grow at 25° to 30°C.

■ **Macroscopic (Colony) Morphology.** On modified SDA at 25°C, after 5 to 10 days, flat colonies appear; they become cottony as they age. *Alternaria* organisms are dematiaceous; the obverse pigment of colonies is dark brown or dark olive-green with a white fringe around the colony. The reverse pigment is black.

■ **Microscopic Morphology** (Figs. 3.9 and 3.10). Hyphae are septate and darkly pigmented. Conidiophores are septate, simple or branched, and darkly pigmented. The poroconidia are also dematiaceous, smooth, or rough. They may occur singly but are usually arranged in chains that are simple or branched. The large (approximately 8 × 28 μm) poroconidia have both transverse (running across the width) and longitudinal septa; that is, the conidia are *muriform.* They are shaped like clubs that taper to a thin, rounded end. When poroconidia are produced in chains they are described as "beaked," with the thin, tapered conidiogenous (germ tube) end of the older conidium attached to the broader rounded blunt end of the newer one. Conidia are produced acropetally; that is, the youngest cell is at the tip of the chain of cells. In older, more deeply pigmented colonies it may be difficult to see the septa in conidia.

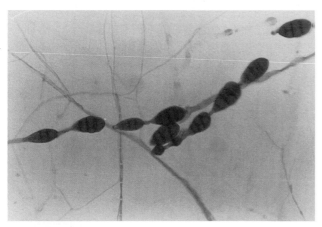

FIGURE 3.9

Alternaria species are difficult to miss because of the dark pigment in the septate hyphae and the characteristic shape and arrangement of the conidia. The knobby geniculate conidiophore characteristic of *Alternaria* runs from the upper right of this photomicrograph. At the top is a chain of club-shaped conidia. The conidia on the upper right of the picture show the horizontal and transverse septa. Note that some of the conidia are elliptical rather than club shaped (*extreme upper right*).

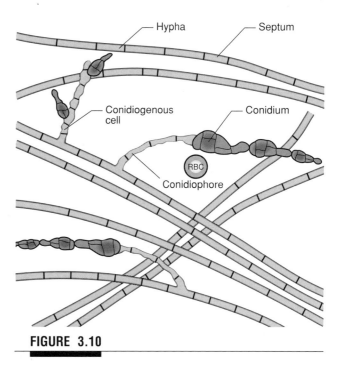

FIGURE 3.10

Hyphae of *Alternaria* are dematiaceous and septate. Conidiophores are also darkly pigmented and have septa; the conidiophores may branch. The conidiophores are knobby, with conidia produced in a zigzag pattern around them. The club-shaped conidia are divided by both horizontal and transverse septa. The broad base of the younger conidium is attached to the smaller tip of the older conidium to form chains. The red blood cell (RBC) of approximately 7 μm is included to indicate the relative sizes of the mycotic elements.

■ **Helpful Features for Identification of *Alternaria* Species**

Dark brown or dark olive-green colony with a white fringe
Dematiaceous hyphae, conidiophores, and conidia
Muriform conidia that are large, club shaped, and beaked

■ **Organisms from Which *Alternaria* Must Be Differentiated.** The microscopic appearance of *Alternaria* species makes them distinctive if not unique. There are no similar organisms from which they must be distinguished.

Contaminant/Opportunistic Pathogen

MONILIACEAE

ASPERGILLUS FUMIGATUS (As-per-jIll-us fume-uh-got'-us)

A. fumigatus is the species of *Aspergillus* that is most frequently isolated from human patients. Rippon, and Kwon-Chung and Bennett, both

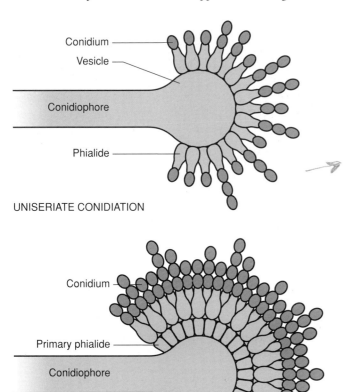

Conidium
Vesicle
Conidiophore
Phialide

UNISERIATE CONIDIATION

Conidium
Primary phialide
Conidiophore
Secondary phialide

BISERIATE CONIDIATION
FIGURE 3.11

Uniseriate species of *Aspergillus* produce one "layer" or set of phialides between the vesicle and the chains of conidia. In biseriate species two rows of phialides form between the vesicle and the conidia. The large swollen vesicle at the end of the conidiophore is an important feature for distinguishing *Aspergillus* species from other fungi that produce chains of conidia.

report that about 167 species and numerous varieties of *Aspergillus* have been identified. Of these, 16 species and 1 variety have been found as etiologic agents of aspergillosis. The genus *Aspergillus* is separated into species (Fig. 3.11) by morphologic differences, including whether the fungus is *uniseriate* (produces one series of structures between the vesicle and the conidium) or *biseriate* (forms two series of intermediate structures).

Many texts place the aspergilli in groups and discuss the characteristics of the group. The authors have elected, instead, to present representative species in this basic text.

■ **Unique Risk Factors.** *A. fumigatus* and the other species are exogenous (literally, "generated outside"—not

part of the normal flora), and are not infectious. Typically, people are at risk only when they are seriously debilitated or weakened as a result of another disease process (or, ironically, as a result of treatment for some life-threatening illness). Injuries or infections that cause scarring of the lung tissue may predispose a person to an aspergillosis, especially aspergilloma.

■ **Human Infection.** The four leading types of aspergillosis are colonization, allergy, disseminated infection, and toxicity. *A. fumigatus* is most often associated with infection, but many *Aspergillus* species have been isolated from infections.

■ **Specimen Sources.** Any type of specimen may contain *Aspergillus*. Those most often submitted for culture are skin or nails, biopsied tissue, blood cultures, and sputa and other secretions from the lung.

■ **Specimen Collection and Handling.** Standard methods for specimen collection and handling are adequate, except that specimens to be cultured for *Aspergillus* should not be refrigerated because this can slow the growth of the organism or kill it.

Direct examination of specimens should include a direct wet mount; 10% potassium hydroxide (KOH) may be needed to clear the specimen. A calcofluor white–fluorescent antibody preparation can also be done.

■ **Immunology.** When aspergillosis is suspected but cultures are negative, and when a fungus cannot be identified by conventional methods, immunologic techniques can be used (Table 3.3). *Skin tests* are useful for detecting allergic aspergillosis. Either immediate- or delayed-type hypersensitivity reactions may occur if specific anti-*Aspergillus* antibodies are present. The Ouchterlony double-immunodiffusion (ID) method is useful for detecting

TABLE 3.3 Serologic Tests for Aspergillosis

Immunologic Method	Component Detected
Complement fixation	Antibody
Counterimmuno-electrophoresis (CIE)	Antibody
Double immunodiffusion	Antibody
Enzyme-linked immunosorbent assay (ELISA)	Antigen
Radioimmunoassay (RIA)	Antigen
Skin tests	Antibody (allergic response)

antibodies to *Aspergillus* species in almost any kind of aspergillosis, unless the patient is anergic. One or more precipitin bands suggests an active infection, if the reference sera yield the proper reactions. Three or more lines of identity with the control sera indicate invasive disease or an aspergilloma. If the culture is also positive, the combination of ID test and culture is diagnostic of active infection. When reference antisera are used, the ID test is 100% specific for aspergillosis. People with titers of C-reactive protein, a nonspecific protein associated with trauma, inflammation, or infection, gives false-positive results in the ID test unless control sera are used. A radioimmunoassay (RIA) method is recommended for detecting antigens in the blood (antigenemia) caused by *Aspergillus*. RIA has a positive predictive value of 82% for antigenemia, with reported 74% sensitivity and 90% specificity. Sensitivity is the conditional probability that the antigen will be detected when it is present. Specificity is the conditional probability that when the test is positive the patient has the infection or disease. Complement fixation (CF) tests and counterimmunoelectrophoresis (CIE) have also been developed for the diagnosis of aspergillosis. CIE is recommended for use only as a screening test because it lacks the desired specificity. CF methods are sensitive but not specific; the patient's serum should be tested against a battery of antigens if CF is done. An enzyme-like immunosorbent assay method detects antigens in the patient; it is not yet considered ready for routine use.

When serologic tests are done first, cultures should generally also be done to attempt to confirm the results of the serologic tests. Immunocompromised patients may have negative tests even when they are actively infected because they are anergic. Immunologic methods using a battery of antigens are preferred to a single antigen. Sera may be concentrated to improve detection of *Aspergillus* species in anergic patients.

■ **Special Precautions.** None are needed, but specimens and cultures should be studied within a biologic safety cabinet. The masses of conidia produced by *Aspergillus* species readily become airborne.

■ **Culture Media.** Modified SDA, modified SDA with chloramphenicol or gentamicin, Czapek's agar, or 2% malt extract agar should be used for morphology studies. Czapek's agar (Czapek-Dox medium) incorporates magnesium and ferrous sulfate with sucrose and potassium salts to enhance pigment production. Malt extract agar contains maltose, dextrin, and glycerol in an otherwise nutritionally poor medium to encourage conidiation.

Some species of *Aspergillus* are sensitive to cycloheximide. A combination of selective and nonselective media should be inoculated and held 3 to 4 weeks before the cultures are discarded as negative if aspergillosis is the tentative diagnosis.

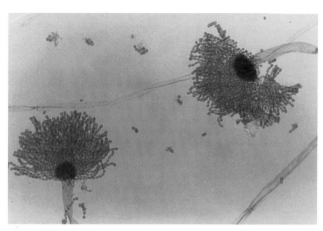

FIGURE 3.12

Aspergillus fumigatus typically has long conidiophores that connect to the hyphae by foot cells (not shown). The swollen, flask-shaped vesicle found at the tip of the conidiophore is visible in the lower left quadrant of this field. Long compact chains of conidia are produced from the phialides that cover the upper one half to one third of the vesicle. The pattern of conidial chains shown, where the mass is almost flat at the base and rounded into a half circle across the top, is typical. *A. fumigatus* is uniseriate.

Temperature Considerations. *A. fumigatus* grows at both 25° and 37°C. The Tmax (maximum temperature at which the organism grows) of *A. fumigatus* is 50°C, a fact that can be helpful in distinguishing this fungus from other *Aspergillus* species.

■ **Macroscopic (Colony) Morphology.** On modified SDA at 25°C a flat white colony typically develops in 3 to 6 days. As it ages and conidia are produced the colony turns bluish green to gray. The reverse remains unpigmented, white, or ivory. The texture is velvety to floccose, or granular; the topography is generally rugose.

■ **Microscopic Morphology** (Figs. 3.12 through 3.14). Hyphae are hyaline, septate, and relatively broad (average diameter 5 μm, range 2.5 to 8 μm), as they are for all aspergilli, with parallel walls. Dichotomous branching occurs at an angle of approximately 45 degrees. Conidiophores are smooth walled, up to 300 μm in length and 3 to 8 μm (average 5 μm) in width. They may be light green or brown. The vesicle, a swelling at the terminal end of the conidiophore, is flask shaped and is approximately 25 μm in diameter (range 20 to 30 μm). Uniseriate flask-shaped phialides bend upward from the upper half of the vesicle; each phialide bears a single chain of conidia. The round phialoconidia are green, echinulate (spiny or prickly), and 2 to 5 μm in diameter. A *foot cell*, a specialized cell that forms in the hyphae where the conidiophore originates, is present. The conidiophore and foot cell appear to be double walled, or to be more refractile than the hyphae. Conidial heads are columnar (arranged in columns) and compact (tightly grouped). The overall conformation of the aspergilli, especially un-

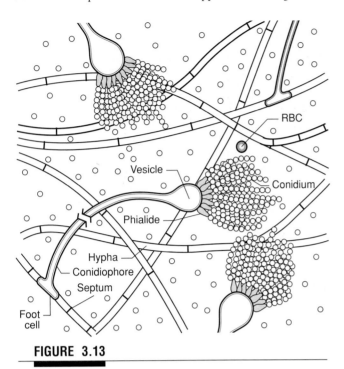

FIGURE 3.13

Conidiophores of *Aspergillus fumigatus* are relatively broad and very long, connecting to the hyphae by "foot cells," which are more refractile than the hyphae. Hyphae are septate, with smooth, parallel walls. The tip of the conidiophore swells into a broad flask-shaped vesicle from which a single band of phialides is produced. Compact chains of conidia are produced from the phialides to form the conidial head. The 7-μm red blood cell (RBC) shows the relative sizes of the mycotic elements.

der low power, reminded one student of Carmen Miranda (a 1950s performer known for wearing a towering hat or turban composed of bananas, pineapples, and other fruits). Another thought it looked more like the head of a child who'd stuck his finger in a live lamp socket.

In *direct examination* of specimens long dichotomous hyphae branching at a 45-degree angle may be seen, indicating a fungus is present. When the patient has an aspergilloma, the sputum may be bloody. Sputum from patients with aspergilloma typically shows hyphae with conidiophores and vesicles bearing conidia. Sometimes knots of twisted hyphae are present, indicating that the fungus has colonized a portion of tissue that was in contact with air.

■ **Helpful Features for Identification of *Aspergillus fumigatus***

Bluish green to gray colonies
Flask-shaped vesicles
Uniseriate arrangement of phialides
Compact columnar arrangement of conidia
Tmax of 50°C
Hyphal foot cell

■ **Organisms from Which *Aspergillus fumigatus* Must Be Differentiated** (Table 3.4 and Fig. 3.15)

Scopulariopsis
Other species of *Aspergillus*

Contaminant/Opportunistic Pathogen

MONILIACEAE

ASPERGILLUS FLAVUS   (As-per-jill-us flay-vus)

Note: Only those features of *A. flavus* that are significantly different from features of most other species of *Aspergillus* are presented.

■ **Human Infection.** *A. flavus* produces toxins. The organism has been reported from cases of allergic pulmonary aspergillosis and in disseminated disease. Occasionally cutaneous, nasal, orbital, and cerebral infections occur in debilitated patients. Charcot-Leyden crystals and increased numbers of eosinophils may be seen in sputa in *A. flavus* infections.

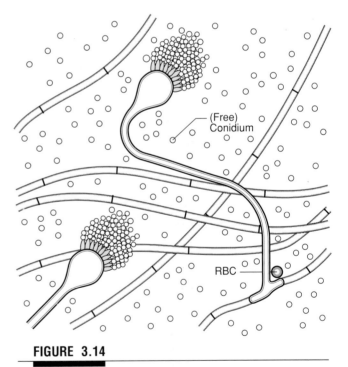

FIGURE 3.14

Even in bad preparations the presence of a foot cell at the base and a swollen vesicle at the tip of a conidiophore suggests *Aspergillus*. Clouds of free conidia are often seen when the preparation has been handled too roughly. A single row of phialides suggests *Aspergillus fumigatus*, but further study is necessary to confirm the species. The pigment, texture, and topography of the colony help differentiate *Aspergillus fumigatus* from other aspergilli. The 7-μm red blood cell (RBC) shows the relative sizes of the mycotic elements.

TABLE 3.4 *Aspergillus fumigatus* and Fungi that Resemble *A. fumigatus*

Fungus	Size of Conidia (μm)	Shape of Conidia	Arrangement of Conidia	Width of Hyphae (μm)	Length of Conidiophore (μm)	Shape of Conidiophore	Vesicle (diameter)	Colony Morphology	Growth Rate	Other Helpful Features
Aspergillus fumigatus	2–5	Round phialoconidia	Compact chains	3–8	150–300	Smooth parallel walls	Flask shaped with phialides over upper half (average 25 μm)	Powdery or granular with blue-green obverse pigment	Rapid	Uniseriate; vesicle is present
Aspergillus flavus	4	Round phialoconidia	Loose divided chains	5–6	≤850	Roughened parallel walls	Globose or sub-globose with phialides over most of surface (average 40 μm)	Yellow or yellow-green surface pigment	Rapid	Uniseriate or biseriate; vesicle is present
Aspergillus niger	4–5	Round echinulate phialoconidia	Compact chains	6	≤3 mm	Broad, with brownish tint in upper half	Spherical (average 60 μm)	Granular black surface with creamy reverse	Rapid	Biseriate, with large black echinulate conidia; vesicle is present
Scopulariopsis	6	Pyriform annelloconidia with flat bases	Long chains	6	≤10–30	Branching, with annellides alone or in clusters	None	Velvety or powdery light brown	Rapid	Echinulate conidia with flattened bases and nipple-like projections at the tip; NO vesicle
Aspergillus terreus	2	Smooth ellipses	Long chains	5	100–250	Smooth parallel walls	Dome shaped (average 13 μm) with biseriate phialides on upper half	Rugose cinnamon with brown reverse	Rapid	Smallest of aspergilli presented

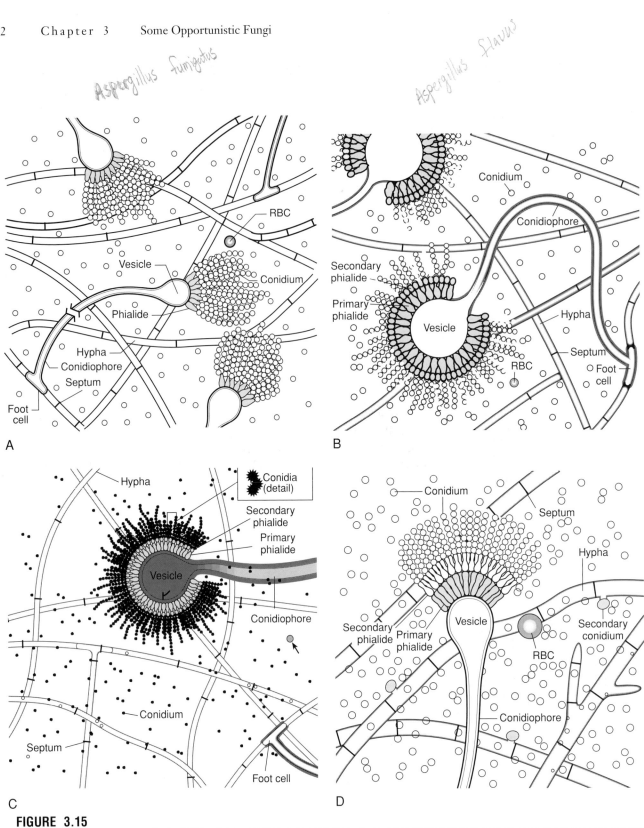

Aspergillus fumigatus

Aspergillus flavus

A

B

C

D

FIGURE 3.15

Aspergilli are differentiated by colony morphology and by the conidial head. This composite of the aspergilli treated in this text allows the reader to compare these species. *Aspergillus fumigatus (A)* has a flask-shaped vesicle and is uniseriate, with compact chains of conidia. *Aspergillus flavus (B)* can be biseriate or uniseriate; the vesicle is globose or subglobose, with loosely formed chains of conidia. *Aspergillus niger (C)* has large black echinulate conidia in chains and is biseriate; the vesicle is globose. The smaller *Aspergillus terreus (D)* is also biseriate, with a dome-shaped vesicle; only the upper half of the vesicle is covered with phialides. The 7-μm red blood cell (RBC) (arrow) shows the relative sizes of the mycotic elements.

■ **Special Precautions.** None are needed, but specimens and cultures should be studied under a biologic safety hood.

Temperature Considerations. *A. flavus* does not grow at 45°C, but growth is enhanced at 37°C.

■ **Macroscopic (Colony) Morphology.** After 3 to 6 days on modified SDA at 25°C the colony is matlike; the topography is flat or rugose. Surface pigment is intensely yellow to yellow-green. The reverse pigment is colorless to a drab pink.

■ **Microscopic Morphology** (Figs. 3.16 through 3.18). Hyphae are hyaline, septate, and relatively broad. Conidiophores are up to 850 μm in length and 5 to 8 μm in width. They are thick walled, hyaline, and coarsely roughened. Vesicles are large and *globose* (round), with an average diameter of 40 μm (range 20 to 65 μm). Phialides are biseriate, or biseriate and radiate; they are produced over most of the vesicle. The phialides produced directly on the vesicle are primary phialides; their average length is 10 μm. In uniseriate strains of *A. flavus* the primary phialides are the conidiogenous cells. In biseriate conidiation secondary phialides averaging 5 μm in length are produced from the primary ones. The secondary phialide is the conidiogenous cell in biseriate strains of *A. flavus*. Phialoconidia are unicellular and typically globose, averaging 4 μm in diameter; they become echinulate as they age. Conidial heads divide into several long, loosely formed, columnar chains. Foot cells attach the conidiophores to the hyphae.

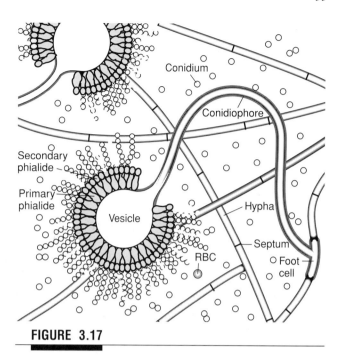

FIGURE 3.17

Aspergillus flavus has relatively broad septate hyphae. The conidiophores are ve-r-r-ry long, with parallel sides and thick, roughened walls; conidiophores end in refractile foot cells. The head of the conidiophore swells into a globose (or subglobose) vesicle, which may bear one or two bands of phialides. When they are present the secondary phialides are short and "stubby" compared with the primary phialides. Conidial heads divide into long, loosely formed, columnar chains of conidia. The 7-μm red blood cell (RBC) shows the relative sizes of the mycotic elements.

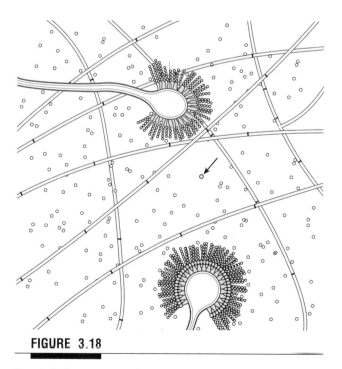

FIGURE 3.18

Even in bad preparations, the presence of a swollen vesicle and a foot cell in the conidiophore suggests *Aspergillus*. Clouds of free conidia are often seen when the preparation has been handled too roughly. A long conidiophore with roughened walls and a globose or subglobose vesicle covered over most of its surface by phialides suggest *Aspergillus flavus*, but further study is necessary to confirm the species. Colony morphology should be considered. The 7-μm red blood cell (arrow) shows the relative sizes of the mycotic elements.

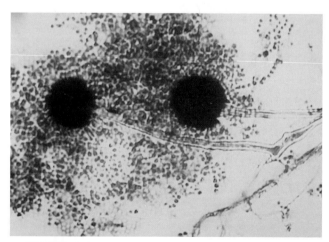

FIGURE 3.16

Typical isolates of *Aspergillus flavus* have very long conidiophores with rough-textured parallel sides that are more refractile than the hyphal walls. A foot cell is present in the conidiophore; one is shown in the center of the right side of the field. Vesicles are globose or subglobose; they are obscured by the masses of conidia in this photomicrograph. The chains of conidia are loosely formed, and they divide into columns. The dark color of the conidia is an artifact caused by the lactophenol–cotton blue stain and the magnification used.

■ **Helpful Features for Identification of** *Aspergillus flavus*

> Yellow to yellow-green colonies
> Globose to subglobose vesicles with uniseriate or biseriate phialides
> Conidial heads that radiate and are loosely formed rather than compact
> Foot cells are present

■ **Organisms from Which** *Aspergillus flavus* **Must Be Differentiated** (see Table 3.4 and Fig. 3.15)

> *Scopulariopsis* species
> Other species of *Aspergillus*

Contaminant/Opportunistic Pathogen

MONILIACEAE

ASPERGILLUS NIGER (As-per-jill-us nigh[5]-jur)

Note: For *A. niger* only those features that are significantly different from features of *Aspergillus fumigatus* are presented.

■ **Reservoirs.** The organism is found worldwide in soil and air, on moldy storage grains, and on decaying vegetation. It is airborne.

■ **Human Infection.** *A. niger* has been reported most often from cases of otomycosis (fungal condition of the ear), aspergilloma, and nasal sinus infections.

■ **Specimen Sources.** Scrapings from tissue, pulmonary fluids, and aspirates and biopsied material from the ear or the sinuses are most likely to be cultured.

■ **Special Precautions.** None are needed, but specimens and cultures should be studied under a biologic safety hood.

Temperature Considerations. *A. niger* grows at 25° to 37°C but does grow at 45°C.

■ **Macroscopic (Colony) Morphology.** After 2 to 6 days the colony on modified SDA at 25°C is flat and white. The surface is quickly covered with the jet black conidia from which the organism gets its species name, giving the culture its typical granular texture. This fungus is not considered dematiaceous because the reverse of the colony is colorless to ivory or pale yellow, not dark

brown or black. Colonies are very distinctive because of the creamy surface texture with the heavy overlay of black "sprinkles" resembling coarsely ground pepper. A distinct musty odor may be present.

■ **Microscopic Morphology** (Figs. 3.19 and 3.20). The morphology of *A. niger* generally resembles that of other *Aspergillus* species except for the black conidia. Hyphae are hyaline and closely septate, averaging 6 μm in diameter (range 3 to 10 μm), with smooth parallel walls and dichotomous branches at a 45-degree angle. As with other *Aspergillus* species, a foot cell is found at the junction of the conidiophore with the vegetative hypha. Conidiophores are wide (15 to 20 μm) and up to 3 mm long; the hyaline appearance changes to a brown tint in the upper half of the conidiophore. Vesicles are spherical, ranging from 45 to 75 μm in diameter with an average diameter of 60 μm. The biseriate conidial head composed of a series of secondary phialides topped with flask-shaped phialides surrounds the vesicle. The conidiogenous phialides bear abundant chaining conidia in compact columns. The large (4 to 5 μm) globose phialoconidia are produced *basipetally*; that is, the newest conidium is at the base and the oldest at the tip of the chain. They have thick echinulate walls and are jet black. In mature forms the vesicles may be completely masked by the black phialoconidia.

■ **Helpful Features for Identification of** *Aspergillus niger*

> Coarse black granules against the creamy colony surface
> Globose vesicles with biseriate phialides
> Large echinulate jet black conidia in chains
> Foot cells are present

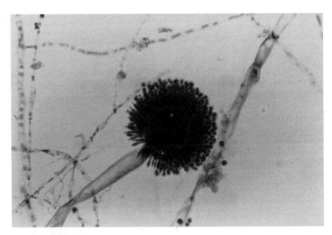

FIGURE 3.19

Aspergillus niger stands out among the aspergilli. The conidia distinguish it from other organisms with vesicles, foot cells, and chains of conidia because the conidia are larger than those of other aspergilli, echinulate, and very dark. This preparation from a young culture shows the broad conidiophore and the very dark conidia. Individual phialides with one or two conidia attached can be seen at the base of the vesicle.

[5]"Nigh" rhymes with rye.

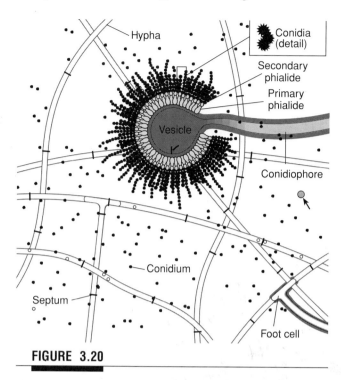

FIGURE 3.20

Aspergillus niger has a globose vesicle at the tip of the conidiophore. Conidiophores are anchored in the hypha by a foot cell. *A. niger* is biseriate, although it may be difficult to see both sets of phialides because of the dark pigment, especially in mature cultures. The outstanding characteristic is the chains of black prickly conidia in compact columns. The 7-μm red blood cell (arrow) shows the relative sizes of the mycotic elements.

■ **Organisms from Which *Aspergillus niger* Must Be Differentiated** (see Table 3.4 and Fig. 3.15)

> *Scopulariopsis* species
> Other species of *Aspergillus*

Contaminant/Opportunistic Pathogen

MONILIACEAE

ASPERGILLUS TERREUS   (As-per-jill-us tare-us)

Note: For *A. terreus* only those features that are significantly different from *Aspergillus fumigatus* are presented.

■ **Human Infection.** *A. terreus* has been found in cases of invasive or disseminated aspergillosis, particularly in cases of meningitis, osteomyelitis, and endocarditis in immunosuppressed patients.

■ **Special Precautions.** None are needed, but cultures should be studied within a biologic safety cabinet.

Temperature Considerations. *A. terreus* does not grow at 45°C. The optimum temperature for growth is 25° to 30°C.

■ **Macroscopic (Colony) Morphology.** The colony appears on modified SDA within 5 to 10 days at 25°C. Initially the texture is cottony to velvety. Heavy sporulation may result in development of a granular texture. Colonies may be rugose or have an irregular topography. The surface pigment varies from cinnamon to buff brown. The reverse pigment is white to brown.

■ **Microscopic Morphology** (Figs. 3.21 through 3.23). The septate hyphae are hyaline and relatively broad (average diameter 5 μm). Conidiophores have an average length of 175 μm (range 100 to 250 μm), and are approximately 5 μm wide. They are smooth walled and colorless. Vesicles are dome shaped, averaging 13 μm in diameter (range 10 to 16 μm). Phialides are produced in a biseriate pattern over the upper half of the vesicle. Conidia are small (2 μm), elliptical, and smooth; they are produced in chains. The conidial head is long and columnar. Foot cells develop where conidiophores originate in the hyphae.

> **Note:** Hyphae growing into the medium may form single globose conidia (approximately 6 μm in diameter).

■ **Helpful Features for Identification of *Aspergillus terreus***

> Smallest of aspergilli studied
> Cinnamon to buff brown colonies
> Dome-shaped vesicles with biseriate phialides
> Long and compact conidial heads
> Submerged hyphae that may form globose conidia

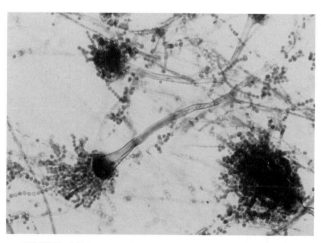

FIGURE 3.21

The biseriate phialides typical of *Aspergillus terreus* cannot be seen at this magnification. The shape of the vesicle is visible, however, with the chains of conidia streaming out from it. One thick-walled refractile conidiophore runs from the lower left of the field to the upper right. Another less mature form extends across the upper half of the field; its foot cell is obscured by the first conidiophore, hyphae, and free conidia. *A. terreus* is the smallest of the aspergilli included in this text.

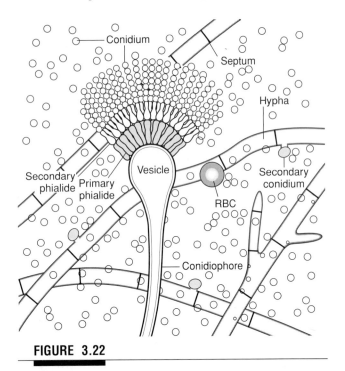

FIGURE 3.22

Aspergillus terreus has broad septate hyphae with refractile foot cells connecting the conidiophores to the hyphae. Two series of phialides form over the upper half of the small dome-shaped vesicles to support long chains of small conidia. Some strains of *A. terreus* occasionally produce secondary conidia directly on the hypha. The 7-μm red blood cell (RBC) shows the relative sizes of the mycotic elements.

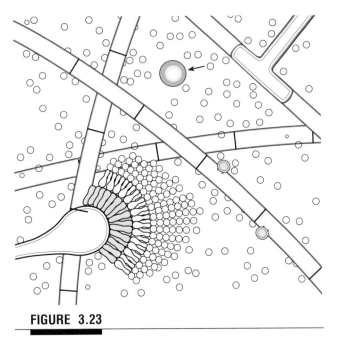

FIGURE 3.23

Even in a bad preparation containing many free conidia, the small conidia should suggest *Aspergillus terreus* when foot cells and vesicles are present. Relatively short conidiophores topped by small, dome-shaped vesicles also suggest *A. terreus*, especially if the phialides are biseriate. Colony morphology provides further clues to the identity of the fungus. The 7-μm red blood cell (arrow) shows the relative sizes of the mycotic elements.

■ **Organisms from Which *Aspergillus terreus* Must Be Differentiated** (see Table 3.4 and Fig. 3.15)

Scopulariopsis species
Other species of *Aspergillus*

Contaminant/Opportunistic Pathogen

DEMATIACEAE

AUREOBASIDIUM PULLULANS (Are-ee-oh-buh-syd'-ee-um pull'-you-lans[6])

■ **Reservoirs.** The fungus is commonly found worldwide in air, soil, foodstuffs, wood, and vegetation.

■ **Unique Risk Factors.** None.

■ **Human Infection.** *A. pullulans* is usually found as a contaminant. It has been reported as a rare agent of human infections, including cases of onychomycosis, pulmonary phaeohyphomycosis, and cutaneous and subcutaneous infections. *Aureobasidium* species occasionally invade deeper tissues (including blood). Dissemination of the infection may occur.

■ **Specimen Sources.** Respiratory secretions, biopsies of infected tissues, blood, scrapings and specimens from the nail and deeper tissues, and aspirates from lesions are most often cultured for *Aureobasidium*.

■ **Special Precautions.** None are needed, but specimens should be handled within a biologic safety cabinet.

■ **Culture Media.** SDA, SDA with antibacterial agents, SDA with cycloheximide.

Temperature Considerations. *A. pullulans* grows at 25° to 37°C.

■ **Macroscopic (Colony) Morphology.** After 6 to 7 days on SDA at 25°C, moist yeastlike colonies appear. They are white to yellow or pink and raised, with a wrinkled or folded topography. As arthroconidia are produced colonies of *A. pullulans* become shiny, mucoid, and dark brown to black. An irregular white fringe of mycelium that is slightly submerged in the medium may develop. Fully mature colonies are leathery, with a black reverse.

■ **Microscopic Morphology** (Figs. 3.24 through 3.26). Colonies of *A. pullulans* in fact may contain two fungi that

[6]"Lans" rhymes with pans.

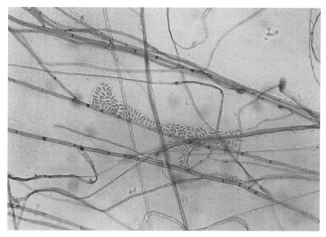

FIGURE 3.24

Typical isolates of *Aureobasidium pullulans* are actually mixtures of two synanamorphs. Microscopic preparations usually contain large, thick-walled dematiaceous arthroconidia and thin hyaline hyphae. Cylindrical conidia on short denticles are also present in most preparations. This photomicrograph shows the hyaline hyphae and conidia, most of which are massed along a hypha in the center of the field. At approximately 6 o'clock two conidia on their short denticles are attached to a hypha. The thick-walled arthroconidia are hinted at by the darkening of the septa in some of the hyphae.

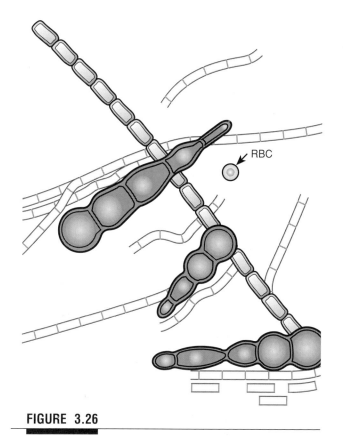

FIGURE 3.26

Even in bad preparations *Aureobasidium* is usually recognizable. If the possibility of a mixed culture can be ruled out, the combination of thick-walled dematiaceous arthroconidia (however distorted they are), delicate, thin-walled hyphae, and elliptical conidia strongly suggests *Aureobasidium pullulans*. Colony morphology is helpful in confirming the identity of the fungus. The 7-μm red blood cell (RBC) (arrow) shows the relative sizes of the mycotic elements.

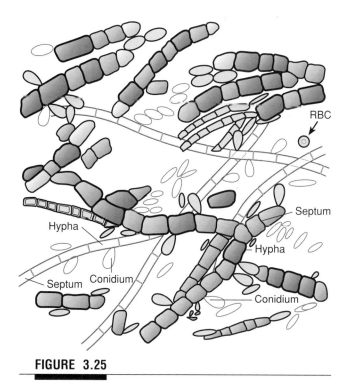

FIGURE 3.25

Scytalidium forms relatively thick dematiaceous hyphae. The cells develop into thick-walled arthroconidia; the arthroconidia become darker as they age so that even within the same hypha, some cells are darker than others. Smaller elliptical phialoconidia may also be present, attached to the arthroconidia. Cultures may also contain the delicate thin-walled hyphae and small elliptical or cylindrical phialoconidia of *Aureobasidium*. The 7-μm red blood cell (RBC) (arrow) shows the relative sizes of the mycotic elements.

are synanamorphs, *Aureobasidium* and *Scytalidium*. Multiseptate dematiaceous, thick-walled hyphae that form arthroconidia are produced by the *Scytalidium* anamorph. Delicate hyaline, thin-walled, septate hyphae are produced by the *Aureobasidium* anamorph.

Both types of hyphae produce unicellular hyaline conidia that are elliptical or cylindrical (approximately 5 × 10 μm); the walls of the conidia may be echinulate. The conidiogenous cells are not differentiated from the hyphae. Conidia are produced blastically from the hyphae on denticles; they may be *intercalary* (formed within the hyphae) or *terminal* (at the end) on the hyphae. Conidia are produced *synchronously* (at the same time) and *nonsynchronously*. They may give rise to secondary conidia (new conidia that bud from the original ones), and conidia can form chains or clusters around the conidiogenous cells. Fortunately, despite this rather confusing discussion, the appearance of the structures is distinctive—elliptical conidia, thin hyaline hyphae, and larger thick-walled dematiaceous hyphae with arthroconidia.

■ **Helpful Feature for Identification of *Aureobasidium pullulans***

> Conidia produced directly from the hyphae or on short denticles
>
> Both thin-walled hyaline and thick-walled dematiaceous hyphae
>
> Absence of conidiophores
>
> Large dematiaceous arthroconidia

■ **Organisms from Which *Aureobasidium pullulans* Must Be Differentiated** (see Table 4.3)

> *Wangiella dermatitidis*
> *Exophiala jeanselmei*
> *Exophiala spinifera*
> *Piedraia hortae*
> *Exophiala werneckii*

Contaminant/Opportunistic Pathogen

DEMATIACEAE

BIPOLARIS SPECIES   (By-pole-air′-us)

■ **Reservoirs.** The fungus is found in soil as a saprophyte.

■ **Unique Risk Factors.** None.

■ **Human Infection.** *Bipolaris* species have been reported as an opportunistic pathogen in cases of sinusitis, chronic pulmonary disease, meningitis and osteomyelitis, and in cutaneous, eye, and nasal infections in immunocompromised or debilitated hosts.

■ **Specimen Sources.** Aspirates from abscesses, cerebrospinal fluid, respiratory secretions, biopsies, and corneal scrapings are most often cultured.

■ **Culture Media.** Modified SDA, modified SDA with antibacterial antibiotics.

Temperature Considerations. *Bipolaris* species grow at 25° to 30°C.

■ **Macroscopic (Colony) Morphology.** The organism produces colonies on modified SDA at 25°C within 5 days. They are dematiaceous and cottony, with a gray to brownish black surface pigment and a black reverse pigment.

■ **Microscopic Morphology** (Figs. 3.27 through 3.29). Hyphae are light brown, septate, and branching. The conidiophores are darkly pigmented and septate; they are

geniculate, resembling a "bent knee," and twisted where poroconidia are borne. Conidia are produced in a *sympodial* pattern, a kind of indeterminate conidiogeny in which the oldest conidium is found at the tip of the conidiophore. As the conidiophore continues to elongate during conidiogeny, each new conidium is produced at the point just behind and to one side of the previous conidium, creating a zigzag pattern. The bent knees result from the growth and swelling of the conidiophore to accommodate conidiogeny. Poroconidia average 9×20 μm[7] in size. The smooth-walled conidia are divided into multiple cells by three to five horizontal septa; the first septum formed is in the approximate center of the conidium. They have rounded ends so that they resemble pea pods. A slightly protruding ***hilum*** (scar) is found at the base of the conidium. Some *Bipolaris* species germinate ("sprout") only at one end of the conidium through the hilum, while other species are able to germinate at both ends of the poroconidium. *Germ tubes,* filamentous outgrowths that are asexual reproductive structures, are formed. These turn to orient themselves parallel to the long axis of the conidium.

■ **Helpful Features for Identification of *Bipolaris* Species**

> Dark brown hyphae, conidiophores, and conidia
> Sympodially produced multicellular conidia shaped like pea pods, with thick walls and horizontal septa

---

[7]Sizes range from 6 to 11×15 to 25 μm, depending on the species of *Bipolaris*.

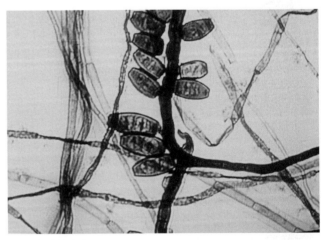

FIGURE 3.27

In typical preparations, *Bipolaris* produces conidia in a zigzag pattern from "bent knees," that is, bends in the conidiophore. The very dark structure that runs into the field from the right, then twists to go straight up, is an example of these geniculate twisted conidiophores. The dark structure running down is a second conidiophore beneath the first one. Isolates of *Bipolaris* species have dematiaceous septate hyphae; in this field some hyphal cells have collapsed. These poroconidia are typical, with three to five cells and a septum in the approximate center of the conidium.

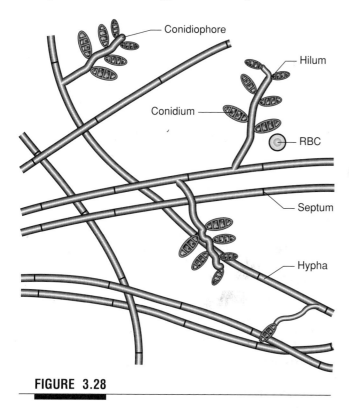

FIGURE 3.28

Bipolaris species have dark macroconidia with three to five cells and septate dematiaceous hyphae; the rounded ends make the condidia resemble pea pods. Conidiophores are geniculate and twisted from producing conidia. A slightly protruding hilum may be visible at the base of conidia. Hypha are septate and dematiaceous. The 7-μm red blood cell (RBC) shows the relative sizes of the mycotic elements.

Conidiophore that are geniculate and twisted where conidia are borne
Prominent hila at both ends of the conidium
Germ tubes parallel to the long axis of the conidium

■ **Organisms from Which *Bipolaris* Must Be Differentiated** (Table 3.5 and Fig. 3.30)

Drechslera
Exserohilum
Helminthosporium

Contaminant/Opportunistic Pathogen

MONILIACEAE

CHRYSOSPORIUM SPECIES (Chris-oh-spore′-ee-um)

■ **Reservoirs.** The organisms are found in soil, air, and water and may be a transient inhabitant of the human skin (especially the feet).

■ **Unique Risk Factors.** None.

■ **Human Infections.** *Chrysosporium* species have been isolated as a rare cause of hyalohyphomycosis, endocarditis, osteomyelitis, and *adiaspiromycosis*. Adiaspiromycosis is the enlargement of conidia in tissue without replication, under the influence of elevated temperatures.

feet

■ **Specimen Sources.** Respiratory secretions, blood, and aspirates and biopsies of bone and skin may be cultured.

■ **Special Precautions.** None are needed, but cultures should be handled within a biologic safety cabinet.

■ **Culture Media.** Modified SDA, modified SDA with antibiotics.

Temperature Considerations. *Chrysosporium* species grow at 25°C. Some species grow at temperatures to 40°C.

■ **Macroscopic (Colony) Morphology.** Colony morphology varies greatly among the species of *Chrysosporium*. On modified SDA at 25°C after 6 days, floccose or flat colonies appear. They become granular or cottony, glabrous or velvety. The topography may remain flat or

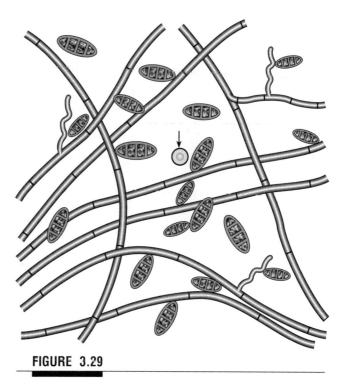

FIGURE 3.29

Even in bad preparations dematiaceous hyphae and conidia suggest *Bipolaris* species as one choice. "Pea pod" conidia with a cental septum, and geniculate twisted conidiophores, increase the possibility of *Bipolaris*. Germ tubes oriented to the length of the conidia confirm the isolate as *Bipolaris*. The 7-μm red blood cell (arrow) shows the relative sizes of the mycotic elements.

TABLE 3.5 Dematiaceous Saprobes with Poroconidia

Fungus	Size of Conidia (μm)	Shape of Conidia	Arrangement of Conidia	Width of Hyphae (μm)	Length of Conidiophore (μm)	Shape of Conidiophore	Arrangement of Conidiophores	Colony Morphology	Growth Rate	Other Helpful Features
Bipolaris	9 × 20	Elliptical with 3–5 septa	Sympodial	5–6	27–40	Geniculate and twisted	Solitary	Dematiaceous	Rapid	Basal hilum on conidium; germ tubes oriented to length of conidium
Exserohilum	17 × 210	Cigar shaped with septa	Sympodial	8–10	Variable	Geniculate but not twisted	Solitary	Dematiaceous	Rapid	Hila at the base of conidia; germ tubes produced adjacent to hila that lie along length of conidium
Curvularia	11 × 25	"Crescent rolls" with ≥3 septa	Sympodial	3	Variable	Slender and geniculate	Solitary with occasional branching	Dematiaceous	Rapid	Scars on conidiophores; dark protruding hilum at base of conidium
Drechslera	9 × 25	"Pea pods" with 3–5 septa	Sympodial	3	55	Geniculate	Solitary	Dematiaceous	Rapid	Scars on conidiophores; unobtrusive hilum at base of conidium
Helminthosporium	5 × 30	Club shaped with >5 septa	Like birds on a fence and in whorls	4	Variable	Smooth parallel walls with pores	Solitary	Dematiaceous	Rapid	Scars on conidiophores; no hilum

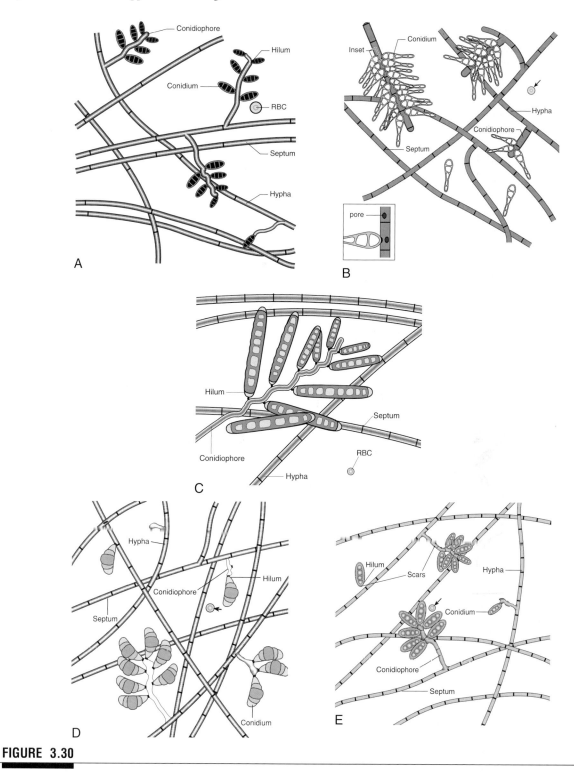

FIGURE 3.30

Several dematiaceous saprobes produce elongated macroconidia. This composite compares these easily confused species. *Bipolaris* species *(A)* have geniculate twisted conidiophores, and the "pea pod" conidia with rounded ends are produced in a sympodial pattern; germ tubes lie along the long axis of the conidium. The swollen central cell of *Curvularia (D)* makes it relatively easy to distinguish; conidiophores are geniculate, with sympodial conidiogeny. Conidiophores of *Drechslera (E)* are geniculate and broader, with sympodial conidia production; conidia also resemble pea pods, but germ tubes are perpendicular to the long axes of the conidia. *Helminthosporium (B)* conidia are club shaped, tapering from the point of attachment to the tip; conidiophores have straight, parallel walls without twisting and without "knees." The conidia of *Exserohilum (C)*, another mould that may be confused with these four fungi, are slender tubes with nearly parallel sides and rounded basal hila. Colony morphology is not helpful in differentiating among these fungi. The 7-µm red blood cell (RBC) (arrows) shows the relative sizes of the mycotic elements.

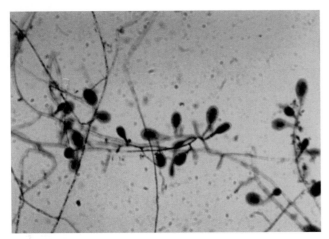

FIGURE 3.31

Characteristic preparations of *Chrysosporium* have hyaline, septate hyphae. The ovoid or club-shaped conidia vary somewhat in size and shape, and they may seem almost too heavy for the delicate hyphae and conidiophores. Conidia are produced directly from the hyphae as well as on micronematous conidiophores. The dark color is an artifact due to the lactophenol–cotton blue stain.

■ **Microscopic Morphology** (Figs. 3.31 through 3.33). Hyaline, septate hyphae may form spiral vegetative structures. Hyaline conidiophores are poorly differentiated from the hyphae. The one-celled ovoid to *clavate* (club-shaped) conidia are broader than the hyphae; they average 6 μm in diameter by 8 μm in length. Sizes vary greatly among species of *Chrysosporium*. Conidia are smooth walled or echinulate to *tuberculate* (having wartlike protuberances). They may be terminal and intercalary, or they may be produced directly on the sides of the hyphae on short pedicles. The base of attachment for conidia is broad. They have *annular frills*, rings of fragments of the conidiophore or hyphae that remain attached to the conidia when the conidia detach from the supporting structure. Numerous large, swollen arthroconidia, broader than the hyphae, are also distributed throughout the hyphae.

■ **Helpful Features for Identification for *Chrysosporium* Species**

> Numerous arthroconidia
> Unicellular conidia on conidiophores or directly on the hyphae
> Conidiophores of varying lengths that are poorly differentiated from the hyphae
> Mould form colonies at 25° to 30°C and 37°C
> Sensitivity to cycloheximide

become raised and folded as the culture ages and conidia are produced. *Chrysosporium* colonies also vary greatly in color, from ivory white to tan to yellow, beige, pink, orange, or lavender. The reverse is white to light brown.

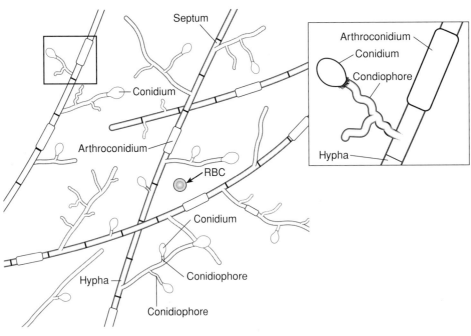

FIGURE 3.32

Chrysosporium species have thin septate hyphae that are hyaline. The conidiophores are somewhat thinner than the hyphae but are poorly differentiated from them. Conidia are ovoid or club shaped and vary in size. They are produced within and along the hyphae as well as on the conidiophores. The conidia may be smooth or echinulate; at the base free conidia have annular frills (*inset*), which may not be visible with a standard microscope. The fringed area at the base of the conidium in the inset shows where annular frills develop when the conidium breaks away. With age, arthroconidia develop in the hyphae. The 7-μm red blood cell (RBC) (arrow) shows the relative sizes of the mycotic elements.

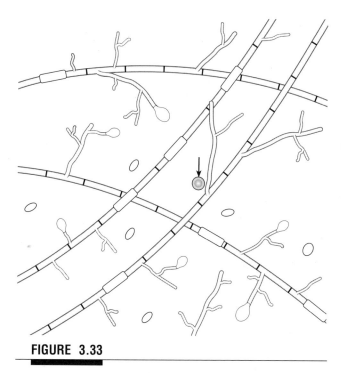

FIGURE 3.33

In bad preparations *Chrysosporium* species are difficult to identify because of the absence of any striking features. Conidia vary in size and shape. The club-shaped conidia and undistinguished conidiophores may suggest *Chrysosporium*, but growth rate and colony morphology are important for confirming the identity of the isolate. The 7-μm red blood cell (arrow) shows the relative sizes of the mycotic elements.

■ **Organisms from Which *Chrysosporium* Must Be Differentiated** (see Table 8.3)

Blastomyces dermatitidis
Histoplasma capsulatum
Scedosporium apiospermum
Paracoccidioides brasiliensis

Contaminant/Opportunistic Pathogen

DEMATIACEAE

CLADOSPORIUM SPECIES

Some species of *Cladosporium* are identified with the subcutaneous fungi as agents of chromoblastomycosis, so the organism is discussed with that group of fungi in Chapter 6. Other species, however, are commonly isolated as contaminants in the clinical laboratory.

Contaminant/Opportunistic Pathogen

DEMATIACEAE

CURVULARIA SPECIES   (Curve-you-lair'-ee-uh)

■ **Reservoirs.** The fungus is commonly found in the air and soil as a saprophyte. It has also been found on and in textiles and decaying vegetation.

■ **Unique Risk Factors.** None.

■ **Human Infection.** *Curvularia* species are usually found as a contaminant but may be found as an opportunistic pathogen. They have been reported as the agent of mycotic keratitis, phaeohyphomycosis, allergies and paranasal sinusitis, *onychomycosis* (fungal condition of the nails), endocarditis, pulmonary and nasal infections, and cutaneous infections.

■ **Specimen Sources.** Aspirates from lesions, respiratory secretions, biopsies of infected tissue, and scrapings and specimens from the nail, skin, and nose are most likely to be submitted for culture.

■ **Special Precautions.** None are needed, but cultures should be manipulated within a biologic safety cabinet.

■ **Culture Media.** Modified SDA, modified SDA with antibacterial agents.

■ **Temperature Considerations.** *Curvularia* species grow at 25° to 30°C.

■ **Macroscopic (Colony) Morphology.** After 5 to 6 days on modified SDA at 25°C, *Curvularia* species are velvety or woolly, with dark brown to black to olive-green pigment. Very young colonies may have a pink tinge on the surface. The reverse of the colony is brown to black.

■ **Microscopic Morphology** (Figs. 3.34 through 3.36). Hyphae of *Curvularia* are dematiaceous and septate, with thin walls. The conidiophores are also darkly pigmented and septate; they are simple or branched, and geniculate when sympodial growth has taken place. Scars are found at the pores where poroconidia have been produced. The conidiogenous cells are *polytridic*; that is, they produce multiple conidia from tiny pores in the cell walls. The large dematiaceous poroconidia (approximately 11 × 28 μm) are produced singly or in whorls. A typical conidium has transverse septa and is shaped like an ellipse or a curve, with three to five cells per conidium. The central cells of the conidia are darker than the end cells and are asymmetrically swollen, causing the conidium to resem-

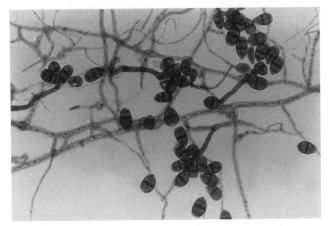

FIGURE 3.34

Typical isolates of *Curvularia* have dark septate hyphae and brown-to-black multicellular conidia. The unequal cells within the conidia are clearly visible, with the swollen central cell(s) and the smaller cells at the base (which may be tapered somewhat) and the tip. In the upper left quadrant a cluster of four conidia is arranged around the tip of a conidiophore that enters the field from the left margin, in a pattern characteristic of this fungus. Three other examples of the dark geniculate conidiophores appear in this field, each with a group of conidia at its tip.

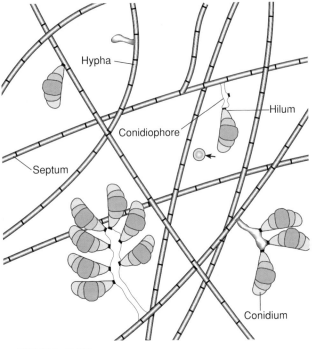

FIGURE 3.35

Curvularia species produce dark, curved, multicellular conidia resembling crescent rolls; the center cell is swollen and darker than the cells lateral to it. Conidia develop in a sympodial pattern around the slender geniculate conidiophores. A dark, protruding hilum is seen at the base of conidia, and scars remain on the conidiophores when conidia are released. The 7-μm red blood cell (arrow) shows the relative sizes of the mycotic elements.

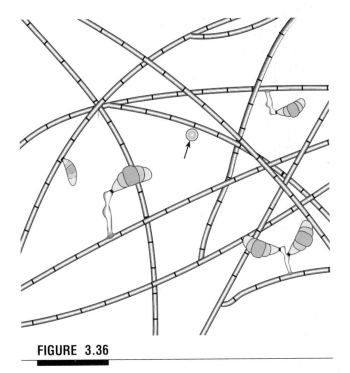

FIGURE 3.36

Even in very bad preparations the dark, curved macroconidia with swollen central cells strongly suggest *Curvularia*. Dark hyphae and slender geniculate conidiophores confirm the identification. The 7-μm red blood cell (arrow) shows the relative sizes of the mycotic elements.

ble a crescent roll. Poroconidia of *Curvularia* have a dark protruding basal hilum at their point of attachment to the conidiogenous cells.

■ Helpful Features for Identification of *Curvularia* Species

> Dematiaceous hyphae
> Sympodial conidiogeny
> Geniculate conidiophores
> Darkly pigmented, multicellular poroconidia with transverse septa, produced in whorls
> Large dark conidia with darker swollen central cells, resembling a crescent roll

■ Organisms from Which *Curvularia* Must Be Differentiated (see Table 3.5 and Fig. 3.30)

> *Exserohilum*
> *Bipolaris*
> *Helminthosporium*
> *Drechslera*

Contaminant/Opportunistic Pathogen

DEMATIACEAE

DRECHSLERA SPECIES (Dresh[8]-lair'-uh)

■ **Reservoirs.** The fungus exists in the soil as a saprobe.

■ **Unique Risk Factors.** None.

■ **Human Infection.** *Drechslera* species have been reported as the agent of mycotic keratitis, phaeohyphomycosis, allergies and sinusitis, meningoencephalitis and peritonitis, and infections of the nasal mucosa.

■ **Specimen Sources.** Aspirates from the peritoneum, respiratory secretions, biopsies of infected tissue, and scrapings and specimens from the skin and nose are most likely to be cultured.

■ **Special Precautions.** None are needed, but cultures should be handled within a biologic safety cabinet.

■ **Culture Media.** Modified SDA, modified SDA with antibacterial agents. Subculture to PDA or PFA to enhance conidiation.

Temperature Considerations. *Drechslera* species grow at 25° to 30°C.

■ **Macroscopic (Colony) Morphology.** The organism is mature in 5 to 6 days on modified SDA at 25°C. In early growth *Drechslera* colonies are flat and spreading with gray or olive-gray surface pigment. As the colony matures it develops a matted black woolly center and a braided fringe. The reverse is gray to black.

■ **Microscopic Morphology.** (Figs. 3.37 through 3.39). Hyphae are dark brown and septate, averaging 4 μm in diameter. The conidiophores are also darkly pigmented and septate; they are simple or branched, and geniculate. The large (approximately 9 × 25 μm) dark brown poroconidia are produced sympodially at the apex of the conidiophores, through pores in the walls; the conidia resemble pea pods. Conidiophores are indeterminate, producing secondary conidia acropetally, with conidia developing on alternate sides of the conidiophore, creating a zigzag pattern. The cylindrical poroconidia are divided into four or five cells by thick transverse septa; in contrast to *Curvularia* all cells of *Drechslera* conidia are approximately equal in diameter. Conidia may occur singly or in small clusters. The dark hila of the poroconidia are continuous with the cell walls and do not noticeably pro-

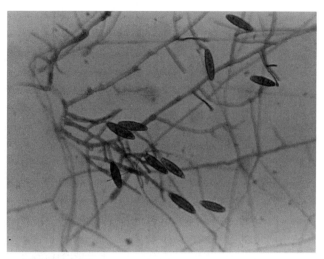

FIGURE 3.37

Typical isolates of *Drechslera* have dark multicellular conidia that resemble pea pods. Hyphae are dematiaceous and septate. The upper right quadrant shows several conidia attached to the geniculate conidiophores. The conidium in the upper right quadrant that lies almost straight up and down shows the thick transverse septa characteristic of this organism. As more conidia develop, they form in a sympodial pattern around the conidiophores.

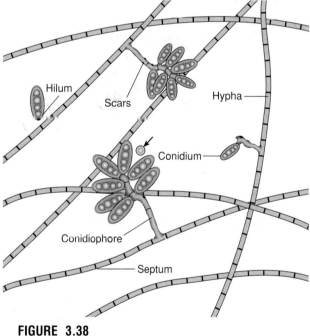

FIGURE 3.38

Drechslera species have dark septate hyphae and broader septate conidiophores that are geniculate. The dark conidia have thick transverse septa dividing them into "pea pods" with four or five cells. The hilum is unobtrusive. Scars (annellations) mark the places where conidia were attached to conidiophores. Germ tubes sometimes form midway between the hilum and the first septum; they grow perpendicular to the long axis of the conidia. The 7-μm red blood cell (arrow) shows the relative sizes of the mycotic elements.

---

[8]"Drech" rhymes with mesh.

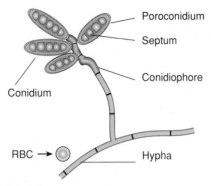

FIGURE 3.39

Even in bad preparation *Drechslera* species should be considered when the isolate has dark septate hyphae and geniculate conidiophores. This identification is supported by the presence of multicellular macroconidia with rounded ends; the thick transverse septa distinguish this mould from *Bipolaris* species, whose macroconidia also resemble pea pods. The absence of obvious hila on the macroconidia further suggests *Drechslera*. The 7-μm red blood cell (RBC) (arrow) shows the relative sizes of the mycotic elements.

trude. Germ tubes are formed at right angles to the conidial axis at the base of the conidium and from other cells of the conidium.

■ **Helpful Features for Identification of *Drechslera* Species**

> Dematiaceous hyphae
> Sympodial conidiogeny
> Geniculate conidiophores
> Darkly pigmented cylindrical poroconidia produced in a zigzag pattern at the apex of the conidiophores
> Multicellular poroconidia with four or five thick transverse septa

■ **Organisms from Which *Drechslera* Must Be Differentiated** (see Table 3.5 and Fig. 3.30)

> *Exserohilum*
> *Bipolaris*
> *Helminthosporium*
> *Curvularia*

Contaminant/Opportunistic Pathogen

TUBERCULARIACEAE

EPICOCCUM SPECIES (Epp-ee-cock'-um)

■ **Reservoirs.** The fungus is found in soil, air, and water and on rotting vegetation.

■ **Unique Risk Factors.** None.

■ **Human Infection.** *Epicoccum* species have occasionally been associated with skin allergies.

■ **Specimen Sources.** Skin scrapings and biopsies may be cultured.

■ **Special Precautions.** None are needed, but cultures should be handled within a biologic safety cabinet.

■ **Culture Media.** Modified SDA, modified SDA with chloramphenicol.

Temperature Considerations. *Epicoccum* species grow at 25°C.

■ **Macroscopic (Colony) Morphology.** The colony that appears on modified SDA at 25°C after 6 to 7 days is initially floccose or velvety. As conidia are produced, the colony becomes irregular in shape with a rough texture. Great variation is possible with a yellow or orange "turf" overlaid by patches of brown to black. Some species also produce a diffusible purple-red pigment on the reverse. *Sporodochia*, tight mats or patches of conidiating conidiophores within the velvety mycelium, appear on the surface of colonies as they mature. The sporodochia give the surface its patchy, mottled appearance.

■ **Microscopic Morphology** (Figs. 3.40 through 3.43). The septate hyphae are bunched together. They may be yellow or orange as pigment develops; eventually they become brown. Conidiophores develop on intertwined hyphae; they are short, thick, and dark, with repeated branching. Conidia are hyaline and nonseptate. As the

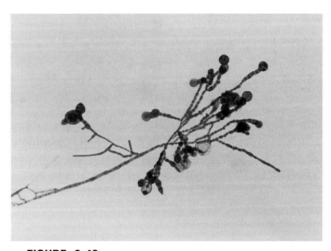

FIGURE 3.40

Characteristically, *Epicoccum* species have septate hyphae that become brown with age. Conidiophores are short and thick, with many branches; in this photomicrograph the conidiophores are lumpy, almost "beaded" looking. The large, multicellular conidia are round, with both lateral and transverse septa. As usual, the conidia vary greatly in size; the septa are more apparent in some conidia than in others.

FIGURE 3.41

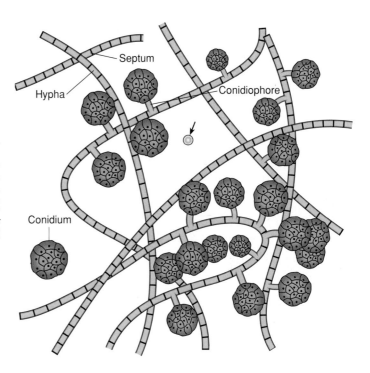

Epicoccum species have septate hyphae that are bunched together and intertwined in older cultures to form sporodochia (see Fig. 3.43). In older cultures hyphae are dark. The simple conidiophores are short, thick, and dark and may branch repeatedly. Immature conidia are clavate, hyaline, and nonseptate. As they mature they "round up," become echinulate, and develop muriform septa. The pigment of the conidia becomes dark brown to black as they age. The 7-μm red blood cell (arrow) shows the relative sizes of the mycotic elements.

FIGURE 3.42

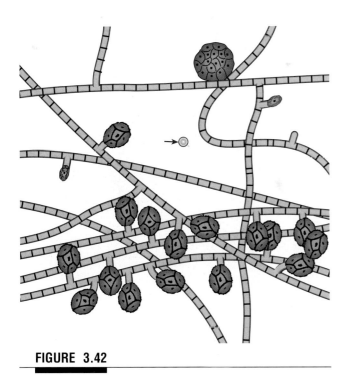

Even in a bad preparation *Epicoccum* should be suspected when bunches of hyphae are seen in the company of short, dark, thick, and branching conidiophores. Suspicion should intensify if the conidia are multicellular, with both lateral and transverse septa; they look somewhat like black basketballs. Colony morphology provides further clues to the possibility of *Epicoccum* species. The 7-μm red blood cell (arrow) shows the relative sizes of the mycotic elements.

FIGURE 3.43

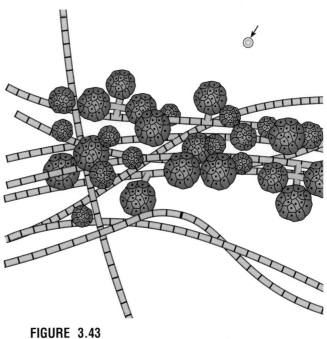

The sporodochia of *Epicoccum* are aggregations of hyphae—far more complex than those shown—that are covered with conidia and branching conidiophores. Colonies with sporodochia have a patchy, mottled appearance because of the thick mats of hyphae. The 7-μm red blood cell (arrow) shows the relative sizes of the mycotic elements.

conidia age they become large (average diameter 20 μm, range 15 to 25 μm) and irregularly globose to *subglobose* (irregularly rounded). Sporodochia are formed by the aggregation of hyphae that are covered with branching conidiophores and conidia.

■ Helpful Features for Identification of *Epicoccum* Species

Rough-textured, irregularly shaped colonies
Great variation in color in the colony surface
Globose muriform conidia that are dark and thick walled
Conidiophores that develop sporodochia

■ Organisms from Which *Epicoccum* Must Be Differentiated (Table 3.6)

Stemphylium
Ulocladium
Nigrospora

Contaminant/Opportunistic Pathogen

TUBERCULARIACEAE

FUSARIUM SPECIES   (Few-sarh[9]-ee-um)

■ **Reservoirs.** *Fusarium* species are found worldwide in soil and on rotting vegetation and ripe fruit. Because of its importance as a plant pathogen, a U. S. Department of Agriculture permit is required to purchase a culture from the American Type Culture Collection.

■ **Unique Risk Factors.** Exposure to dust containing *Fusarium* may result in keratitis, especially in contact lens wearers. Burn patients are peculiarly prone to develop *Fusarium* infections.

■ **Human Infection.** *Fusarium* species have been associated with keratitis, onychomycosis, fungemia, invasive nasal infections that spread to the lungs, skin infections—especially in burn patients, and disseminated disease.

■ **Specimen Sources.** Corneal scrapings, aspirates from lesions, respiratory secretions, blood, biopsies of tissue and skin, nail clippings, cerebrospinal fluid, and gastric secretions are most likely to be submitted for culture.

■ **Special Precautions.** None are needed, but cultures should be handled within a biologic safety cabinet.

---

[9]"Sarh" rhymes with jar.

■ **Culture Media.** Modified SDA, subculture to PFA or PDA.

Temperature Considerations. *Fusarium* species grow at 25° to 30°C.

■ **Macroscopic (Colony) Morphology.** The organism produces colonies after 5 to 6 days on modified SDA at 25°C. Initially colonies of *Fusarium* are white and velvety. As conidia are produced the texture becomes woolly to cottony. A great variety of colors may be produced, from gray on a white surface to yellow on brown, buff pink on violet, or tan on pale green. Colonies are most often pink to violet. Patches of darker pigment appear in the center of the colony, with a lighter periphery. The pigments are water soluble and diffuse into the medium and the hyphae. The reverse of the colony is usually light in color but eventually absorbs the diffusible surface pigment. This is one of the cases where colony morphology is more confusing than helpful (unless violet pigment is present), but the presence of water-soluble pigment is distinctive, suggesting *Fusarium*.

■ **Microscopic Morphology** (Figs. 3.44 through 3.46). The septate hyaline hyphae of *Fusarium* are approximately 4 μm in diameter. Conidiophores are absent. Phialides arise directly from the hyphae. They are hya-

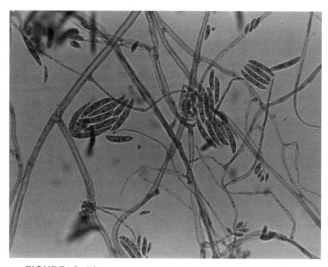

FIGURE 3.44

Characteristically *Fusarium* species have delicate septate hyphae; this feature is not obvious because of the magnification. Two kinds of conidia form; they are more often found free in the preparation than attached to the conidiophores because the attachment is very tenuous. Small oval or cylindrical microconidia are free in this field; at the base of the lower right quadrant you can see four that are attached. The large fusiform macroconidia with their tapered ends resemble bananas when they are slightly curved or—when the curvature is greater—sickles (look at those in the left half of the field at the horizontal midline of the photomicrograph). This "whorl" of macroconidia is typical of *Fusarium*; the palisading of four free macroconidia in the upper right corner is also typical. Few of these macroconidia are attached.

TABLE 3.6 Dematiaceous Saprobes with "Globose" Conidia

Fungus	Size of Conidia (μm)	Shape of Conidia	Arrangement of Conidia	Width of Hyphae (μm)	Length of Conidiophore (μm)	Shape of Conidiophore	Arrangement of Conidiophores	Colony Morphology	Growth Rate	Other Helpful Features
Epicoccum	15–25	Globose or subglobose	Individual	5	8	Short, thick, dark, with branching	Individual	Rough texture with dark patches, with pale reverse	Intermediate	Sporodochia are present; conidia are muriform
Nigrospora	12	Slightly flattened	Individual	4	8–15	Short, with prominent swelling and flared "mouth"	Individual	Gray-to-black surface, with black reverse	Rapid	Black unicellular conidia
*Ulocladium**	11–18	Globose or elliptical	Individual	4	20–60	Erect and geniculate, with branching	Individual	Velvety black, with white-to-gray overgrowth and black reverse	Rapid	Conidia are muriform; conidiophores are septate and zigzag sympodially
*Stemphylium**	15–20	Subglobose	Individual	5	10–14	Swollen tips and branching	Individual	Floccose; brown to black, with black reverse	Rapid	Conidia are muriform, and center is usually constricted

*These fungi appear nowhere else in this text.

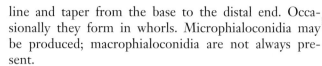

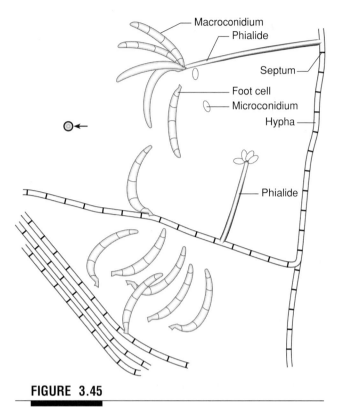

FIGURE 3.45

Fusarium species have delicate, thin-walled septate hyphae. Phialides form directly on the hyphae. The microconidia are small oval or cylindrical forms; they are found alone or in small clusters. The macroconidia are large "canoes" or "sickles" with pointed ends, divided into multiple cells by thin septa. The end of the conidium that attaches to the phialide is a foot cell. Macroconidia are usually found in whorls around a phialide but are easily dislodged. The 7-μm red blood cell (arrow) shows the relative sizes of the mycotic elements.

line and taper from the base to the distal end. Occasionally they form in whorls. Microphialoconidia may be produced; macrophialoconidia are not always present.

Both types of conidia are hyaline, with smooth walls. The *microphialoconidia* are cylindrical unicellular forms and may be found singly or held together in small clusters by a mucoid substance. *Macrophialoconidia* are, logically enough, larger (averaging 5 × 50 μm with a maximum length of 80 μm). They are typically *fusiform* (canoe shaped or sickle shaped with pointed ends) and divided into 2 to 11 cells by septa. The macroconidia of *Fusarium* have a distinct foot cell at the point of attachment to the phialide. Chlamydoconidia are seen in cultures of most species.

In *direct examination* of specimens the presence of *Fusarium* is suggested by fragments of hyaline septate hyphae with dichotomous branching.

■ **Helpful Features for Identification of *Fusarium* Species**

Woolly to cottony colonies in a great variety of diffusible colors—most often pink or purple

Both microphialoconidia and macrophialoconidia, which are crescent shaped with a distinct foot cell

■ **Organisms from Which *Fusarium* Must Be Differentiated** (see Table 3.2)

Acremonium
Cylindrocarpon

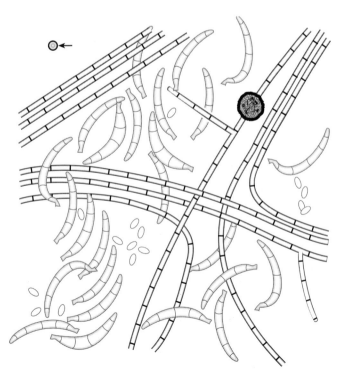

FIGURE 3.46

Even in bad preparations (which are more common than good ones) the combination of microconidia and large fusiform macroconidia with foot cells suggests *Fusarium* species. Chlamydoconidia may develop in the hyphae, as shown within the hypha at the upper right. The connection between the conidium and the phialide is so tenuous that most microscopic preparations contain many free conidia. Colony morphology, especially the pigment, is useful to identify the colony. The 7-μm red blood cell (arrow) shows the relative sizes of the mycotic elements.

Contaminant

MONILIACEAE

GLIOCLADIUM SPECIES   (Glee-oh-clay'-dee-um)

■ **Unique Risk Factors.** None.

■ **Human Infection.** *Gliocladium* species are not known to be a human pathogen.

■ **Specimen Sources.** Occasionally the organism is isolated as a contaminant from a specimen; culture for *Gliocladium* is rarely requested.

■ **Special Precautions.** None are needed, but cultures should be handled within a biologic safety cabinet.

■ **Culture Media.** Modified SDA.

Temperature Considerations. Gliocladium species grow at 25°C.

■ **Macroscopic (Colony) Morphology.** On modified SDA at 25°C, after 3 to 5 days, the colony fills the entire Petri dish or test tube. The appearance of the colony can vary greatly. It is at first white and floccose, then granular and pastel (green, light yellow, pink, or salmon). The topography is level and carpet-like as conidia are produced. The reverse pigment is white to light yellow.

■ **Microscopic Morphology** (Figs. 3.47 through 3.49). The hyaline septate hyphae of *Gliocladium* sometimes produce terminal chlamydoconidia. Conidiophores develop into a ***penicillus,*** a brushlike arrangement due to the branching of the conidiophores to support the primary *metulae,* sterile branches within the reproductive system that bear flask-shaped phialides. Conidia on adjacent phialides mass together in large sticky balls surmounting the group of phialides—as if a small tripod were supporting a popcorn ball. The individual phialoconidia are unicellular and spherical. The ball of conidia may be green or white.

FIGURE 3.47

Typical preparations of *Gliocladium* species contain short, erect branching conidiophores supporting three or four tapering phialides in a penicillus, with clusters of round conidia at the tip of each phialide (arrow). Two or more penicilli may branch from the conidiophore at approximately the same point, with the conidia from each joining to form a single mass. Hyphae are septate. The dark pigmentation is an artifact caused by stain. (From Rippon JW: Medical Mycology: The Pathogenic Fungi and the Pathogenic Actinomycetes, 3rd ed. Philadelphia, WB Saunders, 1988, p 757.)

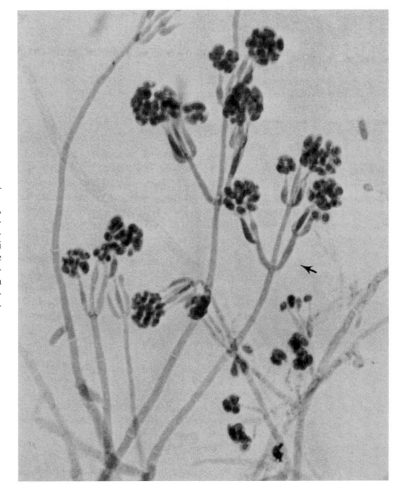

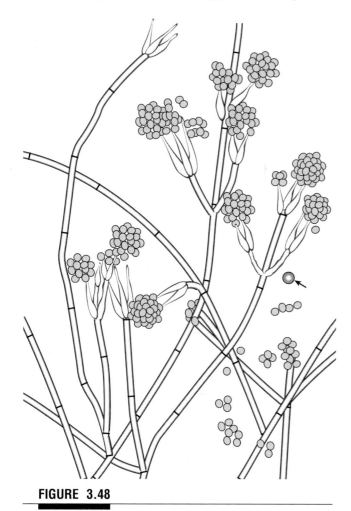

FIGURE 3.48

Gliocladium species have septate hyphae and sticklike conidiophores. Metulae develop from the conidiophores to support flask-shaped phialides arranged in a penicillus. The clumps of spherical conidia on individual phialides mass together at the tip of the penicillus to resemble popcorn balls set on tripods. Chlamydoconidia are sometimes present on the tips of hyphal branches. The 7-μm red blood cell (arrow) shows the relative sizes of the mycotic elements.

■ **Helpful Features for Identification of *Gliocladium* Species**

Pastel colonies that fill the test tube or Petri dish in 3 to 5 days with a carpet-like growth

Erect and branched conidiophores supporting penicilli

Balls of phialoconidia situated on the apices of adjacent flask-shaped phialides (popcorn balls on tripods)

■ **Organisms from Which *Gliocladium* Must Be Differentiated** (see Table 3.2 and Fig. 3.8)

Trichoderma
Verticillium

Contaminant/Opportunistic Pathogen

DEMATIACEAE

HELMINTHOSPORIUM SPECIES   (Hell-minth'-oh-spore'-ee-um)

■ **Reservoirs.** The fungus is found in soil as a saprophyte. It is isolated infrequently as a contaminant in the laboratory.

■ **Unique Risk Factors.** None.

■ **Human Infection.** *Helminthosporium* species have been reported in rare cases of mycotic keratitis and endocarditis. Confusion is rampant in earlier literature about the role of *Helminthosporium* in human infection because review of the cases shows that many infections attributed to *Helminthosporium* were in fact caused by *Drechslera*, *Bipolaris*, or *Exserohilum*.

■ **Specimen Sources.** Blood and scrapings from eye infections are likely specimen sources.

■ **Special Precautions.** None are needed, but specimens should be handled within a biologic safety cabinet.

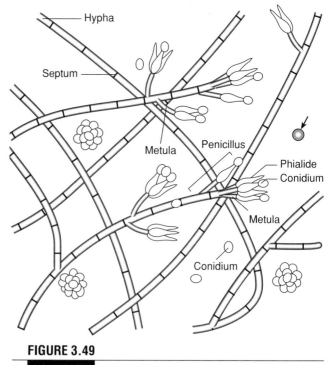

FIGURE 3.49

Even in bad preparations the presence of penicilli and "popcorn balls" suggest *Gliocladium* species, especially when the clusters of spherical conidia are balanced on the tips of phialides. Use colony morphology to help distinguish *Gliocladium* from fungi with similar structures. The 7-μm red blood cell (arrow) shows the relative sizes of the mycotic elements.

FIGURE 3.50

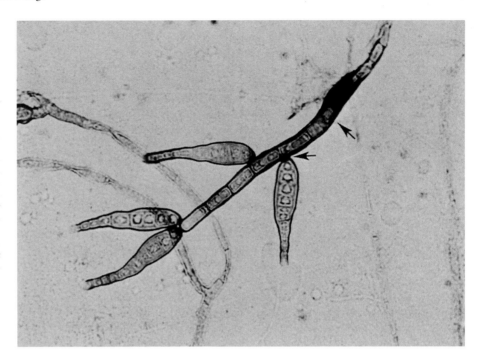

Typical conidia of *Helminthosporium* are shaped like the clubs associated with a cave man; they are attached to the conidiophores at their "heads." Conidia emerge from the hyphae from prominent pores that can often be seen with the light microscope (arrows); the conidia are multicellular with dark pigment and heavy darker walls. Hyphae are dematiaceous and septate and may be somewhat uneven in size. (From Rippon JW: Medical Mycology: The Pathogenic Fungi and the Pathogenic Actinomycetes, 3rd ed. Philadelphia, WB Saunders, 1988, p 769.)

■ **Culture Media.** Modified SDA, modified SDA with chloramphenicol should be used.

Temperature Considerations. *Helminthosporium* species grow at 25° to 30°C.

■ **Macroscopic (Colony) Morphology.** The organism is mature in 5 to 6 days on modified SDA at 25°C. In early growth *Helminthosporium* species are flat and spreading with gray or olive-green pigment. As the colony matures the texture becomes cottony and the pigment intensifies to a brownish black surface pigment with a dark brown to black reverse pigment.

■ **Microscopic Morphology** (Figs. 3.50 through 3.52). Hyphae are dark brown and septate, averaging 4 μm in diameter. The determinate conidiophores are also darkly pigmented and septate. They are simple, unbranched, and slightly curved, with smooth parallel walls. The shape of the conidiophore is a key feature for distinguishing *Helminthosporium* from *Bipolaris*, *Drechslera*, and *Exserohilum*, all of which have geniculate conidiophores. Poroconidia are produced individually through prominent pores in the cell walls of the conidiophores. The dark brown conidia are divided into five or more cells by thick transverse septa. They are long and club shaped (average size 5 × 30 μm), rounded where they attach to the conidiophore, and slightly curved and tapering at the distal ends. The "head" of the club is attached to the conidiophore and tapers to the free "handle." Poroconidia may occur singly along the length of the conidiophores but are often found in whorls.

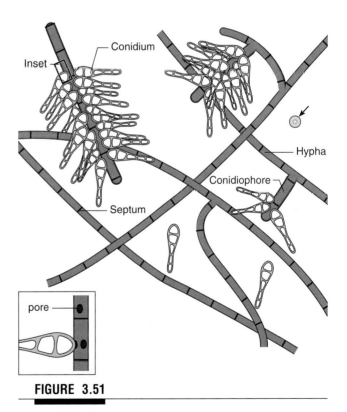

FIGURE 3.51

Helminthosporium species have septate dematiaceous hyphae and dark brown to black macroconidia. The club-shaped macroconidia are attached to the conidiophores at the head of the "club"; they have five or more thick, transverse septa. Conidiophores have straight parallel walls; pores *(inset)* can sometimes be seen on the conidiophores when conidia are released. The 7-μm red blood cell (arrow) shows the relative sizes of the mycotic elements.

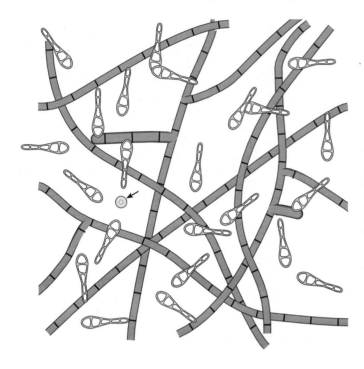

FIGURE 3.52

Even in bad preparations *Helminthosporium* species should be considered if dark septate hyphae and multicellular macroconidia are seen in the preparation. This is supported by conidiophores with parallel walls and macroconidia that are club shaped, attached to the conidiophore at the larger "heads." The 7-μm red blood cell (arrow) shows the relative sizes of the mycotic elements.

■ **Helpful Features for Identification of *Helminthosporium* Species**

Dematiaceous hyphae and dark unbranched conidiophores

Darkly pigmented clavate poroconidia produced laterally through pores along the conidiophores

Multicellular poroconidia with more than five thick transverse septa

■ **Organisms from Which *Helminthosporium* Must Be Differentiated** (see Table 3.5 and Fig. 3.30)

Drechslera
Exserohilum
Bipolaris
Curvularia

Contaminant/Opportunistic Pathogen

HYALINE HYPHOMYCETE/ZYGOMYCETE

MUCOR SPECIES

Mucor is discussed with the other four Zygomycetes at the end of this chapter.

Contaminant/Opportunistic Pathogen

DEMATIACEAE

NIGROSPORA SPECIES   (Nigh[10]-grow-spore-uh)

■ **Reservoirs.** The fungus is found worldwide in soil as a saprobe.

■ **Unique Risk Factors.** None.

■ **Human Infection.** *Nigrospora* species are isolated as contaminants but only rarely cause human infection. It has been reported as a rare agent of mycotic keratitis.

■ **Specimen Sources.** Specimens from the eye are most likely to be cultured.

■ **Special Precautions.** None are needed, but cultures should be handled within a biologic safety cabinet.

■ **Culture Media.** Modified SDA, modified SDA with chloramphenicol.

Temperature Considerations. *Nigrospora* species grow at 25° to 30°C.

■ **Macroscopic (Colony) Morphology.** After 4 to 5 days on modified SDA at 25°C, the colony is compact and woolly and fills the plate. At first the colony is

---

[10]"Nigh" rhymes with rye.

FIGURE 3.53

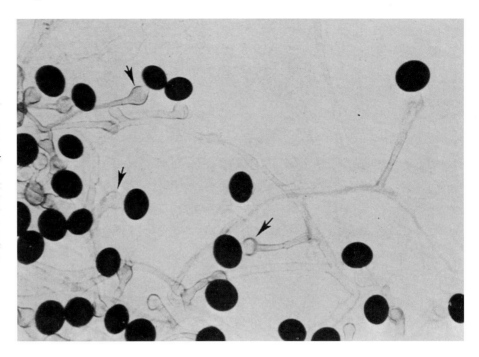

Typical preparations of *Nigrospora* demonstrate large, dark, slightly flattened oval conidia that are attached to the conidiophores at the side rather than the end of the oval, rather as if a ripe olive were attached along the long axis rather than at the tip. The conidiophores of *Nigrospora* have prominent swellings just below the tip (arrows). Hyphae are septate and colorless. (From Rippon JW: Medical Mycology: The Pathogenic Fungi and the Pathogenic Actinomycetes, 3rd ed. Philadelphia, WB Saunders, 1988, p 774.)

white, then it becomes gray with black patches where conidia are produced. The reverse of the colony is black.

■ **Microscopic Morphology** (Figs. 3.53 through 3.55). Hyphae are septate. They initially are hyaline but darken as the colony ages. The hyaline conidiophores are short and rarely branch. They are broad with a prominent globular swelling in the middle and a tapering nipple where the conidium attaches. The large unicellular black conidia of *Nigrospora* are produced individually, one per conidiophore. They average 12 μm in diameter (range 10 to 14 μm). The conidia are ovoid or subglobose, with horizontal flattening that makes them resemble a rubber ball after someone stepped on it. They are *aleuric*, that is, released from the conidiophore by fracturing.

■ **Helpful Features for Identification of *Nigrospora* Species**

Unicellular black ovoid to subglobose conidia that may be horizontally flattened
Short, broad conidiophores that are terminally swollen

■ **Organisms from Which *Nigrospora* Species Must Be Differentiated** (see Table 3.6)

Ulocladium
Stemphylium
Epicoccum

Contaminant/Opportunistic Pathogen

MONILIACEAE

PAECILOMYCES SPECIES   (Pay-sill-oh-my-sees)

■ **Reservoirs.** *Paecilomyces* species are found worldwide in soil and decaying vegetation. The spores are airborne.

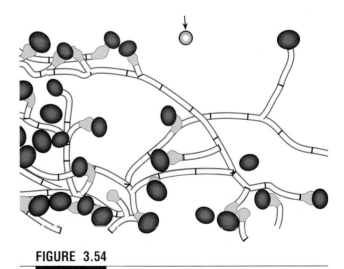

FIGURE 3.54

Nigrospora species have septate hyphae that become dark as they age. The conidiophores are short and stubby with a prominent, slightly darker swelling in the central portion and a flared lip that supports the large, dark conidium. Conidia are slightly oval and rounded, like a balloon that has lost part of its air. The pigmentation of swelling is intensified here to emphasize the swelling. The 7-μm red blood cell (arrow) shows the relative sizes of the mycotic elements.

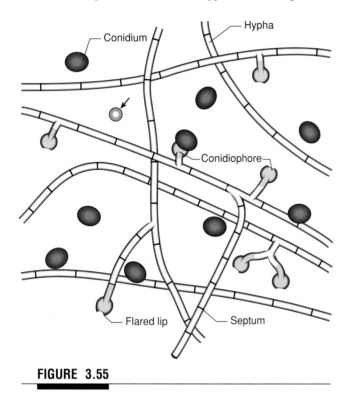

Conidium — Hypha —
Conidiophore —
Flared lip — Septum —

FIGURE 3.55

Even in a bad preparation *Nigrospora* should be suspected when large, slightly flattened, dark conidia are seen. Identification as *Nigrospora* becomes more likely if the conidiophores have a flared lip and a prominent globose swelling. The pigmentation is intensified here to emphasize the swelling. The 7-μm red blood cell (arrow) shows the relative sizes of the mycotic elements.

■ **Unique Risk Factors.** None.

■ **Human Infection.** *Paecilomyces* species are usually present as a contaminant. Occasionally it has been reported as a pathogen in pulmonary infections, endocarditis, and sinusitis. Infections of cutaneous lesions have occasionally occurred after traumatic inoculation of the host, and *Paecilomyces* species have been associated with infections in patients who have had organ transplants.

■ **Specimen Sources.** Respiratory secretions, tissue biopsy specimens, skin scrapings, blood, and aspirates from abscesses are most likely to be submitted for culture.

■ **Special Precautions.** None are needed, but cultures should be manipulated in a biologic safety cabinet.

■ **Culture Media.** Modified SDA.

Temperature Considerations. *Paecilomyces* species grow at 25°C.

■ **Macroscopic (Colony) Morphology.** After 4 to 5 days on modified SDA at 25°C, the colony of *Paecilomyces* is initially flat and floccose. As they age colonies develop a velvety or powdery texture. The color of the colony can vary from ivory white to greenish brown to yellow-brown

to violet, with an ivory white to light brown reverse—in short, almost anything is possible, although some authors insist that *Paecilomyces* species do not develop a true green or greenish blue color.

■ **Microscopic Morphology** (Figs. 3.56 through 3.58). Hyphae of *Paecilomyces* are hyaline and septate. Conidiophores are erect with irregular branching at the apices. In some species conidiophores bear metulae and phialides in a penicillus arrangement resembling *Penicillium* species. In other species of *Paecilomyces* the phialides arise directly from the vegetative hyphae singly and in pairs or whorls. In all species conidia are produced from the tips of the phialides in chains that tend to bend away from the conidiophores. The phialides are long and delicate, and they taper from the relatively large base to slender tubes at their distal ends like bottles with lo-o-o-ong narrow necks. The unicellular phialoconidia are small (approximately 3 μm) and hyaline or lightly pigmented. They are elliptical in shape; the walls may be smooth or rough. The conidia are produced basipetally. Some species of *Paecilomyces* produce chlamydoconidia.

■ **Helpful Features for Identification of *Paecilomyces* Species**

Conidiophores that are irregularly branched at the apices
Chains of conidia bending away from the conidiophores
Long phialides that taper from the base to a narrow tip
Arrangement of phialides in whorls
Production of phialides directly from the hyphae in some species

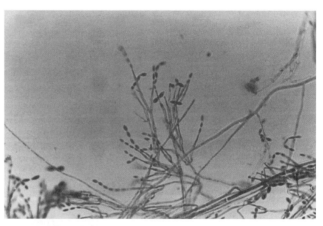

FIGURE 3.56

In characteristic preparations *Paecilomyces* species show septate hyphae and erect branching conidiophores with a penicillus arrangement; in some species the phialides of *Paecilomyces* arise directly from the hyphae. The phialides have a relatively wide base that tapers to a long, slender neck. Conidia are produced in chains from the phialides.

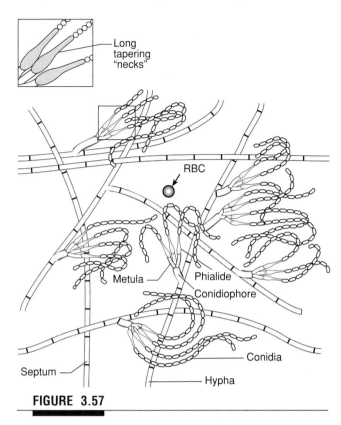

FIGURE 3.57

Paecilomyces species produce long chains of elliptical conidia from phialides that have long, narrow necks. When the phialides develop from metulae at the tips of conidiophores, the "penicillus" arrangement may cause this fungus to be confused with *Penicillium*. Long, tapered tips on the phialides *(inset)* indicate *Paecilomyces*. The chains of conidia typically bend away from the conidiophore. The 7-μm red blood cell (RBC) (arrow) shows the relative sizes of the mycotic elements.

■ **Organisms from Which *Paecilomyces* Must Be Differentiated** (Table 3.7 and Fig. 3.59)

Penicillium

Contaminant/Opportunistic Pathogen

MONILIACEAE

PENICILLIUM SPECIES   (Pen-uh-sill'-ee-um)

■ **Reservoirs.** *Penicillium* species are ubiquitous and omnipresent throughout the world. They are found in soil and decaying vegetation. *Penicillium* species are likely to be found in the kitchen and other areas of the house and occur normally on skin and in some secretions. The fungi are spread by an airborne route. Species of *Penicillium* are one of the most common laboratory contaminants.

■ **Unique Risk Factors.** None.

■ **Human Infection.** *Penicillium* species are usually a contaminant or a secondary invader, but infections do occur. Seven of the approximately 900 species have been isolated as etiologic agents of infection. Pulmonary infections, keratomycosis, onychomycosis, external ear infections, cutaneous lesions, bladder infections, and endocarditis due to *Penicillium* species have been reported with, in some cases, considerable doubt about the reliability of the report. A case of *fungemia* (fungi in the blood) has been reported in a patient with acquired immunodeficiency syndrome.

Penicillium species are not usually invasive. Even when the fungus is isolated mycologists have difficulty determining whether the isolate is simply colonizing the tissue or is actively involved in infection (see Table 3.1). Repeatedly recovering *Penicillium* from body surfaces or secretions is not considered proof of its role in infection unless it is also demonstrated in sections of the tissue. Some species produce a toxin on decaying vegetation that may cause gastrointestinal disturbances if it is ingested.

■ **Specimen Sources.** Respiratory secretions, urine, blood, biopsies of the eye or ear or other infected tissues, and aspirates are most likely to be submitted for culture.

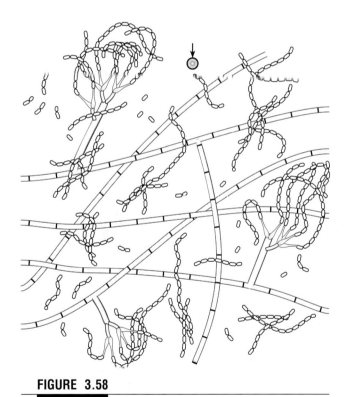

FIGURE 3.58

Even in a bad preparation, the genus *Paecilomyces* is one possible identification when the preparation contains long chains of conidia and phialides arising at the tips of conidiophores. The mould is likely to be *Paecilomyces* rather than *Penicillium* when the phialides arise directly from the septate hyphae. Phialides with long, slender, tapering necks always indicate *Paecilomyces*. Colony morphology may be helpful in confirming the identification. The 7-μm red blood cell (arrow) shows the relative sizes of the mycotic elements.

TABLE 3.7 Hyaline Saprobes with Penicilli

Fungus	Size of Conidia (μm)	Shape of Conidia	Arrangement of Conidia	Width of Hyphae (μm)	Length of Conidiophore (μm)	Shape of Conidiophore	Arrangement of Conidiophores	Colony Morphology	Growth Rate	Other Helpful Features
Paecilomyces	3	Elliptical	Chains	2–3	10–12	Penicillus	Solitary and erect WHEN PRESENT	Velvety or powdery pastel—not green	Rapid	Phialides have lo-o-o-ng necks with tapering tips
Penicillium	2–5	Round	Chains	2–3	45	Penicillus	Solitary and erect	Velvety or powdery pastel	Rapid	Phialides have relatively short necks with blunt tips
Scopulariopsis	6	Pyriform annelloconidia with flat bases	Chains	6	10–30	Branching annellides RESEMBLE penicillus	Solitary or in clusters	Velvety or powdery light brown	Rapid	Echinulate conidia with flattened bases and nipple-like projections at the tip

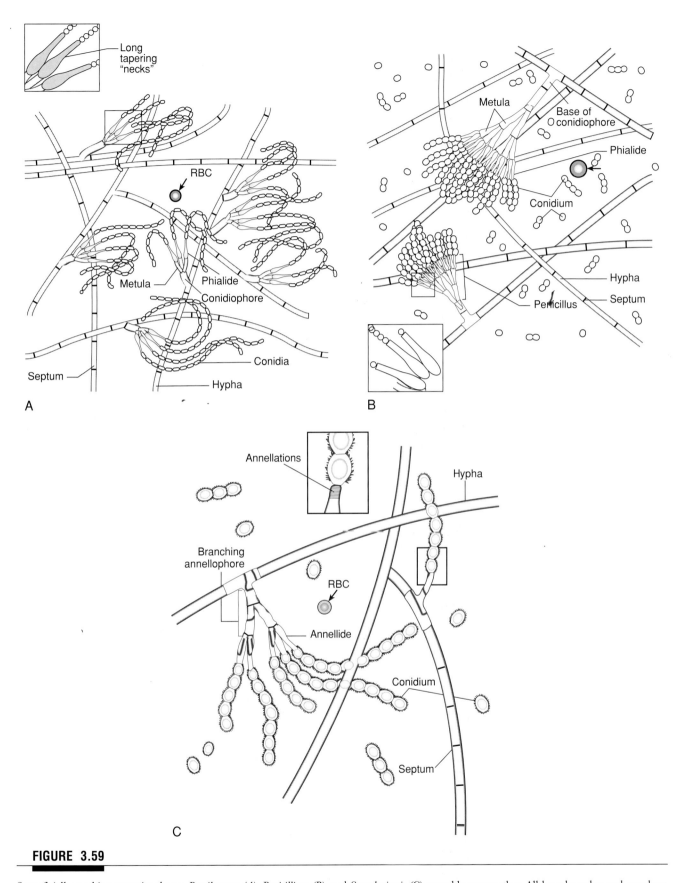

Long tapering "necks"

RBC

Metula

Phialide

Conidiophore

Conidia

Septum

Hypha

A

Metula

Base of conidiophore

Phialide

Conidium

Hypha

Septum

Penicillus

B

Annellations

Hypha

Branching annellophore

RBC

Annellide

Conidium

Septum

C

FIGURE 3.59

Superficially, as this composite shows, *Paecilomyces (A)*, *Penicillium (B)*, and *Scopulariopsis (C)* resemble one another. All have branches and may have arrangements resembling penicilli, and all produce conidia in chains. However, the structures of *Scopulariopsis* are much larger than those of the other two genera and the conidia are definitely echinulate. *Paecilomyces* and *Penicillium* can be differentiated by the different shapes of the tips of the phialides. Most *Paecilomyces* species also have phialides produced directly from the hyphae, or developing on the ends of conidiophores. The 7-μm red blood cell (RBC) (arrow) shows the relative sizes of the mycotic elements.

■ **Special Precautions.** None are needed; specimens should be handled within a biologic safety cabinet.

■ **Culture Media.** Modified SDA, modified SDA with chloramphenicol.

Temperature Considerations. Penicillium species grow at 25° to 45°C.

■ **Macroscopic (Colony) Morphology.** The organisms typically produce colonies on modified SDA at 25°C after 4 days. NOTE that *Penicillium marneffei*, the species most often isolated as a pathogen, takes 2 weeks to produce a mature colony. Colonies have a velvety to powdery texture. The topography is often rugose but may be flat. *Penicillium* colonies are characteristically blue-green with a white periphery and a white reverse, but a great variety of colors (with some combinations of yellow, green, brown, and red) is possible. The pigment of some species may diffuse into the agar surrounding the colony. Colonies of *Penicillium* are sometimes (often?) difficult to distinguish from those of *Aspergillus fumigatus*. Both are typically granular and blue-green to green, and they grow rapidly. The microscopic structures of the two genera, however, are very different, even when the low-power objective is used.

■ **Microscopic Morphology** (Figs. 3.60 through 3.63). Hyphae of *Penicillium* are relatively thin (average diameter 3 μm), hyaline, and septate. The conidiophores are erect, septate, and hyaline to lightly colored. *Penicillium* species typically have a penicillus, that also branches and bears secondary phialides from which chains of conidia grow. Exceptions to this pattern may occur, with simple unbranched conidiophores supporting phialides that arise directly above the conidiophores. The phialides are flask shaped with blunt ends; usually they are aggregated in whorls at the tip of the metula or directly on a branch of the conidiophore. The phialoconidia form basipetally, from the tips of the phialides, in long unbranched chains, with the oldest conidium at the tip. The ovoid to elliptical conidia are small (2 to 5 μm), unicellular, and hyaline or lightly pigmented; the walls may be rough. Differentiation of *Penicillium* to species depends on subtle differences in the shape and arrangement of conidiophores, phialides, and metulae (see Fig. 3.61)—well beyond the scope of this book. If *Penicillium* species are not considered an adequate identification, the culture can be sent to a reference laboratory for *speciation* (identification to species).

Sometimes in a *penicilliosis* (a "condition" of *Penicillium*) small intracellular bodies resembling the yeast form of *Histoplasma capsulatum* are found within macrophages; the two fungi can be differentiated in tissue by the manner in which the yeastlike structures of *Penicillium* divide. Colony morphologies of the two fungi and the microscopic structures produced in culture by *Histoplasma* and *Penicillium* are very different, so the organisms are differentiated quickly when growth appears in culture.

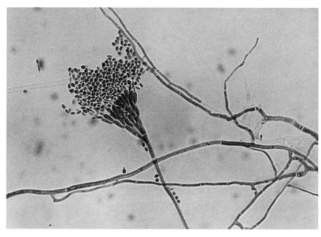

FIGURE 3.60

The hyphae of *Penicillium* are slender and septate. Typically "penicilli" are present; the layers created by branches of the conidiophore, metulae, and phialides make the conidiophores resemble paintbrushes. Conidia are produced in chains from blunt-tipped phialides.

■ **Helpful Features for Identification of *Penicillium* Species**

Flat granular colonies that are typically blue-green
Brushlike penicillus
Phialides with blunt tips
Chains of conidia from the phialides
Phialides may be arranged in whorls

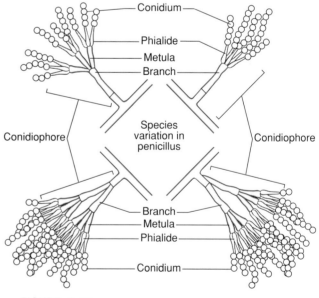

FIGURE 3.61

Differentiation of isolates of *Penicillium* to species depends on subtle differences in the conidia, the arrangement and shape of the phialides and metulae, and the number of "layers" in the penicillus. These variations are presented solely as examples, without the detail necessary to identify isolates to the species level.

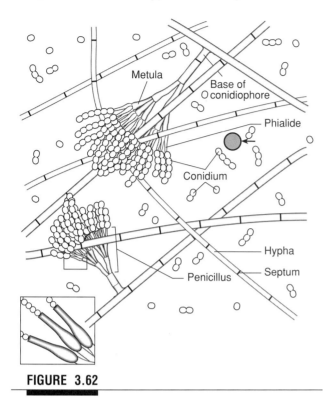

FIGURE 3.62

Penicillium species have slender septate hyphae and erect septate conidiophores. The brushlike penicillus is created by the branching of the conidiophore into metulae, which may also branch and bear phialides. Conidia are produced in chains from the phialides. Phialides have tapering necks that are relatively short with blunt tips *(inset)*. The 7-μm red blood cell (arrow) shows the relative sizes of the mycotic elements.

■ **Organisms from Which *Penicillium* Must Be Differentiated** (see Table 3.7 and Fig. 3.59)

Paecilomyces
Scopulariopsis

Contaminant/Opportunistic Pathogen

HYALINE HYPHOMYCETE/ZYGOMYCETE

RHIZOMUCOR SPECIES

Rhizomucor is discussed with the other four Zygomycetes at the end of this chapter.

Contaminant/Opportunistic Pathogen

HYALINE HYPHOMYCETE/ZYGOMYCETE

RHIZOPUS SPECIES

Rhizopus is discussed with the other four Zygomycetes at the end of this chapter.

Contaminant/Opportunistic Pathogen

MONILIACEAE

SCOPULARIOPSIS SPECIES   (Scope-you-lair-ee-op'[11]-siss)

■ **Reservoirs.** *Scopulariopsis* species are ubiquitous worldwide. They are found in soil and decaying vegetation. The fungus is spread by an airborne route.

■ **Unique Risk Factors.** None.

■ **Human Infection.** *Scopulariopsis* species are usually a contaminant, but they have been recovered on numerous occasions from patients with onychomycosis. It is a rare cause of pneumonia, keratomycosis, otitis, and septicemia.

■ **Specimen Sources.** Respiratory secretions, blood, aspirates and biopsies of the ear, and scrapings of skin and nail are most likely to be submitted for culture.

---

[11]"Op" rhymes with hop.

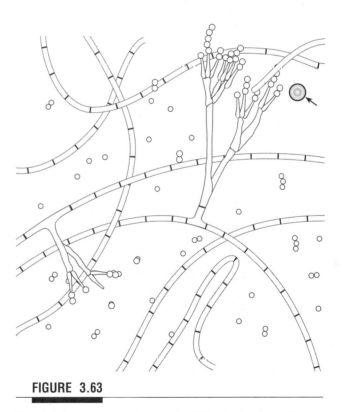

FIGURE 3.63

Even in bad preparations, the genus *Penicillium* (or *Paecilomyces)* is suggested by penicilli and chains of conidia produced from phialides. Identification of the genus as *Penicillium* is confirmed by phialides with relatively short necks and blunt tips, which are produced from conidiophores rather than directly from the hyphae. Colony morphology may be helpful in identification. The 7-μm red blood cell (arrow) shows the relative sizes of the mycotic elements.

■ **Special Precautions.** None are needed, but cultures should be handled within a biologic safety cabinet.

■ **Culture Media.** Modified SDA without cycloheximide.

Temperature Considerations. Scopulariopsis species grow at 25° to 30°C.

■ **Macroscopic (Colony) Morphology.** Colonies of *Scopulariopsis* are mature in 2 to 4 days at 25°C on modified SDA. They are white and membranous at first, becoming velvety or powdery with the production of numerous conidia and aerial hyphae. *Scopulariopsis* colonies are most often light brown with a lighter periphery. The reverse is tan with a brown center. The topography is rugose with irregular folds. Variants may resemble colonies of *Microsporum gypseum*, a dermatophyte presented in Chapter 5.

■ **Microscopic Morphology** (Figs. 3.64 through 3.66). The hyphae of *Scopulariopsis* are relatively broad (average diameter 6 μm, with a range of 2 to 10 μm), hyaline, and septate. The short septate annellophores cannot be distinguished from the hyphae. *Annellophores* are specialized conidiophores that directly support annellides. When the annellophores are branched—especially if clusters of annellides are present—they resemble the brushlike penicillus of *Penicillium*.

The annellides are cylindrical or flask shaped with annellations on their tips. The annellations *may* be seen with oil immersion and a good microscope; usually phase-contrast or interference microscopy is needed. Long unbranching chains of annelloconidia are produced basipetally from the annellides, with the most mature cell

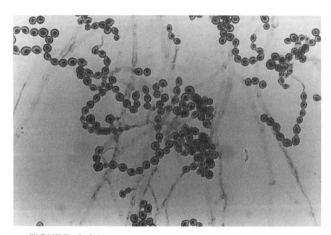

FIGURE 3.64

Typical preparations of *Scopulariopsis* species show septate hyphae and branching conidiophores. The most striking feature is the long chains of large echinulate conidia with the broad base of one conidium attached to the rounded tip of the one below. The denser center of the conidia sometimes stains more intensely than the periphery so that the conidia appear to have thick walls.

at the tip of the chain. The unicellular conidia are relatively large (average diameter 6 μm), hyaline or lightly pigmented, and globose to *pyriform* (pear shaped) with flattened bases. The more mature annelloconidia have thick echinulate walls; small nipple-like projections may be visible on their tips, making them resemble lemons.

In *direct examination* of specimens intact chains of conidia have been seen in cases of onychomycosis.

■ **Helpful Features for Identification of *Scopulariopsis* Species**

> Flask-shaped or cylindrical annellides with annellations
> Large echinulate, lemon-shaped annelloconidia with flattened bases
> Brushlike penicillus
> Mousy brown velvety or granular colonies

■ **Organisms from Which *Scopulariopsis* Must Be Differentiated** (see Table 3.7 and Fig. 3.59)

> *Aspergillus niger*
> *Paecilomyces*
> *Penicillium*

Contaminant

MONILIACEAE

SEPEDONIUM SPECIES   (Sep[12]-uh-doan'-ee-um)

■ **Reservoirs.** *Sepedonium* species are found growing as a parasite on mushrooms and in soil and decaying vegetation.

■ **Unique Risk Factors.** None.

■ **Human Infection.** No infections with *Sepedonium* have been reported in the literature.

■ **Specimen Sources.** *Sepedonium* may be isolated as a contaminant from any specimen, but culture specifically for *Sepedonium* is rarely requested.

■ **Special Precautions.** None are needed, but cultures should be examined within a biologic safety cabinet.

■ **Culture Media.** Modified SDA.

Temperature Considerations. Sepedonium species grow at 25°C, but little or no growth occurs at 37°C.

---

[12]"Sep" rhymes with pep and "doan" rhymes with moan.

FIGURE 3.65

Scopulariopsis species have short, fat, sticklike conidiophores that may branch. The conidiophores support single annellides and clusters of annellides; the annellides are flask shaped or cylindrical. The conidia are large, with a prickly surface and flattened base; they are arranged in chains. Some conidia have small, nipple-like projections on their tips. Annellations may be seen on one or more annellides *(inset)*. The 7-μm red blood cell (RBC) (arrow) shows the relative sizes of the mycotic elements.

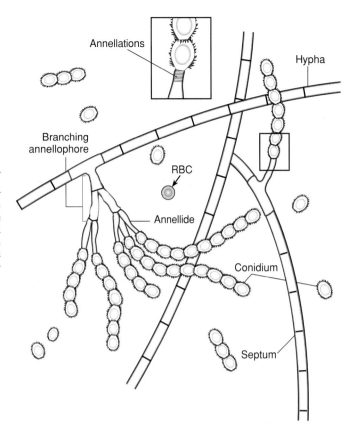

FIGURE 3.66

Even in a bad preparation, chains of large echinulate conidia formed from branching conidiophores should suggest *Scopulariopsis*. The flattened base of the conidia and a small, nipple-like projection from the tip strengthens the probability that the isolate is *Scopulariopsis*. The 7-μm red blood cell (arrow) shows the relative sizes of the mycotic elements.

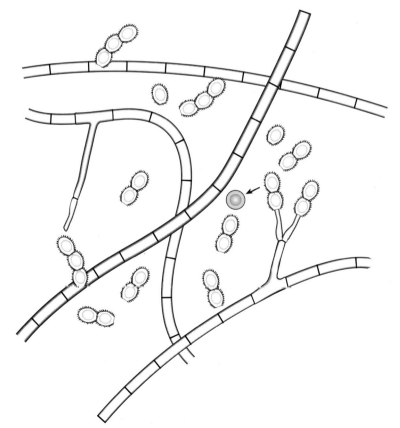

■ **Macroscopic (Colony) Morphology.** On modified SDA at 25°C after 6 to 8 days, the colony of *Sepedonium* is white and cottony. Later it becomes powdery and develops thick white tufts that may become golden yellow. The reverse pigment is white to light brown or yellow.

■ **Microscopic Morphology** (Figs. 3.67 through 3.70). Hyphae of *Sepedonium* are hyaline, septate, and multibranched. Conidiophores are simple; they may have septa, and they may branch. Annellides are produced singly or in a penicillus. The unicellular annelloconidia are at first 7 μm, smooth, thin walled, and elliptical. With age they enlarge to approximately 17 μm and become globose to ovoid (see Fig. 3.67). The surface of the thick-walled conidia[13] may be smooth or rough to tuberculate. Conidia are usually borne singly but may occur in clusters; they may be hyaline or yellow.

■ **Helpful Features for Identification of *Sepedonium* Species**

> Young conidia are globose to ovoid, unicellular, and smooth or rough walled
> Mature macroconidia are large (7 to 17 μm) with rough to tuberculate walls
> Conidiophores resemble vegetative hyphae

■ **Organisms from Which *Sepedonium* Must Be Differentiated** (see Table 8.3)

> *Histoplasma capsulatum*
> *Blastomyces dermatitidis*

───────

[13]Older texts refer to both microconidia and macroconidia. Currently mycologists consider that the microconidia are immature macroconidia.

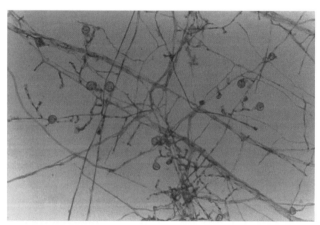

FIGURE 3.67

Typical isolates of *Sepedonium* have septate hyphae and simple conidiophores. Conidia are unicellular. They vary so much in size that this species was thought to form both macroconidia and microconidia until relatively recently. As the conidia mature they develop thick walls that may be vaguely lumpy or obviously tuberculate, creating a resemblance to the dimorphic fungus *Histoplasma*.

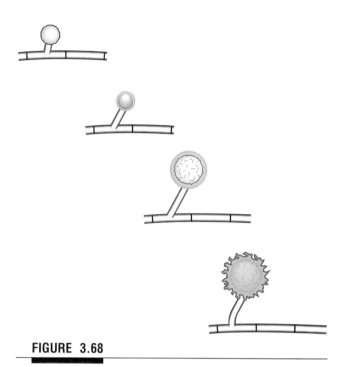

FIGURE 3.68

Older texts may refer to *macro*conidia and *micro*conidia produced by *Sepedonium*. Today *Sepedonium* is recognized as having a *single* type of conidium that looks very different at different stages of growth. The young conidium at the *upper left* is small, with smooth walls, on a short conidiophore. As the conidium matures (moving from *upper left* to *lower right*) it enlarges, and the outer wall develops the rough tuberculate protrusions shown at the *lower right*. During maturation the conidiophore elongates and thickens somewhat.

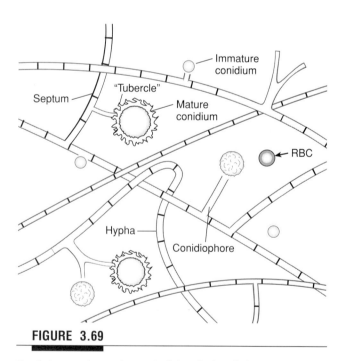

FIGURE 3.69

Sepedonium species produce unicellular, thick-walled conidia on short conidiophores that may branch. The conidia sometimes develop tuberculate extensions of the cell wall, resembling the mould form of *Histoplasma*. Typically conidia in varying stages of growth are present. Hyphae are septate and hyaline. The 7-μm red blood cell (RBC) (arrow) shows the relative sizes of the mycotic elements.

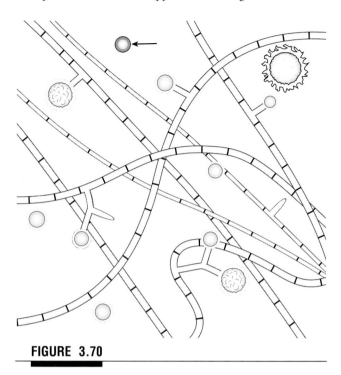

FIGURE 3.70

Even in bad preparations the presence of large tuberculate conidia suggests *Sepedonium* (or *Histoplasma*). The presence of only one kind of conidium in varying sizes strengthens the probability of *Sepedonium*. Relatively rapid growth and thermal monomorphism confirm that the isolate is *Sepedonium*. The 7-μm red blood cell (arrow) shows the relative sizes of the mycotic elements.

Contaminant/Opportunistic Pathogen

HYALINE HYPHOMYCETE/ZYGOMYCETE

SYNCEPHALASTRUM SPECIES

Syncephalastrum species are discussed with the other four Zygomycetes at the end of this chapter.

Contaminant/Opportunistic Pathogen

MONILIACEAE

TRICHODERMA SPECIES (Trick-oh-derm-uh)

■ **Reservoirs.** *Trichoderma* species are found in soil throughout the world. They are spread by an airborne route.

■ **Unique Risk Factors.** None.

■ **Human Infection.** Infections with *Trichoderma* are rare, but increasing numbers are being reported. The fungus has been associated with hyalohyphomycosis and has been reported from *nosocomial* (hospital-acquired) infections traced to contaminated solutions.

■ **Specimen Sources.** Aspirates from lesions, blood, biopsies of tissue and skin are most likely to be cultured.

■ **Special Precautions.** None are needed, but specimens should be handled in a biologic safety cabinet.

■ **Culture Media.** Modified SDA. Subculture to Czapek-Dox, PDA, or PFA to enhance conidiation and pigmentation.

Temperature Considerations. *Trichoderma* species grow at 25° to 30°C.

■ **Macroscopic (Colony) Morphology.** On modified SDA at 25°C after 4 to 5 days, colonies of *Trichoderma* cover the plate with a flat white lawn of hyphal growth. Later the colonies may become velvety to powdery and form concentric rings of growth where conidiation is heavy. The color varies from yellow to yellow-green. The reverse pigment is colorless to light yellow or light orange-tan.

■ **Microscopic Morphology** (Figs. 3.71 through 3.73). Hyphae of *Trichoderma* are thin, hyaline, and septate. They produce short, erect hyaline phialophores that may be smooth or echinulate, with branching at wide angles. The phialides found on the phialophores are short, fat, hyaline structures. They swell from the base to the central portion, then taper to the apex, forming vases. Phialides form at wide angles to the phialophores singly and in clusters that form compact tufts. The small (2 μm) subglobose to elliptical phialoconidia are unicellular. They are hyaline to green.

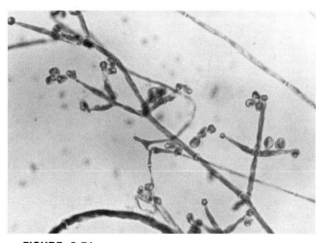

FIGURE 3.71

Delicate septate hyphae are typical of *Trichoderma* species. Conidia are arranged in spherical clusters at the tips of vaselike phialides. The phialides form along the sticklike conidiophores at wide angles to one another. In this photomicrograph most of the conidia are free; at the right of the field a cluster is tilted off center somewhat but remains attached to the phialide.

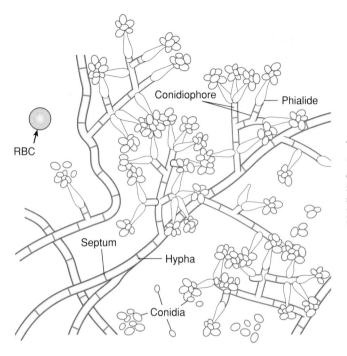

FIGURE 3.72

Trichoderma species have hyaline vaselike phialides from which oval conidia are produced; the conidia remain clustered at the tips of the phialides in spherical groups. The sticklike conidiophores branch at wide angles, and the phialides form at wide angles to one another on the conidiophores. The 7-μm red blood cell (RBC) (arrow) shows the relative sizes of the mycotic elements.

The phialoconidia are produced individually, but a slimy substance holds them together initially in easily disrupted spherical clusters around the tips of the phialides.

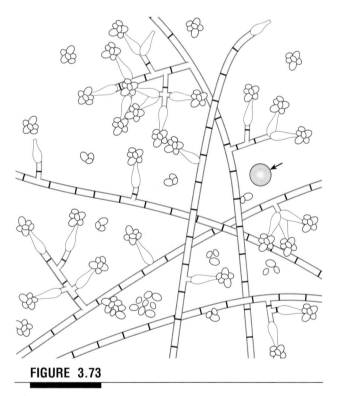

FIGURE 3.73

Even in a bad preparation spherical clusters of oval conidia and vaselike hyaline phialides indicate *Trichoderma* species. Wide angles between the branches of the conidiophores and between adjacent phialides strengthen the presumption that the isolate is *Trichoderma*. Colony morphology can be helpful for identification of the fungus. The 7-μm red blood cell (arrow) shows the relative sizes of the mycotic elements.

■ **Helpful Features for Identification of *Trichoderma* Species**

> Unicellular hyaline phialoconidia on short, plump, flask-shaped phialophores
> Wide angle of branches of the phialophores and phialides
> Clusters of subglobose to elliptical conidia in balls at the tip of the phialides

■ **Organisms from Which *Trichoderma* Must Be Differentiated** (see Table 3.2 and Fig. 3.8)

> *Fusarium*
> *Verticillium*
> *Gliocladium*
> *Acremonium*

Contaminant/Opportunistic Pathogen

Hyaline Hyphomycete

Zygomycetes (Zigh-go-my-seats)

The five organisms listed subsequently all belong to the same Class. They share many similarities in colony morphology and microscopic structures, are found in the same reservoirs, and cause the same kinds of infections. Because of these similarities, and because specimens are collected and handled in the same manner for these five organisms, a general discussion of the Zygomycetes is presented first. Following it, each organism is discussed with emphasis on the features that are important for its identification.

Absidia species (Ab[14]-syd'-ee-uh)
Mucor species (Mhew'-core)
Rhizomucor species (Rye'-zoh-mhew-core)
Rhizopus species (Rye'-zo[15]-puss)
Syncephalastrum species (Sen-seff'-uh-last'-rum)

■ **Reservoirs.** These fungi are found worldwide in soil, leaf mold, and other decaying vegetation and in animal dung. The spores are easily airborne.

■ **Unique Risk Factors.** Immunocompromised, debilitated, and nutritionally deficient hosts are susceptible to infection with Zygomycetes. Patients who are acidotic, such as diabetics, are at particular risk. Other risk factors are hormonal imbalances and trauma to tissues.

■ **Human Infection.** Zygomycoses, or mucormycoses, are usually initiated by inhalation of sporangiospores by susceptible people. Allergic reactions may result, or infection may develop in the lungs or paranasal sinuses. If the spores are introduced by traumatic inoculation, the cornea, ear, and cutaneous or subcutaneous tissues may be infected. Gastrointestinal infection may occur if food contaminated with the fungal toxins is eaten. When the zygomycete enters the blood the lumen of the vessels may be *occluded* (blocked). The primary infection may disseminate through the blood or the nerve trunk to other organs, especially the central nervous system.

Zygomycosis/mucormycosis is a particularly terrifying infection because of the rapid fulminant growth of the fungus and the corresponding tissue destruction.

■ **Specimen Sources.** Respiratory secretions, tissue biopsy specimens, cerebrospinal fluid, gastric washings, scrapings of infected mucosal tissue, and aspirates from abscesses are most likely to be submitted for culture.

■ **Specimen Collection and Handling.** Follow standard procedures, except that if specimens cannot be plated immediately, they should be left at room temperature (25° to 30°C) rather than refrigerated. Special care should be taken, due to the ubiquitous nature of these organisms, to avoid contaminating the specimen. Specimens such as tissue that must be processed before they can be inoculated to media should be minced rather than ground. Grinding destroys the large reproductive structures in the process of pulverizing the tissue. Media should be heavily inoculated with the spec-

imen since only a few of the spores may be viable. Minced tissue should be partially submerged in the medium.

Direct examination of the specimen should follow standard procedures. Wide aseptate hyphae with branches at a 90-degree angle in tissue samples suggest Zygomycetes; this should be confirmed with multiple positive cultures from the same specimen type or by isolation of the fungus from specimens that are normally sterile (see Table 3.1).

■ **Immunology.** Species of zygomycetes share antigens, and cross-reactions occur in immunologic tests. The *Manual of Clinical Laboratory Immunology* describes enzyme immunoassay, ID, and RIA methods for detection of zygomycoses. In the manual, that particular section closes with the statement that "although these tests are useful, additional studies are needed to develop more sensitive and reliable methods for the immunologic diagnosis of zygomycosis" (p. 525).

■ **Special Precautions.** None are needed, other than use of a biologic safety cabinet to prevent contamination of the work area and other cultures.

■ **Culture Media.** Modified SDA is adequate. Antibacterial antibiotics may be added but cycloheximide should not be used. Malt extract agar, PDA, or PFA may be inoculated to enhance sporulation. Sterilized bread can also be used.

Temperature Considerations. Pathogenic species of zygomycetes grow at both 25°C and 35° to 37°C. Some varieties grow at higher temperatures.

■ **Macroscopic (Colony) Morphology.** On modified SDA at 25° to 37°C after 2 to 4 days, colonies typically are floccose and dense. The organism rapidly fills the entire Petri dish or test tube with abundant intertwining aerial mycelium, which looks rather like gray cotton candy. Pigmentation of the isolates varies somewhat with the genus isolated, but pigments are variations of off-white, gray, brown, or beige. Zygomycetes technically are hyaline rather than dematiaceous. Subculture of colonies and microscopic preparations can be difficult to do because the mycelium sticks to the teasing needle. Using two teasing needles and "working" them together in the same way that one spoon is used to scrape cookie dough onto the baking sheet from another spoon can alleviate this problem.

■ **Microscopic Morphology.** The hyphae are predominantly aseptate or very sparsely septate and wider (6 to 15 μm, average 10 μm) than the hyphae of most other fungi isolated from human infections (Fig. 3.74). The ribbon-like hyaline hyphae are thin walled and irregular

---

[14]"Ab" as in absent.
[15]"Zo" rhymes with low.

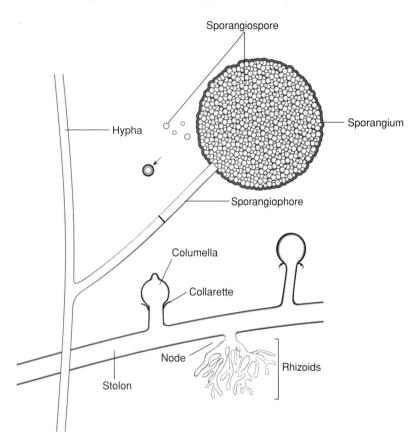

FIGURE 3.74

Zygomycetes have features common to the Family, but no genus has all of the familial characteristics, except that all Zygomycetes have aseptate or sparsely septate hyphae and reproduce asexually through sporangiospores. The genera differ in the size and shape of the sporangia and columellae and the length of the sporangiophores. Other differential features are the presence (or absence) of collarettes, apophyses, and rhizoids. The 7-μm red blood cell (arrow) shows the relative sizes of the mycotic elements.

in width and frequently intertwined, and they branch haphazardly.

The primary asexual reproductive structure for all the zygomycetes is the *sporangiospore*, which is produced in a *sporangium* (a sack). The shape of the sporangium is helpful for differentiation of the zygomycetes; the length of the *sporangiophore* (a specialized conidiophore) that supports the sporangium and whether or not the sporangiophore branches are also useful distinguishing characteristics. Hyphae and sporangiophores are almost indistinguishable unless the columella or sporangium is present on the sporangiophore or unless rhizoids are attached to the hypha.

Sporangiophores of some genera enlarge at the distal end into a **columella,** a sterile domelike structure that extends into and supports the sporangium. The columella may have an **apophysis,** swelling of the sporangiophore at the juncture with the columella. Some genera also have a **collarette,** a ring of fragments of the sporangium that remains attached to the sporangiophore at the base of the columella when the sporangium ruptures or disintegrates.

Zygomycetes may have **rhizoids,** structures that resemble tree roots and that serve approximately the same role—anchoring the fungus to the substrate and absorbing nutrients. When the sporangiophore develops on the hyphae at a point opposite rhizoids, the sporangiophore

is described as *nodal.* Sporangiophores that develop between groups of rhizoids are *internodal.* In some genera the rhizoids are up to 12 μm wide and 350 μm long, while in others they are *rudimentary,* that is, primitive or poorly developed. While sporangiospores are the primary asexual reproductive structures formed by all zygomycetes, some genera also produce other asexual structures such as chlamydoconidia, as well as sexual reproductive structures. The sexual reproductive structures are zygospores.

The features that are most useful for distinguishing among the zygomycetes are the presence and level of development of the rhizoids, the shape of the sporangium, and the nodal or internodal location of the sporangiophores. Because all of the structures of the zygomycetes are relatively large, they can sometimes be distinguished by using a dissecting microscope to examine the original colony. The sizes of the structures do, of course, vary among the genera and between species in addition to the normal differences seen between the mature and immature structures of a single isolate.

The four genera most likely to be found in clinical specimens, and most likely to be confused with one another, are *Absidia, Mucor, Rhizomucor,* and *Rhizopus.* These are compared in Figure 3.75. *Syncephalastrum,* because the shape of its sporangia is so different, is unlikely to be part of any such mix-up.

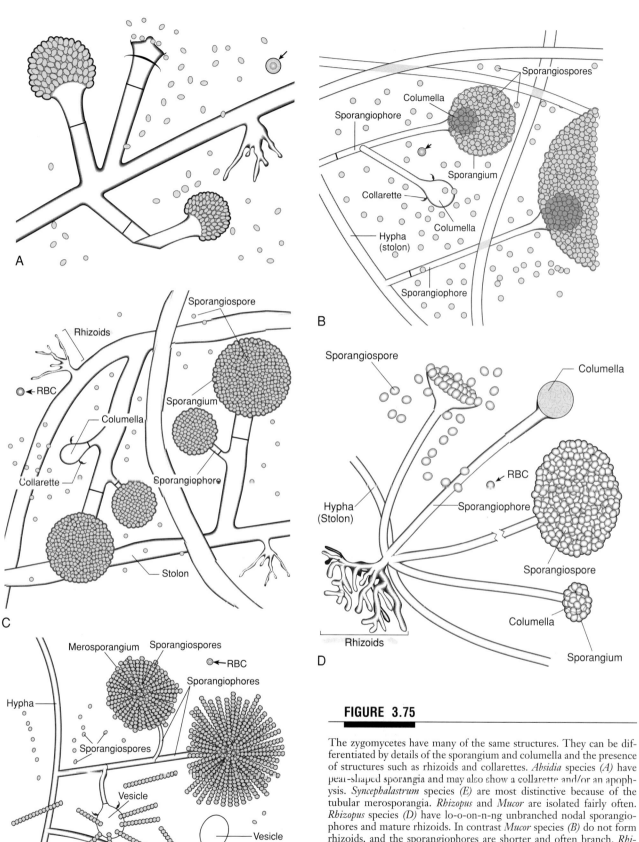

FIGURE 3.75

The zygomycetes have many of the same structures. They can be differentiated by details of the sporangium and columella and the presence of structures such as rhizoids and collarettes. *Absidia* species *(A)* have pear-shaped sporangia and may also show a collarette and/or an apophysis. *Syncephalastrum* species *(E)* are most distinctive because of the tubular merosporangia. *Rhizopus* and *Mucor* are isolated fairly often. *Rhizopus* species *(D)* have lo-o-on-n-ng unbranched nodal sporangiophores and mature rhizoids. In contrast *Mucor* species *(B)* do not form rhizoids, and the sporangiophores are shorter and often branch. *Rhizomucor* species *(C)* are reported much less than any of the others; as the name implies, *Rhizomucor* species look like a hybrid of *Rhizopus* and *Mucor* and may be misidentified. The 7-μm red blood cell (RBC) (arrow) shows the relative sizes of the mycotic elements.

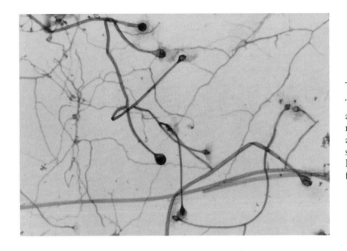

FIGURE 3.76

Typical isolates of *Absidia* have relatively short, straight sporangiophores and pyriform sporangia filled with round or oval spores. When the sporangium ruptures, the details of the columella can sometimes be seen; look at the sporangium near the center. Most of the sporangia in this field are still surrounded by clouds of sporangiospores. Hyphae do not have septa. Rudimentary rhizoids may be visible but are usually difficult to distinguish from hyphal strands.

Contaminant/Opportunistic Pathogen

HYALINE HYPHOMYCETE/ZYGOMYCETE

ABSIDIA SPECIES (Ab[16]-syd'-ee-uh)

■ **Macroscopic (Colony) Morphology.** On modified SDA at 25° to 37°C after 2 to 4 days, the colony of *Absidia* is woolly and dense. It rapidly fills the entire Petri dish or test tube with abundant intertwining, cottony aerial mycelium. The colony is white at first but becomes olive-gray as it matures, and the surface becomes dotted

---

[16]"Ab" as in absent.

with olive-gray sporangia. The reverse is colorless or cream colored.

■ **Microscopic Morphology** (Figs. 3.76 through 3.78). The broad (10 μm) hyaline aseptate hyphae are ribbon-like. They are thin walled and irregular in diameter and frequently are intertwined; branching occurs irregularly at angles of approximately 90 degrees. Sporangiophores up to 70 μm long and 15 μm wide may arise singly or in internodal groups of groups of two to five. The long, straight sporangiophores of *Absidia* are hyaline to light gray, with smooth walls. Sporangiophores broaden into large (approximately 20 μm in diameter, ranging from 16 to 27 μm) columellae that are cone shaped, with a pointed projection at the *apex*—somewhat like a Hershey's Kiss. A conical apophysis is present.

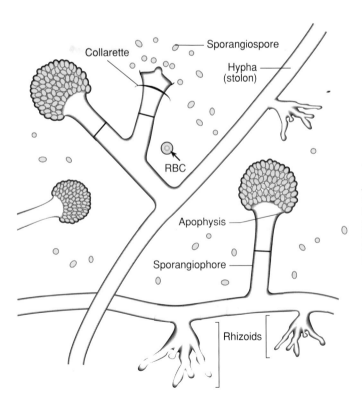

FIGURE 3.77

Absidia species have internodal sporangiophores that may branch. The sporangium is pyriform. After the sporangium ruptures, releasing round or oval spores, an apophysis and a collarette can sometimes be seen at the base of the columella. Columellae are cone shaped, resembling a Hershey's Kiss. Hyphae are aseptate or sparsely septate. The 7-μm red blood cell (RBC) (arrow) shows the relative sizes of the mycotic elements.

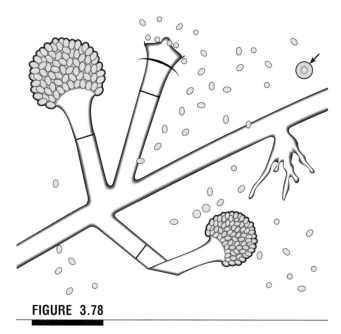

FIGURE 3.78

Even in bad preparations sporangia and broad aseptate hyphae indicate the isolate is a zygomycete. Sporangiophores that are internodal and/or branching suggest *Absidia*. An apophysis or a collarette, and pear-shaped sporangia, help confirm the identification. The 7-μm red blood cell (arrow) shows the relative sizes of the mycotic elements.

Sporangia are pyriform and hyaline, varying in diameter from 20 to 35 μm (average 27 μm); they become brownish gray with age. The unicellular round or oval sporangiospores are 5 to 6 μm in diameter and usually have smooth walls and a flat base. They are hyaline or yellow to greenish. When sporangia mature and rupture or dissolve, the sporangiospores are released. The apophysis remains on the sporangiophore, where it can usually be seen with a small attached collarette, all that remains of the sporangium. Chlamydoconidia may be present in some species. Stolons that curve into arches are present. Rhizoids are present but are often indistinct and are submerged in the medium; sporangiophores are internodal.

■ **Helpful Features for Identification of *Absidia* Species**

> Rapid growth of cottony to woolly olive-gray colonies that are sticky and difficult to transfer
> Broad, irregular hyphae that are aseptate or sparsely septate
> Branching sporangiophores internodal on connecting stolons
> Conical (Hershey's Kiss–shaped) columellae
> An apophysis with collarette
> Rudimentary rhizoids
> Growth at 25° to 42°C

■ **Organisms from Which *Absidia* Must Be Differentiated** (Table 3.8; see also Fig. 3.75)

> *Mucor*
> *Rhizomucor*

Rhizopus
Syncephalastrum

Contaminant/Opportunistic Pathogen

HYALINE HYPHOMYCETE/ZYGOMYCETE

MUCOR SPECIES (Mhew'-core)

■ **Macroscopic (Colony) Morphology.** On modified SDA at 25°C after 2 to 4 days, colonies of *Mucor* are woolly and rapidly fill the entire Petri dish or test tube with an abundant matted or intertwining aerial mycelium. The colony is white at first and becomes gray or yellow. The surface is covered with dark spots when sporangia develop.

■ **Microscopic Morphology** (Figs. 3.79 through 3.81). The hyaline hyphae of *Mucor* are predominantly aseptate or sparsely septate and broad (average 10 μm). They are thick walled and irregular in diameter and frequently are intertwined. The sporangiophores that arise irregularly from the hyphae are long and straight; irregular branching often occurs. *Mucor*'s sporangiophores enlarge at their distal end into columellae of varying shapes; they may be hyaline or darkly pigmented. Globose sporangia vary in size from 60 to 300 μm in diameter (average 180 μm). The sacs are filled with unicellular ovoid or elliptical sporangiospores that are approximately 5 μm in diameter; the spores are yellow to brown. A collarette remains at the base of the columella when the sporangia mature and rupture or dissolve. No rhizoids are produced by *Mucor*. Some species reproduce sexually in culture, forming zygospores. A few chlamydoconidia are found on sporangiophores.

■ **Helpful Features for Identification of *Mucor* Species**

> Cottony to woolly gray colonies that rapidly fill the Petri dish or test tube
> Broad irregular hyphae that are aseptate or sparsely septate
> Branching sporangiophores with columellae-supporting sporangia filled with sporangiospores
> Collarettes
> Absence of rhizoids
> Growth at 25° and 37°C but not at 50°C

■ **Organisms from Which *Mucor* Must Be Differentiated** (see Table 3.8 and Fig. 3.75)

> *Absidia*
> *Rhizomucor*
> *Rhizopus*

TABLE 3.8 Saprobes with "Aseptate" Hyphae

Fungus	Size of Sporangiospores (μm)	Shape of Sporangiospores	Shape of Columella	Size of Sporangium (μm)	Length of Sporangiophore (μm)	Arrangement of Sporangiophores	Colony Morphology	Growth Rate	Other Helpful Features
Absidia	5	Round or oval	Cone shaped (a Hershey's Kiss)	20–30	25–70	Internodal; singly or in groups of ≥2	Cottony to woolly olive-gray	Rapid	Pyriform sporangia; arched stolons; rudimentary rhizoids
Mucor	5	Ovoid or elliptical	Variable	60–300	150–250	Solitary; branching may occur; collarettes form	Woolly gray	Rapid	Globose sporangia; stolons and rhizoids absent; no apophysis
Rhizomucor	3	Oval	Globose	60–70	25–100	Internodal, with branching; collarettes form	Woolly gray to dark brown	Rapid	WIDE hyphae; primitive rhizoids; globose columellae; brown sporangiospores
Rhizopus	7	Varies with species	Hemispherical	100–150	0.5–2 mm	Nodal; singly or in groups of ≥2	Salt-and-pepper "lid lifter"	Rapid	Well-developed rhizoids; columella collapses after spores are released
Syncephalastrum	4	Round	Vesicle is round	5 × 60	—	Straight or branching irregularly	White and cottony	Rapid	Merosporangia radiating from vesicles; rudimentary rhizoids

FIGURE 3.79

Typical isolates of *Mucor* have long, straight sporangiophores that may branch. Columellae vary in shape. Sporangia are round, with ovoid or elliptical spores. Collarettes are formed, but rhizoids are not produced.

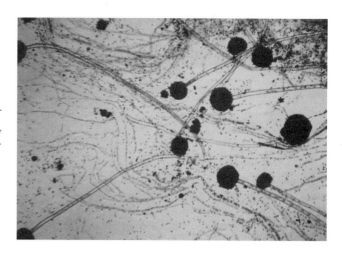

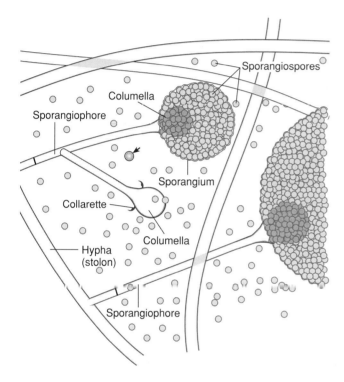

FIGURE 3.80

Mucor species do not form rhizoids. The sporangiophores are straight; branching may occur. The columellae vary in shape from round to ovoid; a collarette remains at the base of the columella when the sporangium ruptures. Sporangiospores are round and hyaline. The 7-µm red blood cell (arrow) shows the relative sizes of the mycotic elements.

FIGURE 3.81

Even in bad preparations broad aseptate hyphae and sporangia suggest a zygomycete. Branching sporangiophores indicate *Absidia* or *Mucor*. The presence of collarettes and the absence of rhizoids rule out *Absidia*. Round-to-ovoid columellae help to confirm the isolate as *Mucor*. The 7-µm red blood cell (arrow) shows the relative sizes of the mycotic elements.

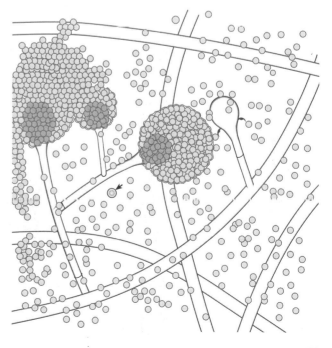

Contaminant/Opportunistic Pathogen

HYALINE HYPHOMYCETE/ZYGOMYCETE

RHIZOMUCOR SPECIES (Rye'-zo[17]-mhew-core)

Rhizomucor has often been misidentified as *Mucor* or *Rhizopus*. It is in fact considered an intermediate between those two genera.

Temperature Considerations. *Rhizomucor* is thermophilic and grows at temperatures up to 55°C.

■ **Macroscopic (Colony) Morphology.** After 1 to 2 days on modified SDA at 30°C, the colony of *Rhizomucor* is woolly. Abundant intertwining aerial mycelium rapidly fills the entire Petri dish or test tube. Colonies are white at first, then become gray to dark brown as they mature; the surface becomes dotted with dark sporangia. The reverse is colorless or cream colored.

■ **Microscopic Morphology** (Figs. 3.82 and 3.83). Hyphae are predominantly aseptate or sparsely septate and *much* wider than the hyphae of most other fungi isolated from human infections. The range is 3 to 25 μm, with an average diameter of 14 μm, but the diameter varies markedly within a single hypha. The ribbon-like hyphae have thin walls and are frequently intertwined. Short sporangiophores arise irregularly from the aerial hyphae,

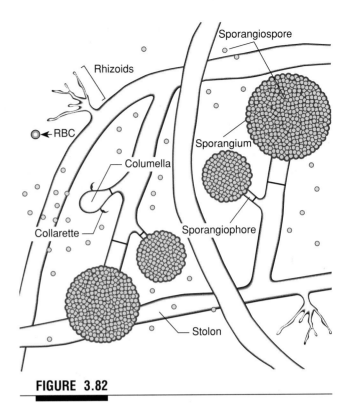

FIGURE 3.82

Rhizomucor has very wide, aseptate hyphae that have thin walls. Sporangiophores are short, with branching; they are internodal. Both sporangia and columellae are round. Sporangia and sporangiospores are relatively small. Collarettes and primitive rhizoids develop, but apophyses are not present. The 7-μm red blood cell (RBC) (arrow) shows the relative sizes of the mycotic elements.

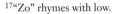

[17]"Zo" rhymes with low.

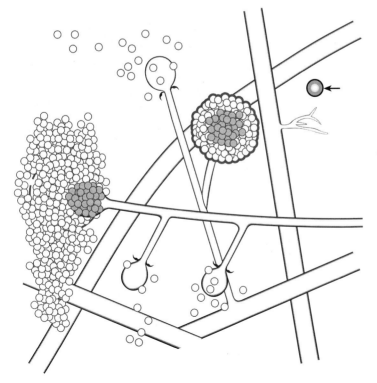

FIGURE 3.83

Even in a bad preparation sporangia and broad aseptate hyphae suggest a Zygomycete. Poorly developed rhizoids, very broad hyphae, and short internodal sporangiophores support the possibility of *Rhizomucor*. Round sporangia and columellae help confirm the identification. The 7-μm red blood cell (arrow) shows the relative sizes of the mycotic elements.

singly or in tufts. Short primitive, that is, poorly developed, rhizoids are produced along the vegetative hyphae.

The dark brown sporangiophores of *Rhizomucor* are internodal and branch repeatedly; they may arise on aerial hyphae. They enlarge distally into smooth, sterile globose columellae that extend into and support round black sporangia. Sporangia vary in diameter from 60 to 70 μm. The sporangiospores within the sporangia are small (approximately 3 μm), unicellular, oval, and brown. When sporangia mature and rupture or dissolve, releasing the sporangiospores, a collarette remains but no apophysis is present. If sexual spores are present, they are found on the aerial hyphae.

■ **Helpful Features for Identification of *Rhizomucor* Species**

Cottony to woolly olive-gray to brown colonies that rapidly fill the Petri dish

Broad, irregular hyphae that are aseptate or sparsely septate

Short, branching sporangiophores with globose columellae

A collarette but no apophysis

Development of primitive rhizoids

Growth at temperatures up to 50° to 55°C

■ **Other Organisms from Which *Rhizomucor* Must Be Differentiated** (see Table 3.8 and Fig. 3.75)

Absidia
Mucor
Rhizopus

Contaminant/Opportunistic Pathogen

HYALINE HYPHOMYCETE/ZYGOMYCETE

RHIZOPUS SPECIES (Rye'-zo[18]-puss)

■ **Macroscopic (Colony) Morphology.** After 2 to 4 days on modified SDA at 25°C, the colony of *Rhizopus* is floccose or woolly. It rapidly fills the entire Petri dish or test tube with abundant matted or intertwining aerial mycelium. *Rhizopus* species have been called a "lid lifter" because it can literally push up the top of a standard plastic Petri dish. The colony is white at first to brownish gray with a colorless or light cream reverse. The surface becomes covered with dark spots when sporangia appear, so that *Rhizopus* species are sometimes described as having a "salt-and-pepper" appearance.

[18]"Zo" rhymes with low.

■ **Microscopic Morphology** (Figs. 3.84 through 3.86). Hyphae resemble those of the other zygomycetes: predominantly aseptate or very sparsely septate, broad (approximately 10 μm), thin walled, and irregular in diameter, with frequent "tangles." Yellow or light brown rhizoids are submerged in the medium. The light brown sporangiophores of *Rhizopus* are long (0.5 to 2 mm) and straight and are usually unbranched. They may arise singly or in groups of two or more from nodes. Sporangiophores enlarge distally into a sterile hemispherical columella with a flattened base that gradually swells as it extends into and supports the sporangium. Sporangia are round and hyaline with flattened bases; they become darker when they are filled with sporangiospores. Sporangia vary in size from 100 to 150 μm in diameter. The unicellular ovoid or elliptical sporangiospores are approximately 7 μm in diameter and have a flat base; the surface may be smooth, *spinulose* (having spines), or *striated* (striped). They are colorless or light brown; details of the features of the spores vary with the species of *Rhizopus*. When sporangia mature and rupture or disintegrate, the columellae often collapse and bend over, like an upside-down umbrella. A barely visible apophysis is found in some species. Some species reproduce sexually in culture, forming zygospores. Chlamydoconidia may be present.

The two species of *Rhizopus* that are most often isolated from infection are *Rhizopus arrhizus* and *Rhizopus oryzae*. They can be differentiated by whether or not zygospores are produced in routine culture.

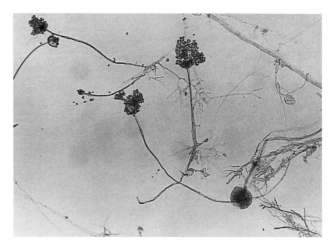

FIGURE 3.84

Characteristic isolates of *Rhizopus* have prominent rhizoids and long, straight nodal sporangiophores. The columella forms a half circle with a flattened base. Sporangia are large and round. Hyphae are aseptate or sparsely septate. The center of the field contains a good example of all these features, from the ruptured sporangium at the top of the field, down the long straight sporangiophore, to the rhizoids at the base. The upper left quadrant shows another complete example; just below it is a sporangium that has ruptured and collapsed into an "umbrella."

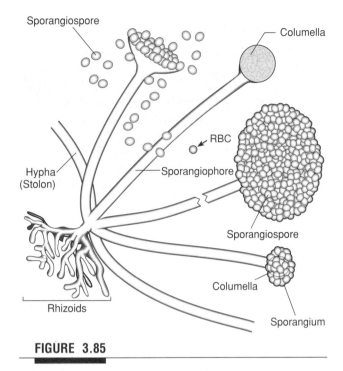

FIGURE 3.85

Rhizopus species all have long nodal sporangiophores that may develop singly or in clumps of two or more; sporangiophores often span several microscopic fields, even at ×10 magnification. Rhizoids are well developed. Intact sporangia are large and round; after one ruptures the columella may collapse into an umbrella-like form. Spores are relatively large; the shape and texture vary with the species. Collarettes are not seen. The 7-μm red blood cell (RBC) (arrow) shows the relative sizes of the mycotic elements.

■ **Helpful Features for Identification of *Rhizopus* Species**

> Cottony to woolly gray colonies that rapidly fill the Petri dish or test tube
> "Salt-and-pepper" colony surface
> Broad irregular hyphae that are aseptate or sparsely septate

Well-developed rhizoids
Branching sporangiophores with hemispherical columellae arising from nodes adjacent to rhizoids
Growth at 25° and 37°C; some species grow at temperatures up to 50°C

■ **Other Organisms from Which *Rhizopus* Must Be Differentiated** (see Table 3.8 and Fig. 3.75)

> *Absidia*
> *Mucor*
> *Rhizomucor*

Contaminant/Opportunistic Pathogen

HYALINE HYPHOMYCETE/ZYGOMYCETE

SYNCEPHALASTRUM SPECIES   (Sen[19]-seff'-uh-last'-rum)

■ **Human Infection.** Infection with *Syncephalastrum* is rare. Dermatomycoses and onychomycoses are more likely than the pulmonary and central nervous system infections associated with other Zygomycetes.

■ **Macroscopic (Colony) Morphology.** After 3 to 4 days on modified SDA at 30°C, the colony of *Syncephalastrum* is cottony or woolly with abundant intertwining aerial mycelia. It is white at first, then becomes gray or black as it ages. Mature colonies of *Syncephalastrum* superficially resemble young colonies of *Rhizopus* or *Mucor*.

---

[19]"Sen" rhymes with den.

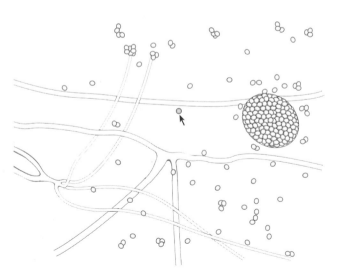

FIGURE 3.86

Even in bad preparations aseptate hyphae and long, straight sporangiophores developing in groups of two or more from well-developed rhizoids suggest *Rhizopus*. The presence of collapsed umbelliferous columellae further suggests *Rhizopus*. Colony morphology may help confirm the identification. The 7-μm red blood cell (arrow) shows the relative sizes of the mycotic elements.

FIGURE 3.87

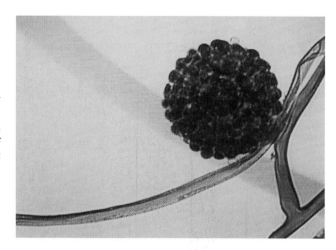

In typical preparations of *Syncephalastrum* aseptate hyphae or sparsely septate hyphae are seen. The long sporangiophores may branch. Long tubular merosporangia filled with round spores radiate from a vesicle at the end of the sporangiophore. Rudimentary rhizoids may develop; they are not shown.

The dotted or speckled surface associated with mature colonies of other Zygomycetes is not typical of *Syncephalastrum*. The reverse of the colony is a pale yellow-brown.

■ **Microscopic Morphology** (Figs. 3.87 through 3.89). Hyphae are predominantly aseptate; sparse septa appear in old colonies. The hyphae are irregularly broad—but not as wide as the other Zygomycetes (range 4 to 8 μm, average 6 μm)—with branching at right angles. The hyaline sporangiophores arise sympodially from the aerial hyphae. They are long and erect, with irregular branching. The side branches of the sporangiophores are short and curved, and they enlarge distally into swollen brown globose vesicles. The brown vesicles are approximately 25 μm in diameter (range 10 to 40 μm). The surface of the vesicle is smooth except for *spicules* (pegs) at the points where the merosporangia are attached. *Merospo-*

rangia are long (up to 60 μm) with an average width of 5 μm. The cylindrical structures resemble tubes or fingers and radiate all around the vesicle. Each ***merosporangium*** contains a line of 2 to 18 unicellular brown ovoid to globose merosporangiospores that are approximately 4 μm in diameter. Overall the reproductive structure of *Syncephalastrum* looks as if someone had filled a series of test tubes with marbles, then stuck one end of each tube into a ball of clay. Rudimentary rhizoids are usually formed.

■ **Helpful Features for Identification of *Syncephalastrum* Species**

Cottony to woolly gray to black colonies that rapidly fill the Petri dish

Broad irregular hyphae that are aseptate or sparsely septate in old cultures

FIGURE 3.88

Syncephalastrum species have the sparsely septate hyphae associated with *Zygomycetes*, but spores are produced in multiple tubular merosporangia that radiate from vesicles. The relatively small merosporangiospores are ovoid to round. Rudimentary rhizoids are often formed. The 7-μm red blood cell (RBC) (arrow) shows the relative sizes of the mycotic elements.

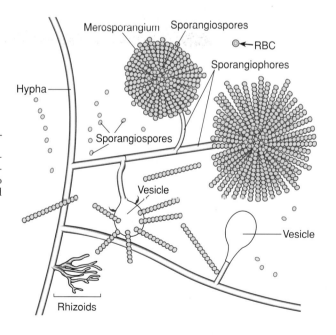

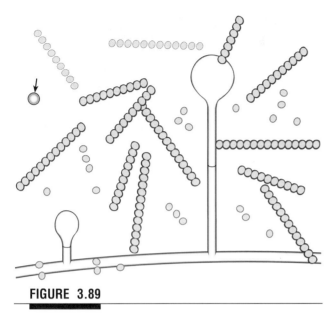

FIGURE 3.89

Even in a bad preparation the long cylindrical merosporangia strongly suggest *Syncephalastrum*. The identification is supported by sparsely septate hyphae and long, erect sporangiophores with irregular branching. The 7-μm red blood cell (arrow) shows the relative sizes of the mycotic elements.

Branching sporangiophores with globose vesicles supporting tubular sporangia filled with sporangiospores

Growth at temperatures up to 40°C

■ **Organisms from Which *Syncephalastrum* Must Be Differentiated** (Fig. 3.90; see also Table 3.8)

Aspergillus

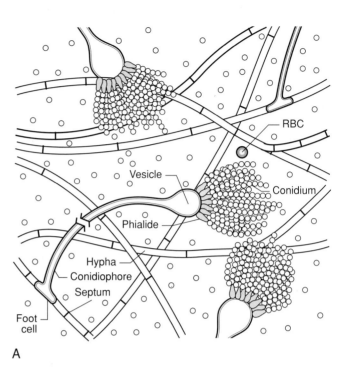

A

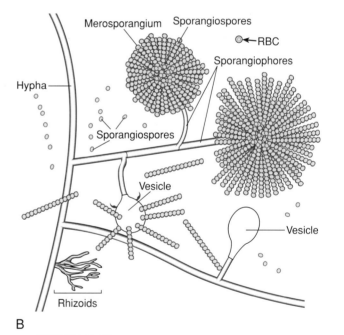

B

FIGURE 3.90

Superficially, *Aspergillus* (especially *Aspergillus niger*) resembles *Syncephalastrum*. A brief look for septa in the hyphae, and at the walls of the spores/conidia, is enough to distinguish these two genera—which are also easily distinguished by the appearance of the colonies. The aspergilli (*A*), represented here by *Aspergillus fumigatus*, have septa and the conidia are free, that is, not enclosed within a casing. In *Syncephalastrum* (*B*), septa are absent and the conidia develop within tubular sacs. The 7-μm red blood cell (RBC) (arrow) shows the relative sizes of the mycotic elements.

SUGGESTED EXERCISES FOR CHAPTER 3

(Some Opportunistic Fungi)

Exercise 5 (1st Session)

Purpose. To practice the method that was demonstrated for transferring a fungus to a new medium, determine the growth rate, study changes in colony morphology, and (incidentally) prepare cultures for the next laboratory.

Suggested Fungus Cultures.[20]

Set 1	**Alternaria,** *Aureobasidium,* **Cladosporium**
Set 2	*Curvularia, Drechslera, Bipolaris*
Set 3	*Fusarium*
Set 4	*Gliocladium*
Set 5	*Paecilomyces,* **Penicillium,** *Scopulariopsis*
Set 6	1 Zygomycete (*Absidia, Mucor, Rhizopus, Syncephalastrum*)
Set 7	1 **Aspergillus** (*A. fumigatus, A. flavus, A. niger, A. terreus*)

Initial Process. Go to the supply table and get three slide culture setups and four plates of PFA or PDA; the fourth plate will be used to do the slide cultures. Select three different cultures from the seven sets available. Do NOT pick the fungus you used for Exercises 2 through 4. Do NOT take more than one from any set. Do CHECK with your laboratory partner first—if you have one—so that you have six different organisms between you. Mark the cultures "Exercise 5" and add the name of the organism to each tube if this has not already been done.

Record names of the organisms, today's date, and the medium used for subculture on three different LABORATORY WORK SHEETS. Remember to bring all your work sheets to the next laboratory session.

Label each plate appropriately with the name of the culture, your name or initials, and today's date. Go to the biologic safety cabinet and transfer the fungus cultures to the new plates, using the directions for "Transferring Fungi" found in Appendix D. Seat the fungus firmly on the new medium, remembering that fungi must have ample oxygen if they are to grow well. Place your cultures in the 25–30°C incubator in an inverted position.

You should also set up slide cultures on each of the three organisms (in the biologic safety cabinet) so that you will have the slides to study during the next laboratory.

All of the slide cultures should have grown adequately within 5 to 7 days. You should visit them every 2 to 3 days to observe the rate of growth and the morphologic changes that occur. During your visit, add sterile water to the container ("water your cultures") if the filter paper appears dry. The water goes on the *filter paper*, not the fungus.

Exercise 5 (2nd Session)

Remove the three culture plates you inoculated last session from the 25–30°C incubator and check them for growth. If they have grown well, continue this exercise by completing the tasks outlined below. If growth is sparse or absent, consult your instructor to determine whether you should (1) reincubate the plate you

---

[20]Organisms in **bold type** were recommended for Exercises 2 through 4.

have; (2) inoculate a fresh plate of the fungus; or (3) use plates of the organism prepared by another student.

Complete all the work on one organism before you go to the next culture. The "assembly line" approach has the advantage of speed, but the study of fungi is not a race. By concentrating on the gross and microscopic morphology of one culture at a time, you will forge a better memory link of the characteristics of one organism.

First, describe the gross colony morphology of the organism, adding the information to the LABORATORY WORK SHEET you started during the previous session. Remember to note the age of the organism as well as the pigment, texture, and topography.

Then, with the same culture, prepare a tease mount and a Scotch tape prep. Label the microscopic preparations with the name of the organism, your name or initials, and the date. Examine the tease mount and the Scotch tape preparation microscopically, and use both preparations to make a composite drawing[21] in the appropriate section of the LABORATORY WORK SHEET. Follow these same steps two more times (assuming that all your cultures grew well).

Fetch your slide cultures from the 25–30°C incubator and examine them. If you are not certain the cultures are mature enough, use a microscope to check the intact cultures. Be *very* careful not to touch the coverslip—having to set the slide culture up again is annoying (and time consuming). This examination process is described in Appendix D.

Work with One Organism at a Time. "Harvest" the slide culture; the process has been demonstrated by your instructor, and the technique is given in Appendix D.

One slide culture results in two preparations. Label both with the name of the organism, the medium on which it was grown, and the age of the culture when it was harvested. This information will be important when the slide is used again. Put both preparations aside in a slide flat to dry before you begin the microscopic examination—you will be less likely to damage the "mount" by dislodging the coverslip.

After the preparations have dried several days (or during the next laboratory), you can seal the edges of the coverslip. Time will be allowed during the next laboratory session to examine the dried preparations and complete your drawings.

Repeat these steps for the two remaining cultures.

Exercise 5 (3rd Session)

If you have not already done so, make the mounts of the slide cultures of the saprobic fungi permanent by sealing the edges of the coverslips. Be sure that each preparation is labeled properly and put them aside to dry before they are examined and added to your slide collection.

ASSESS WHAT YOU HAVE LEARNED

Responses to the questions below are located in Appendix A.

1. Define "opportunistic fungi." Explain why they are increasingly important in diagnostic microbiology laboratories.

---

[21]The details provided by examination of the slide culture will allow you to complete the composite during a later laboratory session.

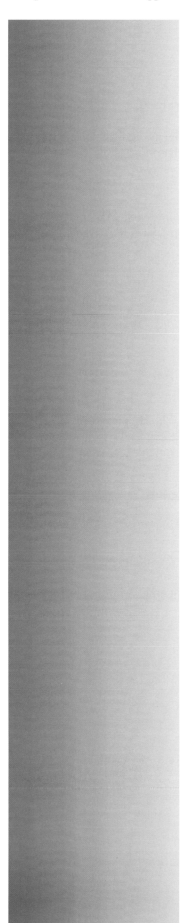

2. What is the difference between a "contaminant" and a "commensal"?
3. Define hyalohyphomycosis and phaeohyphomycosis. Why is it important to identify the etiologic agents of these mycoses?

For questions 4 through 8 **MATCH** the term **(numbered)** with the definition **(lettered).**
4. annellide
5. annelloconidium
6. annellophore
7. conidiogeny
8. determinate

   a. conidium produced by an annellide
   b. conidiogenous cell that continues to lengthen after producing the first conidium
   c. conidiogenous cell that stops elongating after production of the first conidium
   d. hyphal cell that supports an annellide
   e. production or genesis of conidia

9. List four features of the organism and/or the infection that are used to determine whether the fungus isolated is likely to be the agent of a mycosis.
10. Name the three artificial groups into which opportunistic fungi are divided, and state the basis for the groupings.
11. Define the following terms: clavate, elliptical, phialide, pyriform, sporodochia, tuberculate, vesicle.
12. What is the difference between micronematous and macronematous conidiophores?
13. Describe the characteristic microscopic features shared by members of the genus *Aspergillus* and by members of the Zygomycetes.

For questions 14 through 19 **MATCH** the term **(numbered)** with the definition **(lettered). NOTE** that some definitions are not used.
14. acropetal
15. basipetal
16. biseriate
17. internodal
18. poroconidia
19. synchronous

   a. conidia produced through openings in the wall of the conidiophore
   b. conidia produced together at the same time
   c. youngest conidium is found at the tip of the chain of conidia
   d. one series of phialides develops on the vesicle
   e. phialides arising from the vesicle in two series
   f. rhizoids are formed on stolons between the sporangiophores
   g. sporangiophores are produced opposite the rhizoids
   h. youngest conidium is found at the base of the chain of conidia

20. List "helpful features" that differentiate *Absidia, Mucor, Rhizomucor, Rhizopus,* and *Syncephalastrum* from each other.

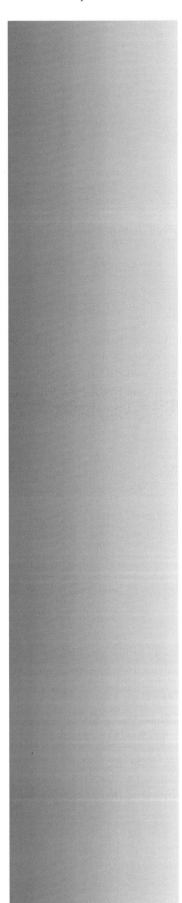

For questions 21 through 25 **MATCH** the microscopic characteristics **(numbered)** with the fungus **(lettered).** NOTE that some fungi are not used.

21. broad aseptate hyphae; branching sporangiophores; collarettes at the bases of columellae; rhizoids are absent
22. brushlike penicillus composed of phialides with blunt tips; chains of small ovoid to elliptical conidia
23. dark brown hyphae with sympodial conidiogeny and geniculate conidiophores; the central cells of the dark multicellular poroconidia are swollen, resembling crescent rolls
24. flask-shaped annellides and large echinulate lemon-shaped conidia with flattened bases in chains from a brushlike penicillus
25. vesicles are dome shaped, with uniseriate phialides and a compact columnar arrangement of conidia; conidiophores end in a foot cell

   a. *Aspergillus*
   b. *Curvularia*
   c. *Drechslera*
   d. *Fusarium*
   e. *Mucor*
   f. *Paecilomyces*
   g. *Penicillium*
   h. *Rhizomucor*
   i. *Scopulariopsis*

For questions 26 through 30 **MATCH** the fungus **(numbered)** with the colony description **(lettered).** NOTE that some descriptions are used more than once.

26. *Aspergillus*
27. *Bipolaris*
28. *Fusarium*
29. *Nigrospora*
30. *Rhizopus*

   a. dark brown velvety surface with a black reverse pigment
   b. gray woolly colony with a cream reverse pigment
   c. granular colony with pastel surface pigment and a white or cream reverse pigment

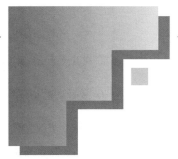

CHAPTER 4

Superficial Fungi

Instructional Objectives

1. Define the following terms: tinea, piedra, pityriasis versicolor, Wood's lamp, lipophilic, fusiform, annellide, annellophore, phialide, phialoconidium, "spaghetti and meatballs," arthroconidia, sympodial.

2. Describe the lesions seen in white piedra, black piedra, tinea versicolor, and tinea nigra. Name the etiologic agent of each of these superficial infections.

3. Outline special precautions (if any) needed to recover each of the superficial fungi in culture.

4. Describe the characteristic appearance of *Exophiala werneckii*, *Malassezia furfur*, *Piedraia hortae*, and *Trichosporon beigelii* in direct microscopic preparations from lesions and in preparations made from cultures.

5. Describe the typical colony morphology of *Exophiala werneckii*, *Malassezia furfur*, *Piedraia hortae*, and *Trichosporon beigelii*.

6. Given a description of the patient's symptoms and history and the characteristics of the fungus, correctly name the etiologic agent of the infection.

INTRODUCTION

Infections of the superficial and cutaneous tissues are "among the most prevalent of human infectious diseases" (Rippon, p. 169). Mycotic infections of the hair and skin fall into two categories. The superficial infections, called *tineas* and *piedras*, are confined to the horny, nonliving layer of the skin and the extrafollicular parts of the hair. Usually the immune system doesn't respond to the presence of the fungus because, says Rippon, the "organisms are so remote from living tissue, or the infection is so innocuous" (p. 154). If the patient seeks treatment, it is because of the way the infected area looks, not because the lesions are painful or debilitating.

Specimens from suspected mycotic infections should be cultured on Emmon's modification of Sabouraud's dextrose agar (modified SDA) with and without antimicrobials. The antimicrobial agents are necessary because they prevent overgrowth of the etiologic agent by the bacteria and saprophytic fungi that are part of the normal flora of the hair and skin. Inoculation of modified SDA without antimicrobials is essential, however, because some of the fungi infecting humans are sensitive to them (especially cycloheximide). Media additives, and special media, are discussed when extra care is required for specific fungi.

Piedra ("stone") is a hair infection, with nodular masses of fungal elements surrounding the hair shaft. The patient suffers no discomfort; hair loss does not occur. The hair is normal except for the nodule, with no involvement of the base of the shaft or the hair follicle. Two kinds of piedra are recognized: black and white (Table 4.1).

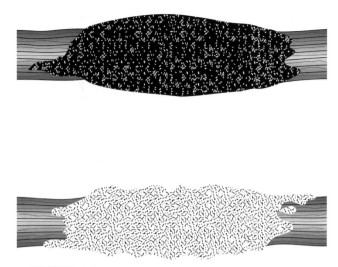

FIGURE 4.1

Upper, The nodules caused by *Piedraia hortae* are stonelike and dark—hard enough to click together; black piedra occurs primarily on the scalp, eyebrows, and eyelashes. *Lower,* The soft white nodules of *Trichosporon beigelii* are shown; this organism most often infects the beard, mustache, axillary, and pubic hair. Approximately ×100.

Black piedra is caused by a mould, *Piedraia hortae* (Fig. 4.1). Scalp hair is primarily affected. Black piedra occurs in tropical areas of the world. It is found more frequently in males, after puberty; long hair seems to increase the possibility of infection. Scalp hair, eyebrows, eyelashes, and pubic hair are most often infected; the hairs of the beard and axilla are more rarely involved. Infected hairs are covered by firmly intertwined, cemented masses of hyphae. The interior of the nodule is a disorganized mass of hyphal strands and conidia, with asci and spores. The nodules are hard enough to make a clicking noise when the hair is combed. Infection begins under the cuticle of the hair, then penetrates between the cuticle and the cortex of the hair. The cuticle is ruptured because of the pressure of the growing nodules; eventually the fungus surrounds the hair shaft if the infection is not checked. This phaeohyphomycotic piedra is best treated by shaving the affected area or cutting the hairs.

White piedra occurs on the temperate periphery of the tropical black piedra zone. Hairs of the beard and mustache, axilla, and groin are most often affected; the scalp is rarely involved. The fungus, *Trichosporon beigelii,* initiates growth below the cuticle of the hair shaft, forming nodular swellings that weaken the hair and cause it to break off. Growth may break out to form a sheath of encapsulated[1] arthroconidia and blastoconidia around the hair shaft. The external growth produces soft, pale

TABLE 4.1 The Piedras

	Black Piedra	White Piedra
Agent	*Piedraia hortae*	*Trichosporon beigelii*
Morphology	Mould	Yeast
Geographic Site	Tropical zones	Temperate zones
Tissue Involved	Scalp hair, eyebrows and eyelashes (and pubic hair)	Mustache, beard, hair of axilla and groin
Texture of Nodule	Hard	Soft
Color of Nodule	Black or dark brown	White or cream

Diagnosis of a typical piedra can frequently be done on the basis of the patient's history and the appearance of the lesion, without recourse to laboratory studies of the organism.

---

[1]The capsule is present on the conidia only when the conidia are associated with the hair shaft; it is not present in cultures.

masses on the infected hairs without causing lesions of the adjacent skin or hair follicles. This piedra is also best treated by shaving the area or clipping the hairs.

An experienced practitioner can diagnose the two piedras simply by the appearance of the nodules and the hair (see Table 4.1). The fungi are also easily distinguished. *Piedraia hortae*, the agent of black piedra, is a dematiaceous mould that grows slowly at 25°C on standard laboratory media. In contrast, *T. beigelii* produces creamy white yeastlike colonies on standard laboratory media; older colonies develop radial furrows and irregular folds.

Infections of the skin (and, confusingly enough, infections of the hair, the nails, and the deeper layers of the epidermis) are called *tineas.* The two superficial skin infections are *tinea nigra* (also known as *tinea nigra palmaris*) and tinea versicolor (Table 4.2). As with the piedras, the infections can usually be diagnosed simply by the appearance of the lesion; the fungi are also easy to distinguish.

Tinea nigra, caused by *Exophiala werneckii*, is generally considered to be a tropical disease, although increasing numbers of cases are being diagnosed in North America. Patients are usually younger than 19 years of age at onset of the disease. The palmar surfaces of the hands and fingers, and occasionally the feet, are affected. The flat and irregularly shaped lesions, called *macular patches*, are not scaly. They are brown to black, darker at

the edges than in the center, resembling stains made by the chemical silver nitrate. Darkly pigmented hyphae and yeastlike cells are found in sections and scrapings of the infected tissues. Typically the infection tends to remain localized but can spread to other cutaneous sites. *E. werneckii* has rarely been reported as an etiologic agent of tinea capitis, tinea pedis, and tinea cruris (see Chapter 5).

Tinea versicolor, also known as **pityriasis versicolor**, is the second superficial skin infection, caused by *Malassezia furfur*. The infection is a transient superficial *furfuraceous* (scaly) infection of the outermost horny epidermal layer of the skin, the *stratum corneum* layer. It is found primarily in young adults and is most likely to be detected after exposure to sunlight. Incidence increases in the summer and fall, prompting Rippon to postulate a relationship between infection with this **lipophilic** (lipid-loving) yeast and the use of tanning lotions. A relationship to the rate of shedding of squamous cells and a genetic predisposition to tinea versicolor have also been suggested by Rippon.

In light-skinned people the fungus causes pink to fawn or dark brown patches that do not tan when exposed to the sun. On dark-skinned people the infection results in depigmented or discolored areas that are lighter than the surrounding unaffected skin. The lesions occur primarily on the upper chest, back, arms, and neck; other areas are more rarely affected. Apparently the distribution of *melanosomes* ("black bodies"), the pigment granules produced by melanocytes in the skin, is rearranged in some way and their size is altered. Lesions are typically scaly and fluoresce golden yellow under a Wood's lamp because of a coproporphyrin produced by *Malassezia*. A **Wood's lamp** is an ultraviolet light used to detect fluorescence.

The typical infection is not painful but causes "cosmetic distress," that is, it looks bad and may itch in hot weather. Pityriasis versicolor can be spread from person to person or by *fomites* such as towels. Fomites are inanimate objects that contain or carry microorganisms and spread disease. Recently *M. furfur* has been identified as the agent of systemic infection in compromised patients receiving solutions intravenously through indwelling catheters to provide nutrition. The frequency with which this infection occurs in patients receiving intralipid therapy is not known.

Young colonies of *E. werneckii* are yeastlike in both colony appearance and microscopic morphology, while mature colonies are mouldlike in both colony appearance and microscopic morphology. Colonies of *Exophiala* develop dark pigmentation as they mature. One difference between *Malassezia* and *Exophiala* is that *M. furfur* cannot be cultured unless olive oil or other fatty acids are added to standard laboratory media. Other species of *Malassezia* (*Malassezia pachydermis*, for example) do not require the addition of oil to culture media. Colonies of *Malassezia* develop slowly into bacteria-like colonies that are white to cream.

TABLE 4.2 The Superficial Tineas		
	Tinea Nigra	**Tinea Versicolor**
Agent	*Exophiala werneckii*	*Malassezia furfur*
Morphology	Mould	Yeast
Geographic Site	Tropical zones	Temperate zones
Tissue Involved	Skin of hands and feet	Skin of chest, arms, and back
Appearance of Lesion	Dark macular patches that do not fluoresce under a Wood's lamp	Skin altered from natural color; lesions may fluoresce under Wood's lamp
Other Differences	Fungus grows slowly on standard mycology media	Yeast requires addition of fatty acids to the medium to grow in culture

When the lesion is typical, tinea nigra and tinea versicolor can often be differentiated from each other and from the dermatophyte infections by the characteristics of the lesion. A Wood's lamp may facilitate the diagnosis.

LABORATORY METHODS FOR SUPERFICIAL FUNGI

Typical superficial mycotic infections are usually easily diagnosed by experienced practitioners from the appearance of the lesion, without culture or microscopic examination. The exception is tinea nigra, when direct examination of skin scrapings is necessary to rule out the diagnosis of *melanoma* ("black tumor") and *nevi*, although a palmar location is uncommon for melanoma. A melanoma is a pigmented mole or tumor that may be cancerous. Nevi are congenital discolorations or vascular tumors of the skin.

Superficial Pathogen

DEMATIACEAE

EXOPHIALA WERNECKII (X-oh-fee-ah[2]-luh were-neck-ee)

Note: A name change for this organism, to *Phaeoannellomyces werneckii*, was proposed by McGinnis. It has not been accepted by all mycologists but is used in the fifth edition of the *Manual of Microbiology*. This text retains the use of *Exophiala* as the genus name.

■ **Reservoirs.** *E. werneckii* is found throughout the world in humid tropical and temperate areas of Central and South America, Africa, Europe, and Southeast Asia and is found with increasing frequency in the United States. It has been found in soil, on trees and rotting wood pulp, in decaying vegetation, in sewage, and as a commensal on normal skin.

■ **Unique Risk Factors.** Infections occur as the result of exposure that allows implantation of the fungus. *E. werneckii* is not believed to be transmitted from person to person. Persons who are related and have this infection are believed to be contaminated in the same way by the same fungus—probably from the same source.

■ **Human Infection.** *E. werneckii* is the etiologic agent of tinea nigra, a superficial infection that occurs primarily on the palmar surfaces of the hands and fingers and on the soles of the feet. Typically the infection tends to remain localized but can spread to other cutaneous sites.

---

[2]"Ah" rhymes with bah, as in "bah humbug."

■ **Specimen Sources.** The most common specimen is skin scrapings from the darkly pigmented cutaneous lesions.

■ **Specimen Collection and Handling.** The scrapings are collected and submitted in the usual manner, taking care to keep the specimen dry.

Direct examination involves study of the skin scrapings in simple wet mounts of (10%) potassium hydroxide (KOH) preparations.

■ **Immunology.** No tests are available; little is known of the antigenic structure of *E. werneckii*.

■ **Special Precautions.** None are needed, but cultures should be handled within a biologic safety cabinet.

■ **Culture Media.** Modified SDA, modified SDA with antibacterial antibiotics and cycloheximide.

Temperature Considerations. Temperatures between 25° and 42°C recover the organism in culture.

■ **Macroscopic (Colony) Morphology.** Colonies on modified SDA at 25° to 30°C first appear after 7 days as young shiny off-white to dark gray yeastlike colonies. After 2 to 3 weeks colonies of *E. werneckii* become very dark olive-green to olive-black and velvety or woolly in texture as short aerial mycelia develop. The reverse of the colony is jet black. The mould colonies are slightly dome shaped initially and become rugose when mature.

■ **Microscopic Morphology** (Figs. 4.2 through 4.5). Young cultures of *E. werneckii* are composed of hyaline to olive-black elliptical yeastlike cells approximately 6 μm in diameter; they are typically two celled. These conidiogenous cells are **annellides,** with one rounded end and one end that tapers slightly. Annellations develop at the tapered end as each new annelloconidium is formed. The annelloconidia are elliptical to subglobose and usually unicellular with smooth hyaline to olive-brown walls. They are typically larger than the original conidiogenous cells.

Septate hyphae are formed in the next stage of development of *E. werneckii*. The hyphae are up to 7 μm in diameter and darkly pigmented, with thick walls. The terminal ends of individual hyphae may be tapered and hyaline. Annellides may be intercalary or they may be produced on erect **annellophores** (a conidiophore that produces annellides) that are thin (approximately 2 μm in diameter and up to 30 μm long). The annellophores may or may not be pigmented, and they may or may not be macronematous, that is, distinctly different from the vegetative hyphae. As successive elliptical conidia form and are released, they leave annellations on the annellophores. These scars are not easily seen with a compound micro-

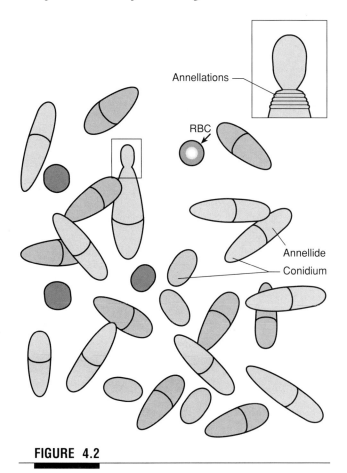

FIGURE 4.2

Exophiala werneckii consists of yeastlike annellides in young cultures. They are typically cylindrical or elliptical and may consist of one or two cells. A conidium buds from the annellide. The *inset* shows the annellations; one of these results each time a conidium is produced. This fungus is actually *Phaeoannellomyces*, an anamorph of *E. werneckii*. The 7-μm red blood cell (RBC) (arrow) shows the relative sizes of the mycotic elements.

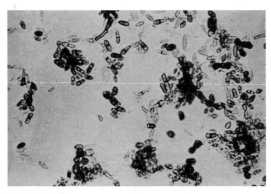

FIGURE 4.3

Typical young cultures of *Exophiala werneckii* contain dark brown budding cells and short hyphae and hyphal fragments. The two-celled yeast vary in size and shape as well as in the intensity of the pigment. ×400. (From Cole G: Conidiogenesis in the black yeasts. *In* The Black and White Yeasts. Pan American Health Organization Science Publication #356, 1978.)

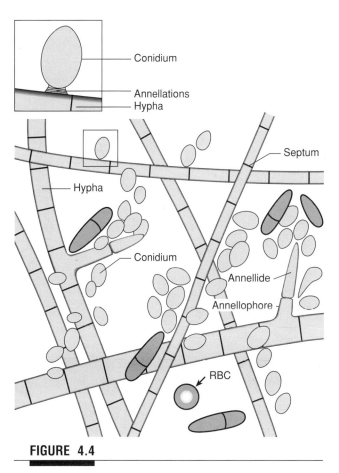

FIGURE 4.4

Exophiala werneckii forms individual elliptical conidia that cluster at the tips of the annellides. Annellides and conidiophores usually resemble hyphal branches. As conidia accumulate they slide down the annellide/annellophore to rest on the hypha. Hyphae are dematiaceous and septate. The 7-μm red blood cell (RBC) (arrow) shows the relative sizes of the mycotic elements.

scope but are distinct when viewed with a scanning electron microscope. The annelloconidia of *E. werneckii* tend to accumulate in clusters around the intercalary annellides or to cluster at the apex of the annellophores and slide down onto the hyphae. Dark thick-walled chlamydoconidia may also be found throughout the colony.

In *direct examination* (see Fig. 4.3) the skin scrapings contain dark budding cells and dark brown branching hyphae and hyphal fragments. All sizes and shapes of cells may be seen; the average diameter is 5 μm. Terminal segments may be hyaline and tapering. When tissue sections are stained with histologic stains, the older hyphae may appear twisted and swollen with thickened cell walls. Dark, elongated budding yeast cells and chlamydoconidia may also be found.

■ Helpful Features for Identification of *Exophiala werneckii*

Typical appearance of the black lesions on the palmar surfaces of the hands and fingers

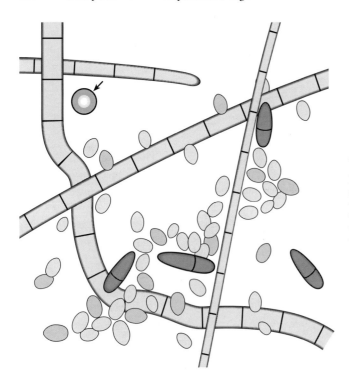

FIGURE 4.5

In bad preparations *Exophiala werneckii* is difficult to identify. Dematiaceous septate hyphae and dark elliptical conidia in clusters, coupled with the absence of distinctive conidiophores, suggest *Exophiala*, as do dark two-celled yeasts, but similar organisms cannot be ruled out without further testing. The 7-μm red blood cell (arrow) shows the relative sizes of the mycotic elements.

Early colonies of black yeast that mature into velvety olive-green mould-form colonies with a black reverse (*y*oung *y*east, *m*ature *m*ould)

Annelloconidia that are intercalary or produced on short annellophores above the darkly pigmented hyphae

■ **Organisms from Which *Exophiala werneckii* Must Be Differentiated** (Table 4.3; see also Fig. 6.19)

Exophiala jeanselmei
Wangiella dermatitidis
Phialophora verrucosa
Aureobasidium pullulans

Superficial Pathogen

Blastomycete

MALASSEZIA FURFUR (Mal-uh-see′-zee-uh fur-fur)

■ **Reservoirs.** The organism is found worldwide as a commensal on normal smooth skin of humans, as well as on domestic animals and birds.

■ **Unique Risk Factors.** Conditions that reduce the rate of *desquamation*, that is, shedding of the epidermal cells, apparently contribute to development of the infection. Other predisposing factors frequently associated with infection are poor nutrition, excessive sweating, pregnancy, and Addison's disease.

■ **Human Infection.** *M. furfur* is the etiologic agent of pityriasis versicolor, also known as tinea versicolor. The lesions occur primarily on the upper chest, back, arms, and neck; other areas are more rarely affected. Recently *M. furfur* has been identified as the agent of systemic infection in compromised patients, especially those receiving intralipid therapy.

■ **Specimen Sources.** Skin scrapings can be collected from discolored areas of skin. Blood or tissue samples should be collected if a disseminated infection with *M. furfur* is suspected.

■ **Specimen Collection and Handling.** Skin scrapings can be collected and submitted in the usual manner, or clear (Scotch) tape can be pressed directly onto affected skin areas and sent to the laboratory. When systemic infection is suspected, blood should be drawn through the catheter used for intralipid therapy into lysis centrifugation tubes. After the specimen is processed, the sediment is placed on media supplemented with olive oil or fatty acids.

A Wood's lamp may be useful in detecting areas to culture by showing yellow to light green fluorescence in the skin, but lack of fluorescence with the Wood's lamp does not mean *M. furfur* is not present.

Direct examination of skin scrapings should include staining the skin scrapings with crystal violet, iodine, or methylene blue.

■ **Immunology.** An immunofluorescent test is available to identify the yeast cells of *Malassezia* in skin scales and in cultures.

TABLE 4.3 Black Yeasts and Fungi that Resemble Them

Fungus	Size of Reproductive Cell (μm)	Shape of Reproductive Cell	Arrangement of Conidia	Width of Hyphae (μm)	Length of Conidiophore (μm)	Shape of Conidiophore	Arrangement of Conidiophores	Colony Morphology	Growth Rate	Other Helpful Features
Aureobasidium	5 × 12	Elliptical or cylindrical	Solitary	6–8	NA	NA—denticles	NA	Dark surface and reverse with white fringe	Intermediate	Dematiaceous arthroconidia; light brown hyphae
Exophiala jeanselmei	3 × 6	Elliptical	Clusters	2–7	10–30	Sticklike or macronematous	Solitary	Velvety surface with black reverse	Intermediate	Young yeast, mature mould
Exophiala werneckii	4 × 6	Elliptical	Pairs	7	≤30	Sticklike	Solitary	Dematiaceous	Intermediate	Young yeast, mature mould
Malassezia furfur	5	Medicine capsules	Clusters	2–3	NA	NA	NA	Cream to beige; bacteria like	Slow	Requires fatty acids for growth
Piedraia hortae	6 × 6	Barrel shaped	Chains	6	NA	NA	NA	Bacteria like, later suede	Intermediate	Asci and ascospores occur (rarely)
Sporothrix schenckii	1.5 × 2 and 2 × 3	Oval to pyriform and spherical to oval	Rosettes or sleeves and singly	1–2	10–20	Tapering toward top with small vesicle at apices	Upright	Mould has dark pigment with age; leathery or velvety texture	Intermediate	Thermal dimorph; two types of conidia, and two arrangements, may be present
Wangiella dermatitidis	2 × 4.5	Oval	Clusters around tip of conidiophore	3–4	Variable	Flask shaped or cylindrical phialides without collarettes	Solitary	Dematiaceous	Slow	Cylindrical phialides without collarettes

"Black yeasts" that cause superficial mycotic infections must be distinguished from similar agents of more serious mycoses.
NA, not applicable.

■ **Special Precautions.** None are needed.

■ **Culture Media.** Modified SDA supplemented with a layer of olive oil or other vegetable oil, supplemented modified SDA with antibacterial antibiotics.

Cycloheximide can be added if the pH of the medium is adjusted to acidity (pH 5.5). Malt extract agar, with the appropriate addition of lipids and antimicrobial agents, can be substituted for modified SDA.

> **Note:** *M. furfur* is a lipophilic yeast that is not usually cultured. This species of *Malassezia* does not grow unless fatty acids are added to the medium.

Temperature Considerations. Temperature of 35° to 37°C is required.

■ **Macroscopic (Colony) Morphology.** Bacteria-like colonies appear in 1 to 2 weeks on modified SDA supplemented with fatty acids and incubated at 37°C. They are shiny or pasty white to cream colored; later the colonies become dull and beige.

■ **Microscopic Morphology** (Fig. 4.6). In culture *M. furfur* rarely produces hyphae. The unicellular yeasts that form are *phialides* with distinct collarettes; these have been variously described as resembling bowling pins, medicine capsules, and bottles. Each produces a single *phialoconidium*, followed by successive budding ("blowing out") at a single locus (site). Budding is the first stage of production of some types of conidia. The phialoconidia are thick walled, round or oval in shape, and approximately 5 μm in diameter; they typically occur in clusters. Each phialoconidium in turn matures into a phialide and produces phialoconidia.

In *direct examination* (Figs. 4.7 and 4.8) *Malassezia* species have septate hyaline hyphae that are usually unbranched. They are approximately 3 μm in diameter and may be short and crescent shaped or long, thin, and straight. Conidia are seen as round budding yeast cells, approximately 3 μm in diameter. Together the hyphae and conidia have been described as resembling *spaghetti and meatballs*.

■ **Helpful Features for Identification of *Malassezia furfur***

The typical appearance of the patient's skin
"Spaghetti and meatballs" in direct smears of infected tissue
Requirement of the organism for added oil and fatty acids in culture

■ **Organisms from Which *Malassezia furfur* Must Be Differentiated** (see Table 7.2)

Candida species

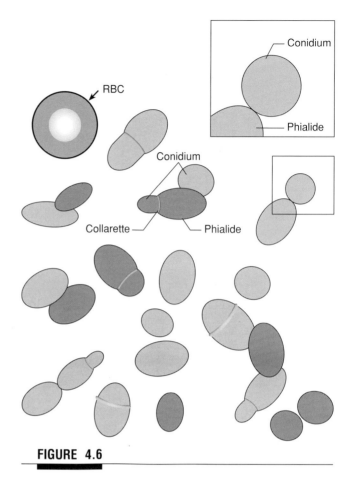

FIGURE 4.6

Malassezia furfur resembles other yeasts until it begins to produce conidia. The yeast cells are unicellular phialides that acquire distinct collarettes during conidiogeny, causing them to resemble bowling pins or bottles. Some cells may be dematiaceous. The 7-μm red blood cell (RBC) (arrow) shows the relative sizes of the mycotic elements.

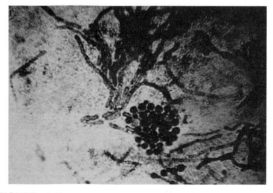

FIGURE 4.7

In tissue preparations such as this skin scraping, *Malassezia furfur* has septate hyphae and round budding conidia resembling yeast. The pattern has been described as resembling spaghetti and meatballs. (Courtesy of M. McGinnis.)

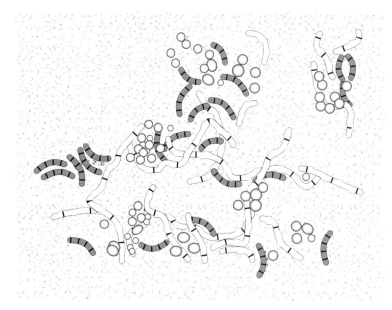

FIGURE 4.8

The spaghetti-and-meatball appearance of *Malassezia furfur* in tissue is caused by the septate hyphae and round budding conidia resembling yeast. The pattern makes it relatively easy for the experienced microscopist to recognize this disease. NOTE that fungi generally do not develop hyphae in tissue.

Superficial Pathogen

ASCOMYCETE

PIEDRAIA HORTAE (Pee-ay-dree-uh harr-tay or hoar-tay)

■ **Reservoirs.** The exact reservoir is unknown, but the organism is probably a plant parasite. Infections are found in hot and wet tropical areas in Africa, South America, and Asia.

■ **Unique Risk Factors.** None. There is no evidence that the infection can be transmitted from person to person.

■ **Human Infection.** Human infections are called *black piedra*. The infection most often occurs on the hair of the scalp where gritty black nodules form on the hair shafts. Nodules usually taper from one end to the other but occasionally may be thicker in the middle, tapering to both ends. The thicker parts are cemented together. The thinner sections clearly show aligned arthroconidia and hyphae.

■ **Specimen Sources.** Infected hairs.

■ **Specimen Collection and Handling.** Hair is clipped or plucked and sent to the laboratory in the usual manner, taking care to keep the specimen dry.

Direct examination involves studying the nodules on the infected hairs.

■ **Immunology.** No tests available; little is known of the antigenic structure of *P. hortae.*

■ **Special Precautions.** None are needed, but cultures should be handled within a biologic safety cabinet.

■ **Culture Media.** Modified SDA, modified SDA with antibacterial antibiotics.

Adding thiamine to the medium increases the production of aerial hyphae.

Temperature Considerations. Temperature of 25°C recovers the organism in culture.

■ **Macroscopic (Colony) Morphology.** The colony on modified SDA at 25°C after 10 days or longer is convex and glabrous at first. Then a cerebriform area develops in the center and becomes covered with short aerial hyphae; the periphery of the colony remains flat. The color of the mature colony varies from greenish black to black, with a black reverse. A rusty pigment may diffuse into the medium surrounding the colony.

■ **Microscopic Morphology.** In culture *P. hortae* has thick-walled, closely septate brown hyphae, with individual cells that are swollen and barrel shaped, averaging 6 μm in diameter. The hyphae frequently fragment into arthroconidia that resemble the arthroconidia of *Coccidioides immitis*, except that they lack disjuncture cells. *Arthroconidia* are asexual conidia produced by blastogenesis; disjuncture cells are cells that release a conidium by fragmentation or lysis. The hyphae show dichotomous branching with many intercalary chlamydospores.

Asci and ascospores are rarely seen in culture. When asci are found they are in locules in the nodules surrounding the hair or in the central cerebriform area of the colony. The asci are approximately 45 μm in diameter, elongated, and elliptical. Asci contain up to eight large (to 30 × 10 μm) *fusiform* ("spindle-shaped") curved ascospores with polar spiral filaments that may be up to 10 μm long.

In *direct examination* the granular nodules vary in size and may be as large as 100 μm in diameter. Fusiform asci, approximately 45 μm in diameter, are cemented tightly together in masses. Ascospores may be seen within the asci.

■ **Helpful Features for Identification of *Piedraia hortae***

Typical appearance of the nodules on the hair
Presence of asci and ascospores in direct preparations of infected hairs

■ **Organisms from Which *Piedraia hortae* Must Be Differentiated** (Table 4.4)

Trichosporon beigelii
Coccidioides immitis
Aureobasidium pullulans

Opportunistic Pathogen

BLASTOMYCETE

TRICHOSPORON BEIGELII[3]   (Trick-oh-spore-un bay-jhuh-lee)

■ **Reservoirs.** These yeastlike organisms are found in soil and lake water in temperate and tropical areas of Asia and South America; they are sporadically found in soil in the United States and Europe. *T. beigelii* may be found in small numbers as part of the normal flora of the human skin and mouth. Domestic animals may be infected.

■ **Unique Risk Factors.** None.

■ **Human Infection.** White piedra is caused by *T. beigelii* and other species of *Trichosporon*. Axillary, facial, and pubic hairs are infected, but the scalp is rarely involved. Soft white or grayish nodular masses are found adhering tightly to the hair shaft. In the right circumstances this yeast can invade deeper tissues to cause other infections. Recently *Trichosporon* species, especially *T. beigelii*, have been reported as the infectious agent in cases of paronychia, an infection of the structures surrounding the nail, and endophthalmitis, inflammation of the eye. Endocarditis, brain abscess, septicemia, and pulmonary infections may also be caused by *Trichosporon* species.

[3]Formerly named *Trichosporon cutaneum*.

■ **Specimen Sources.** In cases of piedra, hair is the appropriate sample. In other infections, aspirates, respiratory secretions, tissue, or blood may be cultured.

■ **Specimen Collection and Handling.** Infected hairs are clipped or plucked and sent to the laboratory. When *Trichosporon* species are suspected in other infections, the appropriate sample of blood, tissue, or exudate should be obtained aseptically, placed in a sterile container, and submitted to the laboratory promptly.

Direct examination involves studying the nodules on the infected hairs in a wet prep.

■ **Immunology.** No tests are available. Patients with systemic *Trichosporon* infection may have a positive reaction in the latex antigen test for *Cryptococcus* because of a cross-reacting antigen.

■ **Special Precautions.** None are needed.

■ **Culture Media.** Modified SDA, modified SDA with antibacterial antibiotics.

T. beigelii is sensitive to cycloheximide.

Subculture to malt extract broth and incubation for 2 to 3 days at 25°C enhance the production of blastoconidia.

Temperature Considerations. The optimal temperature for *T. beigelii* is 25°C. Some species of *Trichosporon* grow only at 37°C, while others grow at temperatures to 41°C.

■ **Macroscopic (Colony) Morphology.** The colony of *Trichosporon* on modified SDA at 25°C after 5 days is white to cream at first. The pigment becomes yellow or yellow-gray with age. The initial colony is smooth; it becomes waxy, wrinkled, and raised as it ages, with central cerebriform folds surrounded by rugose furrows.

■ **Microscopic Morphology** (Figs. 4.9 through 4.11). In culture *Trichosporon* species have hyaline septate hyphae that fragment into arthroconidia approximately 3 μm wide × 6 μm long. The young arthroconidia are rectangular. They may become more spherical after they separate from the main body of the hypha. One-celled blastoconidia of various sizes (ranging from 2 × 4 to 3 × 9 μm) may form ***sympodially*** (i.e., on alternate sides of the hypha or conidiophore in a repetitive zigzag pattern) just below the apex. *Trichosporon* species also form pseudohyphae, chains of blastoconidia that resemble a hypha but lack septa, on cornmeal agar.

Direct Examination. Intertwined hyphae and oval or rectangular arthroconidia, as well as blastoconidia, may be seen in specimens. Arthroconidia on the hair shaft may be encapsulated; arthroconidia are not encapsulated in cultures. The soft whitish nodules from the hair shaft may also contain bacteria or be mixed with *P. hortae*.

TABLE 4.4 Moulds with Yeastlike Colonies and Hyphae

Fungus	Arthroconidia (μm)	Shape of Arthroconidia	Pigment (microscopic)	Disjuncture Cells	Width of Hyphae (μm)	Colony Morphology	Growth Rate	Other Helpful Features
Piedraia hortae	6 × 6	Barrel shaped	Brown	No	4–5	Initially glabrous or cerebriform—becomes velvety with age	Intermediate	Dematiaceous; forms asci and ascospores in nodules on hair
Aureobasidium	7 × 15	Elliptical or cylindrical	Brown to black	No	6–8	Dark surface and reverse with white fringe	Intermediate	Dematiaceous arthroconidia
Trichosporon beigelii	3 × 6	Rectangular, becoming spherical	Hyaline	No	2–3	Smooth and creamy, becoming yellowish and wrinkled with age	Rapid	Pseudohyphae and unicellular blastoconidia also form; arthroconidia in nodules may be encapsulated
Geotrichum candidum	4 × 12	Rectangular; with germ tube resembles a hockey stick	None	No	4	Spreading, dry, and yeast-like initially, then velvety mould with subsurface fringe	2–3 days	Hockey stick arrangement of germinating cells
Coccidioides immitis	3 × 5	Rectangular to barrel shaped	Hyaline	Yes	1.5–3	Variable: initially glabrous and light gray, becoming floccose and white to light brown	Intermediate	Racquet hyphae in young cultures

The superficial fungi must be distinguished from similar yeastlike fungi that develop hypha in older cultures.

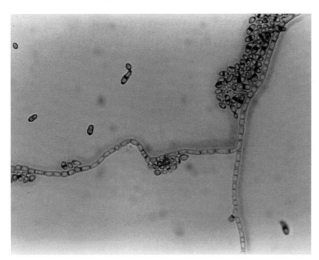

FIGURE 4.9

Microscopic preparations from cultures of *Trichosporon beigelii* contain hyaline septate hyphae and arthroconidia. The distinct cell walls and short arthroconidia in these hyphae make them look almost like strings of beads. Unicellular blastoconidia may also be found, as they are in this photomicrograph, free in the preparation and piled along the hyphae. Notice the new blastoconidium developing from the pair of blastoconidia at 11 o'clock.

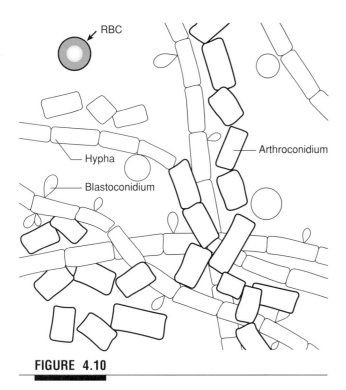

FIGURE 4.10

Trichosporon beigelii forms arthroconidia within the hyphae. These arthroconidia are rectangular at first, and they become more rounded after the hypha fragments. Blastoconidia of varying sizes may form sympodially on the hyphae. The 7-μm red blood cell (RBC) (arrow) shows the relative sizes of the mycotic elements.

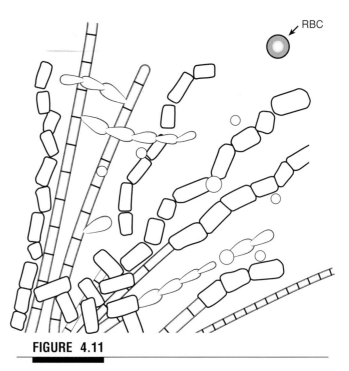

FIGURE 4.11

In cornmeal–Tween 80 agar *Trichosporon beigelii* has hyphae that fragment into arthroconidia. Blastoconidia and occasional chlamydoconidia are also formed. The blastoconidia may remain attached to one another, forming pseudohyphae. The 7-μm red blood cell (RBC) (arrow) shows the relative sizes of the mycotic elements.

■ Helpful Features for Identification of *Trichosporon* Species

Typical appearance of the nodules on hair
Yeastlike colonies at 25°C and, typically, at 37°C
Formation of hyphae and pseudohyphae on cornmeal-Tween 80 agar
Rectangular arthroconidia and blastoconidia
Lack of fluorescence in colony and lesion with a Wood's lamp
Formation of a pellicle in Sabouraud's dextrose broth
Failure to ferment carbohydrates
Positive urease in most strains

■ Related Species from Which *Trichosporon* Species Must Be Differentiated (see Table 4.4; see also Tables 7.1 and 7.2 and Fig. 7.20)

Geotrichum candidum
Candida species
Coccidioides immitis
Piedraia hortae

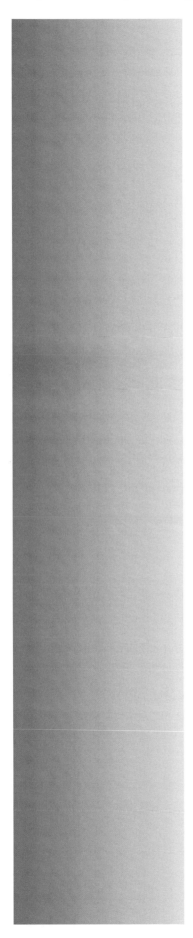

SUGGESTED EXERCISES FOR CHAPTER 4

(S u p e r f i c i a l   F u n g i)

Exercise 6 (1st Session)

Purpose. To practice procedures that you have already done, acquire experience in working with fungi with different textures and rates of growth, and (again) to set up the cultures needed for the next laboratory.

Suggested Fungus Cultures

> *Exophiala werneckii* (2 to 3 weeks old[4])
> *Trichosporon beigelii* on SDA
> *Trichosporon beigelii* in malt extract broth

Initial Process. Pick up four plates of potato flake agar (PFA) or potato dextrose agar (PDA) (one is for the slide cultures) and three slide culture setups from the supply table. At the same time, pick up the three new cultures you are working with today. If you have a laboratory partner you can each do 1½ cultures—you work out the details—or flip a coin to see who will do two organisms this time.

Make a *slide culture* for each of your fungi, following the instructions used during the previous session for Exercise 4. Good aseptic technique is important; the procedure should be done within a biologic safety cabinet. Set these aside to be incubated at 25° to 30°C.

Complete Exercise 6 just as you did Exercise 5; you may want to refer to those directions for details of the process. Essentially you are to record the necessary information on separate LABORATORY WORK SHEETS and *subculture* each fungus to a fresh plate of PFA or PDA.

Incubate all of the new cultures for Exercises 5 and 6 in the 25–30°C incubator. Do not forget to *water your slide cultures* at least once before the next laboratory. Don't wet anything but the filter paper!

Exercise 6 (2nd Session)

Purpose. First (A), you are to become familiar with the morphology of *y*oung cultures of the superficial fungi. Second (B), you are to examine the morphology of *m*ature cultures of the same organisms. Finally (C), you will observe and record the differences in morphology of *y*oung and *m*ature cultures of these fungi.

> *(A) Study of Young Cultures.* Pick up the three cultures of superficial fungi that you inoculated last week, *along with the original cultures used to make the subcultures.*

Complete all the work on one organism before you go to the next culture. Concentrating on the gross and microscopic morphology of one culture at a time makes it less likely that you will confuse the colony morphology of one fungus with the microscopic structures of another.

First, describe the gross colony morphology of your subculture, adding the information to the LABORATORY WORK SHEET you started last week. Re-

---

[4]Using *Exophiala* cultures that are 2 to 3 weeks old allows students to compare the morphology of the young culture that they set up with the morphology of the older culture—a good opportunity to make the point that *y*oung cultures are *y*eastlike and *m*ature colonies are *m*ould forms.

member to note the age of the organism as well as the pigment, texture, and topography.

Then, with the same subculture, prepare a tease mount and a Scotch tape prep. Label the microscopic preparations with the name of the organism, your name or initials, and the date. Examine the tease mount and the Scotch tape preparation microscopically, and make drawings from both preparations in the appropriate sections of the LABORATORY WORK SHEET. If *Trichosporon beigelii* in malt extract broth is available, you should also make a simple wet prep from the culture, examine it microscopically, and make drawings when you are studying this organism. Make a note of any differences you see in the two types of preparations.

Harvest the slide cultures set up during the previous laboratory session and put these aside to dry.

(B) *Study of Mature Cultures.* Complete all the work on one organism before you go to the next culture.

First, observe the gross colony morphology of the mature organism, recording all the necessary information on a new LABORATORY WORK SHEET.

Next, examine the slides of the mature cultures prepared by the instructor and make drawings of the structures on the LABORATORY WORK SHEET.

(C) *The Comparisons.* For each fungus compare the colony morphology of the (*y*oung) subculture to that of the (*m*ature) stock culture and record the differences on the LABORATORY WORK SHEET. In the same manner, compare the microscopic morphology of the *y*oung culture to that of the *m*ature one.

These comparisons are being emphasized to make the point that *Exophiala werneckii* has a distinctive pattern of growth for a monomorphic organism. For most monomorphs the difference between a young colony and a mature one is "more"; that is, more conidia or spores are seen in the mature colony than in the young one. For *Exophiala*, however, and several agents of subcutaneous infections, this different pattern is seen.[5]

Exercise 6 (3rd Session)

Finish work on Exercise 6 by sealing the edges of the coverslips for the slide cultures. Be sure that each slide is labeled properly, and put them aside for the seal to dry before further study.

Complete drawings of each organism in the proper place on the LABORATORY WORK SHEET and, if necessary, finish the comparisons of the gross and microscopic morphologies of the *y*oung and *m*ature superficial fungi. Save the slide culture preparations for your permanent collection.

---

[5]This pattern is related to the complex relationship among the synanamorphs of the fungi, although not all fungi with synanamorphs display such dramatic differences in morphology.

ASSESS WHAT YOU HAVE LEARNED

Responses to the questions below are located in Appendix A.

1. Describe the lesions seen in black and white piedras and the tissues involved. Name the fungi that cause each piedra.
2. Define piedra, tinea, Wood's lamp, lipophilic, glabrous, cerebriform, rugose, fusiform, ascus, ascospore, arthroconidia, annellation, collarette.
3. Compare the colony and microscopic morphologies of *Piedraia hortae* and *Trichosporon beigelii.*
4. Name the fungi that cause tinea nigra and tinea versicolor. Describe the lesions associated with each of these tineas and the tissues involved.
5. Compare the colony and microscopic morphologies of young *Exophiala werneckii* isolates and *Malassezia furfur.*

For questions 6 through 10 **MATCH** the description of the characteristic **(numbered)** with the name of the fungus with which it is associated **(lettered)**. NOTE that some responses will be used more than once, and some may not be used at all.

6. hyphae are dark brown and closely septate; arthroconidia and chlamydospores are present
7. lipids such as olive oil are needed to grow this fungus in culture
8. "spaghetti and meatballs"
9. hyaline hyphae fragment into rectangular arthroconidia that become more spherical after separation from the hyphae
10. *y*oung colonies are *y*eastlike and *m*ature colonies are *m*ould forms

    a. *Exophiala werneckii*
    b. *Malassezia furfur*
    c. *Piedraia hortae*
    d. *Trichosporon beigelii*

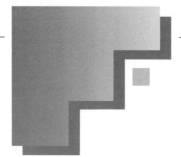

CHAPTER 5

Dermatophytes

Upon completion of this chapter the reader should be able to:

1. Define the following terms: endothrix, ectothrix, tinea, dermatophyte, anthropophilic, geophilic, zoophilic, bullae, kerion, mosaic sheath, *en grappe, en thryses.*

2. Distinguish the dermatophytes to genus, given the microscopic morphology of the fungus and the type of tissue invaded.

3. Describe general characteristics of the gross and microscopic morphology of a culture that suggest the fungus is one of the dermatophytes.

4. Draw or describe the following: pectinate hyphae, racquet hyphae, spiral hyphae, nodular bodies, favic chandeliers.

5. Correctly identify each of the dermatophytes, given a description of the morphology of the organism, patient symptoms and history, and (when pertinent) results of biochemical tests.

6. Describe, in general terms, the characteristics of the ringworm infections: favus, tinea barbae, tinea capitis, tinea corporis, tinea cruris, tinea manuum, tinea pedis, and tinea unguium.

7. Explain how the ingredients in dermatophyte test medium work to detect dermatophytes growing on it.

8. Distinguish between dermato*phytoses* and dermato*mycoses*, black-dot tinea capitis and gray-patch tinea capitis.

INTRODUCTION

The dermatophytes are "among the commonest infectious agents of man and no peoples or geographic area are without them" (Rippon, p. 169). A ***dermatophyte*** is a fungus that invades the keratinized portions of the hair, skin, and/or nails. A dermato*phytosis* is a mycotic infection of the hair, skin, or nails. These infections should not be confused with a dermato*mycosis*, invasion of the cutaneous tissues by other fungi. The dermatophytes are a closely related group of organisms that can use keratin as a nitrogen source. Most of the dermatophytes cause several different clinical manifestations, and most of these clinical states can be caused by more than one dermatophyte.

The dermatophytes are described by Rippon as undergoing "natural evolution from keratin-utilizing soil saprophytes . . . to association with and finally invasion of . . . keratinous tissues of living animals" (p. 176). One loose classification of dermatophytes groups them according to the preferred substrate (Table 5.1). ***Anthropophilic*** ("people-loving") species are believed to have evolved from the ***geophilic*** ("earth-loving") fungi. Rippon says that the dermatophytes are the "only fungi that have evolved a dependency on human or animal infection for the survival and dissemination of the species" (p. 5). In the evolutionary process the patterns of sporulation have changed. ~~As they became more anthropophilic fungi generally ceased to~~ convert to sexual (perfect) forms and produced fewer asexual conidia. They have become host specific. Anthropophilic dermatophytes are more likely to cause chronic infections eliciting relatively mild responses by the host. ***Zoophilic*** ("animal-loving") fungi produce more conidia and cause more severely inflammatory infections in humans. Geophilic dermatophytes are most active in conidiation and cause painful inflamed lesions.

On the basis of clinical, morphologic, and microscopic characteristics three anamorphic genera are recognized as dermatophytes: *Epidermophyton*, *Microsporum*, and *Trichophyton* (Table 5.2 and Fig. 5.1). No sexual (teleomorph) mode of reproduction has been found for *Epidermophyton*. The genus *Arthroderma* contains the perfect stage for many species of *Trichophyton*. Perfect forms of *Microsporum* were assigned to the genus *Nannizzia*. Rippon (1988) reported that there is no clear distinction between *Nannizzia* and *Arthroderma* and lists *Arthro-*

TABLE 5.1 Classification of Dermatophytes by Origin

	Anthropophilic	Geophilic	Zoophilic
Origin	People	Soil	Animals other than humans
Relative number of conidia in culture	Few	Most	Moderate
Human tissue response	Mild	Severe	Moderate
Examples	*Epidermophyton floccosum*	*Microsporum gypseum*	*Microsporum canis* *Trichophyton equinum*

Dermatophytes may be classified by their origin as well as by their taxonomic characteristics and the mycoses they cause.

TABLE 5.2 Classification of Dermatophytes by Morphology

	Epidermophyton	*Microsporum*	*Trichophyton*
Tissue attacked	Skin, nails	Hair, skin	Hair, skin, nails
Microconidia	None	Relatively few	Many
Macroconidia	Smooth thin walls; sparse in number	Thick, rough walls; many present	Smooth thin walls; relatively few present
Teleomorph	Not yet discovered	*Arthroderma* (formerly *Nannizzia*)	*Arthroderma*
Fluorescence in tissue	No	Characteristic of SOME species	No

Identification of the species of dermatophyte can be done, in part, by the kind of tissue attacked and by the appearance of the lesion. Characteristics of the microscopic structures confirm the identity of the species.

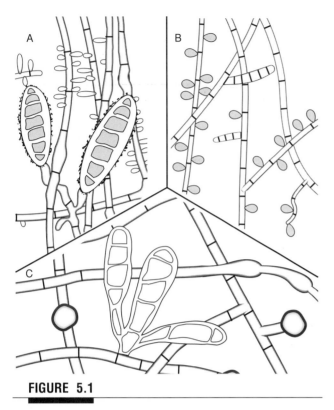

FIGURE 5.1

Cultures of dermatophytes are distinguished by the texture of the cell wall and the shape of the macroconidia and by whether microconidia are present. *Microsporum* species *(A)* have both macroconidia and microconidia; the macroconidia typically have tapered ends and a thick echinulate wall. *Trichophyton* species *(B)* also have both macroconidia and microconidia; the macroconidia are typically cylindrical, with thin, smooth walls. *Epidermophyton* species *(C)* do not have microconidia; the macroconidia have thin, smooth walls.

derma as the teleomorph for both *Microsporum* and *Trichophyton*.

Infections Caused by Dermatophytes. In a world where virtually everyone is exposed to dermatophytes at some time, no one knows why some people are infected and others are not. The resistance of the host is clearly as important as the virulence of the fungus. The kind of lesion that develops is governed by variations in the dermatophyte, by the ability of the host to defend itself, and by the anatomic site and kind of tissue selected for invasion. After the fungus is established in the tissue it must grow at least as fast as the tissue cells are shed if it is to maintain its position and "prosper." For all dermatophytes, the first step in infection is colonization of the horny layer of tissue. Then the fungus spreads in a centrifugal pattern, forming the "ring" that gives the infection the common name "ringworm"; this is most obvious when the affected tissue is skin. The host's response varies from patchy scaling to a toxic eczema-like reaction. Many infections resolve spontaneously.

Dermatophytoses are generally called tineas[1]; *tinea* is Latin for "ringworm." The second part of the name of the dermatophytosis identifies the part of the body infected. For example, tinea corporis is ringworm of the body.

The classic lesion of *tinea corporis* is a reddened, circular, scaly patch with sharply demarcated margins. As the infection advances at the rim the central portion may heal, resulting in a normal-looking patch of skin at the hub of the wheel or ring. In another common manifestation *vesicles* or *pustules* develop near the advancing margin of the ring. Both are small sacs or blisters on the skin. The fluid in vesicles is clear, while pustules contain purulent fluid, that is, pus. Any of the dermatophyte genera can infect the skin; tinea corporis is caused most frequently by *Trichophyton rubrum* or *Trichophyton mentagrophytes*. Dermatophytes look essentially the same in skin scrapings from a lesion (Fig. 5.2). Tinea corporis can be transmitted by direct contact with an infected person, by fomites, or by autoinoculation from another body site. The severity of the response varies with the host and the fungus. It can be diagnosed by examination of a direct

---

[1]Yes, tineas have been discussed already, in Chapter 4. Superficial and cutaneous infections of the hair and skin, and cutaneous mycotic infections of the nails, all are called tineas. It is potentially confusing—but the word *tinea* at least tells you what tissues are likely to be involved in the infection—which can be helpful.

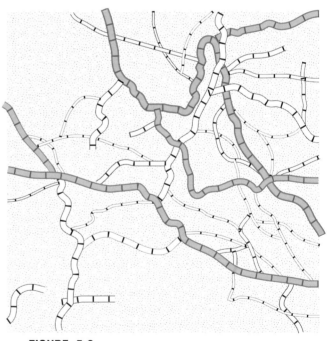

FIGURE 5.2

Dermatophytes cannot be distinguished by their appearance in tissue. All have septate hyphae *without conidia*, with varying widths to the hyphae. Hyphae are sometimes distorted. Arthroconidia in varying shapes and sizes may be present.

preparation of the skin scales. In normal patients the infection usually resolves spontaneously within several months. Sometimes relapse occurs—especially if *T. rubrum* is the agent of the infection.

Tinea cruris, ringworm of the groin ("jock itch"), is a special case of tinea corporis. It occurs most often in the tropics, although it is found throughout the world. Tinea cruris is seen almost exclusively in men, although it can be transmitted by contact to female sexual partners. Moisture, occlusion, and trauma contribute to development of tinea cruris. Generally the lesions resemble those of tinea corporis. In the United States the most common agent of tinea cruris is *T. rubrum. Epidermophyton floccosum* is more often the cause in Europe; *E. floccosum* has been associated with epidemics of tinea cruris in athletic teams and in prisons and barracks.

The third dermatophytosis to be discussed, involving the soles of the feet and the interdigital areas, has been characterized as "a penalty of civilization and the wearing of shoes" (Rippon, p. 219). *Tinea pedis* ("athlete's foot") is found throughout the world and is equally distributed between males and females. It occurs in adults more often than in children. *T. rubrum* tends to cause chronic infections. In contrast, *E. floccosum* causes acute infections that spontaneously resolve. Lesions vary from a chronic *intertriginous* form between skin folds with "peeling, maceration, and fissuring of the skin" (Rippon, p. 220) to a form in which fluid-filled vesicles and bullae are seen. *Bullae* are simply large vesicles. All forms are *pruritic* ("itchy"). Scratching or rubbing can open the way for secondary bacterial infections that are painful.

Dermatophyte infections on the palms and between the fingers are called *tinea manuum*. The most common agents are *T. rubrum, T. mentagrophytes*, and *E. floccosum*. Most cases occur in patients who also have tinea pedis, and the infection is, not surprisingly, usually caused by the same dermatophyte. Symptoms vary somewhat but generally resemble those of tinea pedis.

Tinea barbae ("barber's itch") occurs only on the bearded areas of the face and neck. A superficial form resembles tinea corporis. Another form, a pustular *folliculitis*, is associated with zoophilic dermatophytes. Folliculitis is inflammation of the hair follicles. Tinea barbae is most likely to appear in rural areas in men who work with cattle. *Trichophyton verrucosum* and *T. mentagrophytes* are the usual agents of tinea barbae. The severe tissue response is related first to the fact that hair is involved; such infections tend to be more severe. The other factor is that the usual agents are zoophilic fungi that tend to cause more serious disease in humans. Kerions may develop, and draining sinuses often form. *Kerions* are "boggy tumefactions," that is, spongy swellings. *Alopecia* (hair loss) and permanent scarring are common in untreated infections. Tinea barbae can usually be diagnosed by matching the patient's symptoms with the possibility of contact with animals, especially cattle.

Ringworm of the nail, *tinea unguium*, is seen in as many as 30% of patients with tinea corporis or tinea pedis. Infections may be superficial or severe. In the superficial form whitish patches on the surface of the nail contain the fungus but the nail is not distorted. In the more severe *subungual* form the deep layers of the nail plate are invaded. The nail becomes brittle and thickened and is frequently discolored. Debris from the fungus and from tissue destruction accumulate under the nail, causing distortion and cracking. Tinea unguium is the most difficult of the dermatophytoses to treat because the medication penetrates poorly. Up to a year of systemic medication may be required, and some infections persist despite conscientious adherence to the treatment regimen. Tinea unguium is a specific type of onychomycosis. Many fungi other than dermatophytes, especially *Candida albicans*, are associated with onychomycosis.

Dermatophytosis affecting the hair of the scalp, eyebrows, and eyelashes is called *tinea capitis*. It may be noninflammatory or markedly inflammatory with scarring and alopecia. Epidemic tinea capitis continues to occur, especially in children. Severity is largely determined by the species of fungus and the manner in which the hair is invaded (which is also related to the species of fungus). Arthroconidia are always found in the hair shaft early in the infection. The terms *ectothrix* and *endothrix* refer to the location of the arthroconidia that infect the hair in well-developed infections (Fig. 5.3). Table 5.3 compares three types of tinea capitis.

In *ectothrix* ("ecto," outside; "thrix," hair) invasion, the hyphae fragments into arthroconidia that accumulate around the hair shaft or just beneath the cuticle, destroying it. The arthroconidia that are outside the hair shaft form a *mosaic sheath*, a pattern of arthroconidia resembling a tile mosaic. Hair invaded in ectothrix fashion typically becomes grayish, dull, and discolored; eventually the hair becomes brittle and breaks off. When many hairs have been lost in this fashion, irregular grayish areas are left on the scalp, resulting in the nickname of "gray-patch" tinea capitis. This tinea capitis is not inflammatory, but scaling of the scalp is a prominent feature of the infection. Gray-patch tinea capitis occurs primarily in children. Researchers believe this is because certain fungicidal fatty acids do not appear in the human *sebum*, fatty secretions of the sebaceous glands, until the person has survived puberty. Spontaneous cure of the infection usually occurs when fatty acid production begins.

In *endothrix* ("endo," inside) invasion, arthroconidia form by fragmentation of the hyphae within the hair shaft. The cuticle is not destroyed; arthroconidia are not usually seen outside the hair in well-developed infections. However, the presence of the conidia weakens the hair so that it loses its luster, becomes brittle, and breaks off above the surface of the scalp. As the hair continues to grow the conidia in the shafts of the hair stubs appear as black dots. *Black-dot tinea capitis* is, of course, especially

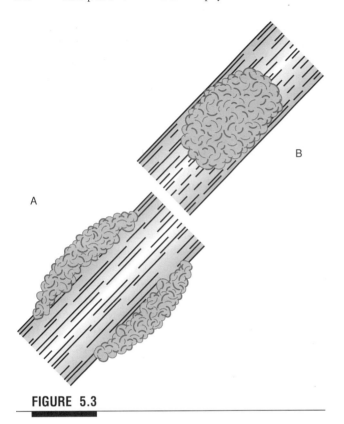

FIGURE 5.3

In *ecto*thrix invasion of the hair (*A*) the arthroconidia of the dermatophyte accumulate around the hair shaft or just beneath the cuticle of the hair. With *endo*thrix invasion (*B*), arthroconidia form within the hair shaft and are rarely seen on the outside of the hair.

visible in blondes. Sometimes the hair curls around beneath the surface of the scalp as it continues to grow after breaking off; these may be removed with a scalpel to obtain a specimen for culture. Alopecia and kerions may develop.

Ectothrix infections usually resolve without therapy, but endothrix infections tend to become chronic unless they are treated with systemic medication, accompanied by daily scrubs to remove the infectious debris.

Another, more severe, tinea capitis causes a pronounced host response with inflammation, kerions, and keloid formation. The typical lesion is a suppurative folliculitis resembling severe tinea barbae. This tinea capitis is painful. Hair falls out, and permanent hair loss may result. It occurs more often in African American children than in children of other races.

Favus, or *tinea favosa*, is also a special variety of tinea capitis, a "clinical entity characterized by the occurrence of dense masses of mycelium and epithelial debris, which forms yellowish, cup-shaped crusts called *scutula*" (Rippon, p. 197). The scutulae consist of "intertwined mycelial masses, scales, sebum, and other debris cemented together" (Rippon, p. 198). Scutulae develop in hair follicles and destroy them, with scarring and alopecia. The hair shaft is filled with long filamentous hyphae but few if any arthroconidia; empty air-filled areas are left in the hair when the hyphae degenerate into fat droplets. Lesions have a "mousy" odor. Unless the lesion is treated promptly the scalp atrophies and scars, resulting in permanent baldness. The infection is found in Africa and the Middle East; it has occurred in only a few endemic zones in North America. Favus is a "family-centered" infection; everyone from Grandma to the baby may have it. Unless it is treated properly it can last a lifetime, with two or three generations of bald people sharing a household.

A *dermatophytid* or "*id*" *reaction* occurs in some people as an allergic response to a dermatophyte infection elsewhere in the body. The id lesions do not contain the fungi causing the dermatophytosis, but they are itchy and sometimes painful.

TABLE 5.3 Mycotic Infections Involving the Hair

Mycosis	Most Common Site	Fungus	Symptoms	Target Population	Pattern of Hair Invasion	Alopecia
"Gray-patch" tinea capitis	Scalp	*Microsporum audouinii*	Itching; dullness of hair	Prepuberty; may be epidemic	Ectothrix	Possible
"Black-dot" tinea capitis	Scalp	*Trichophyton tonsurans*	Hair breaks off	Any age	Endothrix	Possible
Favus	Scalp	*Trichophyton schoenleinii*	Inflammation, kerions, scarring	Any age	Neither	Yes
Black piedra	Scalp, eyebrows, eyelashes, groin	*Piedraia hortae*	None	Both sexes	Hard nodule	No
White piedra	Beard, mustache, axilla, and groin	*Trichosporon beigelii*	None	Both sexes	Soft nodule	No

Both superficial and cutaneous fungi cause infections of the hair. The symptoms caused by these fungi differ markedly.

LABORATORY METHODS
FOR DERMATOPHYTES

Collection of specimens of infected hair, skin, or nails should be done according to your laboratory's procedure manual. Generally the task is to decontaminate the affected area to remove as much of the normal skin flora as possible and to obtain tissues from the area most likely to contain viable organisms. The most important element in transport of specimens believed to contain dermatophytes is to keep the specimen dry. This prevents overgrowth of the tissue and fungus by bacteria and preserves the fungus for culture. Containers such as test tubes that allow moisture to condense around the specimen should not be used.

A Wood's lamp can be useful for detecting dermatophyte infections. Generally tissues infected with *Microsporum* fluoresce bright yellow-green, while other dermatophytes generally do not cause fluorescence. In humans the fluorescence develops only *in vivo* and may persist for years after the infection is resolved. Of course, absence of fluorescence does not mean a dermatophyte is not present. The infection may be developing, or due to a dermatophyte other than *Microsporum*, or caused by a species of *Microsporum* that does not fluoresce. Some medications, and some hair oils, can cause fluorescence and false-positive reactions.

Direct microscopic examination of material from the lesions is not a sensitive test for detecting dermatophytoses, but it is the most rapid method of determining the etiology of an infection when the test is positive. It is most useful in more severe infections and should always be done. Correct selection of the specimen to be examined is critical to successful cultures and microscopic preps. The clinical material should be examined by suspending a portion in a clearing agent such as potassium hydroxide (KOH); 10%$^{w/v}$ is used for skin and hair, but 20%$^{w/v}$ is needed for nails. Dyes or blue-black ink may be added to the fluid to enhance the contrast between the fungal elements and the tissue cells that have not dissolved. Some workers recommend adding dimethyl sulfoxide (DMSO) to the fluid to increase the penetration of the stain into the tissue. DMSO should not be used with hair or thin scales of skin because the specimen dissolves.

Culture of dermatophytes requires media containing antibiotics because specimens from cutaneous sites almost always contain the normal bacterial flora of the skin, hair, and nails in addition to saprobic fungi from the environment and any fungus that may be present as the etiologic agent. We prefer Emmon's modification of Sabouraud's dextrose agar (modified SDA) for isolation of most fungi from clinical specimens, although McGinnis says that the original formula for SDA with 4% glucose is better for the dermatophytes. Antibacterial agents such as chloramphenicol and/or gentamicin may be added to the SDA to prevent overgrowth of the fungus by

bacteria. Cycloheximide must be added to reduce growth of saprobic fungi that may be present. *SDA without antibiotics should always be included in any regimen for culture*, because pathogens sensitive to the antimicrobial agents will otherwise be missed.

Dermatophyte test medium (DTM) was developed by Taplan and associates to screen specimens for the presence of dermatophytes. They incorporated gentamicin or chloramphenicol and cycloheximide into a basal medium to discourage growth of bacteria and saprobic fungi. Phenol red indicator was added to take advantage of the fact that dermatophytes produce alkaline metabolic products; the indicator detects these and the medium changes color from yellow to reddish orange or red. DTM is particularly recommended as a screening medium. It should NEVER be the only medium used. Some pathogenic nondermatophytes[2] are not inhibited by the antibiotics at 25° to 30°C and produce alkaline products that cause the red color to develop.

Potato dextrose agar (PDA) or potato flake agar (PFA) is used for initial culture by some mycologists because the pigmentation of the colony is better than it is on modified SDA and the development of reproductive structures is usually enhanced on PDA or PFA. In some cases additives such as vitamins are needed in isolation media to supply special nutrients when a particular fungus is suspected. Additional media may be used for the identification of specific fungi. These are introduced when the fungi are discussed.

One clue to the identity of the dermatophyte causing the infection is provided initially by considering the kind of tissue attacked. Typically *Microsporum* species invade the hair and skin but not the nail, while *Epidermophyton* species invade the skin and nail but not the hair. *Trichophyton* can typically cause infection in all three kinds of tissue.

Colony morphology has one feature that is helpful for distinguishing the dermatophytes from other pathogenic fungi. Colonies that have one pigment on the surface of the colony and another pigment—other than black—on the reverse are likely to be dermatophytes, although the pattern is found in other hyaline fungi. Not all dermatophytes have this pattern of pigmentation.

In addition, each genus has a distinctive pattern of conidiation that is considered characteristic (see Fig. 5.1 and Table 5.2). Differentiation relies heavily on the kinds of *microconidia* ("micro," small) and *macroconidia* ("macro," large) produced, the size, shape, septation, and attachment to the hyphae of the conidia, and the vegetative hyphal structures present. *Microsporum* can produce both macroconidia and microconidia. Typical macroconidia are fusiform, or *spindle shaped*, that is, they taper

---

[2]For example, *Acremonium, Blastomyces dermatitidis, Chrysosporium, Exophiala jeanselmei, Fonsecaea pedrosoi, Histoplasma capsulatum, Pseudallescheria boydii,* and *Sporothrix schenckii.*

from the center to both ends, like the spindles used to hold wool for weaving. The wall of *Microsporum*'s macroconidia is thick and echinulate with up to 15 septa. Microconidia are less commonly seen; they are pyriform or clavate and are borne directly on the hyphae or on short conidiophores. *Trichophyton* also produces both macroconidia and microconidia. The microconidia are globose, pyriform, or clavate, borne in two patterns (Fig. 5.4). Microconidia **en thryses** form a sleevelike arrangement around the hyphae. Microconidia **en grappe** refers to the arrangement of microconidia in clusters resembling bunches of grapes. Microconidia predominate in *Trichophyton* cultures. The walls of *Trichophyton*'s macroconidia are relatively thin and smooth; the conidia themselves are fusiform or cylindrical, with 2 to 12 cells per conidium. Some species of *Trichophyton* are characterized by unusual vegetative hyphal elements and do not produce macroconidia or microconidia unless a medium enriched with vitamins is used. The genus *Epidermophyton* NEVER produces microconidia. The macroconidia have thin, smooth walls and contain one to five cells. Various authors have described them as resembling beaver tails or snowshoes. These generic characteristics are useful for preliminary identification of a dermatophyte, BUT remember that every species in a genus does NOT have all of the characteristic features, even under optimum conditions.

The third clue to help with identification is that a culture that contains a relatively large number of bizarre structures such as pectinate hyphae, racquet hyphae, nodular bodies, and/or spiral hyphae in the vegetative hyphae (Fig. 5.5) is more likely to be a dermatophyte than to be one of the other pathogenic fungi.

Pectinate hyphae resemble the teeth of a somewhat battered and aged comb. The multiple projections from the hyphae, even though they are uneven in length and only approximately parallel, are the teeth of the comb.

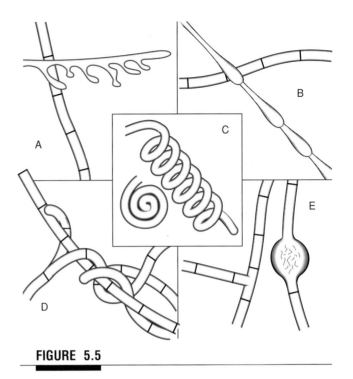

FIGURE 5.5

Bizarre vegetative hyphal structures seen in a microscopic preparation suggest that the fungus is a dermatophyte. These structures are found in cultures of other fungi, but with much less frequency: *A*, pectinate hyphae; *B*, racquet hyphae; *C*, spiral hyphae; *D*, nodular bodies; and *E*, chlamydoconidia.

Racquet hyphae superficially resemble pseudohyphae. In them you will note the walls swell out to form the head of one racquet, then a new racquet begins to form from the apex of the previous one. No septum separates the racquets. *Spiral hyphae* look as if they had been coiled around a pencil and released, resembling ribbon that has been treated that way to produce a curly embellishment for wrapping a present. *Nodular bodies* are formed when two or more hyphae become twisted together to form a roundish structure, as if someone had tied a knot. Chlamydoconidia may also be seen in large numbers.

Biochemical tests, temperature of growth, and the *in vitro* hair perforation test are also used for definitive identification of the dermatophytes, especially the *Trichophyton*s, to species. Nutritional testing involves growing the isolate on basal casein medium and on the basal medium to which supplements have been added. Thiamine and/or inositol are the supplements most often used. After 10 to 14 days of incubation at room temperature all cultures are examined to see which nutritional supplements (if any) enhanced growth of the fungus. The media for nutritional testing are commercially available as *Trichophyton* Agars.

To test the ability of the fungus to perforate hair *in vitro*, a lock of sterile "natural" hair—hair that has not been dyed or permed or treated with hair spray or other chemicals—is placed in a weak aqueous solution of yeast extract in a Petri dish. Many mycologists ask the barber

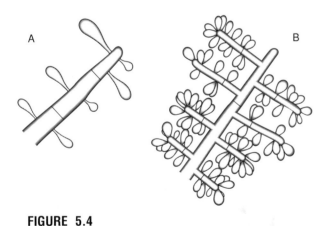

FIGURE 5.4

Microconidia of the dermatophytes, especially *Trichophyton* species, are often found in characteristic patterns or groupings. Microconidia *en thryses* (*A*) resemble a sleeve around the hyphae. Microconidia *en grappe* (*B*) resemble bunches of grapes.

→ Jock itch
athletes foot

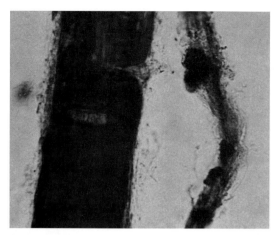

FIGURE 5.6

Penetration of hair *in vitro* is one test for differentiation of dermatophytes. The broad, dark cylinder running from top to bottom in this photomicrograph is a hair shaft at × 440 magnification. On the right side of the straight shaft, approximately one third below the top, is a pale wedge-shaped indentation caused by a dermatophyte penetrating the hair. (From Rippon JW: Medical Mycology: The Pathogenic Fungi and the Pathogenic Actinomycetes, 3rd ed. Philadelphia, WB Saunders, 1988, p 252.)

or beautician for hair from a young child to use for this test. The mixture is inoculated with the culture in question and incubated at room temperature for 10 days to 2 weeks. The step-by-step procedure is included in Appendix D. Dermatophytes can be differentiated in part by their ability to penetrate the hair shaft *in vitro*, causing cone-shaped perforations of the hair shaft (Fig. 5.6).

Cutaneous Pathogens

MONILIACEAE

EPIDERMOPHYTON FLOCCOSUM

skin & nails

(Epp-ee-derm-oh-phy-tun flahk-oh-some)

E. floccosum is the only human pathogen in this genus.

■ **Teleomorph.** None has been identified.

■ **Reservoirs.** The organism is found worldwide, especially in the hot and humid tropical zones. It is an anthropophilic fungus that has not been found in soil or on other species of animals.

■ **Unique Risk Factors.** *E. floccosum* is highly contagious. It has been recovered from clothing, jock straps, towels, rugs, and shower stalls.

■ **Human Infection.** This fungus infects the skin and nails but not the hair in both children and adults. *E. floc-*

cosum is an etiologic agent of tinea cruris, tinea pedis, tinea manuum, and tinea unguium. Infections with *E. floccosum* can become epidemic in athletic teams, in camps and dormitories, and in institutions such as jails.

■ **Specimen Sources.** Scrapings of the skin or nail should be obtained for culture.

■ **Specimen Collection and Handling.** Nail scrapings, material from under the tips of the nails, and skin scrapings should be collected aseptically and transported to the laboratory in a sterile, dry container. Specimens should not be refrigerated because *E. floccosum* is sensitive to cold temperatures.

Direct examination of specimens should include treatment of the material with KOH (plus blue-black ink and/or DMSO, if preferred), or a calcofluor white–KOH preparation may be done.

■ **Differential Methods.** None.

■ **Immunology.** No tests are available.

■ **Special Precautions.** None are needed, but cultures should be handled within a biologic safety cabinet.

■ **Culture Media.** Modified SDA, modified SDA with antimicrobials. DTM may be used for screening. PDA or PFA should be inoculated as soon as growth appears in primary cultures. Production of conidia is enhanced by using media with a low sugar content.

Preferred Temperature. Temperature of 25° to 30°C.

■ **Macroscopic (Colony) Morphology.** The organism appears on modified SDA after 6 to 12 days at 25° to 30°C as a white, downy, perhaps somewhat scanty colony. Later it becomes velvety or powdery, depending on the quantity of macroconidia produced. The center of the colony may be folded, with radiations to a thin, flattened, fringed periphery. The obverse color is mustard-yellow or khaki with a yellow fringe. The reverse pigment is yellow-brown or yellow-orange. Colonies of *E. floccosum* quickly develop a white sterile hyphae that may completely cover the colony.

■ **Microscopic Morphology** (Figs. 5.7 through 5.9). Hyphae of *E. floccosum* are thin, hyaline, septate, and branched. Macroconidia are produced abundantly in young cultures. They occur singly or in small clusters of two or three on the same conidiophore. The clavate macroconidia are sometimes compared to snowshoes, paddles, or beaver's tails. They are large (approximately 30 μm long × 9 μm wide) with blunt bases and rounded distal ends. The walls are smooth and relatively thin; as many as five cells may be found within a macroconidium. *Microconidia are not produced.* Numerous chlamydoco-

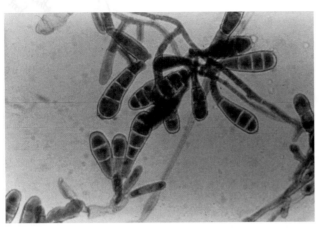

FIGURE 5.7

Microscopic preparations of *Epidermophyton floccosum* show thin, septate, hyaline hyphae and abundant macroconidia. The large macroconidia resemble paddles, or snowshoes, with thin, smooth walls; they are often produced in groups of two or three from the same conidiophore. Microconidia are never present. The dark color is due to the stain. (Courtesy of the Centers for Disease Control and Prevention.)

nidia, and a few spiral hyphae, racquet hyphae, and nodular bodies may be seen.

In *direct examination* of skin and nail scrapings *E. floccosum* is seen as branching hyaline, septate hyphae and/or chains of barrel-shaped arthroconidia.

■ Helpful Features for Identification of *Epidermophyton floccosum*

Abundant characteristic snowshoe or paddle-shaped macroconidia, with thin, smooth walls
Absence of microconidia

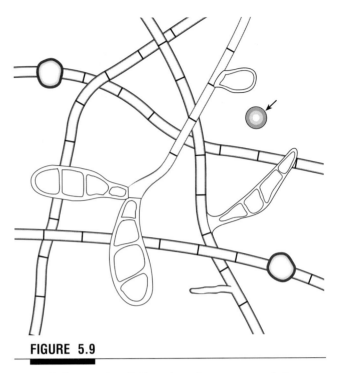

FIGURE 5.9

Even in bad preparations *Epidermophyton floccosum* can usually be recognized by the large, paddle-like macroconidia with thin, smooth walls and the *absence of microconidia.* Colony morphology, and the source of the specimen, should also be considered in making the identification. The 7-μm red blood cell (arrow) shows the relative sizes of the mycotic elements.

Colony morphology, especially the mustard or khaki pigment

■ Organisms from Which *Epidermophyton floccosum* Must Be Differentiated (Fig. 5.10 and Table 5.4)

Some species of *Microsporum*, especially *Microsporum nanum*

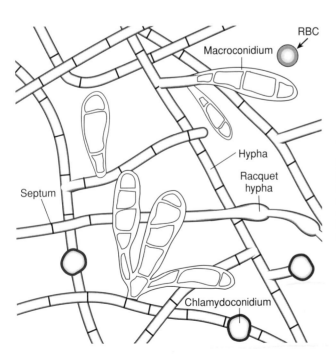

FIGURE 5.8

Epidermophyton floccosum has hyaline, septate hyphae; bizarre vegetative structures such as racquet hyphae may also be present. This figure shows chlamydoconidia within several of the hyphae, as well as a terminal chlamydoconidium. The large, paddle-shaped macroconidia have smooth, thin walls. A typical clustuer of macroconidia appears at the bottom center of the field. *Microconidia are never present.* The 7-μm red blood cell (RBC) (arrow) shows the relative sizes of the mycotic elements.

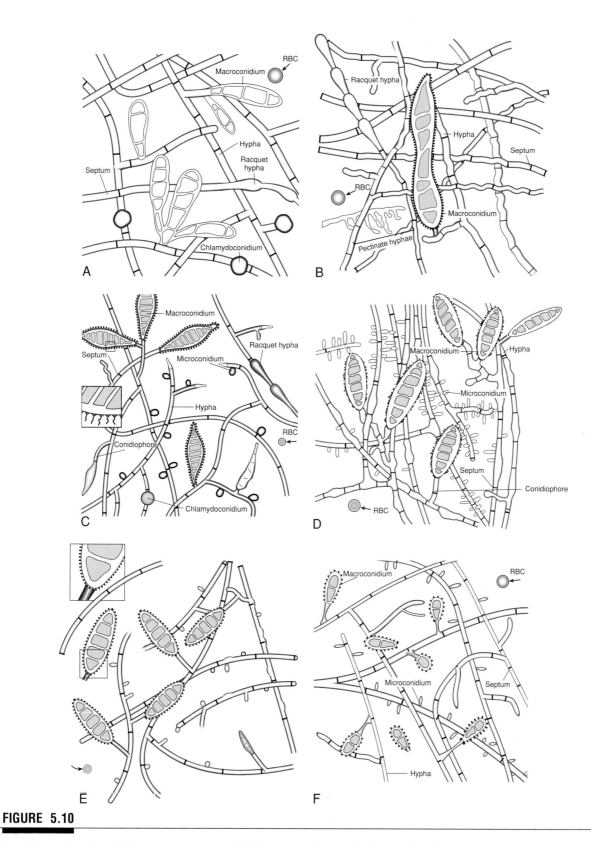

FIGURE 5.10

Epidermophyton and species of *Microsporum* are compared in this composite because both genera have large, broad macroconidia. The absence of microconidia, and the paddle shape and the smooth wall of the macroconidia, identify *Epidermophyton (A)*. Speciation of *Microsporum* depends primarily on the shape of the macroconidia. The genus *Microsporum* is represented here by *Microsporum audouinii (B)*, *Microsporum canis (C)*, *Microsporum cookei (D)*, *Microsporum gypseum (E)*, and *Microsporum nanum (F)*. The 7-μm red blood cell (RBC) (arrow) shows the relative sizes of the mycotic elements.

TABLE 5.4 *Microsporum* and *Epidermophyton* Species

Fungus	Size of Macroconidia (μm)	Shape of Macroconidia	Number of Cells per Macroconidium	Arrangement of Macroconidia	Size of Microconidia (μm)	Shape of Microconidia	Arrangement of Microconidia	Width of Hyphae (μm)	Colony Morphology (SDA)	Growth Rate	Other Helpful Features
Epidermophyton	9 × 30	Snowshoes, paddles or beaver's tails with smooth, thin walls	2–5	Individual or in clusters of 2 or 3	Not applicable	Not applicable	Not applicable	3–4	Velvety or powdery with mustard-yellow obverse and yellowish orange or brown reverse	Intermediate	Microconidia are not produced
Microsporum audouinii	15 × 80	Distorted cylinders or spindles with thick walls	5–7	Individual (rare)	2 × 3	Clavate or ovoid	Solitary	3–5	Rugose, dense, and velvety with light obverse pigment and reddish brown reverse	Intermediate to slow	Vegetative structures are present, including large (25 μm) vesicles
Microsporum canis	11 × 72	Spindle shaped with asymmetrical beaked apex and thick, rough walls	6–15	Individual	3 × 5	Clavate or pyriform	Solitary (sparse)	4–6	Cottony or granular with buff obverse	Rapid	Bright yellow reverse pigment in colonies <5 days old
Microsporum cookei	14 × 60	Ellipsoidal to fusiform with thick, rough walls	6–10	Solitary	3 × 5	Oval to pyriform	Sessile and solitary	3–5	Powdery or coarsely granular with tan surface and deep purple-red reverse	Intermediate	Many conidia
Microsporum gypseum	11 × 42	Ellipsoidal to fusiform with thick, rough walls	2–6	Alone and in clusters	3 × 5	Clavate	Sessile and solitary	3–5	Flat and granular with sterile hyphae. Surface and reverse are tan to cinnamon-pink	Rapid	Resembles *M. cookei*
Microsporum nanum	6 × 15	Clavate to ellipsoidal with relatively thin, rough walls	1–2 (rarely 4)	Solitary	2–5	Clavate to pyriform	Solitary and sessile	3–5	Powdery and rugose, with cream to reddish tan obverse and brownish red reverse	Rapid	Many microconidia

Identification of *Epidermophyton* and *Microsporum* species can usually be done by examination of the microscopic structures of the fungus.
SDA, Sabouraud's dextrose agar.

Cutaneous Dermatophytes

MONILIACEAE

MICROSPORUM AUDOUINII (My-crow-spore-um aw-dough-een-ee or awd-ween-ee)

■ **Teleomorph.** None has been identified.

■ **Reservoirs.** It is found worldwide, especially in Africa, Europe, and the United States. This organism is an anthropophilic fungus.

■ **Unique Risk Factors.** *M. audouinii* is highly contagious. The infection is most often transmitted by contaminated fomites such as hair clippers or barber's shears, combs, hats, linens, towels, and upholstery. *M. audouinii* can also be transmitted from person to person by direct contact.

■ **Human Infection.** *M. audouinii* causes gray-patch tinea capitis in children; epidemics can occur. Infections are rare after puberty. The circular lesions fluoresce when a Wood's lamp is used. Lesions are itchy and uncomfortable but noninflammatory and therefore not painful. Only a small number of infections with *M. audouinii* are now seen each year in the United States, but historically it has been the most important etiologic agent of epidemic tinea capitis in school-age children. Researchers believe that children are the primary targets of *M. audouinii* because of the absence of certain fungicidal ("cidal," lethal) fatty acids in the sebum. The tinea capitis is an ectothrix type of hair infection, with a mosaic sheath of conidia.

M. audouinii also is the agent of tinea corporis in children and, rarely, in adults.

■ **Specimen Sources.** The stubs of hair remaining when the hair breaks off, or skin scrapings, should be cultured. Infected areas can sometimes be identified because of the bright yellow-green fluorescence emitted when a Wood's lamp is used.

■ **Specimen Collection and Handling.** Hair should be plucked from the infected area and sent to the laboratory. Skin scrapings can be collected and submitted in the usual manner.

Direct examination of specimens should include treatment with 10% KOH (blue-black ink may be added), or a calcofluor white–KOH preparation may be done.

■ **Immunology.** No tests are available.

■ **Special Precautions.** None are needed, but cultures should be handled within a biologic safety cabinet.

■ **Culture Media.** Modified SDA, modified SDA with antibacterial antibiotics and cycloheximide. DTM may be used for screening. PDA or PFA should be inoculated as soon as growth appears in the primary cultures. Adding yeast extract to media may improve production of conidia.

Preferred Temperature. Temperature of 25° to 30°C.

■ **Differential Methods:** A colony suspected of being *M. audouinii* can be inoculated onto sterile (cooked) rice, a nutritionally poor medium. The *in vitro* hair test can also be performed. *M. audouinii* is negative in both tests. It either does not grow at all on the rice grains or it grows poorly and produces a brown pigment. Hair is not perforated *in vitro*.

■ **Macroscopic (Colony) Morphology.** *M. audouinii* defies the usual classification as a rapid, intermediate, or slow grower because while colonies first appear on modified SDA at 25°C in 7 to 10 days, they require up to 3 weeks to mature sufficiently to be identified. The initial colony is flat and white. Later it becomes rugose, dense, and velvety, with a tan to light gray surface pigment. On modified SDA the colony's reverse pigment is beige to reddish brown. On PDA, after 2 weeks, the reverse is salmon pink; it later turns orange-brown.

■ **Microscopic Morphology** (Figs. 5.11 through 5.13). The hyphae of *M. audouinii* are hyaline, septate, and branched. Vegetative hyphal structures that may be seen include terminal and intercalary vesicles, pectinate bodies, and racquet hyphae. The vesicles[3] are swollen areas

---

[3]These structures are called "chlamydospores" in older publications.

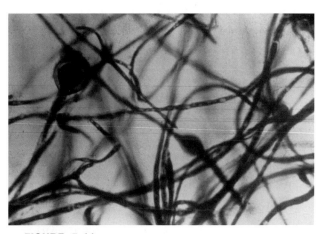

FIGURE 5.11

Typical preparations of *Microsporum audouinii* contain bizarre hyphal structures such as the chlamydoconidia in the upper left quadrant. Macroconidia are *rarely* seen. In the absence of conidia vesicles in the hyphae, like the one at 10 o'clock, suggest this dermatophyte. (Courtesy of the Centers for Disease Control and Prevention.)

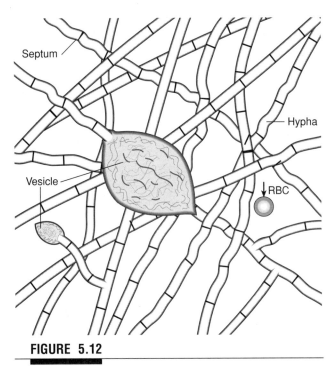

FIGURE 5.12

Microsporum audouinii produces large, swollen vesicles and other bizarre vegetative structures, but conidia are rarely seen. Hyphae are septate. Both colony morphology and growth on sterile rice grains must be considered for a definitive identification of this fungus. The 7-μm red blood cell (RBC) (arrow) shows the relative sizes of the mycotic elements.

of the hyphae that may be pointed or nipple-like; they sometimes resemble chlamydoconidia. Often these vegetative structures are the only structures seen in preparations from *M. audouinii* colonies. They are also in microscopic preparations of other fungi, especially the

dermatophytes. Macroconidia and microconidia are RARELY produced in culture on standard media.

When macroconidia are observed, they are large (approximately 15 × 80 μm) and appear distorted, with irregular cylindrical or spindle shapes. Each macroconidium has thick walls and is divided into multiple cells by septa. The cell wall is echinulate or smooth. Macroconidia are connected to the hyphae by cells that collapse and break away when the conidium is mature. The microconidia, which are *rarely* produced, are clavate or ovoid, approximately 3 μm in diameter. They are borne on short pedicles along the hyphae.

In *direct examination* of skin scrapings, *M. audouinii* is seen as hyaline, septate hyphae and/or chains of barrel-shaped arthroconidia.

■ **Helpful Features for Identification of *Microsporum audouinii*** (Table 5.5; see also Table 5.4)

> Bright yellow-green fluorescence of infected hairs *in vivo*
> Rare appearance of conidia on standard media
> Distorted appearance of macroconidia, when present
> Poor growth (if any) on rice grains, although a brownish tinge may be produced in the grains of rice
> Negative *in vitro* hair perforation test
> Intercalary and terminal vesicles

■ **Organisms from Which *Microsporum audouinii* Must Be Differentiated** (see Fig. 5.10 and Tables 5.4 and 5.5)

> Most dermatophytes, but especially *Microsporum canis*

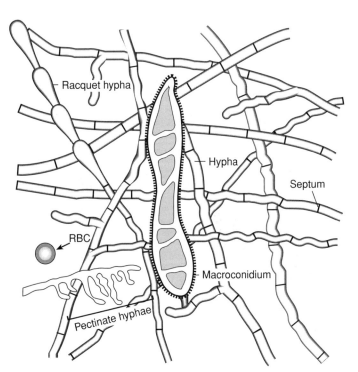

FIGURE 5.13

The macroconidia of *Microsporum audouinii* share the characteristics of other *Microsporum* species, with thick, rough walls and a "spindle" shape, but they are usually twisted and distorted. Bizarre hyphal structures, such as pectinate hyphae and racquet hyphae, are also typically present among the septate hyphae. The 7-μm red blood cell (RBC) (arrow) shows the relative sizes of the mycotic elements.

TABLE 5.5 Additional Tests for Differentiation of Dermatophytes

Fungus	Fluorescence of Infected Area	Growth on Rice Grains	In Vitro Hair Perforation	Urease Hydrolysis	Effect of Thiamine	Effect of Inositol	Vegetative Hyphal Structures	Other Helpful Features
Epidermophyton	NA	NA	NA	NA	NA	NA	—	No microconidia; macroconidia with thin, smooth walls
Microsporum audouinii	Yes	Poor or none (may develop brown pigment)	No penetration	NA	NA	NA	Racquet and pectinate hyphae, nodular bodies, chlamydoconidia	Sparse conidiation; terminal vesicles
Microsporum canis	Yes	Yes (yellow pigment)	Penetration	NA	NA	NA	Racquet and pectinate hyphae.	Asymmetric "beaks" on macroconidia
Microsporum cookei	No	Yes	Penetration	NA	NA	NA	Racquet hyphae	Wine-red reverse pigment in colonies
Microsporum gypseum	Rare	Yes	Penetration	NA	NA	NA	Racquet and pectinate hyphae	Few clavate microconidia
Microsporum nanum	No	Yes	Penetration	NA	NA	NA	NA	Macroconidia with 1–3 cells
Trichophyton mentagrophytes	No	NA	Penetration	Yes (<4 days)	Growth without enhancement	Growth without enhancement	Microconidia *en grappe*; spiral hyphae and nodular bodies	"Rat-tail" conidia may form. Red pigment may develop in colonies on SDA. More conidia in Type I colonies than in Type II colonies
Trichophyton rubrum	No	NA	No penetration	Yes (>6 days)	No effect	No effect	Chlamydoconidia, pectinate hyphae	Two colony types; conidia are most abundant in Type II colonies. Microconidia may form directly on macroconidia
Trichophyton schoenleinii	Rarely (light green)	NA	No penetration	Positive >11 days	No effect	No effect	Nail heads and favic chandeliers	Lesions have "mousy" odor. Microconidia produced on rice grain medium. Arthroconidia in young cultures
Trichophyton tonsurans	No	NA	Penetration	Positive >4 days	Growth is enhanced	Growth of some strains is enhanced	Occasional spiral hyphae and terminal chlamydoconidia	"Ballooning" microconidia. Reverse pigment usually diffuses into medium
Trichophyton verrucosum	No fluorescence in human infections	NA	No penetration	Positive >15 days	Required for growth	Enhanced growth of some strains	Chains of chlamydoconidia; favic chandeliers	Colonies submerged in medium. Conidiation sparse even on enriched media. "Rat-tail" macroconidia
Trichophyton violaceum	No	NA	No penetration	Positive >15 days	Enhanced growth	No effect	Chlamydoconidia; occasional favic chandeliers	Swollen hyphal cells containing cytoplasmic granules Sparse conidiation even on enriched media

Microsporum species except, perhaps, *Microsporum audouinii*) and *Epidermophyton floccosum* can usually be identified by the morphology of the colonies and the microscopic structures. Biochemical reactions and growth patterns are usually needed—especially by inexperienced personnel—to determine the correct species of *Trichophyton*.
NA, not applicable; SDA, Sabouraud's dextrose agar.

Cutaneous Dermatophytes

MONILIACEAE

MICROSPORUM CANIS (My-crow-spore-um cane-us)

- **Teleomorph.** *Arthroderma (Nannizzia) otae.*

- **Reservoirs.** It is found worldwide as a zoophilic pathogen of lower animals and is the most common zoophile in human infections.

- **Unique Risk Factors.** *M. canis* is highly contagious and easily transmitted from animal to animal and from animals to humans. Transmission from person to person is believed to be rare. Children are infected more often than adults.

- **Human Infection.** As with *Microsporum audouinii*, researchers believe that children are the primary targets of *M. canis* because certain fungicidal fatty acids are absent until after puberty. Also, children are more likely to have frequent contact with the family cat or dog. It is an ectothrix-type of infection, resulting in a gray-patch tinea capitis. Hyphae enter the hair shaft at midfollicle and grow within the hair shaft. As the hair emerges from the follicle the fungus breaks out onto the surface of the hair and covers it with arthroconidia. The lesions are more acute, inflammatory, and uncomfortable than the lesions of chronic tinea capitis.

    M. canis also causes tinea corporis, infecting the smooth skin of both children and adults. Rippon says that "an outbreak of tinea capitis in children due to *M. canis* and *M. audouinii* will manifest itself in an associated adult population as tinea corporis" (p. 199).

- **Specimen Sources.** Skin scrapings or the stubs of hair remaining when the hair breaks off should be cultured. Either specimen may be identified by the bright yellow-green fluorescence emitted when a Wood's lamp is used; however, as noted previously, the absence of fluorescence does not mean that infection is not present.

- **Specimen Collection and Handling.** Hair should be plucked from the infected area and sent to the laboratory. Skin scrapings can be collected and submitted in the usual manner.

    Direct examination of skin scrapings should include treatment of the skin with 10% KOH (with blue-black ink), or a calcofluor white–KOH preparation may be done.

- **Immunology.** No tests available.

- **Special Precautions.** None are needed, but cultures should be handled within a biologic safety cabinet.

- **Culture Media.** Modified SDA, modified SDA with antibacterial antibiotics and cycloheximide. Adding yeast extract to media enhances the production of macroconidia. DTM may be used for screening. PDA or PFA, or modified cornmeal agar (CMA) with 0 to 1% dextrose should be inoculated as soon as growth appears in the primary cultures. CMA, like PDA and PFA, is a starchy medium that enhances pigmentation and conidiation of fungi.

Preferred Temperature. Temperature of 25° to 30°C.

- **Differential Methods:** A colony suspected of being *M. canis* can be inoculated onto sterile cooked rice, a nutritionally poor medium. The *in vitro* hair test can also be performed. *M. canis* grows well on sterile rice grains, producing a yellow pigment and characteristic conidia. The hair perforation test is positive for *M. canis*.

- **Macroscopic (Colony) Morphology.** The colony on modified SDA at 25°C after 4 to 6 days is at first flat with radial grooves, white to yellow, and cottony. Later it may become buff colored with a feathery periphery. The texture may remain cottony or become granular, depending on the number of macroconidia produced. On modified SDA the reverse pigment of colonies less than 5 days old is bright yellow; later the pigment becomes yellow-orange or brownish yellow. This pigmentation is readily seen on PDA or PFA.

- **Microscopic Morphology** (Figs. 5.14 through 5.16). The hyphae of *M. canis* are hyaline, septate, and branched. Abundant macroconidia are produced. They are large (averaging 11 × 72 μm) and spindle shaped, often with an asymmetrical beaked apex. The outer walls are thick and echinulate, while the inner septa are thin; the roughness is

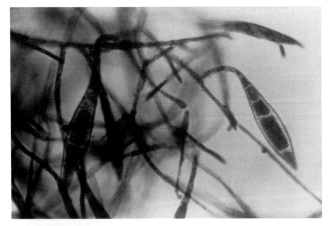

FIGURE 5.14

Microsporum canis produces large macroconidia with thick, rough walls; the roughness of the walls is not evident in this photograph. The macroconidia are spindle shaped with pointed ends, and often the apex of the conidium is knobby and asymmetrical. Microconidia (shown in the center of the field) are clavate or pyriform, with thin, smooth walls. (Courtesy of the Centers for Disease Control and Prevention.)

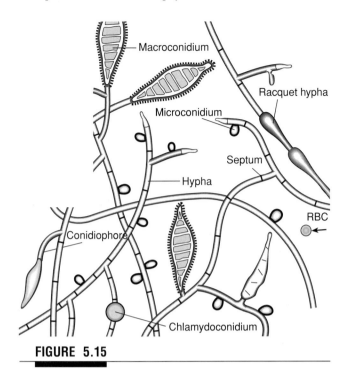

FIGURE 5.15

In microscopic preparations *Microsporum canis* typically has many large, spindle-shaped macroconidia with thick, rough walls and eccentric knobs on the ends. Microconidia resemble clubs, with smooth walls. Hyphae are septate, and bizarre vegetative structures may also be present. The 7-μm red blood cell (RBC) (arrow) shows the relative sizes of the mycotic elements.

more evident on the beaked end. From 6 to 15 cells develop within individual macroconidia. Macroconidia are attached to the hyphae by cells that collapse and break away when the conidia mature, leaving an annular frill at the base of the conidium. Only a few microconidia are produced by *M. canis* in culture on routine media. They are one-celled clavate or pyriform structures with smooth walls, approximately 3 × 5 μm in diameter. Microconidia are borne singly along the hyphae. Production of microconidia is enhanced by growth on PDA, PFA, or CMA. Vegetative hyphal structures that may be seen include pectinate bodies, nodular bodies, racquet hyphae, and chlamydoconidia.

■ Helpful Features for Identification of *Microsporum canis* (see Tables 5.4 and 5.5)

> Bright yellow-green fluorescence under a Wood's lamp
> Rare microconidia on standard media
> Characteristic spindle-shaped macroconidia with beaked tips
> Good growth and conidiation on rice grains, with production of a yellow pigment
> Positive *in vitro* hair perforation test
> Yellow pigment on reverse of young colonies (5 days)
> Typical vegetative structures

■ Organisms from Which *Microsporum canis* Must Be Differentiated (see Fig. 5.10 and Tables 5.4 and 5.5)

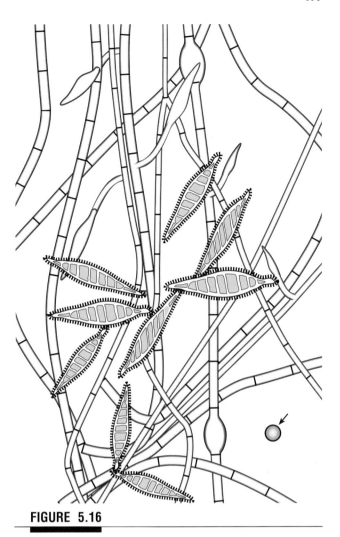

FIGURE 5.16

Even in bad preparations *Microsporum canis* is strongly suggested by the distinctive shape of the macroconidium with its thick echinulate outer walls, relatively thin septa, and asymmetrical "beaked" tip. Smooth-walled microconidia, and vegetative hyphal structures, may also be seen. Colony morphology—especially of young cultures—helps confirm the identity of this dermatophyte. The 7-μm red blood cell (arrow) shows the relative sizes of the mycotic elements.

Most dermatophytes, but especially *Microsporum audouinii*

Cutaneous Dermatophytes

MONILIACEAE

MICROSPORUM COOKEI (My-crow-spore-um cookie-eye)

■ **Teleomorph.** *Arthroderma (Nannizzia) cajetani.*

■ **Reservoirs.** This geophilic dermatophyte is found worldwide as a soil saprophyte. It has been isolated from asymptomatic animals but rarely from humans.

■ **Unique Risk Factors.** *M. cookei* is considered to be an infrequent pathogen. Colonization is believed to be related to contact with contaminated soil.

■ **Human Infection.** *M. cookei* has been isolated from rare cases of tinea corporis, scalp infections, and onychomycosis in humans. It does not invade hair *in vivo*, although it is positive in the *in vitro* hair perforation test. The fungus should be identified because (1) it can generally be ruled out as the cause of infection and (2) when symptoms are present the search for the etiologic agent of the tinea should be continued.

■ **Specimen Sources.** Nail and skin scrapings are most likely to be submitted for culture.

■ **Specimen Collection and Handling.** Nail and skin scrapings can be collected and submitted in the usual manner.

 Direct examination of skin scrapings should include treatment of the specimen with KOH, or a calcofluor white–KOH preparation may be done. Blue-black ink and/or DMSO can be added to the KOH. For the nail, 20% KOH should be used; 10% KOH is recommended for hair and skin.

■ **Immunology.** No tests are available.

■ **Special Precautions.** None are needed, but specimens should be handled within a biologic safety cabinet.

■ **Culture Media.** Modified SDA, modified SDA with antimicrobials. DTM may be used for screening. PDA or PFA should be inoculated when growth appears in the primary cultures.

 Preferred Temperature. Temperature of 25° to 30°C.

■ **Differential Tests.** The *in vitro* hair perforation test can be done. *M. cookei* is positive.

■ **Macroscopic (Colony) Morphology.** *M. cookei* grows moderately fast, producing colonies on modified SDA at 25°C after 6 to 7 days. They are at first white and downy; with age, colonies become powdery to coarsely granular and spreading. The surface pigment deepens to yellowish tan to dark tan, and a distinctive deep burgundy (purple-red) or wine-red color develops in the reverse of the colony.

■ **Microscopic Morphology** (Figs. 5.17 through 5.19). The hyphae of *M. cookei* are hyaline, septate, and branched. Many macroconidia are produced. They are large (approximately 14 × 60 μm), with an ellipsoid to fusiform shape; 6 to 10 cells are produced in each macroconidium. The walls are moderately thick (approximately 4 μm) and echinulate. Microconidia are also numerous.

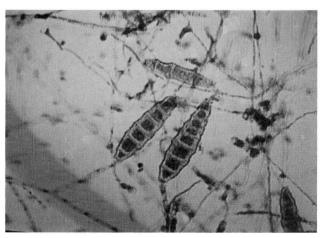

FIGURE 5.17

Typical microscopic morphology of *Microsporum cookei* includes hyaline septate hyphae, numerous microconidia, and large ellipsoid or fusiform macroconidia with rough, thick walls. The thickness of the macroconidium's walls means that they are often distorted in stained preparations, as these are, so that the wall seems to sink in between the septa of the macroconidium.

They are oval to pyriform, approximately 3 × 5 μm wide and are *sessile*, that is, produced directly on the hyphae without conidiophores or pedicles. Racquet hyphae are also found.

■ **Helpful Features for Identification of** *Microsporum cookei* (see Tables 5.4 and 5.5)

 Abundant thick-walled fusiform macroconidia
 Numerous oval or pyriform microconidia
 Colonies with powdery to granular texture, pale surface pigment, and wine-red reverse pigment
 Perforation of hair *in vitro*

■ **Organisms from Which** *Microsporum cookei* **Must Be Differentiated** (see Fig. 5.10 and Table 5.4)

 Most dermatophytes, but especially *Microsporum gypseum*

Cutaneous Dermatophytes

MONILIACEAE

MICROSPORUM GYPSEUM (My-crow-spore-um gip-see-um)

■ **Teleomorph.** *Arthroderma (Nannizzia) incurvulata* and *Arthroderma (Nannizzia) gypseum*.

■ **Reservoirs.** The dermatophyte is found worldwide in rich soil. It is a geophilic fungus.

FIGURE 5.18

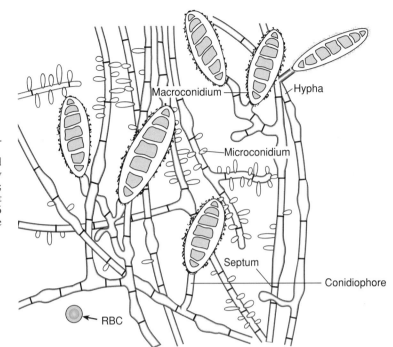

Microsporum cookei has septate hyphae of irregular width and numerous smooth-walled microconidia produced directly from the hyphae. The macroconidia have thick rough walls; the shape is more rounded and less spindle-like than most other species of *Microsporum*. Mature macroconidia contain 6 to 10 cells. The 7-μm red blood cell (RBC) (arrow) shows the relative sizes of the mycotic elements.

■ **Unique Risk Factors.** *M. gypseum* is not considered to be transmitted from person to person. Infection is usually believed to be contacted from contaminated soil.

■ **Human Infection.** *M. gypseum* often causes infections in animals. Tinea capitis and tinea corporis have been re-

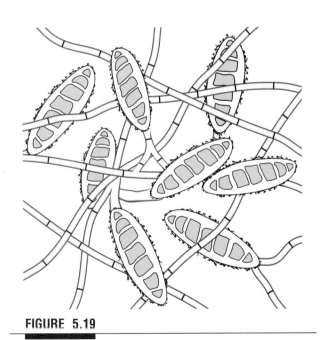

FIGURE 5.19

Even in bad preparations large numbers of ellipsoid or fusiform macroconidia with thick echinulate walls suggest *Microsporum cookei*. The identity is supported by the presence of 6 to 10 cells per macroconidium, septate hyphae, and many microconidia. The distinctive colony morphology further distinguishes *M. cookei* from other species of *Microsporum*.

ported sporadically in humans. Both children and adults have been infected, particularly those who garden and dig or play in the dirt. Solitary skin lesions are usually found on the extremities but can occur anywhere on the body. The lesions are raised and boggy (spongy) and are accompanied by inflammation. The infection usually develops and resolves rapidly. Hair invasion is the large arthroconidia-ectothrix type, but typically only a few chaining arthroconidia are seen. Nails are not often infected.

■ **Specimen Sources.** Skin scrapings or the stubs of hair remaining when the hair breaks off should be taken for culture. Infected hairs can rarely be identified by the dull yellow-green fluorescence emitted from the lesion when a Wood's lamp is used.

■ **Specimen Collection and Handling.** Hair should be plucked from the infected area and sent to the laboratory. Skin scrapings can be collected and submitted in the usual manner.

Direct examination of specimens should include treatment with 10% KOH plus blue-black ink, or a calcofluor white–KOH preparation should be done.

■ **Immunology.** No tests are available.

■ **Special Precautions.** None are needed, but cultures should be handled within a biologic safety cabinet.

■ **Culture Media.** Modified SDA, modified SDA with antimicrobials. DTM may be used for screening purposes. PDA or PFA should be inoculated as soon as growth appears in the primary cultures

Preferred Temperature. Temperature of 25° to 30°C.

■ **Differential Tests.** The *in vitro* hair test may be done. *M. gypseum* perforates hair *in vitro*.

■ **Macroscopic (Colony) Morphology.** The colony on modified SDA at 25°C after 5 to 6 days is at first white and downy. Later it becomes flat and granular as numerous macroconidia are produced. The colony may have fringed edges or be entire (unbroken). *M. gypseum* quickly develops white sterile hyphae[4] in the center of the colony. The surface pigment of the colony is tan to cinnamon-pink to brown. The reverse is tan to orange-brown or modified cinnamon-pink on PDA.

■ **Microscopic Morphology** (Figs. 5.20 through 5.22). Hyphae of *M. gypseum* are hyaline, septate, and branched. Macroconidia are produced abundantly, sometimes occurring in clusters. They are large (25 to 60 μm long × 8 to 15 μm wide, averaging 42 × 11 μm), and ellipsoid to cucumber shaped. They have moderately thick echinulate walls, 1 to 3 μm wide, and contain two to six cells. The macroconidia are borne by cells of the conidiophores that subsequently collapse, leaving a ragged annular fringe on the conidia that have broken away. The scar can usually be seen by a diligent microscopist using a standard microscope. Free macroconidia are rounded on the tip end and somewhat flattened at the base.[5]

---

[4]See Mycelia Sterilia, Chapter 2.

[5]McGinnis (1980, p. 82) says there is a tendency for the outer wall of the macroconidia to collapse slightly between the septa. This becomes more pronounced in preparations from old cultures.

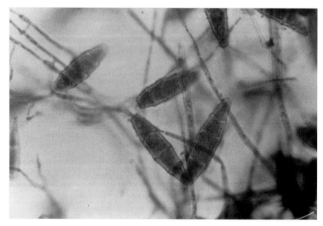

FIGURE 5.20

In typical preparations *Microsporum gypseum* has septate hyphae, clavate sessile microconidia, and large echinulate macroconidia with thick walls. The macroconidia are ellipsoid to fusiform and contain up to six cells. In this field the roughness of the walls is best seen on the tip of the macroconidium poking its nose into the field at the upper right. No microconidia are shown. (Courtesy of the Centers for Disease Control and Prevention.)

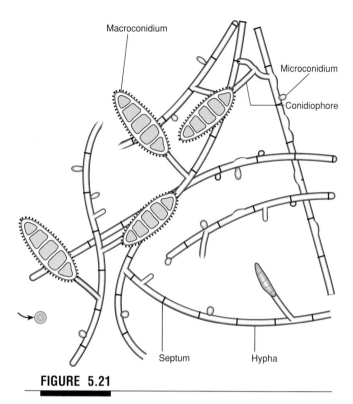

FIGURE 5.21

Microsporum gypseum produces septate hyphae. The club-shaped microconidia are sessile on the hyphae. Macroconidia are large and echinulate, with thick walls. The base of free macroconidia sometimes shows a ragged annular fringe, a remnant of the wall of the conidiophore. The 7-μm red blood cell (arrow) shows the relative sizes of the mycotic elements.

Thin filaments may extend from the apices of the macroconidia. Microconidia are usually fewer in number. They are clavate, 2 to 3 μm × 4 to 6 μm, and are sessile.

In *direct examination* of skin scrapings, *M. gypseum* is seen as hyaline, septate hyphae, and/or chains of barrel-shaped arthroconidia.

■ **Helpful Features for Identification of *Microsporum gypseum*** (see Tables 5.4 and 5.5)

Dull yellow-green fluorescence of infected hair[6]
Abundant fusiform macroconidia with thick echinulate walls
Ellipsoid or cucumber-shaped macroconidia
Annular fringes on macroconidia
Few (sessile) microconidia
Flat, granular, fringed colonies with a tan to brown obverse pigment and orange-brown to cinnamon-pink reverse
Perforation of hair *in vitro*

---

[6]Fluorescence is less common with *M. gypseum* than with other species of *Microsporum*, and it is less pronounced. Rippon says that some strains fluoresce only on actively growing hairs.

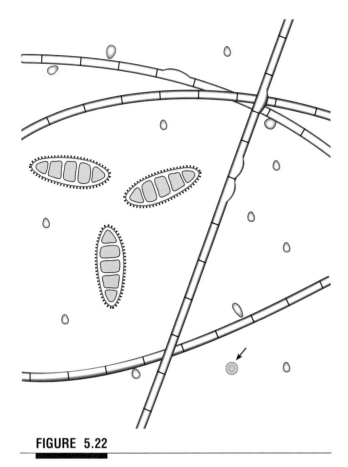

FIGURE 5.22

Even in a bad preparation large echinulate macroconidia indicate a *Microsporum* species. The ellipsoid shape, with two to six cells per macroconidium, suggests *Microsporum gypseum*. Annular fringes on the macroconidia, and the presence of microconidia, also point to *M. gypseum*. Colony morphology helps confirm the identification of the fungus. The 7-μm red blood cell (arrow) shows the relative sizes of the mycotic elements.

■ **Organisms from Which *Microsporum gypseum* Must Be Differentiated** (see Fig. 5.10 and Table 5.4)

Most dermatophytes, but especially *Microsporum canis*

Cutaneous Dermatophytes

MONILIACEAE

MICROSPORUM NANUM (My-crow-spore-um nan[7]-um)

■ **Teleomorph.** *Arthroderma (Nannizzia) obtusum.*

■ **Reservoirs.** *M. nanum* is geophilic and zoophilic. It has been found in the United States, Mexico, Cuba, Canada, and Australia as a soil saprophyte. It has also been recovered from the soil in pig lots.

[7]"Nan" as in banana.

■ **Unique Risk Factors.** *M. nanum* infections are believed to be most often contacted from contaminated soil or infected pigs.

■ **Human Infection.** *M. nanum* is primarily the agent of tinea in pigs. Rare cases of tinea corporis and tinea capitis have been reported in humans. Hair invasion by *M. nanum* is similar to that due to *Microsporum gypseum*. It follows the ectothrix pattern, with only a few arthroconidia found on the hair. *M. nanum* is important, in part, for teaching programs because it grows relatively rapidly and demonstrates most of the characteristic features of the genus *Microsporum*.

■ **Specimen Sources.** Hair stubs and skin scrapings should be submitted for culture.

■ **Specimen Collection and Handling.** Hair should be plucked from the infected area and sent to the laboratory. Skin scrapings can be collected and submitted in the usual manner.

Direct examination of skin scrapings should include treatment of the skin with 10% KOH plus blue-black ink and DMSO, or a calcofluor white–KOH preparation may be done.

■ **Immunology.** No tests are available.

■ **Special Precautions.** None are needed, but cultures should be handled within a biologic safety cabinet.

■ **Culture Media.** Modified SDA, modified SDA with antimicrobials. DTM may be used for screening. PDA or PFA should be inoculated when growth appears in the primary cultures.

Preferred Temperature. Temperature of 25° to 30°C.

■ **Differential Tests.** *M. nanum* perforates hair in the *in vitro* hair perforation test.

■ **Macroscopic (Colony) Morphology.** *M. nanum* grows moderately fast (7 days), producing colonies on modified SDA at 25°C that are at first white to yellow and downy. With age colonies become cream to deep tan with a reddish tint and a brownish red reverse. The texture becomes powdery. Colonies are flat, with a rugose and spreading topography. Colonies of *M. nanum* bear some resemblance to typical colonies of *M. gypseum*.

■ **Microscopic Morphology** (Figs. 5.23 through 5.25). The hyphae of *M. nanum* are hyaline, septate, and branched. Macroconidia are produced abundantly. They are smaller than those of *M. gypseum* (average 15 × 6 μm; range 12 to 18 μm long × 4 to 8 μm wide), and clavate to

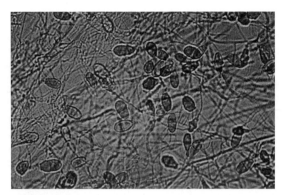

FIGURE 5.23

Typical slide preparations of *Microsporum nanum* show two-celled macroconidia with echinulate, relatively thin walls, and septate hyphae. Microconidia are often present. (From Rippon JW: Medical Mycology The Pathogenic Fungi and the Pathogenic Actinomycetes, 3rd ed. Philadelphia, WB Saunders, 1988, p 244.)

ellipsoidal in shape. The walls of the macroconidia are relatively thin but echinulate. Most macroconidia have two cells; rarely four cells are produced. The microconidia are smooth walled and clavate to pyriform, with diameters of 2 to 5 μm. They are born sessile on the hyphae.

■ **Helpful Features for Identification of *Microsporum nanum*** (see Tables 5.4 and 5.5)

Abundant clavate two-celled macroconidia with rough walls

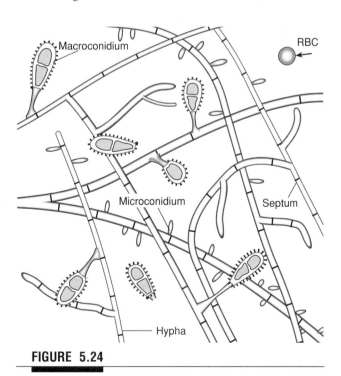

FIGURE 5.24

Microsporum nanum has septate hyphae and clavate microconidia sessile on the hyphae. The macroconidia are smaller than those of other *Microsporum* species, with relatively thin, relatively smooth walls. Most of the echinulate macroconidia contain two cells, a distinctive feature. The 7-μm red blood cell (RBC) (arrow) shows the relative sizes of the mycotic elements.

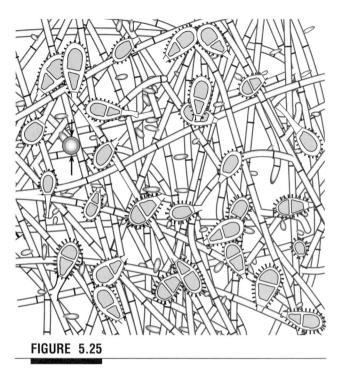

FIGURE 5.25

Even in bad preparations echinulate macroconidia indicate the fungus is a species of *Microsporum*. Relatively thin walls and the predominance of two-celled forms suggest *Microsporum nanum*. Colony morphology can help confirm the identity of the fungus. The 7-μm red blood cell (arrows) shows the relative sizes of the mycotic elements.

Colony morphology
Perforation of hair *in vitro*
Infected hair is not fluorescent

■ **Organisms from Which *Microsporum nanum* Must Be Differentiated** (see Fig. 5.10 and Table 5.4)

Most dermatophytes, but especially *M. gypseum*

Cutaneous Dermatophytes

MONILIACEAE

TRICHOPHYTON MENTAGROPHYTES (Trick-oh-phy'-tun or Try-koff'-uh-tun men-ta-grow-phy'-tees)

■ **Teleomorph.** *Arthroderma (Nannizzia) benhamiae* and *Arthroderma (Nannizzia) vanbreuseghemii*

■ **Reservoirs.** The organism is found throughout the world. According to Rippon, *T. mentagrophytes* is the most common agent of dermatophyte infections in humans and animals. It is both anthropophilic and zoophilic. Although it has also been found in soil contaminated with animal debris, it is not considered geophilic.

■ **Unique Risk Factors.** *T. mentagrophytes* is contagious. It can be transmitted between animals, from animals to humans, and from person to person.

■ **Human Infection.** This fungus can infect the stratum corneum layer of skin and the hair and nails in both children and adults. It has been associated with tinea manuum, tinea cruris, tinea corporis, tinea pedis, tinea capitis, tinea barbae, and tinea unguium (invading the nail plate). The zoophilic strain contacted from animals is called *T. mentagrophytes* var. *mentagrophytes*; it tends to cause more severe inflammatory reactions that are of relatively short duration. The anthropophilic agent, *T. mentagrophytes* var. *interdigitale*, causes a tinea that is less inflammatory but more chronic. As the name implies, the *interdigitale* variety is often associated with cases of tinea pedis.

■ **Specimen Sources.** Scrapings of the skin, scrapings from under the nail, and hairs that have been plucked should be obtained for culture.

■ **Specimen Collection and Handling.** Infected hairs—the intact hair, not clippings—nail scrapings and material from under the tips of the nails, and skin scrapings should be collected aseptically and transported to the laboratory in sterile dry containers.

Direct examination of specimens should include treatment of the material with KOH (blue-black ink and DMSO may be added), or a calcofluor white–KOH preparation may be done. Use 20% KOH for nails and 10% for hair and skin.

■ **Immunology.** No tests are available.

■ **Special Precautions.** None are needed, but cultures should be handled within a biologic safety cabinet.

■ **Culture Media.** Modified SDA, modified SDA with antimicrobials. DTM may be used for screening. Subculture to PDA and PFA slants, or to CMA with 1% dextrose, when growth appears in the primary cultures.

Preferred Temperature. Temperature of 25° to 30°C. Growth also occurs at 37°C.

■ **Differential Methods** (see Table 5.5). The *in vitro* hair test, *Trichophyton* nutritional media, and urease tests may be helpful in definitive identification of suspected *T. mentagrophytes*. It penetrates the hair *in vitro*. Growth is not enhanced by either thiamine or inositol. The urease test is positive in less than 4 days. Tests that are positive after 4 days are not significant; the delayed result does not indicate *T. mentagrophytes*.

■ **Macroscopic (Colony) Morphology.** *T. mentagrophytes* can develop two types of colonies. Either may appear on modified SDA after 6 to 8 days at 25° to 30°C. Type I colonies are formed by *T. mentagrophytes* var. *mentagrophytes*, the zoophilic agent. They are flat, granular, creamy yellow to tan or reddish brown with a buff, yellow-brown, or reddish brown reverse. The dark red pigment does not appear in cultures on PDA or CMA. Concentric rings of growth can sometimes be seen in the topography of the colony. The periphery of the colony is raylike. Type II colonies, seen with the anthropophilic form, *T. mentagrophytes* var. *interdigitale*, are flat and downy. The surface pigment is cream to light yellow with white feathery fringes that may become pink, and the reverse is light yellow to yellow-orange.

■ **Microscopic Morphology** (Figs. 5.26 through 5.28). The hyphae of both varieties of *T. mentagrophytes* are hyaline, septate, and branched. Macroconidia are more abundant in the zoophilic Type I colonies than in the anthropophilic Type II colonies, where they are sparse or absent. In both varieties the macroconidia average 6×35 μm (range 4 to 7 μm wide $\times$ 20 to 50 μm long). They are clavate to cigar shaped, with three to six cells per macroconidium; the walls are thin and smooth. Macroconidia are attached to the hyphae by narrow pedicles; a ragged edge remains on the conidium and the pedicle when the conidium breaks away from the attachment. A thin tail-like appendage may be present on the macroconidia, causing them to be called "rat tail" conidia.

As with the macroconidia, microconidia are usually abundant in Type I (var. *mentagrophytes*) colonies and sparse in Type II (var. *interdigitale*) colonies. The microconidia in Type I colonies are globose and unicellular. They are produced singly along the hyphae on short pedicles or *en grappe*. This arrangement, with the branching of the conidiophores at right angles, is characteristic of both varieties of *T. mentagrophytes*. As might be expected, the pattern is more prevalent in the variety with the most abundant microconidia, var. *mentagrophytes* (Type I). In Type II colonies the few microconidia that are seen are clavate or pyriform in shape, unlike the Type I microconidia, and are attached to the hyphae by pedicles. Arthroconidia are also seen in both varieties of *T. mentagrophytes*.

Other structures on the vegetative hyphae that may be found in both types of *T. mentagrophytes* colonies (see Fig. 5.5) are chlamydoconidia, hyphae that resemble reindeer antlers ("favic chandeliers") (Fig. 5.29), well-developed spiral hyphae in clusters, and racquet hyphae. Nodular bodies are frequently found in Type II colonies.

In *direct examination* of skin and nail scrapings *T. mentagrophytes*, like other dermatophytes, is seen as hyaline, septate hyphae. Arthroconidia are often seen in specimens of skin. Hair is infected in the ectothrix type of invasion with a sheath of small (2 to 3 μm) conidia surrounding the hair shaft. Some arthroconidia are also found within the hair shaft.

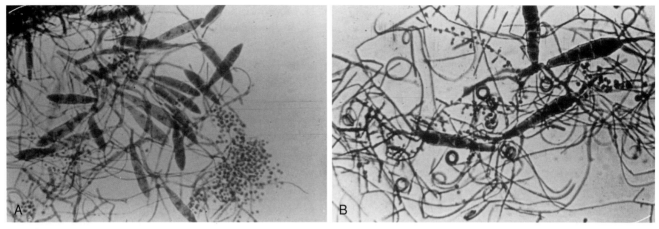

FIGURE 5.26

Characteristic lactophenol–cotton blue preps of *Trichophyton mentagrophytes* contain septate hyphae and bizarre vegetative hyphal structures. The shape and arrangement of the microconidia vary with the Type of *T. mentagrophytes*, but the macroconidia are the same for Types I and II: clavate to cigar shaped with thin, smooth walls and three to six cells per macroconidium. In Type I *(A)* the microconidia are *en grappe*, that is, in clusters resembling grapes. In Type II *(B)* microconidia are arranged *en thryses*, that is, singly in sleeves along the hyphae. Spiral hyphae are present in the center and the lower left quadrant of this field. *(A and B courtesy of the Centers for Disease Control and Prevention.)*

■ **Helpful Features for Identification of *Trichophyton mentagrophytes*** (Fig. 5.30 and Table 5.6; see also Table 5.5)

Lack of dark red pigment on PDA or CMA with 1% dextrose

Penetration of the hair in the *in vitro* test
Positive urease after less than 4 days of incubation
No effect of special nutrients on growth
Ectothrix invasion of the hair
Cigar-shaped macroconidia with thin, smooth walls
Typical shapes and *en grappe* arrangements of microconidia

■ **Organisms from Which *Trichophyton mentagrophytes* Must Be Differentiated** (see Table 5.6)

Other species of *Trichophyton*, especially *Trichophyton rubrum*.

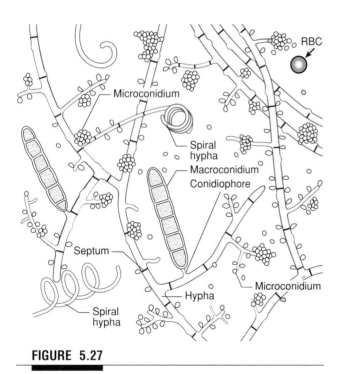

FIGURE 5.27

Trichophyton mentagrophytes, Types I and II, produce large cigar-shaped or clavate macroconidia with thin, smooth walls and three to six cells per macroconidium. Microconidia and vegetative hyphal structures are often present as well. The *en thryses* and *en grappe* arrangements of microconidia are shown, but typically an isolate of *T. mentagrophytes* produces microconidia in one pattern or the other, but not both. Hyphae are hyaline and septate. The 7-μm red blood cell (RBC) (arrow) shows the relative sizes of the mycotic elements.

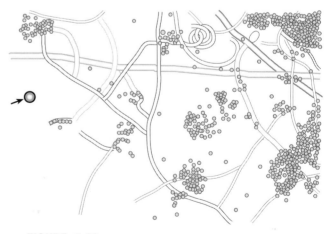

FIGURE 5.28

In bad preparations, even at ×10 magnification, thin septate hyphae with bizarre vegetative structures and many microconidia suggest some species of *Trichophyton*, but biochemical tests and colony morphology are generally necessary to confirm the identification. The 7-μm red blood cell (arrow) shows the relative sizes of the mycotic elements.

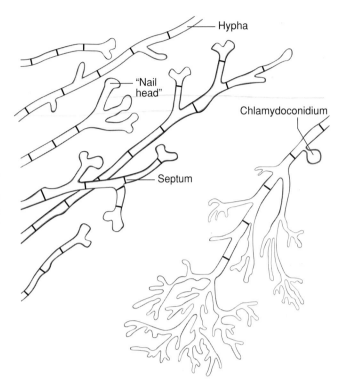

FIGURE 5.29

Favic chandeliers are configurations of the vegetative hyphae that resemble reindeer antlers. "Nail heads," which are blunt, rounded tips to the hyphae, may also be present. Favic chandeliers suggest *Trichophyton mentagrophytes*, *Trichophyton schoenleinii*, or *Trichophyton verrucosum*.

Cutaneous Dermatophytes

MONILIACEAE

TRICHOPHYTON RUBRUM (Trick-oh-phy'-tun or Try-koff'-uh-tun rube'-rum)

- **Teleomorph.** None has been identified.

- **Reservoirs.** The organism is found throughout the world. It is anthropophilic and, rarely, zoophilic. According to Kwon-Chung and Bennett, *T. rubrum* is the most frequent agent of dermatophyte infections in humans.

- **Unique Risk Factors.** *T. rubrum* is contagious. It can be transmitted by contact with the lesions of infected people.

- **Human Infection.** This fungus can infect the hair and skin of both children and adults, but the nail is not invaded. The most frequent infections due to *T. rubrum* are tinea corporis, tinea cruris, tinea pedis, and tinea manuum. Tinea capitis is rarely caused by this organism. Ectothrix infections, with a mosaic sheath of conidia around the hair shaft, are characteristic when tinea capitis does occur; endothrix infections have also been reported. Zoophilic strains contacted from animals tend to cause more severe inflammatory reactions than do the more chronic anthropophilic strains.

- **Specimen Sources.** Scrapings of the skin and hair stubs that have been plucked should be used for culture.

- **Specimen Collection and Handling.** Intact hairs and skin scrapings should be collected aseptically and transported to the laboratory in a sterile dry container.
  Direct examination of specimens should include treatment of the material with KOH (blue-black ink may be added), or a calcofluor white–KOH preparation may be done. Skin scrapings and hair require 10% KOH (without DMSO).

- **Immunology.** No tests are available.

- **Special Precautions.** None are needed but cultures should be handled within a biologic safety cabinet.

- **Culture Media.** Modified SDA, modified SDA with antimicrobials. DTM may be used for screening. PDA or PFA should be inoculated as soon as growth appears in primary cultures. CMA should be inoculated when *T. rubrum* is suspected to enhance the production of conidia and for pigmentation studies.

Preferred Temperature. Temperature of 25° to 30°C.

- **Differential Tests** (see Table 5.5). The fungus can be tested for its ability to perforate hair in the *in vitro* test (it cannot) and for urease production (negative after 5 to 7

Red Pigment

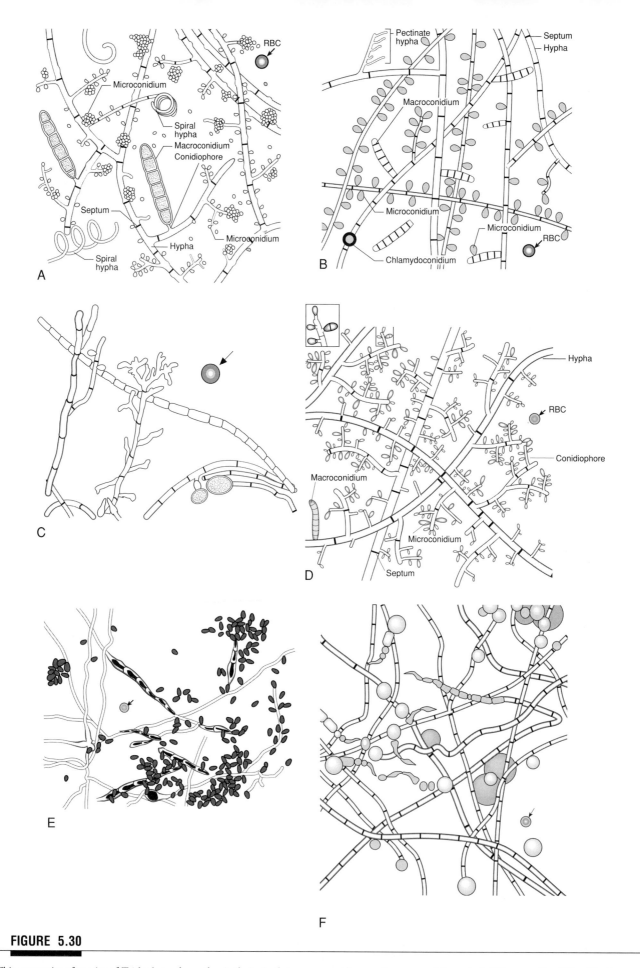

FIGURE 5.30

This composite of species of *Trichophyton* shows the similarity in their macroconidia as well as some of the typical differences. Final identification usually rests on the results of biochemical tests. The species depicted here are *Trichophyton mentagrophytes (A)*, *Trichophyton rubrum (B)*, *Trichophyton schoenleinii (C)*, *Trichophyton tonsurans (D)*, *Trichophyton verrucosum (E)*, and *Trichophyton violaceum (F)*.

TABLE 5.6 _Trichophyton_ Species

Fungus	Size of Macroconidia (μm)	Shape of Macroconidia	Number of Cells per Macroconidium	Arrangement of Macroconidia	Size of Microconidia (μm)	Shape of Microconidia	Arrangement of Microconidia	Width of Hyphae (μm)	Colony Morphology (SDA)	Growth Rate	Other Helpful Features
Trichophyton mentagrophytes	6 × 35	Clavate to cigar shaped with thin, smooth walls	3–6	Solitary	3 × 5	Varies with type	_En grappe_ or singly	3–5	Flat and granular or downy, with varying pigments	Intermediate	"Rat-tail" conidia may form. Red pigment may develop in colonies on SDA. More conidia in Type I colonies than in Type II colonies
Trichophyton rubrum	5 × 22	Narrow cylinders with thin, smooth parallel walls	3–8	Single or in small groups, directly on hyphae	2 × 4	Thin clavate or tear-drop shapes	_En thryses_ or in small clusters	3–5	Most common form is white and downy with yellow to blood-red reverse pigment	Slow	Two colony types; conidia are most abundant in Type II colonies. Microconidia may form directly on macroconidia
Trichophyton schoenleinii	NA	NA—Rarely seen	NA	NA	Varying sizes	Clavate	Sessile and solitary	3–5	Glabrous; white to tan; heaped to folded	Slow	Lesions have "mousy" odor. Microconidia produced on rice grain medium. Arthroconidia in young cultures
Trichophyton tonsurans	4 × 25	Short, blunt, irregular clubs with moderately thick, smooth walls	3–8	Solitary	3 × 5	Truncate, of varying shapes; typically numerous	Singly along hyphae or in clusters on conidiophores	3–5	Most common type is flat and powdery with yellow obverse and yellow-brown to reddish brown reverse pigment	Intermediate to slow	"Ballooning" microconidia. Reverse pigment usually diffuses into medium
Trichophyton verrucosum	>35	Slender elongate and irregular with thin, smooth walls	3–5	Solitary	Large	Clavate or ovoid to pyriform; sessile	Solitary	3–5; distorted	Most common form is thin and white, 1–3 mm wide, with glabrous texture and colorless or salmon reverse	Slow	Colonies submerged in medium. Conidiation sparse even on enriched media. "Rat-tail" macroconidia
Trichophyton violaceum	???	Elongate, with thin, smooth walls	2–5	Solitary	Small	Clavate	Solitary	3–5; distorted	Lavender or purple with verrucose surface and waxy texture	Slow	Swollen hyphal cells containing cytoplasmic granules. Sparse conidiation even on enriched media

The genus _Trichophyton_ can usually be identified by examination of the microscopic structures of the organism, but further testing is often needed to determine the species of the isolate.
NA, not applicable; SDA, Sabouraud's dextrose agar.

days). Neither thiamine nor inositol enhances growth, but the fungus does produce brown pigment on sterile rice grains.

■ **Macroscopic (Colony) Morphology.** *T. rubrum* develop two types of colonies; only the first type is common. Typical Type I colonies appear on modified SDA after 10 to 14 days at 25° to 30°C as white downy to fluffy colonies. The reverse is yellow to blood-red. Type I colonies are usually isolated from tinea pedis. In Type II colonies the surface pigment becomes tan, yellow, or tinged with red, and the texture is granular due to the production of macroconidia. The colony may develop rugose folds. The reverse pigment may be colorless, tan, or yellow to brown; eventually a deep wine-red color appears. Type II colonies of *T. rubrum* are usually isolated from inflammatory tinea corporis and tinea capitis.

On PDA or CMA with 1% to 2% dextrose *T. rubrum* produces colonies after 1 to 2 weeks of incubation that have a velvety texture and a white obverse pigment tinged with pink or red at the periphery. The reverse of the colony may be yellow at first but eventually develops the deep wine-red to purple-red color that is responsible for the species name *rubrum*.

■ **Microscopic Morphology** (Figs. 5.31 through 5.33). The hyphae of *T. rubrum* are hyaline, septate, and branched. Macroconidia are sparse or absent in Type I colonies but are produced abundantly in Type II. The macroconidia are large (4 to 6 μm wide × 15 to 30 μm long, averaging 5 × 22 μm), narrow, and cylindrical, with blunt distal ends and thin, smooth parallel walls. The shape is sometimes compared to pencils or cigars. Each macroconidium contains three to eight cells. They are borne directly on the hyphae with broad bases of attach-

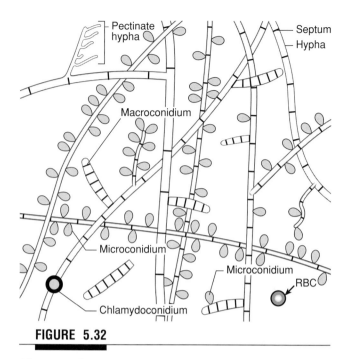

FIGURE 5.32

All variants of *Trichophyton rubrum* have septate hyphae, clavate or tear-drop–shaped microconidia, and pencil-shaped macroconidia with thin, smooth walls. The abundance of conidia varies with the colony type. Macroconidia typically have three to eight cells and broad bases of attachment directly to the hyphae. Microconidia typically develop from the hyphae, but they can form directly on a macroconidium. The 7-μm red blood cell (RBC) (arrow) shows the relative sizes of the mycotic elements.

ment, developing singly or in small groups. The hyphae and macroconidia may fragment into arthroconidia.

As with the macroconidia, microconidia are usually sparse in Type I colonies and more numerous in Type II colonies. The microconidia in both colony types are thin

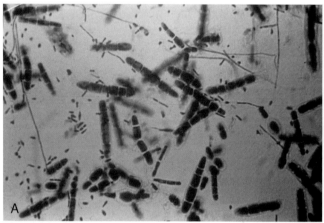
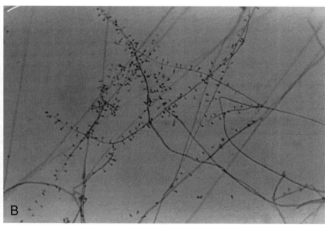

FIGURE 5.31

Characteristically *Trichophyton rubrum* has thin septate hyphae, and bizarre hyphal structures may be seen. *A*, The macroconidia are narrow and pencil shaped, with thin, smooth parallel walls, and are borne directly on the hyphae. In this field the macroconidia are free rather than attached. Both macroconidia and microconidia are produced in large numbers by the granular (Type II) variety of *T. rubrum*. Microconidia are clavate or tear-drop shaped, *en thryses*, or in small clusters. *B*, More commonly *T. rubrum* produces many of the clavate microconidia *en thryses* and few (if any) macroconidia in the downy (Type I) variety. (*A* and *B* courtesy of the Centers for Disease Control and Prevention.)

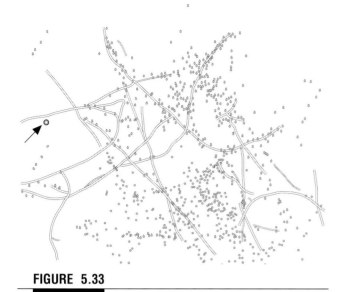

FIGURE 5.33

Even in a bad preparation with the low-power (×10) objective, the presence of microconidia and of macroconidia with thin, smooth walls indicates *Trichophyton* species. Without macroconidia the many clavate microconidia and thin septate hyphae suggest *Trichophyton*, but the exact species cannot be determined. Colony morphology can be helpful in confirming the identity of the dermatophyte. Biochemical tests may be required. The 7-μm red blood cell (arrow) shows the relative sizes of the mycotic elements.

clavate or "tear-drop" forms, approximately 2 × 4 μm. They are borne *en thryses* or in small clusters. *Microconidia may also form directly on the macroconidia.* On PDA or CMA both macroconidia and microconidia are well developed and pigment production is enhanced. Chlamydoconidia, nodular bodies, pectinate hyphae, and racquet hyphae may also be found in colonies of *T. rubrum*.

In *direct examination* of skin and nail scrapings, *T. rubrum* is seen as hyaline, septate hyphae. Chaining chlamydoconidia may be seen, especially in specimens from deeper areas of the skin or nail. Infected hair is surrounded by large arthroconidia.

■ **Helpful Features for Identification of *Trichophyton rubrum*** (see Fig. 5.30 and Tables 5.5 and 5.6)

    Characteristic red pigment that is enhanced by CMA
        or PDA
    Increased conidia production on PDA or CMA
    Failure to perforate hair in the *in vitro* test
    Negative urease after 5 to 7 days of incubation
    No effect of special nutrients on growth

■ **Organisms from Which *Trichophyton rubrum* Must Be Differentiated** (see Table 5.6)

    Other species of *Trichophyton*, especially *Trichophyton mentagrophytes*
    Microsporum cookei colonies

Cutaneous Dermatophytes

MONILIACEAE

TRICHOPHYTON SCHOENLEINII (Trick-oh-phy'-tun or Try-koff'-uh-tun show-en-leen-ee or shane-line-eye)

■ **Teleomorph.** None has been identified.

■ **Reservoirs.** *T. schoenleinii* is found throughout the world but is considered endemic in the European, African, and Asian countries around the Mediterranean Sea. It is also found in several South American countries and occasionally in the Appalachian region of the United States. This fungus is anthropophilic.

■ **Unique Risk Factors.** *T. schoenleinii* is contagious. Transmission is generally directly from person to person. Infection may also be acquired by contact with fomites such as infected hair, hair clippers and combs, hats, linens, towels, and upholstery. The infection is carried in families from generation to generation by people with low-grade infections.

■ **Human Infection.** *T. schoenleinii* is the etiologic agent of tinea favosa or favus, an infection of the scalp characterized by formation of scutulae. Lesions have a mouselike odor. Unless the lesion is treated promptly permanent alopecia may result. Hair is invaded in an endothrix pattern, but fragments of degenerated hyphae, oil droplets, and air rather than conidia fill the hair shaft.

T. schoenleinii also causes tinea corporis, tinea barbae, and tinea unguium. Infections with *T. schoenleinii* usually require prolonged treatment; spontaneous cure rarely occurs. Both children and adults are infected.

■ **Usual Specimen Sources.** Skin and nail scrapings, and stubs of hair from beneath the surface of the scalp.

■ **Specimen Collection and Handling.** Stubs of infected hair, nail scrapings and material from under the tip of the nail, and skin scrapings should be collected aseptically and transported to the laboratory in a sterile dry container. Infected hairs fluoresce a dull green. NOTE that colonies of *T. schoenleinii* and *Trichophyton tonsurans* fluoresce a dull green, but tissues do not fluoresce; tissues infected by some species of *Microsporum* fluoresce a bright green.

Direct examination of specimens should include treatment of the material with KOH (blue-black ink may be added), or a calcofluor white–KOH preparation may be done. DMSO should *not* be used for thin skin scrapings or hair.

■ **Immunology.** No tests are available.

■ **Special Precautions.** None are needed, but cultures should be handled within a biologic safety cabinet.

■ **Culture Media.** Modified SDA, modified SDA with antimicrobials. DTM may be used for screening. Boiled rice grain medium should be inoculated when growth occurs in the primary cultures to enhance production of microconidia.

Preferred Temperature. Temperature of 25° to 37°C.

■ **Differential Tests** (see Table 5.5). The organism is negative in the *in vitro* hair perforation test. Growth is not enhanced by adding thiamine and/or inositol to the medium. Urease production is slow (>11 days).

■ **Macroscopic (Colony) Morphology.** Colonies of *T. schoenleinii* appear after 2 to 3 weeks' incubation on modified SDA at 25° to 30°C. The colonies are small and white to tan with a glabrous texture and heaped or folded topography. After transfer, and with prolonged incubation, colonies may become velvety. The reverse pigment may be colorless or light yellow. Colonies of *T. schoenleinii* are often submerged into the surrounding agar. With age they become brittle and may crack or split the medium. A characteristic mousy odor typically develops in the culture.

■ **Microscopic Morphology** (Figs. 5.34 and 5.35). Hyphae of *T. schoenleinii* are hyaline, septate, branched, and sterile. The characteristic microscopic features are the branched hyphae called "favic chandeliers." The tips of the hyphal branches are swollen to resemble nail heads, that is, the heads of nails such as carpenters use. Spherical arthroconidia can be observed in young cultures of *T. schoenleinii*.

Neither macroconidia nor microconidia are produced on routine culture media, although production of

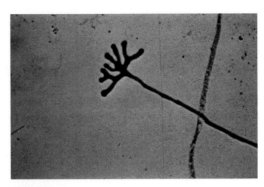

FIGURE 5.34

Typical preparations of *Trichophyton schoenleinii* are unremarkable. The hyphae are septate and sterile. This favic chandelier is characteristic of *T. schoenleinii* but is found in other species. Conidia generally are not produced on standard media. The dark color is due to the stain. (From Rippon JW: Medical mycology: The pathogenic fungi and the pathogenic actinomycetes. *In* Freeman M: Textbook of Microbiology, 22nd ed. Philadelphia, WB Saunders, 1985, p 901.)

microconidia can be enhanced by growth of the culture on rice grain medium. The microconidia are sessile along the hyphae; they are unicellular and clavate and vary greatly in size.

In *direct examination* of skin and nail scrapings *T. schoenleinii* appears as swollen fragments of septate, hyaline hyphae. The favic-type invasion of hair is characterized by development of filaments of fungi in the hair that degenerate to leave tunnels containing air and oil droplets. If KOH is added to the infected hairs, bubbles form when the air in the hair shafts mixes with the KOH.

■ **Helpful Features for Identification of *Trichophyton schoenleinii*** (see Fig. 5.30 and Tables 5.5 and 5.6)

Favus-type endothrix invasion of hair
Very slow growth rate that is not improved by adding thiamine or inositol

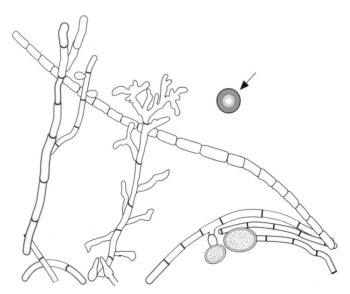

FIGURE 5.35

Trichophyton schoenleinii has hyaline septate hyphae but neither macroconidia nor microconidia in routine cultures. Chlamydoconidia, favic chandeliers, and "nail head" hyphae are present. Characteristics of the colony and nutritional testing are required to confirm the identity of the isolate. The 7-μm red blood cell (arrow) shows the relative sizes of the mycotic elements.

Variation in size of microconidia grown on rice grains
Negative *in vitro* hair perforation test
Nail heads/favic chandeliers/antler hyphae and numerous chlamydoconidia, in vegetative hyphae

■ **Organisms from Which** *Trichophyton schoenleinii* **Must Be Differentiated** (see Table 5.6)

Most dermatophytes, especially *Trichophyton tonsurans*, *Trichophyton violaceum*, and *Trichophyton verrucosum*

Cutaneous Dermatophytes

MONILIACEAE

TRICHOPHYTON TONSURANS (Trick-oh-phy'-tun or Try-koff'-uh-tun tohn-sir-anns)

■ **Teleomorph.** None has been identified.

■ **Reservoirs.** *T. tonsurans* is found throughout the world but is considered endemic to the United States, Canada, Mexico, the Caribbean area, and northern South America. This fungus is anthropophilic.

■ **Unique Risk Factors.** *T. tonsurans* is highly contagious, although most transmission is indirect rather than from person to person. It is believed to be acquired by contact with fomites such as infected hair, hair clippers and combs, hats, linens, towels, and upholstery.

■ **Human Infection.** Epidemic black-dot tinea capitis is caused by *T. tonsurans*; it is the leading cause of this infection in the United States and Canada. Children are the primary target population, but adults—especially those caring for the infected children—may also be infected. The tinea capitis caused by *T. tonsurans* may only involve scattered hairs. Little inflammation or itching occurs, a pattern to be expected from an anthropophilic organism. Rippon says that infections with these mild symptoms are especially prevalent in ethnic groups where black-dot tinea capitis is endemic. Black-dot tinea capitis is more likely to become chronic than is the gray-patch ectothrix type, and it may continue into adulthood. Because the lesions do not fluoresce, a population cannot easily be screened to detect subclinical infection.

Hair is invaded in an endothrix pattern and the infected hairs break off next to the scalp. Alopecia and kerions may develop. The alopecia is rarely permanent except in African American children.

T. tonsurans also occasionally causes tinea corporis, tinea unguium, and tinea pedis in children and adults. Skin lesions are red and scaly but usually are not inflam-matory. Infections with *T. tonsurans* usually require prolonged treatment; spontaneous cure at puberty is rare.

■ **Usual Specimen Sources.** Skin and nail scrapings and stubs of hair from beneath the surface of the scalp.

■ **Specimen Collection and Handling.** Stubs of intact hairs, nail scrapings and material from under the tip of the nail, and skin scrapings should be collected aseptically and transported to the laboratory in a sterile dry container.

Direct examination of specimens should include treatment of the material with 10% to 20% KOH (depending on the kind of specimen). Blue-black ink and DMSO may be added, or a calcofluor white–KOH preparation may be done. DMSO should *not* be used with hair or thin skin scrapings.

■ **Immunology.** No tests are available.

■ **Special Precautions.** None are needed, but cultures should be handled within a biologic safety cabinet.

■ **Culture Media.** Modified SDA, modified SDA with antimicrobials. DTM may be used for screening specimens. Growth from the primary culture should be transferred to PDA or polished rice grains to enhance conidiation.

Preferred Temperature. Temperature of 25° to 30°C.

■ **Differential Tests** (see Table 5.5). The urease test, the *in vitro* hair perforation test, and nutritional testing should be done.

T. tonsurans produces urease and penetrates hair. Its growth is enhanced by the addition of thiamine; growth of some strains is also enhanced by inositol.

■ **Macroscopic (Colony) Morphology.** *T. tonsurans* can develop several types of colonies with a variety of colors and surface textures. Any of them may appear on modified SDA after 7 to 14 days at 25° to 30°C. The colony type isolated most commonly in the United States is flat and off-white to yellow initially with a powdery texture. As the colony develops radial grooves may appear, followed by folds and, eventually, a crateriform or cerebriform topography. The texture becomes dense and velvety, while the color changes to sulfur yellow. The reverse on SDA is yellow-brown to reddish brown; the reverse pigment usually diffuses into the surrounding medium.

■ **Microscopic Morphology** (Figs. 5.36 and 5.37). The hyphae of *T. tonsurans* are hyaline, septate, and branched and often have terminal swellings. Macroconidia are rarely produced in culture on routine media. When they appear they are short and blunt, with an irregularly

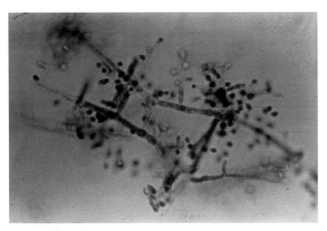

FIGURE 5.36

Standard preparations of *Trichophyton tonsurans* contain septate hyphae that may have terminal swellings. Macroconidia are rare; they resemble the macroconidia of *Trichophyton rubrum*. Numerous microconidia in varied sizes and shapes predominate. The *en thyses* arrangement of microconidia is shown at 12 o'clock as pale ovals in the "sleeve" arrangement. Many of the microconidia in this field are free in the preparation. (Courtesy of the Centers for Disease Control and Prevention.)

clavate or cylindrical shape. The walls of the macroconidia are moderately thick; each macroconidium contains three to eight cells.

Microconidia are numerous. The pronounced variety of sizes and shapes of the microconidia is characteristic of *T. tonsurans*. They are predominantly unicellular, but microconidia with septa may be seen. The usual microconidium is *truncate* ("cut off"; square at the tip) but they may be clavate, elongate, or pyriform. The size

ranges from 2 to 5 μm × 3 to 7 μm. Swelling of microconidia into balloons is characteristic of *T. tonsurans*. Microconidia may be borne directly on the sides of the hyphae (which may be slightly swollen at this point), or they may develop in clusters on conidiophores of varying lengths. When the conidiophores are long, the combination of single conidium and conidiophore resembles a match stick. Conidiophores may branch at right angles to the vegetative hyphae.

Terminal and intercalary chlamydoconidia can be observed throughout cultures of *T. tonsurans*. Occasionally racquet hyphae, large arthroconidia, and spiral hyphae are also seen.

In *direct examination* of skin and nail scrapings, *T. tonsurans* is seen as hyaline, septate hyphae. Large (4 to 7 μm) barrel-shaped arthroconidia may be seen in chains in infected hair. Barrel-shaped arthroconidia are also seen in skin and nail scrapings.

■ **Helpful Features for Identification of *Trichophyton tonsurans*** (see Fig. 5.30 and Tables 5.5 and 5.6)

Noninflammatory black-dot pattern of infection
Slow growth rate
Variation in size and shape of microconidia
Rare irregularly shaped macroconidia and abundant irregularly shaped microconidia (with balloons)
Lack of fluorescence of infected hair
Lack of pigment on CMA or PDA
Ability to penetrate hair in the *in vitro* test
Positive urease after 4 days of incubation
Thiamine and inositol enhance growth and conidiation of some strains

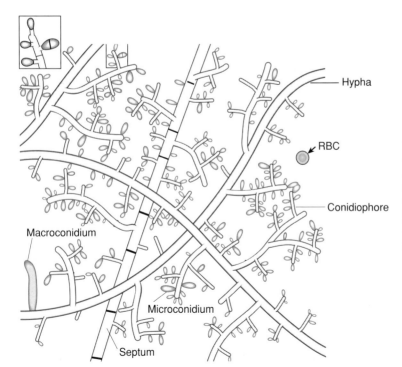

FIGURE 5.37

Trichophyton tonsurans has septate hyphae and numerous microconidia that vary in size and shape; two-celled microconidia are occasionally produced. The rare macroconidia are cylindrical or irregularly clavate, with broad bases of attachment to the hyphae; the tips of the macroconidia may be lopsided. Vegetative hyphal structures may also be present. The 7-μm red blood cell (RBC) (arrow) shows the relative sizes of the mycotic elements.

■ Organisms from Which _Trichophyton tonsurans_ Must Be Differentiated (see Table 5.6)

Most dermatophytes, especially _Trichophyton mentagrophytes_ and _Microsporum audouinii_

Cutaneous Dermatophytes

MONILIACEAE

TRICHOPHYTON VERRUCOSUM (Trick-oh-phy'-tun or Try-koff'-uh-tun verr-uh-kose[8]-um)

■ Teleomorph. None has been identified.

■ Reservoirs. This fungus is found throughout the world as a common cause of ringworm in cattle. It is zoophilic.

■ Unique Risk Factors. _T. verrucosum_ is contagious and can be transmitted by contact with infected cattle or by fomites such as fences or milking machines.

■ Human Infection. Most often infections with _T. verrucosum_ result from direct contact with infected cattle by farmers, dairymen, or ranchers. However, both children and adults have been infected. _T. verrucosum_ causes highly inflammatory infections in humans. Tinea corporis lesions typically are suppurative (producing pus) and involve the deep layers of the skin and the hair follicles. In tinea capitis the hair is infected by an ectothrix type of invasion. The scalp is involved and kerions are often formed. In tinea barbae the hairs of the beard are involved; the skin of the face and neck may also be infected. Tinea manuum infections are predominantly on the back of the hand and the wrist.

■ Specimen Sources. Skin scrapings, stubs of hairs, and exudate from lesions.

■ Specimen Collection and Handling. Intact hair stubs and skin scrapings should be collected aseptically and transported to the laboratory in a sterile dry container. Exudate from lesions can be aspirated and placed in sterile tubes for transport to the laboratory. Refrigeration kills this fungus.

Hair of infected cattle may fluoresce, but infected human tissue and hair do not fluoresce. Like _Trichophyton schoenleinii_, _T. verrucosum_ sometimes produces colonies with a dull green fluorescence under a Wood's lamp.

Direct examination of specimens should include treatment of the material with 10% to 20% KOH. Blue-black

ink and DMSO may be added, or a calcofluor white–KOH preparation may be done. DMSO is _not_ recommended for examination of hair or thin skin scrapings.

■ Immunology. No tests are available.

■ Special Precautions. None are needed, but cultures should be handled within a biologic safety cabinet.

■ Culture Media. _T. verrucosum_ has an absolute requirement for thiamine; many strains also require inositol in the culture medium. When _T. verrucosum_ is suspected, these vitamins (or yeast extract) can be added to brain-heart infusion medium or to modified SDA with antimicrobials. Alternatively, tubes of _Trichophyton_ test medium (#1 to #4) can be inoculated. Cultures should be incubated at 37°C for optimum recovery of the organism in culture. DTM with thiamine may be used for screening purposes, in addition to standard isolation media.

Preferred Temperature. Growth is best at 37°C, although _T. verrucosum_ grows at 25° to 30°C.

■ Differential Tests (see Table 5.5). Nutritional testing is important. _T. verrucosum_ does not grow without thiamine; growth of some strains is also enhanced by inositol. Hair is not penetrated in the _in vitro_ test.

■ Macroscopic (Colony) Morphology. _T. verrucosum_ grows poorly at 25° to 30°C. On modified SDA supplemented with thiamine and inositol 3 to 4 weeks of incubation may be needed before colonies appear. The initial colony of the variety _albeum_ is thin, white, and 1 to 3 mm in diameter. The center is knobby or heaped up and slightly folded, with a glabrous texture. Colonies of other varieties become velvety, with short aerial mycelia; they are white, gray, or yellow. The reverse of the colonies is usually colorless or salmon colored. Typical colonies are deeply submerged in the medium.

■ Microscopic Morphology (Figs. 5.38 and 5.39). Hyphae of _T. verrucosum_ are hyaline, septate, and distorted. Characteristic chains of intercalary chlamydoconidia and favic chandeliers may be present. Macroconidia do not appear on routine SDA without added vitamins.

Even on media that have been enriched with thiamine and inositol, macroconidia are not numerous. They have three to five cells and are elongated, slender, and irregularly shaped, with thin, smooth walls. Macroconidia taper at the distal end so that they have been called rat-tail conidia. Many sessile microconidia are produced; they are large and clavate or ovoid to pyriform. Many chlamydoconidia are produced at 37°C.

In _direct examination_ hyaline, septate hyphal fragments, and/or chaining chlamydoconidia, are characteristic of _T. verrucosum_ in exudate from lesions and in skin.

---

[8]"Kose" rhymes with close.

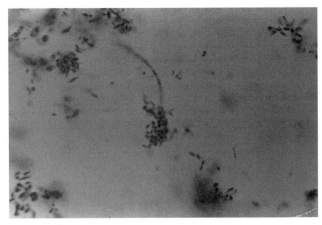

FIGURE 5.38

Growth of *Trichophyton verrucosum* is usually sparse, especially on standard media. The hyphae of *Trichophyton verrucosum* are septate and typically are distorted. Favic chandeliers and chains of intercalary chlamydoconidia may be present, but conidia are not produced in routine cultures.

A mosaic of large arthroconidia (5 to 10 μm in diameter) is seen around infected hair shafts.

- **Helpful Features for Identification of *Trichophyton verrucosum*** (see Fig. 5.30 and Tables 5.5 and 5.6)

  Fluorescence in infected hair from cattle (infected human hair does not fluoresce)
  Distinctive pattern of growth at 25° to 30°C and 37°C

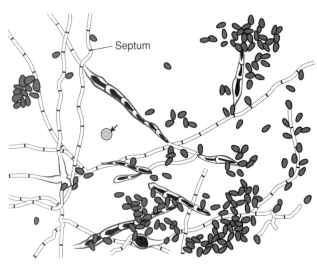

FIGURE 5.39

Trichophyton verrucosum is characterized by the absence of conidia in routine cultures, although chlamydoconidia and favic chandeliers form on the vegetative hyphae at 37°C. On enriched media the microconidia are sessile and large, with varied shapes. The rare macroconidium is an irregular cylinder with thin smooth walls. The tapering distal end of the macroconidium has led to its description as "rat-tailed." The 7-μm red blood cell (arrow) shows the relative sizes of the mycotic elements.

Different growth patterns on media with and without inositol
Increased conidiation on supplemented media

- **Organisms from Which *Trichophyton verrucosum* Must Be Differentiated** (see Table 5.6)

  Other species of *Trichophyton*, especially *Trichophyton tonsurans* and *Trichophyton schoenleinii*

Cutaneous Dermatophytes

MONILIACEAE

TRICHOPHYTON VIOLACEUM (Trick-oh-phy'-tun or Try-koff'-uh-tun vi-oh-lay'-see-um)

- **Teleomorph.** None has been identified.

- **Reservoirs.** *T. violaceum* is found throughout the world. It is considered endemic to countries bordering the Mediterranean Sea, as well as in Mexico and South America, but it is rarely found in the United States or Canada. This fungus is anthropophilic.

- **Unique Risk Factors.** *T. violaceum* is highly contagious, although most transmission is indirect rather than from person to person. Infection is believed to be acquired by contact with fomites such as infected hair, hair clippers and combs, towels, and upholstery. The fungus may be transmitted by direct contact within a group of people.

- **Human Infection.** *T. violaceum* causes black-dot tinea capitis; both children and adults are affected. The pattern of tinea capitis caused by *T. violaceum* resembles the condition caused by *Trichophyton tonsurans*, from which it must be differentiated. The infection is usually noninflammatory. It is more likely to become chronic than is gray-patch tinea capitis, and it may continue into adulthood. As with *T. tonsurans*, hair is invaded in an endothrix pattern. Alopecia and kerions may develop; the alopecia may be permanent.

  T. violaceum also causes tinea corporis and tinea unguium. Crusted lesions known as favus may develop. Skin lesions are red and scaly but usually are not inflammatory. As with *T. tonsurans* infections, spontaneous cure rarely occurs.

- **Usual Specimen Sources.** Skin and nail scrapings, and stubs of hair from beneath the surface of the scalp.

- **Specimen Collection and Handling.** Intact hairs, nail scrapings and material from under the tip of the nail, and skin scrapings should be collected aseptically and transported to the laboratory in a sterile dry container. Infected hairs do not fluoresce.

Direct examination of specimens should include treatment of the material with 10% to 20% KOH. Blue-black ink and DMSO may be added, or a calcofluor white–KOH preparation may be done. DMSO is not recommended for hair or thin skin scrapings.

■ **Immunology.** No tests are available.

■ **Special Precautions.** None are needed, but cultures should be handled within a biologic safety cabinet.

■ **Culture Media.** Modified SDA, modified SDA with antimicrobials. DTM may be used for screening purposes. Growth is enhanced by thiamine.

Preferred Temperature. Temperature of 25° to 30°C.

■ **Differential Tests** (see Table 5.5). The *in vitro* hair perforation test and nutritional testing should be done. *T. violaceum* does not penetrate the hair. Growth is enhanced by thiamine.

■ **Macroscopic (Colony) Morphology.** *T. violaceum* produces colonies on modified SDA after 14 to 21 days at 25° to 30°C. At first they are cream colored, glabrous, heaped, and cone shaped. As they age colonies develop a lavender or deep purple color and become verrucose, folded, and waxy. Very old cultures may be covered with short aerial hyphae, creating a velvety texture; the surface pigment becomes a lighter purple, and mutations of white sterile mycelia form and cover the colony. The reverse pigment of cultures is lavender to purple. Subcultured colonies of *T. violaceum* may fail to develop the characteristic pigment.

■ **Microscopic Morphology** (Fig. 5.40). On standard mycology media the hyphae of *T. violaceum* are hyaline, septate, and branched. They are also distorted, tangled, and full of twists and turns and are sterile. The characteristic microscopic features are chains of intercalary and terminal chlamydoconidia and swollen hyphal cells containing cytoplasmic granules.

Conidia are rarely produced in culture on routine media. When the colony is subcultured to SDA that has been supplemented with thiamine, conidiation remains sparse, but a few macroconidia and microconidia can usually be seen. Macroconidia have smooth walls and are elongate, with two to five cells. The microconidia of *T. violaceum* are unicellular and clavate. Occasionally favic chandeliers are also seen.

In *direct examination, T. violaceum* demonstrates hyaline, distorted septate hyphae in skin and nail scrapings. Large (4 to 7 μm) barrel-shaped arthroconidia may be

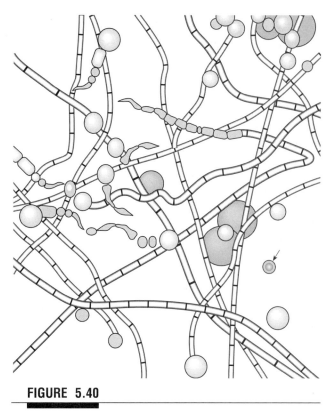

FIGURE 5.40

The hyphae of *Trichophyton violaceum* are septate and sterile, with distortions, tangles, and twists. Only chlamydoconidia and swollen hyphal cells containing cytoplasmic granules are seen. Characteristically conidia are absent; when they are produced they resemble the conidia of other *Trichophyton* species. The problem with identification of *T. violaceum* is, essentially, that it has no remarkable distinctive characteristics. The 7-μm red blood cell (arrow) shows the relative sizes of the mycotic elements.

seen in chains in infected hair. Barrel-shaped arthroconidia are also seen in skin and nail scrapings.

■ **Helpful Features for Identification of *Trichophyton violaceum*** (see Fig. 5.30 and Tables 5.5 and 5.6)

Endothrix hair invasion
Violet or purple pigment in the colonies
Noninflammatory black-dot pattern of infection
Slow growth rate
Few macroconidia or microconidia (even) on enriched media
Distorted twisted hyphae
Chaining chlamydoconidia with cytoplasmic granules in swollen hyphal cells
Inability to penetrate hair in the *in vitro* test
Partial requirement for thiamine

■ **Organisms from Which *Trichophyton violaceum* Must Be Differentiated** (see Table 5.6)

Most dermatophytes, especially *Trichophyton tonsurans* and *Trichophyton schoenleinii*

SUGGESTED EXERCISES FOR CHAPTER 5   °

(The Dermatophytes)

Exercise 7 (1st Session)

Purpose. To practice the procedures and (again) to set up the cultures needed for the next laboratory.

Suggested Fungus Cultures

Set 1   *Epidermophyton floccosum*
Set 2   *Microsporum canis, Microsporum gypseum, Microsporum nanum, Microsporum cookei, Microsporum canis*
Set 3   *Trichophyton mentagrophytes, Trichophyton rubrum, Trichophyton tonsurans*

Initial Process. Get four plates of DTM, PFA, or PDA and three slide culture setups from the supply table; three agar plates are for your subcultures and the fourth will be used to make the slide cultures. At the same time, pick up the three new cultures you are working with today. Take only one organism from each set. Coordinate the selection with your laboratory partner, if you have one, so that you don't both have the same fungus from sets 2 and 3.

Make a *slide culture* for each of your fungi, following the instructions used in previous sessions.

Complete Exercise 7 just as you did Exercise 5 by making *subcultures*; you may want to refresh your memory about the process. Incubate all of the new cultures in the 25–30°C incubator. Do not forget to *add water to your slide cultures* at least once before the next laboratory.

Exercise 7 (2nd Session)

Remove the slide cultures and the subcultures of the dermatophytes from the 25–30°C incubator and examine them. *Harvest* all the mature slide cultures, and put the slides aside in a slide flat to dry until the next laboratory session; you will have time then to examine them. Be sure that all preparations are properly labeled.

After all the slide cultures have been harvested, turn your attention to the subcultures. Remember, now, WORK WITH ONE ORGANISM AT A TIME, record the *colony descriptions* on the correct LABORATORY WORK SHEET. Pay particular attention to the reverse pigment as well as the obverse pigment, then do a *tease mount* and a *Scotch tape preparation* of the fungus. Examine these preparations, and record what you see (with composite drawings). If you need a refresher, the procedures can be found in Appendix D.

NOTE any unusual vegetative hyphal structures such as racquet hyphae or nodular bodies, as well as the presence of septa in the hyphae, the size, shape, and relative number of conidia, and so forth. These structures provide a clue that the fungus is a dermatophyte as well as information about which dermatophyte it is likely to be.

Exercise 7 (3rd Session)

If you have not already done so, make permanent mounts of the slide cultures of the dermatophytes harvested in the last session by sealing the edges of the coverslips. Label them correctly, and be sure they are dry before you attempt to examine them. Save the slide to add to your personal collection.

Exercise 8 (1st Session)

Purpose. To practice some of the differential methods used for differentiation of the dermatophytes. These are especially helpful for differentiation of species of *Trichophyton*, which can be hard to identify when morphology alone is used. You will perform the tests on several fungi so that you can see positive and negative results for the procedures.

Procedures to be Completed

> Growth on sterile rice grains
> Hair perforation test
> Urea utilization
> Growth on *Trichophyton* agars

Initial Process. Use the methods given in Appendix D, and any "tips" your instructor provides, to set up the differential tests. If you are working with a laboratory partner, you should coordinate your work so that, between you, you have a dermatophyte culture that is positive and another that is negative for each test (see Table 5.5).

Be *very* careful not to carry over nutrients from the initial cultures to the tests or your results may be false positive, which will confuse you and result in misidentification of the fungi.

You should record results of the DTM cultures for the dermatophytes with which you are working on the appropriate LABORATORY WORK SHEET.

Exercise 8 (2nd Session)

If the fungi have grown enough, read the differential tests for each of the dermatophytes you cultured and record the results properly on the LABORATORY WORK SHEET. Using "growth" and "no growth" or "perforated" and "not perforated" is recommended (instead of "positive" and "negative"); you are less likely to be confused later about what a positive really indicates. Note the relative amount of growth as +/− to 4+ so you can compare the relative amount of growth for the various nutrients.

Reincubate any tests that do not have adequate growth.

Exercise 8 (3rd Session)

Complete Exercise 8 by reading any tests that had to be reincubated and recording the results on the LABORATORY WORK SHEET. Enter the actual reaction, for example, "perforation" rather than "positive," to make your records as clear as possible. Then use the tables in the text to "identify" the fungi; use the test results as if you did not know the name of the organisms and see if your results are typical. If you have atypical results, attempt to determine the cause(s).

ASSESS WHAT YOU HAVE LEARNED

Responses to the questions below are located in Appendix A.

1. Compare dermato*phytosis* and dermato*mycosis*.
2. What is the difference between *gray-patch* tinea capitis and *black-dot* tinea capitis?
3. Define folliculitis, kerion, alopecia, sebum, scutula, echinulate.
4. Name the three dermatophyte genera. What tissues are infected by each genus? Describe the microscopic morphology characteristic of each genus.

For questions 5 through 10 **MATCH** the tinea **(lettered)** with the tissues infected **(numbered).** NOTE that some responses will not be used.

5. bearded areas of the face
6. dorsal aspect of the hands
7. skin of the body
8. feet
9. groin
10. scalp

    a. tinea barbae
    b. tinea capitis
    c. tinea corporis
    d. tinea cruris
    e. tinea manuum
    f. tinea pedis
    g. tinea unguium

11. Describe the three patterns by which dermatophytes invade hair *in vivo*.
12. Draw or describe the following vegetative hyphal structures: pectinate hyphae, racquet hyphae, spiral hyphae, nodular bodies, favic chandeliers.
13. What is the difference between the *en grappe* and *en thryses* arrangements of microconidia of *Trichophyton*?
14. Which dermatophyte genus causes infected human tissues to fluoresce? How is this detected? Name two substances that may cause a false-positive result.

For questions 15 through 20 **MATCH** the term **(numbered)** with the definition **(lettered).** NOTE that some responses will not be used.

15. bulla
16. fomite
17. "id" reaction
18. intertriginous
19. onychomycosis
20. pruritus

    a. allergic reaction to a dermatophyte
    b. between the folds of the skin
    c. infection of the fingernail or toenail
    d. inflammation of tissues surrounding the nail
    e. inanimate objects that transmit infection
    f. itching
    g. large blister filled with clear fluid
    h. small sac containing purulent material

21. What are the key ingredients of dermatophyte test medium (DTM)? What is the expected reaction to growth of a dermatophyte on DTM?

For questions 22 through 30 **NAME** the organism described.

22. **Lesion:** tinea barbae

    Colony: poor growth on SDA; *slow* growing; colony is thin, white, and small, with a knobby center and a glabrous texture; colony reverse is salmon colored

    Microscopic: distorted hyaline septate hyphae with intercalary chlamydoconidia and favic chandeliers on unsupplemented media

    Other: zoophilic; growth is enhanced by thiamine and/or inositol, with better conidiation

23. **Lesion:** tinea corporis

    Colony: tan granular, fringed colony with cinnamon-pink reverse; white sterile hyphae appear in the center of the colony

    Microscopic: abundant large fusiform macroconidia with moderately thick echinulate walls and annular fringes; microconidia are clavate and sessile

    Other: geophilic

24. **Lesion:** tinea manuum

    Colony: flat, granular, creamy yellow colony with a buff reverse and a ray-like fringe

    Microscopic: abundant, long cigar-shaped macroconidia with thin, smooth walls. Abundant globose unicellular microconidia are also present, predominantly *en grappe*. Conidiophores branch at right angles. Vegetative structures, including favic chandeliers, are also present

    Other: zoophilic; positive urease in <4 days; good growth on all *Trichophyton* agars; *in vitro* penetration of hair

25. **Lesion:** tinea cruris

    Colony: velvety khaki colony with yellow fringe and yellow-orange reverse; sterile hyphae appear in the center of the colony

    Microscopic: moderate numbers of macroconidia with thin, smooth walls that resemble snowshoes; no microconidia are present

    Other: anthropophilic

26. **Lesion:** tinea capitis; endothrix

    Colony: flat off-white powdery colony that develops radial grooves and folds; reverse is a yellow-brown diffusible pigment

    Microscopic: rare macroconidia are short, blunt, and irregular in shape, with moderately thick, smooth walls; terminal swellings on some hyphae. Microconidia are sessile on hyphae and in clusters on conidiophores. They are irregular in size and shape; some resemble balloons

    Other: anthropophilic; penetration of hair *in vitro*; urease positive after 4 days; thiamine enhances growth

27. **Lesion:** tinea capitis (fluorescing); ectothrix

    Colony: flat white velvety surface with beige to reddish brown reverse

    Microscopic: numerous vegetative structures, especially terminal and intercalary vesicles; rare large, twisted macroconidium with thick echinulate walls

    Other: anthropophilic; little or no growth on rice grains

28. **Lesion:** tinea pedis

    Colony: white fluffy surface with blood-red reverse

    Microscopic: Rare macroconidia, which are pencil shaped with blunt distal ends and thin, smooth parallel walls. Microconidia are also sparse; they are clavate and tear-drop shaped, *en thyrses,* and in small clusters

    Other: anthropophilic; no penetration of hair *in vitro*; no effect of special nutrients; negative urease after 5 to 7 days

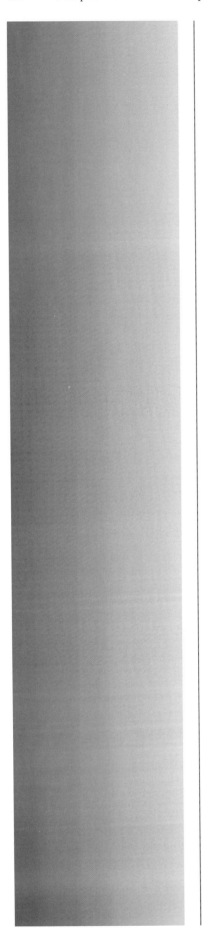

29. **Lesion:** tinea favosa
   Colony: slow-growing glabrous tan colonies with light yellow reverse
   Microscopic: neither microconidia nor macroconidia on SDA; numerous favic chandeliers and nail head hyphae are present
   Other: anthropophilic; neither inositol nor thiamine enhances the slow growth rate; no penetration of hair *in vitro*

30. **Lesion:** tinea capitis (fluorescing); ectothrix
   Colony: buff granular surface with yellow-orange reverse
   Microscopic: many large spindle-shaped macroconidia, some with an asymmetrical beaked apex; outer wall is thick and echinulate, but inner septa are thin. Annular frills on macroconidia. Few microconidia
   Other: zoophilic; reverse of young colonies is bright yellow; good growth on rice grains

CHAPTER 6

Subcutaneous Fungi

Upon completion of this chapter the reader should be able to:

Instructional Objectives

1. Define the following terms: autoinoculation, mycetoma, chromoblastomycosis, phaeohyphomycosis, sporotrichosis, primary, secondary, tertiary, shield cells, sclerotic bodies, synnemata, verrucoid.

2. Recognize or describe the distinguishing characteristics of the gross and microscopic morphology of both forms of *Sporothrix schenckii.*

3. Draw or describe cladosporium-, phialophora-, and rhinocladiella-type conidiogeny.

4. Recognize or describe the distinguishing characteristics of the gross and microscopic morphology of the subcutaneous fungi (*Cladosporium carrionii, Exophiala jeanselmei, Fonsecaea compacta, Fonsecaea pedrosoi, Phialophora verrucosa, Pseudallescheria boydii/Scedosporium apiospermum, Wangiella dermatitidis,* and *Xylohypha bantiana*).

5. Describe the usual route of infection for subcutaneous mycoses and the populations at risk for each infection.

6. Describe the symptoms and appearance of each of the subcutaneous mycoses, including the types of subcutaneous tissues involved.

7. Correctly identify the subcutaneous fungi studied, given pertinent background information such as descriptions of microscopic and gross morphology and the patient's history and symptoms.

8. Outline a procedure for positive identification of an organism as *Sporothrix schenckii* versus *Sporothrix* species.

9. When relevant, list *special* safety precautions that must be taken in working with specimens or cultures believed to contain subcutaneous mycotic agents. Consider each fungus.

■

INTRODUCTION

All of the fungi that cause subcutaneous infections in humans are found as saprobes throughout the world. They exist naturally in soil, on plants, and in decomposing vegetation and wood. The list of subcutaneous fungi varies a little from text to text. This discussion is confined to fungi that are recognized by most authors as predominant: *Cladosporium, Exophiala, Fonsecaea, Phialophora, Pseudallescheria/Scedosporium, Sporothrix schenckii, Wangiella,* and *Xylohypha.*

Infection with these organisms can usually be traced to traumatic inoculation. The injury may be as simple as a splinter or a prick from a thorn, and it may have occurred months or years before the lesion appears. Subcutaneous mycoses are most frequently seen in residents of the tropics and subtropics. The typical patient works outdoors, usually without shoes, in shorts and other lightweight clothing that provides little protection.

The interesting interplay between the host's ability to resist infection and the relative virulence of the fungus is discussed at some length by Rippon. He believes that people who develop a subcutaneous mycosis have some defect in their defenses. The most common defect is lowered resistance of the host that is often the result of poor nutrition.

Because the subcutaneous fungi are all saprobes in the environment, the physician must ascertain whether the isolate is causing the infection or is simply present. The first step is to determine that the symptoms are consistent with a mycotic infection. The fungus must be seen in specimens of material from the lesions. The morphology of the fungus must be consistent with the patient's symptoms, and it must be cultured and identified properly.

The subcutaneous mycoses include four kinds of infections: mycetoma, sporotrichosis, phaeohyphomycosis, and chromoblastomycosis (Table 6.1). Some of the fungi to be studied cause more than one kind of infection. The infections all can be traced to similar routes of inoculation, but symptoms of the infections differ and different tissues are involved.

Infections caused by dematiaceous fungi are technically *phaeohyphomycoses.* Three of these, mycetoma, chromoblastomycosis, and sporotrichosis, are usually referred to by name because they are distinct, recognizable syndromes. The general term **phaeohyphomycosis** is reserved for miscellaneous infections caused by fungi other than the subcutaneous fungi, which are recognized as consistent pathogens. Phaeohyphomycosis is described more fully in Chapter 3.

Mycetoma ("oma," tumor; "myco," fungus) is a chronic granulomatous infection; the typical site is on one of the extremities. Approximately one half the mycetomas are *eumycotic* ("eu," true), caused by several different true fungi. The remaining half are *actinomycotic* ("actino," ray) mycetomas, caused by the bacteria *Nocardia* and *Actinomyces*[1] and related organisms. All mycetomas are subcutaneous infections characterized by swollen, tumor-like areas with sinuses that drain through multiple sinus tracts. "*Granules,*" small flecks of matter that are actually a combination of microcolonies of the causative organism and proteinaceous materials from the host, are present in the drainage from sinus tracts (Fig. 6.1). Infections tend to remain localized at the site of the initial injury, usually on the feet and legs, although any part of the body can be involved. The lymphatic system is not involved in mycetomas.

Sporotrichosis is caused by a single organism, *S. schenckii.* It is a "chronic infection characterized by nodular lesions of the cutaneous or subcutaneous tissues and adjacent lymphatics that suppurate, ulcerate, and drain" (Rippon, p. 325). Sporotrichosis can be separated into five types of infection: lymphocutaneous, fixed cutaneous, mucocutaneous, disseminated, and pulmonary. The portal of entry of the fungus, the dose, and the effectiveness of the host's response determine which type of infection develops.

Lymphocutaneous sporotrichosis, affecting the skin and lymphatic system, is the most common infection. It

---

[1]Anaerobic transport devices should be used for specimens from mycetomas because *Actinomyces* species are anaerobic bacteria.

dimorphism due to temp not age

TABLE 6.1   Subcutaneous Mycotic Infections

Mycosis	Most Common Site	Representative Organism	Appearance of Lesion	Microscopic Elements in Specimen	Lymphatic Involvement
Chromoblastomycosis	Lower limbs	*Fonsecaea pedrosoi, Phialophora verrucosa*	Warty crusted nodules, micro-abscesses	Sclerotic bodies	Possible
Mycetoma	Lower limbs	*Pseudallescheria boydii, Exophiala jeanselmei*	Tumefaction, draining sinuses	Granules	No; localized
Sporotrichosis	Upper and lower limbs	*Sporothrix schenckii*	Ulcers and smooth, painless nodules	Asteroid bodies	Spreads along lymphatic channels
Phaeohyphomycosis	Any area	Any dematiaceous fungus	Diverse symptoms	No specific element	Possible

In the subcutaneous mycoses—especially when the infection is well established—the symptoms and appearance of the lesion are typical enough for the diagnosis (but not necessarily the identification of the fungus) to be made easily.

usually occurs on the feet and legs or on the hands and arms. Following implantation of the fungus, the infection may appear as soon as 5 days after implantation (Rippon, p. 328), or it may incubate as long as 6 months before the primary lesion develops. First, a small, hard, painless, *fluctuant* nodule—one that is movable, not attached to adjacent tissues—develops near the surface. Eventually it attaches to the overlying skin, which becomes black and necrotic. Later, a second ulcer develops at another lymph node proximal to the first one; the two ulcers—one healing, one developing—are typically separated by normal healthy tissue. Rippon states that the clinical picture of an ulcer on the hand associated with swollen lymph nodes extending in a chain up the arm "is so pathognomonic[2] as to be an 'over the telephone' diagnosis" (Rippon, 1988, p. 330). Lymphocutaneous sporotrichosis, despite involvement of the lymph channels, is localized without fever or malaise and without involvement of the regional lymph nodes—those in the axilla or groin. Fixed cutaneous sporotrichosis occurs if the person has been previously sensitized by exposure to *S. schenckii*. The infection remains localized at the point of entry. For information about the remaining three forms, consult a more comprehensive text, such as Rippon.

Asteroid bodies (Fig. 6.2) in the infected tissue are characteristic of sporotrichosis, although they are not always present. An asteroid body is approximately star shaped, with rays of an eosinophilic material radiating from a central yeastlike cell or cells. The yeastlike cell is basophilic, 3 to 5 μm in diameter; the entire complex may be 10 to 15 μm in diameter. Asteroid bodies represent the host's immune response. The eosinophilic mate-

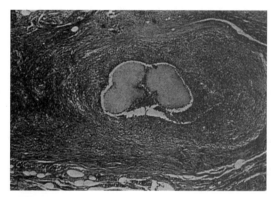

FIGURE 6.1

The single bilobed granule in the center of this figure from a mycetoma caused by *Pseudallescheria boydii* is mostly smooth and homogeneous looking, with darker, rough-looking patches from hyphae and vacuoles. The granule rests in a sinus tract and is surrounded by an area of fibrosis. At the edge of the picture are signs of the granulomatous response associated with these infections. (From Rippon JW: Medical Mycology: The Pathogenic Fungi and Pathogenic Actinomycetes, 3rd ed. Philadelphia, WB Saunders, 1988, p 90.)

rial is a complex of antigenic material from the fungus and antibody protein from the host.

The third distinct clinical entity, **chromoblastomycosis,**[3] is characterized by **verrucoid** (wartlike) crusted nodules on the skin. When the infection is not treated, the lesions may eventually become elevated 1 to 3 cm above the surrounding tissue and begin to resemble a cauliflower. Sometimes microabscesses resembling black dots or cayenne pepper develop on the surface. The infection

---

[2]"Pathognomonic" means characteristic of the infection or disease.

[3]Chromoblastomycosis is the same disease state as the "chromomycosis" described in older texts. The mycosis is characterized by pigmented ("chromo") elements in the infected tissues.

can do direct smear

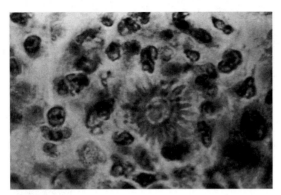

FIGURE 6.2

Asteroid bodies are sometimes present in tissues infected with *Sporothrix schenckii.* One or more tissue forms of the fungus occupies the center of the body. Proteinaceous substances produced by the host surround the fungus in raylike arrangements that create the starlike appearance seen here in the lower right quadrant. Hematoxylin and eosin stain. ×1000. (Courtesy of F. Mariat.)

may spread to surrounding tissue through the lymphatic system or by **autoinoculation,** that is, transfer of the organisms from one area of the body to another, generally through contact. Apparently chromoblastomycosis is not painful unless a bacterial *secondary infection* (infection by a second microorganism that takes advantage of host conditions) occurs. *Elephantiasis* is an increase in size in the skin and subcutaneous tissues—especially those in the scrotum and legs—as a result of the accumulation of lymph due to blocked lymphatic vessels. It may also develop in persons with chromoblastomycosis after a secondary bacterial infection. Specimens from patients with chromoblastomycosis may contain pleomorphic spheri-

cal brown forms, approximately 8 μm in diameter. Muriform septa divide them into two to four cells. These *sclerotic* (hard) *bodies,* sometimes called "copper pennies," may be in clusters or chainlike arrangements (Fig. 6.3).

Most agents of subcutaneous mycoses resemble one another. The exception—one fungus that does not fit the pattern—is *Pseudallescheria boydii. P. boydii* is the most common cause of eumycotic mycetoma in the United States and Europe. It has several unique features. First, *Pseudallescheria* species grow rapidly on standard mycology media. Second, they are hyaline, producing colonies that are initially white and fluffy. Although the colonies later become "house mouse" gray, they are hyaline rather than dematiaceous; microscopic structures are not pigmented; the reverse of the colony becomes gray or black. Slide preparations of material from cultures shows broad septate hyphae and two kinds of asexual conidia. Third, it is a perfect fungus. The sexual (perfect) stage is *P. boydii,* and the asexual (imperfect) form is *Scedosporium apiospermum.* The sexual forms consist of ascocarps that are relatively large, so that the colony may look as if it has been sprinkled with black pepper. Sexual reproduction must be demonstrated for positive identification of a fungus as *P. boydii.*

All of the remaining subcutaneous mycotic agents are dematiaceous. They all have a moderately slow growth rate, requiring at least 10 days to produce mature colonies. Some of them require up to 30 days to produce colonies with typical conidia. Colonies are darkly pigmented when mature, with a velvety texture, and may be heaped or slightly folded.

S. schenckii, the agent of sporotrichosis, is unique among the dematiaceous subcutaneous fungi because it is

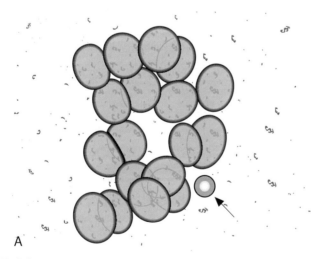
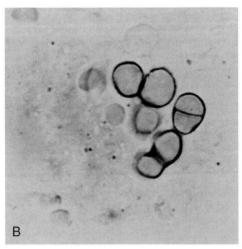

FIGURE 6.3

A and *B,* Sclerotic bodies, also known as "copper pennies," may be found in the material discharged from chromoblastomycotic lesions. They indicate chromoblastomycosis without indicating which fungus is the etiologic agent of the infection. Sclerotic bodies consist of two to four cells with muriform septa. They may be arranged in pairs and clusters, as shown, or chains. *B,* A *Wangiella dermatitidis* phaeohyphomycotic cyst shows the heavy walls and cross-walls of these structures. The details of sclerotic bodies are seen more easily in *A* than in *B.* You can see a larger group of copper pennies in *A,* with a 7-μm red blood cell (arrow) added to show the relative sizes of these structures. (*B* from Greer KE, Gross GP, Cooper PH, Harding SA: Cystic chromomycosis due to *Wangiella dermatitidis.* Arch Dermatol 1979; 115 [12]: 1433–1434. Copyright 1979 American Medical Association.)

dimorphic—the only dematiaceous dimorphic fungus infecting humans. A yeast form develops in infected tissues and in cultures incubated at body temperature (35° to 37°C), while at 25°C the colony is a mould. Young colonies are typically light in color; darker pigment is only seen in old cultures. Yeast colonies may remain predominantly white with black *striations* (stripes). Dimorphism must be demonstrated for definitive identification of *S. schenckii*.

The remaining fungi, *Cladosporium*, *Xylohypha*, *Exophiala*, *Wangiella*, *Phialophora*, and *Fonsecaea*, cause mycetoma or chromoblastomycosis or both—not in the same patient, of course. These fungi all are monomorphic moulds that are dematiaceous and slow growing. Colonies are velvety, with dark reverse and surface pigments. Three patterns of anamorphic conidiation are associated with these fungi: the cladosporium, phialophora, and rhinocladiella types.

In *cladosporium-type* conidiation (Fig. 6.4) conidiophores are of various sizes and may be septate. They are pale greenish black and slightly swollen at the distal ends. Long chains of oval, smooth-walled blastoconidia are produced in a "treelike" fashion; that is, the chains branch wherever a conidium produces two buds rather than one. Blastoconidia may have dark disjuncture scars or hila where they have broken off from the conidio-

phore or from another conidium. Blastoconidia from a branching point may have three disjuncture scars and are called *shield cells* (see Fig. 6.4). The length of the chain, the presence of disjuncture scars, the kinds of tissue attacked, and the posture of the conidiophores—whether they are upright or leaning—are used to distinguish between *Cladosporium*, *Xylohypha*, and *Wangiella (Exophiala) dermatitidis*.[4]

In the second type of conidiation, the *phialophora type*, the conidiogenous cells are phialides produced from conidiophores along the sides and tips of the hyphae (Fig. 6.5). The classic phialide is vase shaped with a rounded base that narrows into the neck, then flares to form a collarette (lip). In some cases the vase shape is less pronounced and the collarette is absent. Phialoconidia are formed within the phialide and extruded blastically into the environment, where they tend to cluster around the tip of the phialide.

In the *rhinocladiella type*[5] of conidiation (Fig. 6.6) the conidia are produced sympodially on short denticles around the tip of the conidiophores. In the early stages this type of conidiation looks like *Sporothrix* that has been "body building" at a fitness center (Fig. 6.7). The arrangement approximates the rosettes produced by *Sporothrix*,

---

[4]This organism was initially placed in the genus *Exophiala*, but McGinnis and others consider it belongs to the genus *Wangiella*. Both genus names are used in this text, with the older name placed in parentheses: *Wangiella (Exophiala) dermatitidis*.
[5]Rhinocladiella-type conidiation was formerly called *acrotheca-type* conidiation.

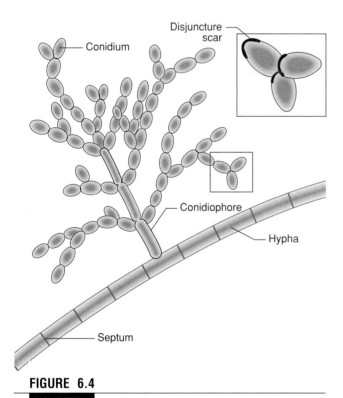

FIGURE 6.4

Cladosporium-type conidiation resembles a tree, where the conidiophore is the trunk and the chains of the conidia are the branches. The chains of conidia also branch, contributing to the treelike appearance. Blastoconidia may have dark disjuncture scars *(inset)* at the point where they were connected to the conidiophore or another conidium. Conidia with three disjuncture scars are called "shield cells."

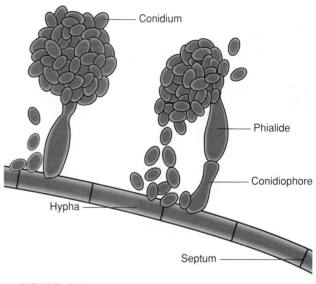

FIGURE 6.5

In phialophora-type conidiation the conidiophores are short, stubby cells that support the conidiogenous cell, the phialide. The phialides may be obviously vase shaped with a distinct collarette, as shown, or they may be slender and tubelike, without the collarette. In phialophora-type conidiation the conidia are extruded through the mouth of the phialide and they cluster around the tip of the phialide.

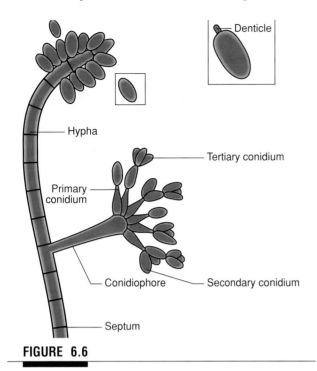

FIGURE 6.6

Conidiophores in rhinocladiella-type conidiation are simple stalks that become knobby as conidia are produced. Initially conidia are produced sympodially from short denticles *(inset)* at the tip of the conidiophore. As the fungus matures rhinocladiella-type conidiation becomes more complex. Secondary conidia are produced from the primary conidia, and tertiary conidia form in branching chains from the secondary conidia, causing the pattern to resemble cladosporium-type conidiation.

but in *Fonsecaea* all of the structures, including the hyphae, are bigger and coarser than those of *Sporothrix*. As rhinocladiella-type conidiation continues, the blastoconidia form a third *(tertiary)* level of branching chains; the conidiation begins to resemble cladosporium-type conidiation. In rhinocladiella-type conidiation conidia are also

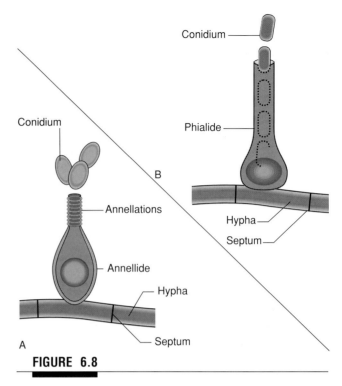

FIGURE 6.8

Distinguishing the annellides and phialides is hard to do with a standard brightfield microscope. In annellidic conidiation *(A)*, the annelloconidia are produced at the tip of the annellide, leaving a ring or annellation (scar); the annellide lengthens as each new annelloconidium is produced. Phialides *(B)* attain their full growth before production of conidia begins. Phialoconidia are produced within the phialide and extruded through the neck, where they tend to remain clustered.

produced from erect sympodial conidiophores of varying sizes and lengths that are slightly swollen at the distal ends.

Annellides and annelloconidia may be produced by the subcutaneous fungi. The annellides may be individual

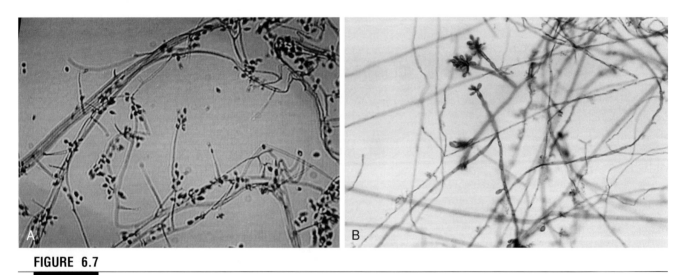

FIGURE 6.7

Superficially *Sporothrix schenckii (A)* and *Fonsecaea pedrosoi (B)* resemble one another, as this composite shows. Both have septate, branching hyphae, and both produce upright conidiophores that swell at the apices. Both also have a pattern of conidiation in which oval conidia are produced individually around the tips of the conidiophores. The differences are that structures of *Fonsecaea* are larger, darker, and coarser, and *Fonsecaea* also produces cladosporium- and phialophora-type conidiation. *Sporothrix schenckii* has delicate, slender structures, and although conidia may be arranged in daisy and rosette patterns, and a second darker conidium may be present, *Sporothrix* has only one type of conidiation.

cells, they may be incorporated into the hyphae, or they may develop on short denticles or annellophores on the hyphae. They are flask shaped or cylindrical when they are integrated with the supporting annellophores and extend above them; the flask-shaped annellides look like phialides. Technically the annellides can be distinguished from phialides by two characteristics. They are narrow at their apices, and they become longer as each annelloconidium is produced, leaving a scar called an *annellation*. Annellophores and phialophores are compared in Figure 6.8.

LABORATORY METHODS FOR SUBCUTANEOUS FUNGI

Specimens for culture should be obtained by aspiration whenever possible. This provides a larger amount of material to be examined and cultured, reduces the chance that the specimen will dry out, and—if actinomycotic mycetoma is a possible diagnosis—provides some protection from oxygen for the anaerobic *Actinomyces*.[6]

The size, color, shape, and consistency of any granules in the aspirate should be recorded to help in identification. Description is facilitated if the granules are first washed in sterile water or a solution of antibacterial antibiotics. For microscopic preparations (and to determine their consistency) granules should be crushed between the slide and the coverslip. Gram's staining method should be used if actinomycotic mycetoma is suspected; lactophenol–cotton blue is used for eumycotic mycetomas.

Cultures for the subcutaneous mycoses should be plated initially on Emmon's modification of Sabouraud's dextrose agar (modified SDA) with and without antibiotics and cycloheximide. Selective SDA should never be used alone because some of the fungi are sensitive to the antimicrobials. *S. apiospermum*, for example, is susceptible to cycloheximide. Additional media such as potato flake agar (PFA), potato dextrose agar (PDA), cornmeal agar (CMA), or malt extract agar may be used for subculture to enhance conidiation of the isolates.

Biochemical methods are available for differentiation of the subcutaneous fungi. Generally the methods involve determining whether the fungus produces enzymes to break down various substrates: gelatin, serum, milk, casein, starch, and tyrosine. Tests for nitrate reduction and resistance to cycloheximide may also be helpful, and the temperatures at which the fungus grows can be tested. These procedures are rarely done in clinical laboratories.

---

[6]Anaerobic methods for collection and transport should be used if actinomycotic mycetoma is a possible diagnosis—and the diagnosis is always possible when granules are present in the specimen.

Subcutaneous Pathogens

DEMATIACEAE

CLADOSPORIUM CARRIONII (Clad-o-spore′-e-um care-ee-own′-ee)

- **Teleomorph.** None has been identified.

- **Reservoirs.** *C. carrionii* is found in soil, on rotting wood, and in decaying vegetation. It is found worldwide, more often in tropical and subtropical areas, but it is occasionally found in the United States, a temperate zone.

- **Unique Risk Factors.** Infections with *C. carrionii* most often occur in people who work outdoors without even such minimal protective clothing as shoes and gloves. The fungi enter the skin through some wound or minor trauma, such as a cut or scrape, with an infected thorn or splinter of wood as the inoculating instrument. Repeated exposure and poor general health may contribute to development of the infection.

- **Human Infection.** *C. carrionii* is one of the etiologic agents of chromoblastomycosis. The fungus may remain dormant for months or years before a second injury occurs, causing fungi that have acclimated to human tissue to be distributed and create an active infection.

  The symptoms of chromoblastomycosis are the same, whether the infection is caused by *C. carrionii* or another fungus. Lesions are wartlike, verrucoid, and crusted. In advanced cases the affected area is grossly swollen and cauliflower-like. The lymphatics are usually not involved, and bone is not invaded. Untreated or poorly treated infections become chronic. Surprisingly, the patient usually reports feeling little or no discomfort unless a secondary bacterial infection develops.

- **Specimen Sources.** Crusts, scrapings, biopsied tissue from verrucous lesions, and aspirates of pus from microabscesses are most likely to be submitted for culture.

- **Specimen Collection and Handling.** No special measures are needed, *except that* anaerobic transport is necessary for specimens if actinomycotic mycetoma is being entertained as part of the differential diagnosis.

  Direct examination of material from crusted areas should include treatment with 10% potassium hydroxide (KOH) (to which stain or ink may be added) prior to microscopic examination. Purulent aspirates can be studied with simple wet mounts in KOH.

- **Immunology.** Complement fixation (CF), precipitin, fluorescent antibody, immunodiffusion (ID), and electroimmunodiffusion tests have been researched, but many cross-reactions occur between *C. carrionii* and

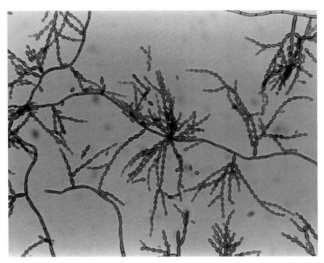

FIGURE 6.9

Typical isolates of *Cladosporium carrionii* have pale greenish brown co-nidiophores and hyphae. Septa can be seen, as in the hyphal fragment snaking through the extreme upper right of this photomicrograph. Long chains of conidia with occasional branches complete the picture. A few detached conidia, singly and in pairs and short chains, can also be seen.

other fungi. The tests that are presently available are nei-ther well standardized nor specific enough for routine diagnostic work.

■ **Special Precautions.** None are needed, but cultures should be handled within a biologic safety cabinet.

■ **Culture Media.** Modified SDA, modified SDA with antimicrobials.

Preferred Temperature. Grows at temperatures of 25° to 37°C.

■ **Differential Methods** (Table 6.2). A colony sus-pected of being *C. carrionii* can be tested for its ability to grow at 35° to 37°C. Other tests that may be helpful in assigning the fungus to the correct species are liquefac-tion of gelatin (negative), liquefaction of Loeffler's serum medium (negative), and hydrolysis of casein (negative).

■ **Macroscopic (Colony) Morphology.** Colonies of *C. carrionii* after 10 to 30 days on modified SDA at 25° to 30°C are gray-green or olive-green to grayish lavender with a jet black reverse pigment. Older colonies may be-come dark gray or black on the surface as well as the re-verse. The surface is covered with a short aerial mycelium, creating a velvety or cottony texture. The topography may be spreading, heaped, or folded.

■ **Microscopic Morphology** (Figs. 6.9 through 6.11). Hyphae of *C. carrionii* have a greenish brown pigment in unstained preparations. They are septate and approxi-mately 4 μm wide. The cladosporium-type conidiation is observed. Conidiophores are of various sizes and often have septa. They are lateral or terminal and pale greenish brown. The distal ends of the conidiophores are slightly swollen. Long branching chains of 12 to 15 blastoconidia are produced. Conidia are oval and slightly pointed with

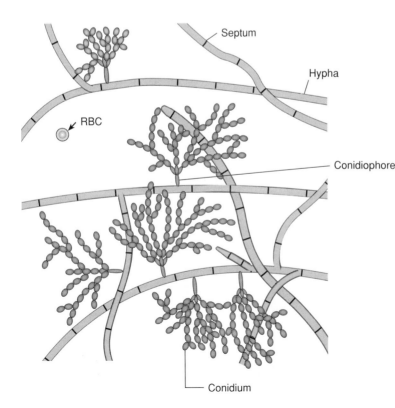

FIGURE 6.10

Cladosporium carrionii produces dark hyphae, conidia, and conidiophores, with septa in the hyphae. Chains of 12 to 15 conidia are produced from the conidiophores, with branch-ing of the chains. Conidia are oval and slightly pointed; dark flattened scars are sometimes visible. Shield cells help to identify the organism. The 7-μm red blood cell (RBC) (arrow) shows the relative sizes of the mycotic elements.

TABLE 6.2 Biochemical Tests for Subcutaneous Fungi

Fungus	Gelatin Liquefaction	Loeffler's Serum Medium	Casein Hydrolysis	Tyrosine Hydrolysis	Nitrate Reduction	Cycloheximide	Starch Hydrolysis	Coagulation of Milk	Growth Temperatures
Cladosporium carrionii	Negative	Negative	Negative	—	—	—	—	—	37°C
Exophiala jeanselmei	Variable	Variable	Negative	Positive	Positive	Sensitive	—	—	37°C
Phialophora verrucosa	Negative	Negative	—	—	—	—	Negative	Negative	37°C
Wangiella dermatitidis	Negative	Negative	Negative	Positive	Negative	Resistant	—	—	37°C
Xylohypha bantiana	Negative	Negative	Negative	—	—	—	—	—	Growth at 42–43°C

Growth patterns and reactions in biochemical tests are necessary for species identification of some of the subcutaneous mycoses.

smooth walls. They are approximately 3×5 μm, with little variation in size. Blastoconidia have dark disjuncture scars or hila where they have broken off from the conidiophore or from another conidium. The shield cells—conidia with three disjuncture scars—readily break off in slide preparations of *C. carrionii* and are helpful in identifying the fungus to genus.

In *direct examination* look for dark brown hyphal fragments (average diameter 4 μm) with branching. Sclerotic bodies (copper pennies) may be seen in chains or clusters.

■ **Helpful Features for Identification of *Cladosporium carrionii*** (Fig. 6.12)

Characteristic dark olive-green to black colonies
Slo-o-o-o-w growth of the fungus
Only cladosporium-type conidiation in cultures
Pigmented brown-green hyphae and sclerotic bodies in specimens
Characteristic appearance of the lesion in well-developed infections

■ **Organisms from Which *Cladosporium carrionii* Must Be Differentiated** (Table 6.3)

Other dematiaceous fungi that produce conidia in branching chains, especially *Xylohypha* and other species of *Cladosporium*

Subcutaneous Pathogens

DEMATIACEAE

CLADOSPORIUM TRICHOIDES

Most mycologists have accepted the new name for this organism, *Xylohypha bantiana*, the name used in this text.

Subcutaneous Pathogens

DEMATIACEAE

EXOPHIALA DERMATITIDIS

The name *Wangiella dermatitidis* was proposed by McGinnis and is used in the fourth edition of the *Manual of Microbiology*. Rippon uses *Wangiella* in *Medical Mycology*, Third Edition, but Kwon-Chung and Bennett, and Emmons, have retained the original name, *Exophiala dermatitidis*. In this text McGinnis's terminology has

been used, with the former genus name in parentheses, as *Wangiella (Exophiala) dermatitidis*.

Subcutaneous Pathogens

DEMATIACEAE

EXOPHIALA JEANSELMEI   (X′-oh-fee-ah′-lah jean-sell-me′-eye)

■ **Teleomorph.** None has been identified.

■ **Reservoirs.** *E. jeanselmei* is found worldwide in soil, on trees and rotting wood, and in decaying vegetation.

■ **Unique Risk Factors.** Infection is usually considered to result from repeated minor trauma (such as pricks and scratches) with contaminated fomites (such as thorns and twigs).

■ **Human Infection.** *E. jeanselmei* may cause mycetoma or phaeohyphomycosis. Both are chronic mycotic infections of the cutaneous and subcutaneous tissues resulting from introduction of the fungus into a wound in the host. For a more complete description of the disease process, refer to the Introduction in this chapter.

■ **Specimen Sources.** Aspirated pus from microabscesses and tissue removed from subcutaneous cysts or nodules are most likely to be submitted for culture.

■ **Specimen Collection and Handling.** Specimens should be collected aseptically into sterile containers and transported to the laboratory without delay. Anaerobic methods should be used if actinomycotic mycetoma is being considered as a possible diagnosis. Tissue specimens should be minced or ground before they are placed on the culture media.

Direct examination of material from crusted areas should include treatment with 10% KOH (to which stain or ink may be added) prior to microscopic examination. Purulent aspirates can be studied with simple wet mounts. Tissue specimens should be sectioned and stained by the histology laboratory before they are examined.

■ **Immunology.** CF and ID tests have been studied. The ID test is used most extensively and is particularly helpful in distinguishing eumycotic mycetoma from actinomycotic mycetoma. CF tests may be helpful in determining the patient's prognosis. Serologic methods for diagnosis of phaeohyphomycosis are not yet refined enough to be helpful for diagnosis of the infection. An

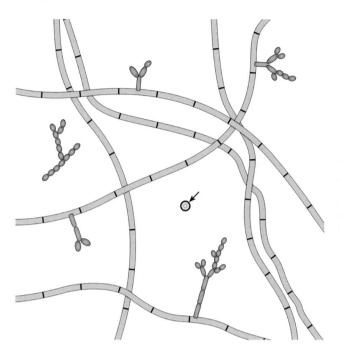

FIGURE 6.11

Even in a bad preparation *Cladosporium* can usually be recognized by the dark pigment in the hyphae and conidiophores, the "Mickey Mouse" ears at the tips of some conidiophores, and the branching chains of conidia. Relatively short chains of conidia suggest *Cladosporium carrionii*; biochemical tests may be needed to confirm the species. The 7-μm red blood cell (arrow) shows the relative sizes of the mycotic elements.

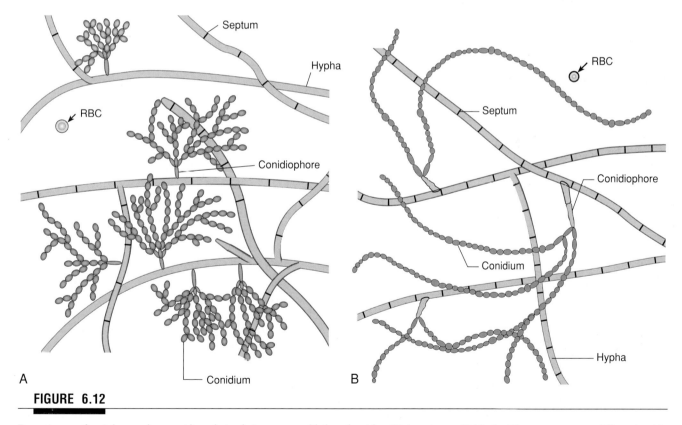

FIGURE 6.12

Dematiaceous fungi that produce conidia only in chains are most likely to be either *Cladosporium* or *Xylohypha*. The two genera are differentiated in part by the number of conidia in the chains and the size of the conidia. In *Cladosporium (A)* the conidia are uniform in size and chains are relatively short (≤15 conidia). In contrast *Xylohypha* species *(B)* typically have shorter conidiophores, with 20 or more conidia in a chain, and the conidia vary in size. Colony morphology is not helpful, but biochemical tests can be used to confirm the identification. The 7-μm red blood cell (RBC) (arrow) shows the relative sizes of the mycotic elements.

TABLE 6.3 Dematiaceous Fungi with Chains of Conidia

Fungus	Size of Conidia (μm)	Shape of Conidia	Arrangement of Conidia	Width of Hyphae (μm)	Length of Conidiophore (μm)	Shape of Conidiophore	Arrangement of Conidiophores	Colony Morphology	Growth Rate	Other Helpful Features
Cladosporium carrionii	3 × 5	Oval and slightly pointed	Branching chains of 12–15 conidia	4	10–12	Short and stocky, with septa	Solitary; right angle to hyphae	Velvety gray-green or olive-green with jet black reverse	Slow	Disjuncture scars may be visible; shield cells may be present
Fonsecaea species	3 × 5	Oval to elliptical	Varies with type of conidiation	2–3	Variable	Variable	Solitary	Velvety gray-green or olive-green with jet black reverse	Slow	At least two patterns of conidiation
Xylohypha bantiana	Variable	Elliptical	Branching chains of ≥20 conidia	4	10	Sticklike	Solitary; oblique angle to hyphae	Dematiaceous velvety	Slow	Conidia lack disjuncture scars

The dematiaceous fungi that produce conidia in chains may be identified to genus by the details of their microscopic morphology.

exoantigen test has been reported for identification of the mature form of *E. jeanselmei*, but it is not yet available commercially.

■ **Special Precautions.** None are needed, but specimens should be handled within a biologic safety cabinet.

■ **Culture Media.** Modified SDA, modified SDA with antimicrobials. Granules found in specimens should be washed in sterile water or an aqueous solution of antibiotics before they are planted on the agar surface.

Preferred Temperature. Grows at temperatures of 25° to 37°C; on SDA 25° to 30°C is the optimum temperature. At 37°C *E. jeanselmei* grows slowly on SDA, with more rapid growth on PDA.

■ **Differential Methods** (see Table 6.2). A colony suspected of being *Exophiala jeanselmei* can be tested for its ability to grow at differing temperatures, and for its effect on casein (o), tyrosine (+), and nitrate (+), as well as its reaction to cycloheximide (sensitive). Microscopic morphology is also important in identification.

■ **Macroscopic (Colony) Morphology.** On modified SDA at 25° to 30°C colonies of *E. jeanselmei* initially resemble colonies of black yeast. After 10 to 14 days the organism begins to develop short aerial mycelia, creating a velvety texture. Surface pigment becomes olive-gray to brownish black with a jet black reverse. The topography is typically dome shaped, folded, and spreading.

■ **Microscopic Morphology** (Figs. 6.13 through 6.17). Yeast cells predominate in young cultures; these technically belong to the genus *Phaeoannellomyces*, a synanamorph of *E. jeanselmei*. As cultures age they develop septate branched hyphae. Sometimes the hyphae have swellings and tortuous bends and turns. Hyphae are relatively broad (average width 4 μm) with a greenish brown pigment.

The conidiogenous cells are annellides. They may be almost imperceptible on individual cells such as we see with "budding yeasts"; they may be incorporated within the hyphae; or the annellides may develop on short denticles or annellophores on the hyphae. The annellides and annellophores may be hyaline or lightly pigmented; distinguishing them from the hyphae can be difficult. Annellides that are integrated with their supporting conidiophores and extend above them are flask shaped or cylindrical, resembling phialides. The annellides become longer and more narrow at their apices as each annelloconidium is produced, leaving an annellation.

Annelloconidia are small (approximately 3 μm wide by 4 to 5 μm long) elliptical to subglobose forms with smooth walls; the unicellular structures may be hyaline or light brown. The conidia tend to accumulate in clusters

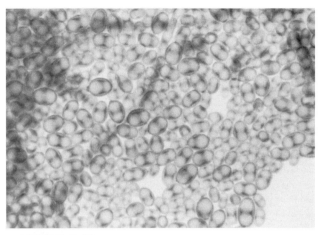

FIGURE 6.13

*Young cultures of *Exophiala jeanselmei* are actually the synanamorph *Phaeoannellomyces*. In typical cultures the cells generally resemble other yeasts except for the light brown pigment. Some cells show a pinched look or a bruise where annellides are beginning to form: look at the lower right quadrant.*

at the apex of the annellide and slide down the annellophore onto the hypha.

In *direct examination* (Fig. 6.18) of specimens the granules formed by *E. jeanselmei* resemble flecks of black pepper. Microscopically the granules are seen to be vermiform, 0.2 to 0.3 mm in diameter, with hollow centers. They are often associated with giant cells. The granules are microcolonies of the fungus, composed of thick-walled hyphae and moderately large (5 to 10 μm) chlamydoconidia-like cells.

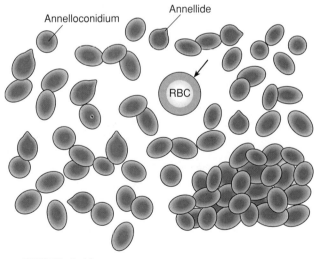

FIGURE 6.14

Exophiala jeanselmei produces yeastlike cells in younger cultures. The cells are difficult to distinguish from other yeasts except for the light brown pigment. Some cells have almost imperceptible buds or protrusions, the annellides. The 7-μm red blood cell (RBC) (arrow) shows the relative sizes of the mycotic elements.

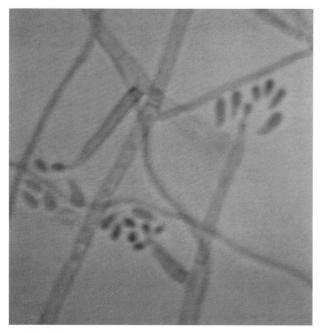

FIGURE 6.15

Typical cultures of *m*ature *Exophiala jeanselmei* are the *m*ould form, with septate brown hyphae. Conidiophores are sticklike, tapered at the tip, and topped at the apices with clusters of elliptical conidia. Septa, and the swollen areas of the hypha associated with this mould, are clearly shown.

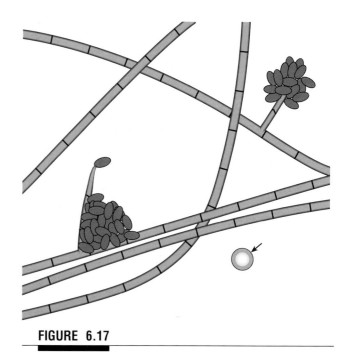

FIGURE 6.17

In bad preparations *Exophiala* should be considered if the hyphae and other structures are dematiaceous and clusters of elliptical conidia are seen at the tips of sticklike conidiophores with tapering tips. Colony morphology is not helpful in distinguishing the species, but careful examination of the annellophores may suggest the species' identity. Biochemical tests can be done to confirm the identification. The 7-μm red blood cell (arrow) shows the relative sizes of the mycotic elements.

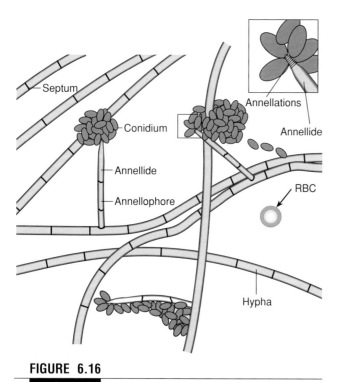

FIGURE 6.16

Exophiala jeanselmei, in the *m*ature *m*ould form, has brown septate hyphae that may have swollen areas, bends, and turns. Annellides may be produced on sticklike conidiophores or on short denticles, or they may form directly on the hyphae. Annellides that form on annellophores are flask shaped or cylindrical, resembling phialides somewhat. The annellides taper at their apices *(inset)*, and annellations are created as each annelloconidium is produced. The 7-μm red blood cell (RBC) (arrow) shows the relative sizes of the mycotic elements.

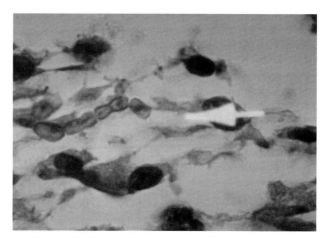

FIGURE 6.18

In tissue *Exophiala jeanselmei* appears as dark brown thick-walled hyphal fragments and cells resembling chlamydoconidia; in this photomicrograph the chain starts at the left edge and extends toward the center. Unchecked, these components aggregate into black, relatively large vermiform granules that are visible macroscopically in exudate from the infected area.

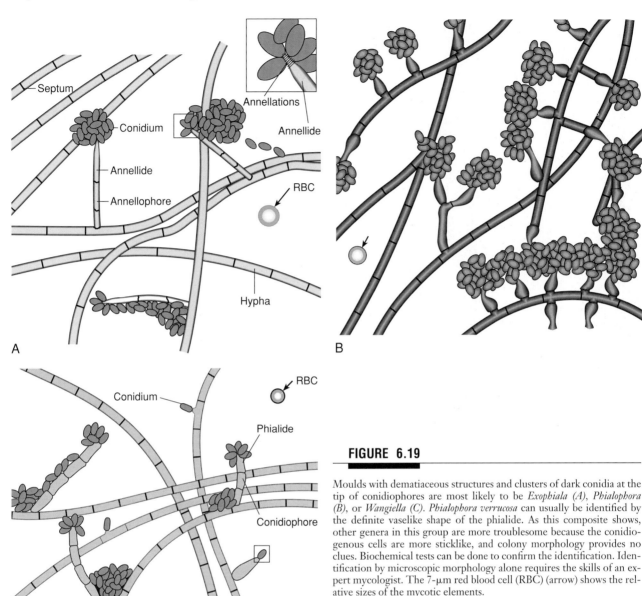

A

B

C

FIGURE 6.19

Moulds with dematiaceous structures and clusters of dark conidia at the tip of conidiophores are most likely to be *Exophiala (A)*, *Phialophora (B)*, or *Wangiella (C)*. *Phialophora verrucosa* can usually be identified by the definite vaselike shape of the phialide. As this composite shows, other genera in this group are more troublesome because the conidiogenous cells are more sticklike, and colony morphology provides no clues. Biochemical tests can be done to confirm the identification. Identification by microscopic morphology alone requires the skills of an expert mycologist. The 7-μm red blood cell (RBC) (arrow) shows the relative sizes of the mycotic elements.

■ **Helpful Features for Identification of *Exophiala jeanselmei*** (Fig. 6.19)

   *Y*oung black *y*east colonies
   *M*ature olive-gray to brownish black *m*ould-form colonies with a black reverse
   Pigmented annellides and annelloconidia
   Brown hyphae and black vermiform granules in tissue samples and aspirates
   Characteristic lesions with localized subcutaneous cysts or nodules, usually on the extremities
   Effect on nitrate (+), casein (o), and tyrosine (+)
   Sensitivity to cycloheximide

■ **Organisms from Which *Exophiala jeanselmei* Must Be Differentiated** (Table 6.4; see also Table 4.4)

   Other dematiaceous fungi that cause subcutaneous infections, especially those that produce annelloconidia

---

TABLE 6.4 Dematiaceous Fungi that Produce Conidia in Clusters

Fungus	Size of Conidia (μm)	Shape of Conidia	Arrangement of Conidia	Width of Hyphae (μm)	Length of Conidiophore (μm)	Shape of Conidiophore	Arrangement of Conidiophores	Colony Morphology	Growth Rate	Other Helpful Features
Exophiala jeanselmei	3 × 5	Elliptical to subglobose	Clusters on tips of annellophores	4	30–40	Sticklike, with tapering at the tips; annellations may be visible	Solitary	Dematiaceous	Intermediate	Hyphal swellings and bends; young yeast, **mature mould**. Annellides
Exophiala werneckii	2.5 × 6	Elliptical	Pairs	7	≤30	Sticklike annellides	Solitary	Dematiaceous	Intermediate	**Young yeast, mature mould** with annellides
Phialophora verrucosa	3 × 5	Ovoid to elliptical	Clusters around tip of phialide	3	10–15	Vase-shaped phialides with collarettes	Solitary	Dematiaceous	Slow	Conidiation resembles vases of flowers
Wangiella dermatitidis	2 × 4.5	Oval	Clusters around tip of phialide	3–4	10–20	Flask-shaped or cylindrical phialides without collarettes	Solitary	Dematiaceous	Slow	Cylindrical phialides without collarettes; **young yeast, mature mold**

A study of microscopic structures is essential if the dematiaceous fungi that produce conidia in clusters are to be identified.

Subcutaneous Pathogens

DEMATIACEAE

EXOPHIALA WERNECKII

E. werneckii, an agent of the superficial mycotic infection tinea nigra, is discussed in Chapter 4. It is listed here also because *E. jeanselmei* and other subcutaneous fungi, especially those that produce annelloconidia, may be confused with it.

Subcutaneous Pathogens

DEMATIACEAE

FONSECAEA PEDROSOI   (Fahn-seek-uh puh-drow-soy)

Note: Common sense has overruled rigid adherence to alphabetical order, and *Fonsecaea compacta* has been placed after *F. pedrosoi* because much of the description of *F. compacta* involves comparison to the more commonly encountered species, *F. pedrosoi*.

- **Teleomorph.** None has been identified.

- **Reservoirs.** *F. pedrosoi* is found in soil, on rotting wood, and in decaying vegetation. It is found worldwide, more often in tropical and subtropical zones than in the United States.

- **Unique Risk Factors.** Infections with *F. pedrosoi* most often occur in farmers and others who work in the soil barefooted in lightweight clothing that doesn't protect them. Repeated exposure and poor general health may contribute to development of the infection.

- **Human Infection.** *F. pedrosoi* can cause chromoblastomycosis or phaeohyphomycosis. The fungi are apparently introduced into host tissues through some minor injury where a contaminated splinter or thorn penetrates the skin. The infection spreads by autoinoculation and through the lymphatic system. The organism may be dormant for a long time until a second injury, occurring after the fungus has adjusted to survival in human tissue, initiates an active infection. A secondary infection with bacteria may occur, blocking lymph channels and resulting in elephantiasis.

    The symptoms of chromoblastomycosis and phaeohyphomycosis caused by *Fonsecaea* resemble infections caused by other fungi. For a more detailed discussion, refer to the Introduction to this chapter.

- **Specimen Sources.** Superficial crusts, skin scrapings, tissue from lesions, and aspirates of pus from microabscesses are most likely to be submitted for culture.

- **Specimen Collection and Handling.** No special measures are needed. Specimens should be collected aseptically and placed in sterile containers, then transported promptly to the laboratory. Tissue to be cultured should be minced or ground before the medium is inoculated.

    Direct examination of material from crusted areas should include treatment with 10% KOH (to which stain or ink may be added) prior to microscopic examination. Purulent aspirates can be cleared with 10% to 15% KOH and studied with simple wet mounts. Submit a request to the histology laboratory to fix and stain tissue specimens for microscopic examination.

- **Immunology.** CF, precipitin, fluorescent antibody, ID, and immunoelectrophoresis tests have been researched but many cross-reactions occur among the agents of chromoblastomycosis and phaeohyphomycosis. Despite the cross-reactions, the rise and fall of precipitin titers may be helpful in determining the prognosis following treatment.

- **Special Precautions.** None are needed, but work should be done in a biologic safety cabinet.

- **Culture Media.** Modified SDA, modified SDA with cycloheximide and antibacterial agents.

Preferred Temperature. Grows at temperatures of 25° to 37°C.

- **Macroscopic (Colony) Morphology.** Within 2 to 3 weeks at 25° to 30°C colonies of *F. pedrosoi* appear on modified SDA. They are olive-green to olive-gray to black, with a jet black reverse pigment. The surface is spreading and flat, or it may be slightly heaped in the center, or folded. A short aerial mycelium results in a velvety or woolly texture. Colonies may be slightly embedded in the medium.

- **Microscopic Morphology** (Figs. 6.20 and 6.21). The dark brown hyphae of *F. pedrosoi* are 2 to 5 μm wide, with septa and branching. Three types of anamorphic conidiation may be seen. At least two different patterns of conidiation must be present if the fungus is to be identified as a *Fonsecaea*. Rhinocladiella and cladosporium types predominate. Rhinocladiella type is characterized by the formation of **primary** (first level) conidia on denticles on erect septate conidiophores. The conidiophores are swollen at their apices after the sympodial production

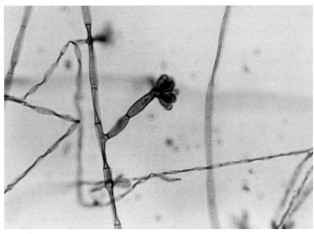

FIGURE 6.20

Typical cultures of *Fonsecaea pedrosoi* have dematiaceous septate hyphae. This dark septate conidiophore, with oval conidia produced sympodially from the tip, is a rhinocladiella-type of conidiation. At least two of the three types of anamorphic conidiation (rhinocladiella, phialophora, cladosporium) must be seen. A cautious mycologist keeps looking even if the rhinocladiella type, which is not found in other genera, is found first; this could be the beginning of a beautiful *Cladosporium*.

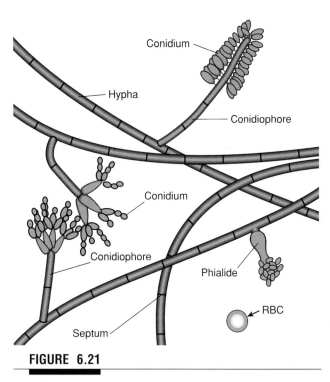

FIGURE 6.21

Fonsecaea pedrosoi has dark brown septate branching hyphae. Conidia are oval to elliptical and dark brown. Phialophora-type conidiation *(lower right quadrant)* is least common. Well-developed rhinocladiella-type conidiation, with tertiary conidiogeny, may be confused with cladosporium-type conidiation. Generally the chains of conidia are longer in cladosporium-type conidiation; a careful search should be made for shield cells and disjuncture scars. Well-developed rhinocladiella-type sporulation is shown in the upper right quadrant. The cladosporium-type is suspended from the hyphae on the lower left half of the drawing. The conidiation in the extreme lower left could be either rhinocladiella or cladosporium type; it is most likely to be cladosporium type because the conidia at the ends are about the same size, suggesting chaining.

of the conidia. These conidia are hyaline or light brown, elliptical, and smooth walled. **Secondary** conidia are sometimes produced by these primary conidiogenous cells, forming complex, multilevel conidial heads. Cladosporium-type conidiation is also present. All the conidia in the chains have hila at the point where they connect to other blastoconidia. Both primary and secondary conidia are approximately 2 × 5 μm. Shield cells, with three dark disjuncture scars, are formed where the chains branch.

Phialides resembling those of *Phialophora verrucosa* may develop directly on the hyphae, but they are found infrequently, and few details of their structure are given in standard texts. The phialoconidia are approximately 2 × 3 μm (Fig. 6.22).

In *direct examination* look for brown yeastlike cells and dark brown pigmented hyphal fragments (average diameter, 4 μm) with branching. Sclerotic bodies may be found in the tissue and exudates.

■ Helpful Features for Identification of *Fonsecaea pedrosoi*

Characteristic olive-black colonies with black reverse
Slo-o-o-o-w growth of the fungus
Presence of two or more types of anamorphic conidiation

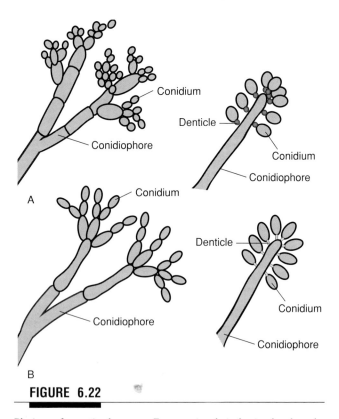

FIGURE 6.22

Placing a fungus in the genus *Fonsecaea* is relatively simple when the colony is mature. Identifying the isolate to species requires expert assistance and is probably unnecessary. *Fonsecaea compacta (A)* is described as more compact than *Fonsecaea pedrosoi (B)*, but "more compact" is difficult to determine even when known typical isolates are used for comparison.

Predominance of cladosporium- and rhinocladiella-type conidiation, with occasional phialophora-type forms

Characteristic appearance of the lesion in well-developed infections

■ **Organisms from Which *Fonsecaea pedrosoi* Must Be Differentiated** (Table 6.5; see also Table 6.3)

Other dematiaceous fungi that cause chromoblastomycosis and phaeohyphomycosis, especially *F. compacta*

Subcutaneous Pathogens

DEMATIACEAE

FONSECAEA COMPACTA (Fahn-seek'-uh komm-pack'-ta)

Debate continues as to whether *F. compacta* is a separate species or a strain of *Fonsecaea pedrosoi*.

■ **Teleomorph.** None has been identified.

■ **Reservoirs.** *F. compacta* is found in soil, on rotting wood, and in decaying vegetation. It has been found in Martinique, Liberia, Russia, and Cuba but is rarely seen in the United States.

■ **Unique Risk Factors.** See the discussion for *F. pedrosoi*.

■ **Human Infection.** *F. compacta* has rarely been isolated in the United States from cases of chromoblastomycosis; only three cases have been officially confirmed. The disease process parallels that for *F. pedrosoi*.

■ **Specimen Sources.** Superficial crusts, skin scrapings, tissue from lesions, and aspirates of pus from microabscesses are most likely to be submitted for culture.

■ **Specimen Collection and Handling.** No special measures are needed. Specimens should be collected aseptically and placed in sterile containers, then transported promptly to the laboratory. Tissue specimens should be fixed and stained by the histology laboratory.

Direct examination of material from crusted areas should include treatment with 10% KOH (to which stain or ink may be added) prior to microscopic examination. Purulent aspirates can be studied with simple wet mounts after treatment with 10% KOH to clear them.

■ **Immunology.** No tests are available except as related to *F. pedrosoi*.

■ **Special Precautions.** None are needed, but work should be done in a biologic safety cabinet.

■ **Culture Media.** Modified SDA, SDA with antimicrobials.

Preferred Temperature. Grows at temperatures of 25° to 37°C.

■ **Macroscopic (Colony) Morphology.** After 3 to 4 weeks at 25° to 30°C on modified SDA, colonies of *F. compacta* are olive-green to black, with a jet black reverse pigment. The surface may be flat, or it may have radial folds with a brittle texture. Several weeks later the surface is covered with tufts of short brown aerial mycelium, which gives the colony a velvety texture. Colonies may be slightly embedded in the medium.

■ **Microscopic Morphology** (Fig. 6.23). The microscopic morphology of *F. compacta* closely resembles that of *F. pedrosoi*—so closely, in fact, that debate continues in some circles about whether these are two species or one species with two variants. Stay tuned for further bulletins. One difference between the species is that the conidial heads, especially those produced in cladosporium-type conidiation, are more complex and compact than those of *F. pedrosoi*. Another difference is that *F. compacta* grows more slowly, and the primary conidiogenous cells are somewhat smaller, less elliptical, and more ovoid than those of *F. pedrosoi*. A third difference is that the denticles seen in rhinocladiella-type conidiation are *cask shaped* (resembling small barrels—microscopic ones, in this case) and are characteristically broader than *F. pedrosoi*. For more information about the microscopic morphology of *F. compacta*, read the Microscopic Morphology section for *F. pedrosoi*. The fact is that differences between the two species are unlikely to be noted unless the unknown organism is compared to known *typical* examples of both species of *Fonsecaea*.

In *direct examination* the picture is similar to that for *F. pedrosoi*.

■ **Helpful Features for Identification of *Fonsecaea compacta*** (see Fig. 6.22)

Characteristic olive-black colonies with black reverse

Slo-o-o-o-w growth of the fungus

Presence of more than one type of anamorphic conidiation

Predominance of cladosporium- and rhinocladiella-type conidiation, with occasional phialophora-type forms

Characteristic appearance of the lesion in well-developed infections

■ **Organisms from Which *Fonsecaea compacta* Must Be Differentiated** (see Tables 6.3 and 6.4)

Other dematiaceous fungi that cause chromoblastomycosis and phaeohyphomycosis, especially *F. pedrosoi*

TABLE 6.5 Fungi with Multiple Arrangements of Conidia

Fungus	Size of Conidia (μm)	Shape of Conidia	Arrangement of Conidia	Width of Hyphae (μm)	Length of Conidiophore (μm)	Shape of Conidiophore	Arrangement of Conidiophores	Colony Morphology	Growth Rate	Other Helpful Features
Fonsecaea pedrosoi	3 × 5	Oval to elliptical	Varies with type of conidiation	2–3	Variable	Variable	Solitary	Velvety gray-green or olive-green with jet black reverse	Slow	At least two types of conidiation
Fonsecaea compacta	Closely resembles *Fonsecaea pedrosoi*, but structures are "more compact."									
Sporothix schenckii	1.5 × 2 and 2 × 3	Oval to pyriform and spherical to oval	Rosettes or sleeves and singly	1–2	10–20	Tapering toward center with small vesicles at apices	Upright	Mould develops dark pigment with age; leathery or velvety texture	Intermediate	Thermal dimorph; two types of conidia and two arrangements of conidia may be present
Acremonium	3 × 6	Elliptical phialoconidia at tips of conidiophores	Slimy balls	3	30–35 from base to tip	Tapers smoothly roughly right	Solitary, at pastel surface angles to hyphae	Cottony texture; pigment	Rapid	Hyaline

The fungi that produce conidia in more than one arrangement are differentiated by attention to the size of the microscopic structures as well as the patterns and shapes.

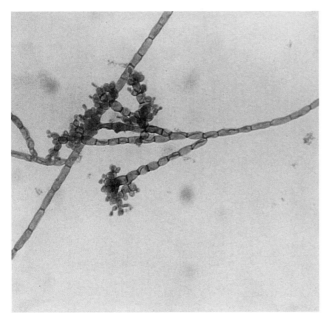

FIGURE 6.23

Fonsecaea compacta resembles *Fonsecaea pedrosoi* closely, with dark brown hyphae and the same patterns of conidiation (cladosporium, phialophora, and rhinicladiella types). The decision about whether the structures are "more compact" is difficult to make.

Subcutaneous Pathogens

CRYPTOCOCCACEAE

PHAEOANNELLOMYCES SPECIES

Phaeoannellomyces species are the black yeasts most frequently isolated in the clinical laboratory. They occur as a synanamorph associated with *Exophiala* species (see Figs. 6.13 and 6.14).

Subcutaneous Pathogens

CRYPTOCOCCACEAE

PHAEOCOCCOMYCES SPECIES

Phaeococcomyces species are black yeasts that may occur as the synanamorph associated with species of *Wangiella* and other genera (see Fig. 6.39). Conidiophores and hyphae are absent in the young colonies. Conidia, blastoconidia, and annelloconidia are also absent. Unicellular yeast cells are pale brown to black; pseudohyphae may be present. Blastoconidia are multilateral; that is, they develop on several sides of the parent cell. When the fungus grows on PDA, it rapidly pro-

duces hyphae and conidiogenous cells typical of the mature synanamorph.

Subcutaneous Pathogens

DEMATIACEAE

PHIALOPHORA VERRUCOSA (Fy-uh-loff-ore-uh verr-uh-kose-uh)

■ **Teleomorph.** None has been identified.

■ **Reservoirs.** *P. verrucosa* is found in soil, on wood and wood pulp, and in decaying vegetation. It is found worldwide but more often in tropical and subtropical areas and in the temperate zone of the United States.

■ **Unique Risk Factors.** Infections with *P. verrucosa* most often occur in people who work outdoors without protective clothing such as shoes and gloves. Repeated exposure and poor general health may contribute to development of the infection.

■ **Human Infection.** *P. verrucosa* can cause chromoblastomycosis or phaeohyphomycosis. The fungi are apparently introduced into host tissues through some minor injury where a contaminated splinter or thorn penetrates the skin. The infection spreads by autoinoculation and via the lymphatic system. The organism may be dormant for a long time until a second injury to the host, after the fungus has adjusted to survival in human tissue, initiates an active infection. Secondary infections with bacteria may occur; this sometimes leads to blockage of the lymph channels and elephantiasis. For a more detailed discussion of chromoblastomycosis and phaeohyphomycosis, consult the Introduction to this chapter.

■ **Specimen Sources.** Superficial crusts, skin scrapings, tissue from lesions, and aspirates of pus from microabscesses are most likely to be submitted for culture.

■ **Specimen Collection and Handling.** No special measures are needed. Specimens should be collected aseptically and placed in sterile containers, then transported promptly to the laboratory. Tissue specimens should be minced or ground before they are placed on the culture media.

Direct examination of material from crusted areas should include treatment with 10% KOH (to which stain or ink may be added) prior to microscopic examination. Purulent aspirates can be studied with simple wet mounts; 10% to 15% KOH can be used to clear the specimen if necessary. Tissue samples should be given to the histology laboratory to be fixed and stained.

■ **Immunology.** CF, precipitin, fluorescent antibody, ID, and electroimmunodiffusion tests have been researched, but many cross-reactions occur among the agents of chromoblastomycosis and phaeohyphomycosis. The rise and fall of precipitin titers may be helpful in determining the prognosis following treatment.

■ **Special Precautions.** None are needed, but work should be done in a biologic safety cabinet.

■ **Culture Media.** Modified SDA, modified SDA with cycloheximide and antibacterial antibiotics. Some variants of *P. verrucosa* are sensitive to chloramphenicol.

Preferred Temperature. Grows at temperatures of 25° to 37°C.

■ **Differential Tests** (see Table 6.2). Tests that are helpful for differentiation of *P. verrucosa* are starch hydrolysis (o), gelatin liquefaction (o) and coagulation of milk (o).

■ **Macroscopic (Colony) Morphology.** Within 2 to 3 weeks colonies of *P. verrucosa* on modified SDA at 25° to 30°C are olive-green to black, with a gray-black to jet black reverse pigment. The surface is spreading and flat with radial folds; the covering of short aerial mycelium results in a velvety texture. Colonies may be slightly embedded in the medium.

■ **Microscopic Morphology** (Figs. 6.24 through 6.26). The hyphae of *P. verrucosa* are approximately 3 μm wide, with septa and branching. In unstained preparations they have a brown pigment. Only phialophora-type conidiation is seen. Phialides develop laterally or terminally from conidiophores on the hyphae or directly along the

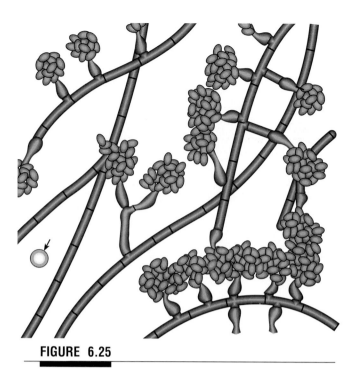

FIGURE 6.25

Phialophora verrucosa has dark brown hyphae, conidia, conidiophores, and phialides. The phialides form directly on the hyphae or on intermediate conidiophores. They are obviously vase shaped, with a flared collarette at the apex. Conidia are oval or elliptical, arranged in clusters at the mouth of the phialide or, in older cultures, resting on the hyphae. The 7-μm red blood cell (arrow) shows the relative sizes of the mycotic elements.

hyphae itself. The conidiophores also have a light brown pigment. The flask-shaped or cylindrical phialides have flared brown collarettes at their apices. The phialoconidia are unicellular ovoid to elliptical structures that are hyaline or pale brown. These relatively small (average 3 × 5 μm) conidia tend to accumulate at the apices of the phialides in balls held together by a sticky substance.

In *direct examination* look for yeastlike cells that are hyaline to brown and dark brown hyphal fragments (average diameter, 4 μm) with branching. In well-developed chromoblastomycosis the tissue and exudates also contain *sclerotic bodies* (see Fig. 6–3). These are about 8 μm in diameter, with muriform septa dividing them into one to four cells. These sclerotic bodies, sometimes called "copper pennies," may be in clusters or chainlike arrangements.

■ **Helpful Features for Identification of *Phialophora verrucosa*** (see Fig. 6.19)

Characteristic dark olive-green to black colonies with black reverse
Slo-o-o-o-w growth of the fungus
Phialophora-type conidiation with flask-shaped phialides
Pigmented brown-green hyphae and sclerotic bodies in specimens

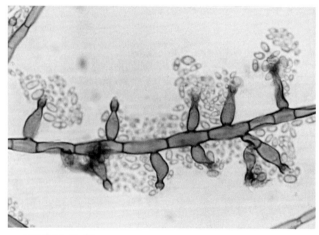

FIGURE 6.24

Typical preparations of *Phialophora verrucosa* show septate dematiaceous hyphae and dark, distinctly vase-shaped phialides with flared openings. Clusters of paler oval conidia surmount the phialides or rest on the hyphae adjacent to the phialide.

FIGURE 6.26

Even in bad preparations *Phialophora verrucosa* can usually be recognized by the distinct shape of the conidiogenous cell with its swollen center, tapered neck, and flared collarette *(inset)*. When this is seen with darkly pigmented structures, and clusters of oval conidia, *Phialophora verrucosa* is the probable identity even when the conidia are scattered instead of clustered in a well-mannered way at the mouth of the phialide. Biochemical tests can be used to confirm the identity, but this is usually unnecessary. The 7-μm red blood cell (RBC) (arrow) shows the relative sizes of the mycotic elements.

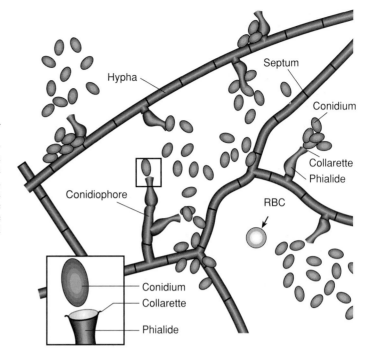

Characteristic appearance of the lesion in well-developed infections

Negative for starch hydrolysis, gelatin liquefaction, and coagulation of milk

- **Organisms from Which *Phialophora verrucosa* Must Be Differentiated** (see Table 6.4)

Other dematiaceous fungi that cause chromoblastomycosis and phaeohyphomycosis, especially *Fonsecaea pedrosoi*, *Fonsecaea compacta*, *Cladosporium carrionii*, and *Xylohypha bantiana*

Subcutaneous Pathogens

PLECTOMYCETES

PSEUDALLESCHERIA BOYDII (Sued-al[7]uh-sheer-ee-uh boy-dee)

- **Teleomorph.** *Pseudallescheria boydii.*

  P. boydii is unique among fungi pathogenic for humans because it is a perfect fungus, able to produce both sexually and asexually in culture on standard media. The sexual form (teleomorph) and the holomorph (the whole fungus, including the anamorphic forms) are both called *P. boydii*. It has two anamorphs or asexual forms, *Scedosporium apiospermum* and *Graphium* species; these are synanamorphs of each other.

- **Reservoirs.** *P. boydii* is found worldwide in temperate and subtropical zones in soil, manure, water from polluted streams, and sewage sludge.

- **Unique Risk Factors.** There are no risk factors other than exposure to the organism in circumstances in which a minor injury could introduce the fungus into tissue.

- **Human Infection.** *P. boydii* is the major etiologic agent of eumycotic mycetoma in the United States and Europe. This mycetoma is characterized by white or light-colored granules in drainage from the infection. For a more complete description of mycetomas, including the difference between eumycotic and actinomycotic mycetomas, refer to the introduction for this chapter.

  P. boydii has also been found in infections of immunocompromised and debilitated patients. In these circumstances the fungus may spread to other tissues or, more rarely, disseminate into systemic infection. It has been reported as the cause of infections of the lung, nasal sinuses, ear, eye, central nervous system, and brain. In the lungs *P. boydii* may form a tumor-like mass, a *fungoma*, that resembles an aspergilloma.

  In contrast with the other subcutaneous fungi *P. boydii* grows rapidly, is hyaline, and is a perfect fungus.

- **Specimen Sources.** Aspirated pus from nodules or sinuses, tissue removed from subcutaneous cysts or nodules, and respiratory specimens are most likely to be submitted for culture.

- **Specimen Collection and Handling.** Specimens should be collected aseptically into sterile containers and

---

[7]"Al" as in al-ligator.

transported to the laboratory without delay. Granules in specimens should be washed in sterile water or a solution of antibacterial agents—*not* cycloheximide—before they are planted on the surface of the agar. Tissue should be ground or minced before it is inoculated to the medium.

Direct examination of material from crusted areas should include treatment with 10% KOH (to which stain or ink may be added) prior to microscopic examination. Purulent aspirates can be studied with simple wet mounts, with 10% to 15% KOH as a clearing agent if this is necessary. Tissues should be fixed and stained in the histology laboratory.

■ **Immunology.** CF tests have not been found to be useful. Gel ID with precipitin bands is currently used, especially if the diagnosis of *P. boydii* infection cannot be confirmed with a positive culture. The precipitin bands that appear during an active infection disappear following adequate treatment and healing. A screening test, using a carbohydrate antigen (antigen I) made from culture filtrates of different strains of *Pseudallescheria* species, and an exoantigen test, are available.

■ **Special Precautions.** Specimens should be handled within a biologic safety cabinet.

■ **Culture Media.** Modified SDA, modified SDA with antimicrobials. While *P. boydii* is not susceptible to cycloheximide, *S. apiospermum* and other agents of mycetoma are. PDA, PFA, 2% water agar, or CMA should be used to enhance conidiation.

Phenoethyl alcohol (PEA) agar, potato-carrot agar, or plain water agar can be used to encourage production of cleistothecia. Tomato juice agar or oatmeal agar can also be used.

Preferred Temperature. Grows at temperatures of 30° to 37°C.

■ **Macroscopic (Colony) Morphology.** After 7 to 10 days on modified SDA at 30°C colonies of *P. boydii/S. apiospermum/Graphium* species appear white and fluffy. They soon spread across the agar surface and become brownish gray to black with a woolly texture as conidia develop. The reverse of the colony is gray to black. With some isolates, and on some types of media, the colony eventually becomes sprinkled with dark gray to black flecks resembling pepper—the cleistothecia indicative of the sexual or teleomorph form, *P. boydii*. Cleistothecia are most often found at the periphery of the colony; they may be slightly submerged so that the agar needs to be scraped for microscopic preparations and subcultures.

■ **Microscopic Morphology.** For *P. boydii* the teleomorph (Figs. 6.27 and 6.28), the characteristic feature is the presence of the sexual ascocarps, the cleistothecia. The cleistothecia are large (50 to 200 μm) dark brown to

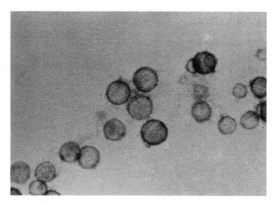

FIGURE 6.27

Typical preparations of *Pseudallescheria boydii* are mixed with structures of one of the anamorphs. The large globose cleistothecia lying from lower left to upper right across the field must be present for identification as *Pseudallescheria boydii*; the ascospores are seen here only as a graininess within the cleistothecia. At this magnification anamorphic structures are not visible. Colony in agar. ×50. (From Rippon JW: Medical Mycology: The Pathogenic Fungi and the Pathogenic Actinomycetes, 3rd ed. Philadelphia, WB Saunders, 1988, p 674.)

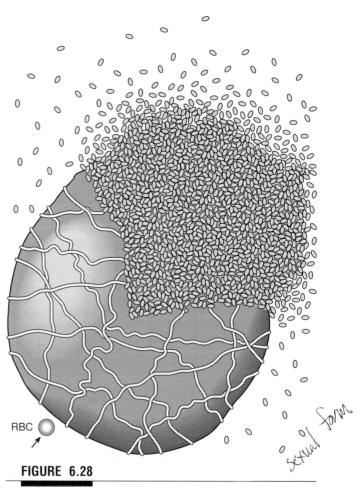

RBC

FIGURE 6.28

Pseudallescheria boydii has large, dark, rounded cleistothecia with thick walls, bound into the hyphae of an anamorphic fungus. Free asci are clavate to subglobose. In this figure individual light brown ascospores are being released from a mature cleistothecium. The 7-μm red blood cell (RBC) (arrow) shows the relative sizes of the mycotic elements.

black globes with thick walls (average 5 μm). The walls are composed of two or three layers of septate hyphae about 3-μm wide that are interwoven. The cleistothecia are invariably found enmeshed in the hyphae of one of the anamorphs. They contain clavate to subglobose asci that are released when the cleistothecia rupture. Each ascus produces up to eight oval to elliptical light brown ascospores that are approximately 4 × 8 μm.

For anamorphs of *P. boydii* (*S. apiospermum*, *Graphium*), the hyphae are 1 to 3 μm wide, hyaline, and septate; they may branch. The conidiogenous cells are annellides that develop on the hyphae or on erect annellophores of varying lengths. The annelloconidia are unicellular, subglobose to ovoid, and colorless, with truncate bases. They are approximately 6 by 8 μm. The microscopic morphology of the anamorphs of *P. boydii* is unremarkable when the cleistothecia are not present. The pyriform or lemon-shaped conidia develop singly on the annellophores, like lollipops on a stick.

In *S. apiospermum* (Figs. 6.29 and 6.30) the annellides that are integrated with and extend above their annellophores are hyphae-like and cylindrical. They narrow at their apices and are elongated by annellations as successive elliptical to subglobose annelloconidia are produced.

For *Graphium species* the annellophores are found in bundles or tufts called **synnemata,** which are borne on the hyphae. The long, narrow, erect annellophores are dark and hyphae-like; they appear to be glued together along the conidiophore, then to separate and radiate out at the tips. In *Graphium* species the pattern of annellophores grouped with their annelloconidia in synnematic tufts creates the appearance of a large ball.

In *direct examination* yellow or whitish granules are seen grossly in material from the lesion. They are small (1 to 2 mm) and usually are oval. Microscopic examination of the granules demonstrates septate hyphae (1.5 to

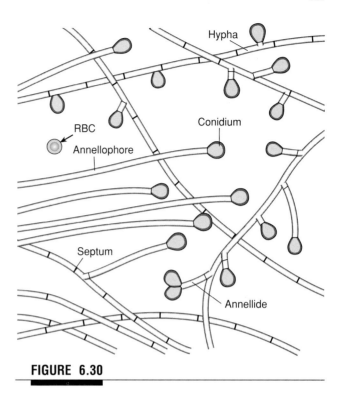

FIGURE 6.30

Scedosporium apiospermum has broad, hyaline, septate hyphae and sticklike annellophores. The brownish conidia are unicellular and pyriform, with truncate bases and a heavy cell wall. *S. apiospermum* does not produce striking or unique structures—just a bunch of lollipops on sticks of varying lengths. The 7-μm red blood cell (RBC) (arrow) shows the relative sizes of the mycotic elements.

5 μm) that are loosely intertwined. Numerous swollen cells may also be present.

■ Helpful Features for Identification of *Pseudallescheria boydii* and Its Synanamorphs

Colony morphology
Dark brown or black cleistothecia
Presence of asci and ascospores
"Lollipop" appearance of annellides and annelloconidia
White to yellow granules in specimens
Appearance of microscopic structures of the anamorphs, especially the synnemata of *Graphium*
Characteristic lesions with localized subcutaneous cysts or nodules, usually on the extremities

■ Organisms from Which *Pseudallescheria boydii* and Its Synanamorphs Must Be Differentiated (see Table 8.4)

Other fungi that cause subcutaneous infections, especially those that produce annelloconidia
Mould-form *Blastomyces dermatitidis*
Mould-form *Paracoccidioides brasiliensis*
Chrysosporium species

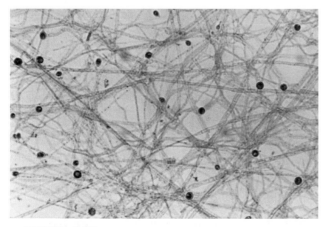

FIGURE 6.29

Typically *Scedosporium apiospermum* has broad hyaline hyphae with septa. Unicellular brownish conidia (appearing as dots) develop on the hyphae or on erect annellophores.

Subcutaneous Pathogens

MONILIACEAE[8]

SPOROTHRIX SCHENCKII   (Spore-oh-thricks schenck-ee)

■ **Teleomorph.** None has been identified.

■ **Reservoirs.** *S. schenckii* is found worldwide in both temperate and tropical zones, predominantly in Central and South America, Mexico, eastern Europe, and the north-central United States. The fungus is found in soil, vegetable debris, moist wood, wood pulp, and sphagnum moss and in some fertilizers.

■ **Unique Risk Factors.** Infection is associated with gardening and working in soil. It has been nicknamed "rose gardener's disease" because infections have often resulted from contact with the sphagnum moss used to mulch roses and other plants. Increasing numbers of infections have also been seen in people who maintain aquaria as a hobby.

■ **Human Infection.** *S. schenckii* is the etiologic agent of sporotrichosis, a chronic cutaneous and subcutaneous mycosis characterized by development of ulcers and abscesses along the lymphatic channels. Most infections are initiated by traumatic inoculation of the fungus into the host's tissues, but the infection can be contracted by inhalation. Swelling is NOT a significant feature of sporotrichosis. The lymphatic system *is* involved. Typically, ulcers form in succession along the lymph channel in the infected limb as the infection moves up the limb toward the regional lymph nodes. Five forms of sporotrichosis have been identified; the type of infection that develops depends on the portal of entry of the fungus, the dose, and the immunocompetence of the host.

■ **Specimen Sources.** Exudates and pus aspirated from draining lesions, respiratory secretions, and tissue and bone biopsy specimens are most likely to be submitted for culture. The use of swabs to obtain specimens for culture should be avoided whenever possible.

■ **Specimen Collection and Handling.** No special measures are needed. Specimens should be collected aseptically and placed in sterile containers, then transported promptly to the laboratory. Tissues should be minced or ground before they are placed on culture media.

Direct examination of material should include treatment with 10% KOH (to which stain or ink may be added) prior to microscopic examination. Purulent aspirates can be studied with simple wet mounts. KOH can be used as the mounting fluid, to clear the specimen, if this is necessary.

■ **Immunology.** A direct fluorescent antibody method may be useful for detecting *S. schenckii* in specimens when cultures are negative. The fluorescent antibodies are prepared by the immunization of rabbits with whole yeast cells of *S. schenckii*. The false-positive results that occur can be eliminated by diluting the specimen, but dilution requires that many microscopic fields be studied because dilution reduces the sensitivity of the method. The tests are available at the Centers for Disease Control and Prevention and in some reference laboratories.

A skin test similar to the tuberculin test for *Mycobacterium tuberculosis* can be used to determine whether the patient has been exposed to *S. schenckii*. The antigen is *sporotrichin*, made from heat-killed yeast cells. Specimens for other immunologic tests should be obtained before the sporotrichin skin test is performed. Patients with cutaneous sporotrichosis usually have a positive skin test, but those with disseminated sporotrichosis may be anergic.

CF, ID, latex agglutination (LA), tube agglutination (TA), and enzyme immunoassay (EIA) have also been developed. The LA, EIA, and TA tests are regarded as the most sensitive, specific, and reliable tests for extracutaneous or systemic sporotrichosis. The CF and ID tests lack sensitivity and are generally not useful for diagnosis; false-positive results are common due to cross-reactions with other fungi. An exoantigen test has been developed but it is not yet commercially available.

Generally both serum and cerebrospinal fluid can be tested; positive tests on cerebrospinal fluid provide strong evidence of meningeal sporotrichosis. When cerebrospinal fluid is tested, the EIA may be positive when the LA test is negative. The LA test will usually be positive for serum drawn at the time the cerebrospinal fluid is positive.

■ **Special Precautions.** None are needed but cultures should be handled within a biologic safety cabinet.

■ **Culture Media.** Modified SDA, modified SDA with cycloheximide and antibacterial agents. Brain-heart infusion agar (BHIA) with blood, for isolation of yeast-form colonies.

Preferred Temperature. Grows at temperatures of 25° to 37°C. Campbell reported that *S. schenckii* from fixed cutaneous and lymphocutaneous lesions may fail to grow at 37°C.

S. schenckii is thermally dimorphic, that is, the fungus has two different colony and microscopic morphologies

---

[8]This is an important exception to note: *Sporothrix schenckii* is classified in the Family Moniliaceae despite its ability to develop dark pigment on the surface and reverse of colonies. Perhaps this makes it easier to remember that colonies, especially the yeast form, often have dark patches or stripes instead of being uniformly dark.

that vary with the temperature at which it grows. Cultures grown at room temperature (25° to 30°C) develop the mould-form colony, while those incubated at body temperature (35° to 37°C) produce yeast-form colonies. Isolates can be converted from one phase to another by inoculating a new plate or tube of medium and incubating it at the "opposite" temperature. A yeast-phase colony, for example, can be produced by subculturing a mould colony of suspected *S. schenckii* to BHIA with 5% to 10% blood or BHI broth containing 0.1% agar and incubating the new culture at 35° to 37°C in 5% to 10% CO_2.

■ **Macroscopic (Colony) Morphology.** At 25° to 30°C a mould colony of *S. schenckii* appears within 3 to 5 days on modified SDA. Young colonies are cream to white, with a glabrous texture. Most colonies develop dark pigment as they age, although this varies somewhat with the isolate; some isolates remain mottled perpetually. Typical mature mould colonies are flat, leathery to velvety, and black with a black reverse pigment.

At 35° to 37°C colonies appear on modified SDA within 3 to 5 days as smooth yeastlike colonies resembling those of *Candida albicans*. The pigment is typically white, beige, or tan; black pigment rarely appears in yeast colonies except as streaks or striations.

■ **Microscopic Morphology.** At 25° to 30°C (Figs. 6.31 through 6.34) *S. schenckii* produces delicate, thin (1 to 2 μm) septate hyphae that are hyaline. Frequently the hyphae are found in parallel strands in a ropelike fashion. Conidiophores usually arise at right angles to the vegetative hyphae. They are slender (1 to 2 μm) and hyaline, and they taper to half their basal width before they swell into small vesicles at the apices. The vesicles are *denticulated*, that is, the surface is toothlike.

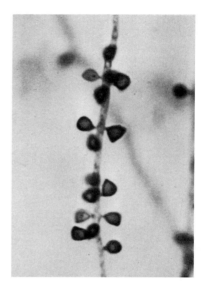

FIGURE 6.32

Older cultures of *Sporothrix schenckii* often also have a sprinkling of somewhat larger, darker conidia, sometimes (erroneously) called macroconidia, along the hyphae and around the conidiophores. These conidia probably help the mould survive hard times. ×2060. (Courtesy of R. Garrison.)

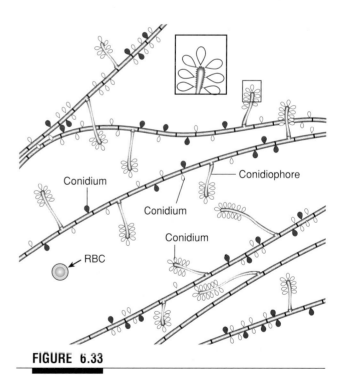

FIGURE 6.33

Sporothrix schenckii moulds have thin septate hyaline hyphae that sometimes intertwine into ropelike strands. The predominant conidia are clear pyriform cells produced on denticles around the tips of upright conidiophores forming rosettes or formed along either side of the hyphae to create sleeves for the hyphae. In older cultures dark, slightly larger conidia with thicker walls are seen among the sleeves and rosettes. The 7-μm red blood cell (RBC) (arrow) shows the relative sizes of the mycotic elements.

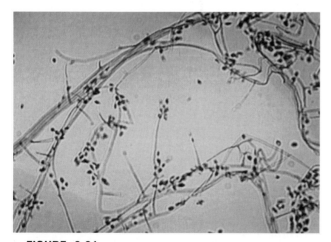

FIGURE 6.31

In typical preparations of mould-form *Sporothrix schenckii* very delicate septate hyphae are seen, with small, clear pyriform conidia. The conidia may be arrayed in a "sleeve" along the hyphae or, as you see in the center of the field, conidia may surround the tip of the conidiophore to form a rosette.

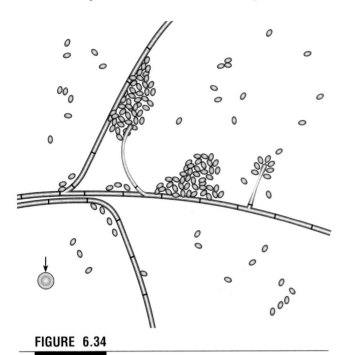

FIGURE 6.34

In bad preparations identification of *Sporothrix schenckii* is difficult. Frequently the conidia are dislodged from their delicate attachments. Small pyriform conidia and delicate septate hyphae in ropelike strands suggest *Sporothrix*. This suggestion is heightened if slender conidiophores with a small vesicle at the tip are present. The 7-μm red blood cell (arrow) shows the relative sizes of the mycotic elements.

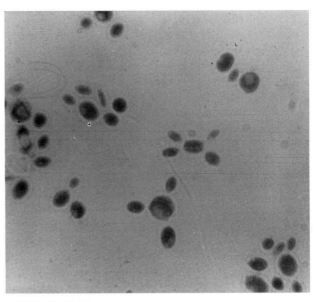

FIGURE 6.35

Sporothrix schenckii yeast typically have a variety of shapes. In preparations from colonies oval shapes predominate but "cigar shapes" and fusiform or globose cells as well as more bizarre forms may be seen. A cigar shape is included between two round cells in the group of five cells at 10 o'clock; it is pointing to the upper left corner of the field. The slender, threadlike connection between the mother and the daughter cell is not visible. (Courtesy of the Centers for Disease Control and Prevention.)

Two kinds of conidia are produced in mould colonies of *S. schenckii*. The first (smaller) type is hyaline, oval to pyriform, and unicellular, with thin walls. Two patterns of conidiation develop with the smaller conidia, a daisy-like or rosette pattern, and a sleevelike arrangement. In the *daisy* (rosette) pattern the conidia are produced sympodially on the vesicle at the apex of the conidiophore, attached to the conidiophore by delicate threadlike denticles. Later, when conidiation reaches its peak, the *sleevelike* appearance is produced by formation of the smaller hyaline conidia on threadlike denticles along the vegetative hyphae.

The second type of conidium is also unicellular, but it is dark brown and thick walled, with a spherical to oval (or, rarely, triangular) shape. These conidia are found singly along the conidiophores and vegetative hyphae, on short denticles. Their black pigment gives the dematiaceous look characteristic of *S. schenckii* colonies. The smaller hyaline conidium appears first, remains present as the dark brown type begins to develop, and typically predominates.

At 35° to 37°C (Figs. 6.35 and 6.36) colonies contain yeast cells that typically vary somewhat in size and shape, from globose to fusiform or oval. The average size is 2 × 6 μm. They are characterized as cigar shaped, with a delicate point of attachment between the mother and the daughter cells.

In *direct examination* of specimens (Fig. 6.37) the picture is similar to that for yeast colonies of *S. schenckii*.

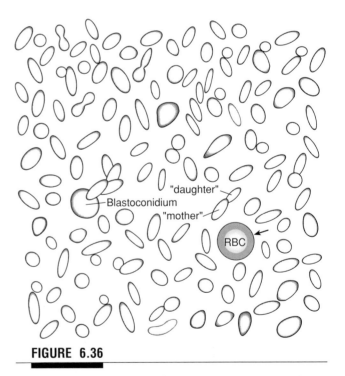

FIGURE 6.36

Yeast cultures of *Sporothrix schenckii* have varied shapes. The most common are oval but they may be globose or fusiform or somewhat bizarre in shape. Occasionally multiple budding cells are seen. Attachments between mother and daughter cells are easily disrupted in the process of preparing the slide. The 7-μm red blood cell (arrow) shows the relative sizes of the mycotic elements.

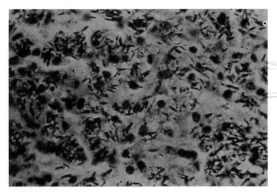

FIGURE 6.37

Sporothrix schenckii is most likely to demonstrate the characteristic cigar-shaped forms in preparations of infected tissue *if* any yeast cells can be seen. The fungus usually does not stain well in tissue unless special methods are used. ×400. (From Rippon JW: Medical Mycology: The Pathogenic Fungi and the Pathogenic Actinomycetes, 3rd ed. Philadelphia, WB Saunders, 1988, p 339.)

Yeast cells are rarely seen in specimens obtained from patients with sporotrichosis because they don't take up most stains. The methenamine silver nitrate stain works well. Specimens can be treated with a mixture of enzymes that converts starch to simple sugars, *malt diastase*, to enhance staining with other methods.

■ **Helpful Features for Identification of *Sporothrix schenckii*** (Fig. 6.38; see also Fig. 6.7)

Thermal dimorphism—the only dematiaceous fungus infecting humans that is thermally dimorphic

At 25° to 30°C

Leathery black or mottled black-and-white colonies
Thin septate hyphae
Tapering sympodial conidiophores with delicate attachments for conidia
Rosette/daisy-like and sleevelike arrangements of conidia
Both hyaline pyriform and black triangular conidia

At 35° to 37°C

Cream to tan yeastlike colony
Hyaline unicellular budding yeast forms, with a variety of shapes
Delicate connection between mother and daughter cells
Resistance to cycloheximide

■ **Organisms from Which *Sporothrix schenckii* Must Be Differentiated** (see Table 6.5)

Other *Sporothrix* species, and dematiaceous fungi with rhinocladiella-type sporulation

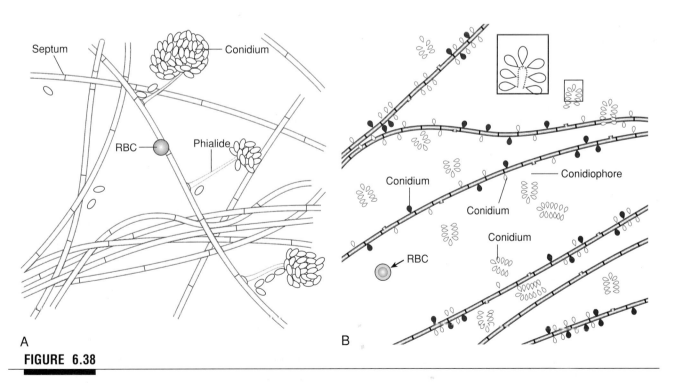

A   B

FIGURE 6.38

Superficially *Sporothrix schenckii* and *Acremonium* species resemble one another in microscopic preparations because of the slender conidiophores and concentration of conidia at the tips of the conidiophores. Obvious distinguishing characteristics are the dark pigment associated with colonies of *Sporothrix* and its thermal dimorphism. In addition, the conidia of *Acremonium (A)* are arranged in loose clusters, while *S. schenckii (B)* has an orderly "rosette" arrangement of conidia at the tip of the conidiophore plus "sleeves" of conidia along the hyphae, and sometimes, a second larger dark type of conidium. The 7-μm red blood cell (RBC) (arrow) shows the relative sizes of the mycotic elements.

Subcutaneous Pathogens

DEMATIACEAE

WANGIELLA DERMATITIDIS[9] (Wang-ee-ell-uh derm-ah-tid-duh-dis)

■ **Teleomorph.** None has been identified.

■ **Reservoirs.** W. dermatitidis is found worldwide in soil and wood as a plant parasite.

■ **Unique Risk Factors.** Infection is usually considered to result from repeated minor trauma such as pricks and scratches with contaminated thorns and twigs.

■ **Human Infection.** W. dermatitidis is one of the etiologic agents of phaeohyphomycosis, an infection characterized by the presence of darkly pigmented hyphae and yeastlike cells, pseudohypha-like elements, moniliform hyphae, or cystlike cells in tissue; a combination of these forms may be present. The infection in subcutaneous and cutaneous tissues tends to remain localized on the extremity at the site of inoculation. W. dermatitidis has been recovered from cases of endocarditis, septic arthritis, phaeomycotic cyst, and brain disease. For a more complete description of phaeohyphomycosis refer to the Introduction to Chapter 3.

■ **Specimen Sources.** Aspirated pus from microabscesses, tissue removed from subcutaneous cysts or nodules, and blood are most likely to be cultured.

■ **Specimen Collection and Handling.** Specimens should be collected aseptically into sterile containers and transported to the laboratory without delay. Anaerobic precautions are necessary if actinomycotic mycetoma is one of the possible diagnoses. Tissues to be cultured should be minced or ground before they are placed on the medium.
    Direct examination of material should include treatment with 10% KOH (to which stain or ink may be added) prior to microscopic examination. Purulent aspirates can be studied with simple wet mounts, after treatment with 10% to 15% KOH if this is indicated. Tissue specimens should be fixed, sectioned, and stained by the histology laboratory.

■ **Immunology.** No tests are available for diagnostic use.

■ **Special Precautions.** None are required, but specimens should be handled within a biologic safety cabinet.

─────────

    [9]*Wangiella dermatitidis* is identified as *Exophiala dermatitidis* in some of the literature.

■ **Culture Media.** Modified SDA, modified SDA with antibacterial agents.

■ **Preferred Temperature.** Grows at temperatures of 25° to 42°C.

■ **Differential Methods** (see Table 6.5). A colony suspected of being W. dermatitidis can be tested for its ability to grow at differing temperatures, and for its effect on casein (o), tyrosine (+) and nitrate (o), as well as its resistance to cycloheximide. Microscopic anatomy is also useful in identification.

■ **Macroscopic (Colony) Morphology.** On modified SDA at 25° to 37°C young colonies of W. dermatitidis initially resemble colonies of yeast; they are mucoid and shiny, and black. After 10 to 25 days Wangiella species mature into a mould colony that may become velvety in texture as short aerial mycelia develop, or the culture may become glabrous. Surface pigment becomes olive-gray to gray-black with a jet black reverse. The topography is typically flat.

■ **Microscopic Morphology** (Figs. 6.39 through 6.42). Young cultures contain yeast cells of a fungus that technically belongs to the genus *Phaeococcomyces*, an anamorph of *W. dermatitidis*. As cultures age they develop hyphae that are septate and branched and that may contain tortuous twists and turns. Hyphae are approximately 4 μm in diameter with a greenish brown pigment and are of varying lengths.
    The conidiogenous cells are phialides that develop laterally or terminally from the hyphae, on conidiophores that are indistinguishable from the vegetative hyphae unless conidia are attached. The phialides are flask shaped or cylindrical and rounded at the ends without collarettes. They can be hyaline or lightly pigmented. The

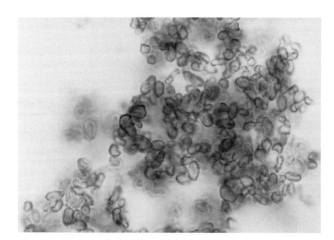

FIGURE 6.39

Typical preparations of young cultures of *Wangiella dermatitidis* contain yeast cells—the anamorph *Phaeococcomyces*. The cells are oval and darkly pigmented.

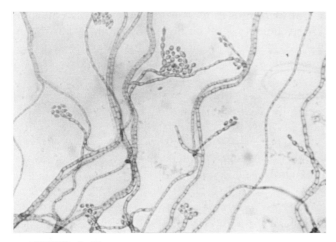

FIGURE 6.40

Characteristic preparations of *Wangiella dermatitidis* have dematiaceous hyphae and conidiophores that cannot be distinguished from the hyphae unless conidia are attached. The conidiogenous cells are phialides that are flask shaped or cylindrical without a distinctive vase shape or collarette. Oval conidia tend to cluster at the apex of the phialide; this is best seen at the bottom center of the field.

conidia produced from the phialides are <u>relatively small</u> <u>(2 × 6 μm) ovoid to subglobose unicellular forms with</u> <u>smooth walls</u>; they may be hyaline or light brown. Phialoconidia tend to accumulate in clusters at the apex of the phialide and slide down it to rest on the hypha. Annellides are rarely produced by this fungus.

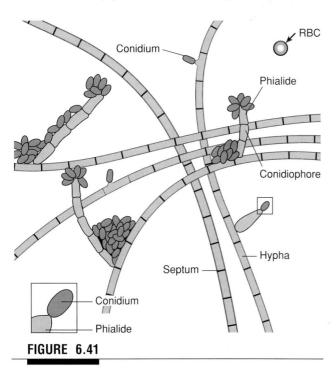

FIGURE 6.41

Wangiella dermatitidis, in the **m**ature **m**ould form, has dark septate, branched hyphae that may be twisted. Conidiophores resemble hyphal branches; the phialides are also unremarkable cylindrical or flask-shaped structures. Clusters of oval conidia form at the mouth of the phialide, then slip down to the base of the conidiophore. Phialides do not have a collarette. The 7-μm red blood cell (RBC) (arrow) shows the relative sizes of the mycotic elements.

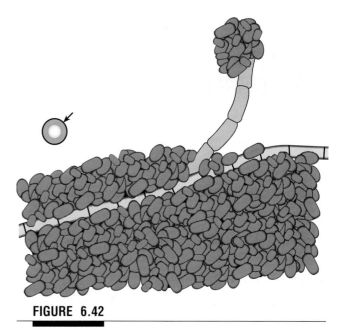

FIGURE 6.42

In bad preparations *Wangiella dermatitidis* is difficult to identify definitively. The genus is suggested when the dematiaceous fungus has a **y**east phase when **y**oung and a **m**ature **m**ould form, but distinguishing it from *Exophiala* species is difficult unless the conidiogenous cells are shown to be phialides rather than annellides. Colony morphology is not helpful, but biochemical tests can be done to confirm the identification. The 7-μm red blood cell (arrow) shows the relative sizes of the mycotic elements.

You can see the characteristic shapes and arrangements of conidia and conidiogenous cells of *W. dermatitidis* with a standard light microscope, but the details of conidiation may not be detectable without special devices such as an electron microscope or greater magnification than is usually available in the clinical laboratory.

In *direct examination* of specimens dark hyphal fragments of many sizes and shapes may be seen, together with dark yeast cells, intact hyphae, and swollen intercalary cells.

■ **Helpful Features for Identification of *Wangiella dermatitidis*** (see Fig. 6.19)

> **Y**oung black **y**east colonies
> **M**ature olive-gray to brownish black **m**ould colonies with a black reverse
> Pigmented hyphae and phialoconidia, with pale brown phialides
> Pigmented brown hyphal fragments—*without* granules or sclerotic bodies—in tissue samples and aspirates
> Characteristic lesions with localized subcutaneous cysts or nodules, usually on the extremities
> Neurotropism

■ **Organisms from Which *Wangiella dermatitidis* Must Be Differentiated** (see Tables 4.3 and 6.4)

> Other dematiaceous fungi that cause subcutaneous infections, especially those that produce phialides

Subcutaneous Pathogens

DEMATIACEAE

XYLOHYPHA BANTIANA[10]   (Zy-lo-hi-fah bann-tee-ann-uh)

■ **Teleomorph.** None has been identified.

■ **Reservoirs.** *X. bantiana* is found in soil and can be airborne. It has been found in North and South America, Europe, India, Japan, and Africa.

■ **Unique Risk Factors.** The organism typically infects debilitated or immunocompromised patients. It should be considered a pathogen because it is highly contagious by the airborne route, and the resulting infection is potentially life threatening.

■ **Human Infection.** *X. bantiana* is an etiologic agent of cerebral phaeohyphomycosis. The organism has been isolated as a rare cause of other conditions, such as respiratory or cutaneous infections. Researchers believe that *X. bantiana* causes infection by a somewhat indirect route. Apparently the fungus is first inhaled into the lungs or enters the body in a mild or asymptomatic primary cutaneous infection. It moves into the bloodstream at a later time, then disseminates to involve the brain.

The symptoms of cerebral phaeohyphomycosis include headache, weakness, and paralysis, followed by coma and seizures. There may be multiple lesions, suggesting hematogenous spread. The fungus has also been recovered from a foot, the skin of the abdomen, and the ear. These sites may have been the primary foci of the infections.

■ **Specimen Sources.** Respiratory secretions, biopsied tissue, aspirates of pus from brain abscesses, and blood are most likely to be cultured. Cerebrospinal fluid should not be cultured; these cultures are always negative.

■ **Specimen Collection and Handling.** Specimens should be collected aseptically into sterile containers and transported to the laboratory without delay. Mince or grind tissues to be cultured before the media are inoculated.

Direct examination of material may require treatment with 10% KOH (to which stain or ink may be added) prior to microscopic examination. Purulent aspirates can be studied with simple wet mounts. The histology laboratory should be asked to process tissues when microscopic examination is done (as it always should be).

---

[10]Formerly known as *Cladosporium trichoides* and, before that, *Cladosporium bantianum.*

■ **Immunology.** Rippon describes a fluorescent antibody technique, developed by Doory and Gordon, that is useful for distinguishing between *X. bantiana* and *Cladosporium carrionii.*

■ **Special Precautions.** Specimens suspected of harboring *X. bantiana* should be handled with GREAT CAUTION within a biologic safety cabinet!!

■ **Culture Media.** Modified SDA, modified SDA with antimicrobials.

Preferred Temperature. Grows at temperatures of 25° to 36°C. Tmax is 42° to 43°C.

■ **Differential Methods** (see Table 6.2). A colony suspected of being *X. bantiana* can be tested for its ability to grow at 35° to 36°C (+) and 42° to 43°C (+). Other tests that may be helpful in assigning the fungus to the correct species are liquefaction of gelatin (o), liquefaction of Loeffler's serum medium (o), and hydrolysis of casein (o).

■ **Macroscopic (Colony) Morphology.** The colony of *X. bantiana* after 14 to 30 days on modified SDA at 25° to 30°C is olive-gray to olive-brown with a dark gray–to–black reverse pigment. Older colonies may become dark gray or black on the surface as well as the reverse. The surface may be covered with a short aerial mycelium, creating a velvety texture, or it may be cottony. The topography is typically flat.

■ **Microscopic Morphology** (Figs. 6.43 through 6.45). Hyphae are septate and may be branched; they are relatively broad (average diameter, 4 μm; range, 2 to 6 μm) with a brown pigment. *X. bantiana* has only one type of

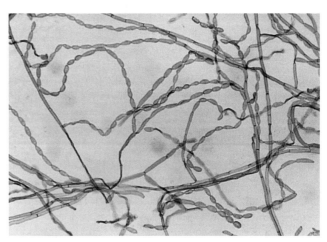

FIGURE 6.43

Characteristic slide preparations of *Xylohypha bantiana* show relatively broad, dark hyphae with septa and cladosporium-type sporulation. The oval brown conidia form long chains, which branch from sticklike conidiophores. Some of the hyphae in this field have collapsed so that they resemble ribbons rather than tubes.

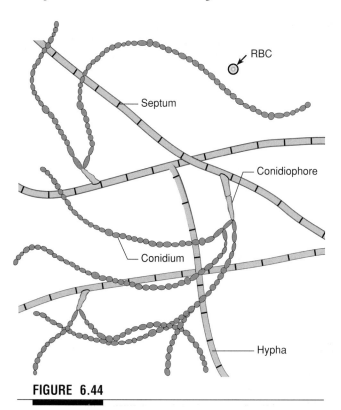

FIGURE 6.44

Xylohypha bantiana has cladosporium-type sporulation, with long branching chains of brown elliptical conidia that vary markedly in size. The conidiophores are sticklike, at oblique angles with the dark septate hyphae. Conidia do not have disjuncture scars. The 7-μm red blood cell (RBC) (arrow) shows the relative sizes of the mycotic elements.

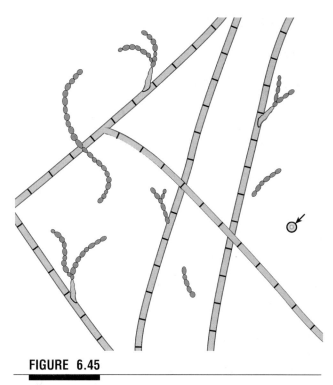

FIGURE 6.45

Even in bad preparations *Xylohypha bantiana* can usually be recognized by the long chains of dematiaceous conidia, the variable sizes of the conidia, the oblique angle that conidiophores form with the hyphae, and the absence of disjuncture scars on the conidia. Biochemical tests can be used to confirm the identification. The 7-μm red blood cell (arrow) shows the relative sizes of the mycotic elements.

sporulation, the cladosporium type. The conidiophores vary in size; they are septate and have poor posture; that is, they are not erect. Conidiophores are brown, like the vegetative hyphae, and are indistinguishable from it. Long chains of 35 to 40 blastoconidia are produced acropetally in a "treelike" fashion, with a small number of points where branching occurs. The blastoconidia are oval with smooth walls and vary greatly in size, from 2 × 7 μm to 3 × 20 μm. Disjuncture scars do not occur at the sites where the blastoconidia break away from the conidiophore or from other conidia.

In *direct examination* look for dark brown hyphal fragments (average diameter, 4 μm), with branching. *X. bantiana* may form chains of round cells.

■ Helpful Features for Identification of *Xylohypha bantiana* (see Fig. 6.12)

Characteristic olive-brown to olive-black colonies with dark reverse

Slo-o-o-o-w growth of the fungus

Only cladosporium-type sporulation in cultures, with elliptical blastoconidia

Long chains with few branches

Poor posture of the conidiophores

Pigmented brown hyphae

Growth at 35° to 37°C and at 42° to 43°C

Neurotropism (invasion of neural tissue) in animal studies

Negative for gelatin liquefaction, liquefaction of Loeffler's serum medium, and casein hydrolysis

■ Organisms from Which *Xylohypha bantiana* Must Be Differentiated (see Table 6.5)

Other dematiaceous fungi that produce conidia in branching chains, especially agents of chromoblastomycosis: *Cladosporium carrionii, Fonsecaea pedrosoi, Fonsecaea compacta, Wangiella dermatitidis,* and *Phialophora verrucosa*

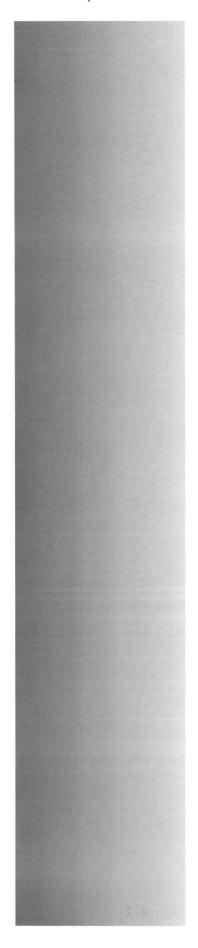

SUGGESTED EXERCISES FOR CHAPTER 6

(S u b c u t a n e o u s   F u n g i)

Exercise 9 (1st Session)

Purpose. To practice the procedures and (again) to set up the cultures needed for the next laboratory.

Suggested Fungus Cultures

Set 1   *Exophiala jeanselmei, Wangiella dermatitidis* (2 to 3 weeks old[11])
Set 2   *Cladosporium carrionii, Fonsecaea pedrosoi, Phialophora verrucosa*
Set 3   *Pseudallescheria boydii, Scedosporium apiospermum*

Initial Process. Pick up four plates of PFA or PDA and three slide culture setups from the supply table. One PFA/PDA plate is for the slide cultures. At the same time, pick up the two new cultures needed for this exercise.

You will study a total of three of the subcutaneous fungi. One of the three must be *Sporothrix schenckii* (Exercise 10). Select the other two fungi from the three sets listed, one organism from a set. Again, if you have a laboratory partner, coordinate your choices so that each of you is working with different organisms.

Make a *slide culture* of each of your fungi and incubate these, as usual, at 25–30°C. *Subculture* each of the two fungi to a plate of PFA/PDA medium. These are also to be incubated at 25–30°C.

Do not forget to *water your slide cultures* at least once before the next laboratory.

Exercise 9 (2nd Session)

Remove the slide cultures and the subcultures of the subcutaneous organisms from the 25–30°C incubator and take them to your desk. Slide cultures should be examined within the biologic safety cabinet to see if enough conidia are present for the culture to be harvested. If so, continue this exercise; if not, reincubate the slide cultures. Harvest all mature slide cultures and put the slides aside in flats to dry while you complete the remainder of today's exercises. Label all preparations properly.

After all the mature slide cultures have been harvested turn your attention to the subcultures. Remember, again, to WORK WITH ONE ORGANISM AT A TIME. Record the *colony descriptions* on the correct LABORATORY WORK SHEET. Then do a *tease mount* and/or a *Scotch tape preparation* of the fungus. Examine these preparations, and record what you see—with drawings, of course. Use the slides you have to make the best composite drawings possible; the drawings can be completed during the next session with the information provided by the permanent mounts of the slide cultures.

Compare the colony morphology and the microscopic picture for each subculture with the original cultures, especially if you selected *Wangiella* or *Exophiala*.

---

[11]Using *Exophiala* cultures that are 2 to 3 weeks old allows students to compare the morphology of the young culture that they set up with the morphology of the older culture—a good opportunity to make the point that *y*oung cultures are *y*eastlike and *m*ature colonies are *m*ould forms

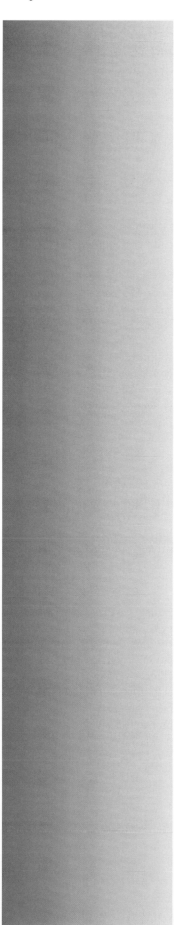

Exercise 9 (3rd Session)

Complete Exercise 9 by sealing the preparations and checking to ensure that the labels are correct. Lay them aside to dry.

When they have dried, examine them and finish your composite drawings.

Exercise 10 (1st Session)

Purpose. To compare the morphology of colonies of *Sporothrix schenckii* grown at two different temperatures.

Fungus Culture

Sporothrix schenckii

Initial Process. You need two plates of PFA or PDA (or, preferably, one plate of PFA/PDA and one plate of BHIA with blood) and a slide culture setup from the supply table. Use the plate you used to make slide cultures for Exercise 9 as the agar source for the slide culture you will make for this exercise.

Transfer the *Sporothrix schenckii* culture to each of the agar plates and make a slide culture in the usual manner. The incubation is the tricky part of this exercise. Incubate the BHIA plate, if the medium was used, or one of the PFA/PDA plates in a 35–37°C CO_2 incubator. Place the (second) PFA/PDA plate and the slide culture in the 25–30°C incubator as usual.

Check the slide culture at least once before the next session, and add sterile water if necessary.

Exercise 10 (2nd Session)

Take the cultures of *Sporothrix schenckii* to your desk. Work with the plate incubated at 25–30°C first. Follow the familiar path of making a *tease mount* and a *Scotch tape preparation* from the colony. Enter a description of the colony on the LABORATORY WORK SHEET for dimorphic fungi and begin your composite *drawing* from the tease mount and Scotch tape prep. *Harvest* the slide culture of *Sporothrix schenckii* if the culture is mature. Label both slides and put them in your slide flat to dry.

If good growth occurred on the plate incubated at 35–37°C, record a *description* of its morphology on the LABORATORY WORK SHEET for dimorphic fungi. Then do a simple *wet prep* from the culture, using saline or water as the mounting fluid. Examine this preparation; record the results and make a drawing.

Exercise 10 (3rd Session)

Wrap up Exercise 10 by sealing the two slides from the slide culture and examining them when the seal has dried. Complete the composite drawing of the mould form of *Sporothrix*.

Your last task for Exercise 10 is to compare the cultures grown at the two different temperatures—the microscopic and gross morphology—and record the similarities and the differences.

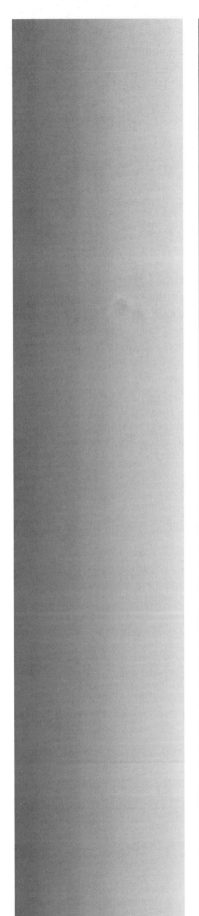

Optional Exercise (1st Session)

Purpose. To study the methods available for the differentiation of subcutaneous fungi. This is not generally found in a basic text such as this one, but is it included because the reactions are presented in Chapter 6 (see Table 6.2).

Suggested Fungus Cultures. Use those studied for Exercise 9.

Procedures to Be Completed

> nitrate reduction
> casein hydrolysis
> tyrosine hydrolysis
> Loeffler's serum medium
> starch hydrolysis
> hydrolysis of milk
> temperature of growth

Initial Process. Set up the *differential tests* listed above. If you are working with a laboratory partner, you should coordinate your work so that, between you, you have a subcutaneous fungus that is positive and one that is negative for each test (see Table 6.2).

You should also note whether the initial colonies of each were in the yeast or the mould form when they were young. Record the results of all the tests, including temperature(s) of growth, on the appropriate LABORATORY WORK SHEET.

Optional Exercise (2nd Session)

If the fungi have grown enough, read the differential tests for each of the subcutaneous organisms you cultured and record the results properly on the LABORATORY WORK SHEET. Using "growth" and "no growth," or "hydrolysis" and "no hydrolysis," is recommended (instead of "positive" and "negative"). You are less likely to be confused later about what a positive really indicates.

Optional Exercise (3rd Session)

Reincubate any tests that do not have adequate growth.

Complete the Optional Exercise by reading any tests that had to be reincubated and recording the results on the LABORATORY WORK SHEET. Enter the actual reaction rather than "positive" or "negative" to make your records as clear as possible. Then use Table 6.2 in the text to "identify" the fungi; that is, use the test results as if you did not know the name of the organisms and see if your results are typical. If you have atypical results, attempt to determine the cause(s).

ASSESS WHAT YOU HAVE LEARNED

Responses to the questions below are located in Appendix A.

1. Define autoinoculation, primary conidiation, secondary infection, shield cell, sclerotic bodies, synnemata, verrucoid.
2. Name the usual route of infection for subcutaneous mycoses, the geographic areas most frequently involved, the population at risk, and the factors that make the hosts susceptible.
3. Compare the subcutaneous mycoses (mycetoma, chromoblastomycosis, sporotrichosis) in terms of symptoms, appearance of the lesions, specific tissues infected, and agent(s) of infection.
4. Name at least three characteristics of colonies and/or microscopic morphology shared by most "subcutaneous fungi."
5. Describe the three major types of anamorphic conidiation associated with the subcutaneous fungi (excluding development of annellides).

For questions 6 through 13 **MATCH** the name of the characteristic **(numbered)** with the name of the fungus **(lettered)**. Responses will be used more than once.

6. conidia uniform in size
7. conidiophores not erect
8. chains of more than 30 blastoconidia
9. neurotropic
10. elliptical conidia
11. has prominent disjuncture cells
12. shield cells
13. thermotolerant (to 43°C)

    a. *Cladosporium carrionii*
    b. *Xylohypha bantiana*

For questions 14 through 18 **MATCH** the name of the characteristic **(numbered)** with the name of the fungus **(lettered)**. Responses will be used more than once.

14. conidiogenous cells are annellides
15. grows up to 37°C
16. neurotropic
17. resistant to cycloheximide
18. sclerotic bodies and granules absent from tissue specimens

    a. *Exophiala jeanselmei*
    b. *Wangiella dermatitidis*

For questions 19 through 22 **MATCH** the name of the fungus **(lettered)** with its synanamorph **(numbered)**. The lettered responses may be used more than once.

19. *Graphium*
20. *Phaeoannellomyces*
21. *Phaeococcomyces*
22. *Scedosporium apiospermum*

    a. *Exophiala jeanselmei*
    b. *Pseudallescheria boydii*
    c. *Wangiella dermatitidis*

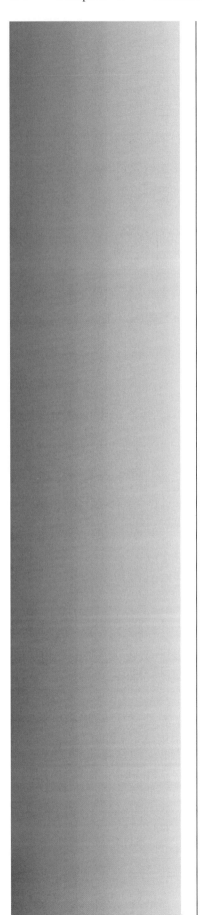

For questions 23–28 **MATCH** the name of the fungus **(lettered)** with the characteristic **(numbered).** Responses will be used more than once.

23. conidiophores swell into denticulated vesicles at their apices
24. fungoma may develop in the lungs
25. hyphae very thin, with conidiophores that taper at the apices
26. perfect fungus
27. sensitive to cycloheximide
28. thermal dimorph

   a. *Pseudallescheria boydii*
   b. *Sporothrix schenckii*

NAME the organism described in each of the items below.

29. **Lesion:** ulcers ascending along the lymph channels of the forearm
    Colony: glabrous creamy colonies that become black and velvety as they age, with black reverse pigment
    Microscopic: delicate, thin hyphae in parallel strands; slender conidiophores at right angles to the hyphae that are tapered from the base, then widen again into denticulated vesicles. Small oval conidia arranged in a rosette pattern and forming sleeves along the vegetative hyphae

30. **Lesion:** tumor-like swellings with draining sinuses; pepper-like granules are present in the drainage
    Colony: creamy yeastlike colonies that mature into dome-shaped velvety colonies with olive-gray obverse and jet black reverse pigments
    Microscopic: hyphae are relatively broad, with greenish brown pigment. Annellides form on annellophores and directly on the hyphae; they are narrower at the tip than at the base, with scars at the apex. Small elliptical conidia accumulate on the hyphae at the base of the annellophores

31. **Lesion:** tumor-like swellings with draining sinuses; pale granules are present in the drainage
    Colony: white fluffy colonies that become woolly and brownish gray as they mature, with black "pepper" flecks on the surface; reverse pigment is dark gray
    Microscopic: broad septate hyphae with sticklike conidiophores and unicellular conidia with truncate bases, resembling lollipops. Occasionally very large black globes, with thick walls of intertwined hyphae, are enmeshed in the hyphae

32. **Lesion:** wartlike crusted lesions with some swelling
    Colony: velvety folded dematiaceous colonies
    Microscopic: relatively broad septate greenish brown hyphae with lateral and terminal conidiophores on which branching chains of conidia are produced. Conidia are oval and slightly pointed, in chains of 12 to 15 conidia; shield cells are present

33. **Lesion:** crusted verrucoid nodules on the skin of the foot and ankle, with "copper pennies" in the exudate
    Colony: velvety olive-green surface with jet black reverse
    Microscopic: dark brown septate hyphae with branching. Primary conidia form on denticles on erect septate conidiophores that are swollen at their apices and secondary conidia are produced from some primary conidia, forming multileveled conidial heads. Cladosporium-type conidiation is also present

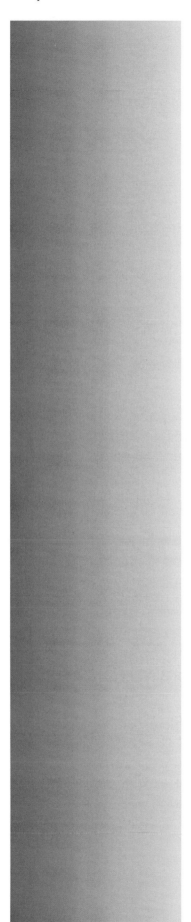

34. **Lesion:** warty verrucoid nodules resembling cauliflower
    Colony: spreading flat black velvety colony with radial folds and a jet black reverse
    Microscopic: dark brown septate hyphae, with vaselike conidiogenous cells laterally and terminally from conidiophores and from the hyphae. The conidiogenous cells have flared collarettes. Conidia are ovoid to elliptical, forming clusters at the apices of the conidiogenous cells
35. **Lesion:** localized ulcer with darkly pigmented yeastlike cells, moniliform hyphae, and swollen cells in tissue sections
    Colony: shiny black yeast colonies that eventually become velvety and flat, with gray-black surface pigment and jet black reverse
    Microscopic: septate dark brown branched hyphae with tortuous twists and turns. Sticklike conidiophores support cylindrical conidiogenous cells that lack collarettes. Clusters of small ovoid conidia are seen at the apices of the conidiogenous cells and resting on the hyphae at the bases of conidiophores

CHAPTER 7

Yeasts and Yeastlike Organisms

Upon completion of this chapter the reader should be able to:

1. Define the following terms: assimilation, candidiasis, colonization, cryptococcosis, geotrichosis, micrometer, ascus (asci), ascospores.

2. Explain how to judge whether the yeast isolated is (presumptively) the etiologic agent of the infection.

3. Describe the clinical symptoms of thrush and cryptococcal meningitis.

4. Outline a general process for primary culture of yeast and for identification of any yeast isolated.

5. Identify the organisms studied (*Candida albicans, Candida* species, *Cryptococcus neoformans, Cryptococcus* species, *Rhodotorula, Geotrichum, Hansenula, Pneumocystis, Trichosporon, Torulopsis,* and *Saccharomyces*) on the basis of information such as patient history, microscopic and colony morphology of the isolate, and biochemical reactions in key tests.

6. For each of the methods used for identification of yeasts, name the reagent or substrate used, positive and negative reactions, and the general technique. State the organism(s) for which the test is primarily used.

7. Explain the difference between the following pairs of terms: yeast versus yeastlike, pseudohyphae versus germ tubes, chlamydospores versus chlamydoconidia, colonization versus infection.

■

INTRODUCTION

Yeasts are important to humans for many reasons. Of course they do cause infections, both major and minor, but they are also very helpful. They ensure that beer is foamy, champagne is bubbly, and bread is "light" rather than unleavened. Within the field of medicine the important yeasts are fungi that are primarily unicellular. These eukaryotic cells produce disease in humans and animals or they contribute to the infection. Yeast reproduce primarily by budding; when the buds remain attached, they form chains called *pseudohyphae* (Fig. 7.1). Fewer than 30 of the recognized species of yeast fall into the category of "yeasts of medical importance."

Yeasts are a significant part of the normal flora of humans, particularly on the skin and mucous membranes. Most infections are endogenous. When the host's de-

(handwritten annotation: Pseudohyphae Sign of true infection)

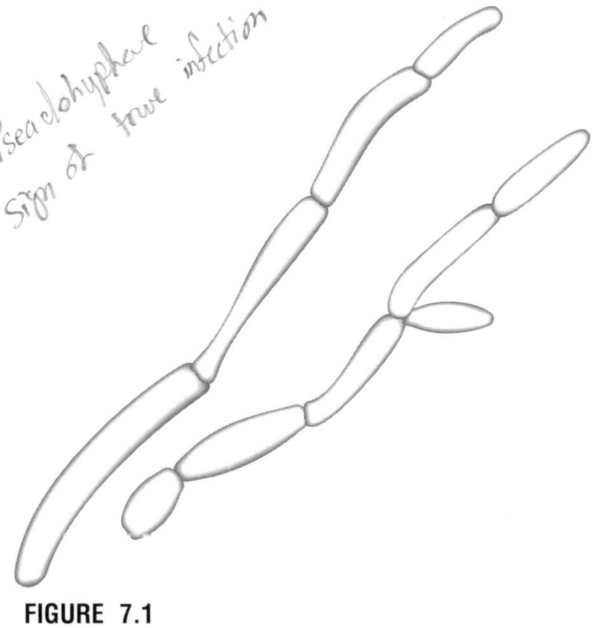

FIGURE 7.1

Pseudohyphae are chains of yeast buds that elongate and remain attached after budding has occurred. Usually the cells are of different sizes because they bud and divide at different rates. Pseudohyphae sometimes branch.

fenses are weakened in some way, the yeast of the normal flora, unchecked by natural immunity, cause disease. The infection typically starts as a localized lesion on a mucous membrane and disseminates. The severity of the infection depends on how the defenses were weakened and how long the condition exists. For example, a person who takes large doses of an antibiotic may develop an intestinal infection because the normal bacteria that maintain the balance of power are killed and the yeast in the normal intestinal flora proliferate. When therapy is stopped, the patient usually recovers without complications. Increases in immunosuppressive diseases such as acquired immunodeficiency syndrome (AIDS), prolonged treatment with antibiotics, immunosuppressive drugs and steroids, and the increased use of invasive procedures such as cardiac catheterization, are reflected in the increasing number of severe yeast infections.

Most yeasts are opportunists rather than pathogens; because they lack offensive properties such as the ability to penetrate skin, they must wait for their chance to cause infection. The severity of the infection is governed more by the underlying condition of the patient and the patient's response to the challenge than by the pathogenic characteristics of the yeast.

The technical distinction between "yeast" and "yeastlike" organisms is that *yeasts* are perfect fungi with a sexual and an asexual method of reproduction, while *yeastlike* organisms are imperfect fungi that reproduce only by asexual means. In this chapter "yeast" is used impartially, simply to identify predominantly unicellular fungi that reproduce by budding.

Yeasts are the most frequently isolated fungus. A study by Silva-Hunter and Cooper showed as many cultures were positive for yeast as were positive for fungi of all other types. However, less than 10% of the people with positive yeast cultures actually had yeast infections. Remember—yeast are normal flora. One step in proving a yeast is a pathogen is to isolate the same yeast in significant numbers from multiple specimens from the same body site (see Table 3.1).

Any tissue or organ may be infected with *Candida*. Rippon describes *Candida albicans* as "probably the most protean[1] infectious agent that inflicts man" (p. 541). Kwon-Chung and Bennett say most studies find that *C. albicans* constitutes at least 60% of the *Candida* species isolated from infections. *Candida* infections include intertriginous candidiasis, paronychia, onychomycosis, vulvovaginitis, thrush, pulmonary infections, eye infections, endocarditis, meningitis, fungemia, and disseminated infections. While *C. albicans* is the most common cause of candidiasis, other species also cause infection. Other important *Candida* species are *Candida tropicalis, Candida parapsilosis, Candida krusei, Candida guilliermondii, Iorulopsis (Candida) glabrata*, and *Candida kefyr*. Some species are regularly associated with a specific clinical disease. Candidiasis may be the primary condition, or it may develop secondary to another condition.

Thrush, an infection of the mucous membranes of the mouth, is one common form of localized candidiasis. It occurs in newborns as a consequence of low oral pH and the absence of normal flora. The infection can occur in any neonate; it is most often seen when the mother has vulvovaginal candidiasis. In older children and adults thrush indicates a defect in host defenses. It occurs in patients with AIDS and avitaminosis, in diabetics, and in patients undergoing antibiotic treatment, radiation therapy, or chemotherapy. Initially white or creamy patches appear on the mucous membranes and the tongue. As the infection progresses the patches become confluent. The pseudomembranous material that constitutes the patches consists of masses of pseudohyphae and blastoconidia. Removal of the pseudomembrane leaves a raw, red, moist base.

Balanitis (inflammation of the penis) and vaginitis are other common localized forms of candidiasis. Diabetes, pregnancy, antibiotic therapy, and oral contraceptives all increase susceptibility to vaginal candidiasis. Other factors that lower the pH of the vagina, such as diet,[2] also contribute to candidiasis by favoring *Candida* over the other normal flora. Balanitis is probably a sexually transmitted disease.

Paronychia, an infection of tissues surrounding the nails, is the most common cutaneous candidiasis. People such as bartenders and dishwashers whose hands are frequently immersed in water are most vulnerable to this form of candidiasis. Localized infections of the skin also occur.

Localized infections sometimes disseminate to cause pulmonary infection, septicemia, endocarditis, or meningitis. Dissemination of yeast and systemic involvement are rare except in severely debilitated or immunocompromised patients and in those receiving therapy that suppresses the immune response. Any organ system may be infected, but the most common systemic candidiasis is

endocarditis, generally after replacement of a heart valve. A species other than *C. albicans* is usually responsible. Typically the yeast accumulates on the valves of the heart, creating vegetations that may form emboli. Candidal endocarditis is also seen in intravenous drug users and in patients with a preexisting heart defect.

Cryptococcosis may be an acute or chronic infection. Infections can usually be traced to exposure to pigeons and their droppings in soil. The alkaline pH of the droppings favors survival of *Cryptococcus*.

Typically cryptococci are inhaled. The lung is the primary site of infection. People with competent immune systems can rapidly clear the yeasts from the lung tissue so infection doesn't develop, but cryptococci spread rapidly within the immunocompromised host. Infection of the brain and meninges is the most commonly diagnosed infection and the most common cause of death. Skin lesions may also develop in about 10% of patients with cryptococcosis. Many of these patients develop meningitis if the cutaneous lesions are not treated.

No one has yet explained why *Cryptococcus* prefers the central nervous system. A typical case begins with a prolonged subclinical period of general irritability and mental changes. In the acute phase patients have severe headaches and fever, perhaps linked to *nuchal rigidity*, a stiff neck in less formal terms—or a sore throat. Host response to cryptococcal infection is minimal, because the yeast is protected by an immunologically inert polysaccharide capsule. Antibody production by the host is poor, especially in the central nervous system. Tissues are usually not affected unless the presence of large numbers of encapsulated yeast causes physical displacement of the tissues.

Because of the low antibody response, no one has developed a useful skin test for diagnosis of cryptococcosis. However, several immunologic tests are available for measuring antigen and antibody titers in patient serum. These are helpful in tracing the course of the disease and the patient's response to treatment.

LABORATORY METHODS FOR YEASTS AND YEASTLIKE ORGANISMS

Methods for specimen collection and handling, media for primary culture, microscopic methods, and biochemical tests for identification differ little for the various yeast and yeastlike organisms. For convenience, and to avoid unnecessary repetition, those that are common to all the fungi in this chapter are presented first. Specific information is presented with the organism when a yeast differs significantly from the general rule.

Any yeast isolated from blood, cerebrospinal fluid, closed lesions, and surgical specimens—any specimen that is normally sterile—should be completely identified.

---

[1]Changeable in terms of form or shape
[2]Heavy consumption of citrus fruits, tomatoes, and other foods that are acidic may lower the vaginal pH.

The significance of yeasts isolated from other specimens should be evaluated carefully after considering the source of the specimen and the patient's symptoms and probable immunocompetence.

The number of yeast recovered is of the greatest importance because small numbers of endogenous yeast are normally present in specimens from the alimentary tract and the mucocutaneous tissues. When infection is suspected at such sites, *C. albicans* or *Candida* species should be recovered in significant numbers in multiple specimens from the same site before the diagnosis of candidiasis is accepted. Opinions differ as to the number of recovered colonies that is significant.

Specimen Source. Yeast have been found in virtually all kinds of specimens. Sputa and other respiratory specimens are most often cultured, but scrapings of the skin and nails, biopsy specimens of tissue and mucocutaneous lesions, corneal scrapings, vaginal discharges, urine, blood, bone, or cerebrospinal fluid may be submitted for culture.

Specimen Collection and Handling. No special procedures are needed to obtain a specimen or to transport the specimen to the laboratory for culture *other than* the standard requirements that the specimen container be sterile and the specimen be transported promptly. Rapid transport is not important because the yeast may die. Rather, rapid transport is important so that the direct microscopic examination of the specimen can be done before the organisms have time to multiply or change morphology. Why not allow multiplication? First, multiplication of the organisms in the specimen gives an erroneous picture of the number of organisms in the host, creating a false idea of the magnitude of the infection. Second, yeasts should not be given time to change morphology because the kinds of structures present provide valuable clues to the identity of the yeast and to its role in the host. Pseudohyphae and hyphae are the growth forms of yeast. On body surfaces and in body fluids unicellular forms without pseudohyphae and hyphae suggest *colonization* of the host, that is, the yeast is "hanging out" in the tissues without causing infection. The presence of the mycelial forms—pseudohyphae and hyphae—in a *fresh* specimen (Fig. 7.2) indicate that the yeast is causing infection, especially if unusually large numbers of neutrophils are present.

Direct examination of specimens can generally be done by a wet mount or gram-stained smear; the technique used depends on the kind of material to be examined. Tenacious or opaque specimens such as mucoid secretions, skin, or nail scrapings may need to be cleared with potassium hydroxide (KOH) before they are examined. A wet prep is convenient for fluids and some mucoid materials. The preparation can be done without stain, a stain such as Parker's blue-black ink can be added, or India ink can be used when an encapsulated yeast is

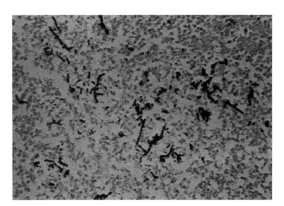

FIGURE 7.2

When yeast infects tissue, the fungus forms pseudohyphae and sometimes hyphae. A small number of unicellular forms may be present. In this photomicrograph the yeast are the darker structures with definite shapes. Neutrophils can be recognized by their rounder, less distinct nuclei. Their presence in this section of cerebral tissue signals the pyogenic response typical of yeast infections. (From Rippon JW: Medical Mycology: The Pathogenic Fungi and Pathogenic Actinomycetes, 3rd ed. Philadelphia, WB Saunders, 1988, p 561.)

suspected. The Gram's stain demonstrates bacteria as well as yeast (Fig. 7.3). All fungi are dark blue-black (gram positive). This, plus the large size of yeast (approximately equivalent to the diameter of a normal red blood cell) make yeast very distinctive in gram-stained smears. Unfortunately yeast cells are often dismissed by novices as artifacts.

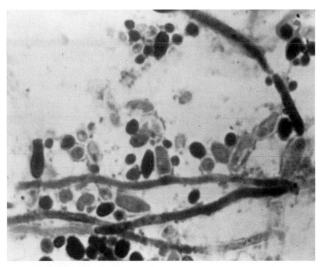

FIGURE 7.3

The long, slender dark structures running across the bottom half of this photomicrograph are pseudohyphae in a gram-stained smear. The fatter and more rounded structure in the center of the extreme right margin, nestled next to the end of a pseudohypha, is an individual yeast cell; more cells are scattered through the field. Yeast stains a very dark blue-black or purple, in contrast with the much smaller bacterial forms that may be (lighter) purple or red. White blood cells are also present. Although the dark blue color is not seen in a black-and-white photograph, the morphology of the pseudohyphae and the large individual yeast cells is evident. (Courtesy of the Centers for Disease Control and Prevention.)

The size and shape of the yeast are helpful; using a *micrometer*, a calibrated device that fits into one of the oculars of the microscope, eliminates any need to guess the size. The number of buds, and the way the buds are attached, sometimes gives good hints about the identity of the organism.

Special Precautions. Because yeasts are generally opportunistic pathogens, special precautions are not needed. Handling cultures—especially respiratory specimens—within a biologic safety cabinet is sensible, however, until the organism is identified as a yeast rather than one of the dimorphic pathogens or some other pathogenic bacterium or fungus.

Temperature Considerations. The yeasts generally grow well at 25° to 30°C. Those that cause infection also grow at 35° to 37°C. Temperature studies are sometimes done, using a standard medium such as Emmon's modification of Sabouraud's dextrose agar (SDA), to help identify a yeast by its temperature tolerance.

Culture Media. Numerous media can be used for primary culture for yeasts. Modified SDA supports growth of the yeasts of medical importance. Cycloheximide inhibits some of these organisms, so media containing this and other antibiotics should be used in conjunction with noninhibitory media. Yeasts grow well on plain blood agar plates (BAPs); they are frequently isolated in bacterial culture and may be referred to the mycologist for identification. SABHI, a combination of SDA and brain-heart infusion (BHI), and BHI agar (BHIA) can also be used. A medium such as thistle medium or niger seed agar that contains *caffeic acid* is frequently used for primary inoculation of cultures from specimens such as cerebrospinal fluid that are likely to contain *Cryptococcus neoformans*. This yeast consistently produces the enzyme *phenoloxidase*, which converts the caffeic acid to melanin (Fig. 7.4). The development of brown-to-black pigment in the colony indicates *C. neoformans* is present. The medium is commercially available as plates or tubes, and as part of many of the rapid systems for identification of yeast. Caffeic acid discs can also be prepared or purchased to provide a 4-hour test for identification of *C. neoformans*.

Additional media are recommended to enhance the microscopic morphology of the yeast and reduce the time needed for identification. Cornmeal-Tween 80 (CMT) agar, rice agar, or another starchy medium enhances production of characteristic microscopic structures such as chlamydospores. Both oxidative *assimilation* and anaerobic *fermentation* methods can be used to determine carbohydrate utilization by *Candida* species because they metabolize carbohydrates by both routes. *Cryptococcus*, on the other hand, cannot ferment carbohydrates but can assimilate them. Since any organism that can ferment a carbohydrate can also assimilate it most laboratories use only assimilation tests.

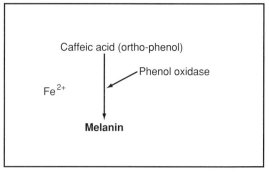

FIGURE 7.4

The metabolism of caffeic acid is a simple, rapid test for identification of *Cryptococcus neoformans*. The method is included in many test kits for identification of yeastlike fungi.

Macroscopic (Colony) Morphology. Colonies of most yeast are white or cream colored and bacteria like. Many people describe them as "looking like a coagulase-negative staph, only drier." Gross morphology is important because the seemingly minor differences in pigment are important clues for identification. The texture is also helpful. Colonies are usually pasty and somewhat dry, but some yeasts produce mucoid colonies. A feathery filamentous fringe may develop in the agar around colonies, especially if the cultures are old.

Microscopic Morphology. Hyphae, pseudohyphae, and individual blastoconidia (Fig. 7.5) all can be present in yeast colonies—sometimes in the same colony. Pseudohyphae are chains of blastoconidia that have remained attached, forming a structure that resembles a string of sausages. No septa develop in pseudohyphae, but there is a constriction where the "daughter" blastoconidium emerges from the "mother." Blastoconidia are unicellular round or oval forms. The daughters may remain attached to the mother cell, but usually the blastoconidia are released, leaving a scar on the mother at the point of attach-

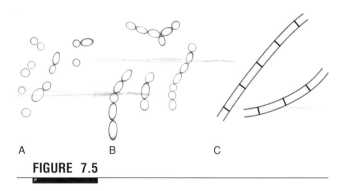

FIGURE 7.5

Yeast form blastoconidia *(A)* by simple budding. The buds may separate from the mother cell or remain attached and elongate to form pseudohyphae *(B)*. Pseudohyphae differ from true hyphae *(C)* in that the individual cells of pseudohyphae differ in width and length and are "pinched off" between cells in contrast with the parallel walls and straighter septa found in most true hyphae.

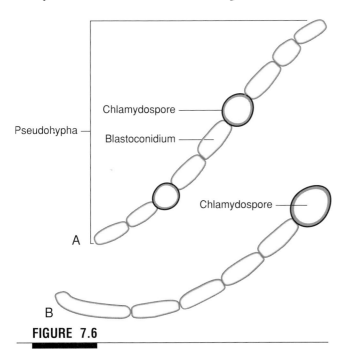

FIGURE 7.6

Chlamydospores are large, thick-walled vesicles with dense protoplasm that help the fungus survive under harsh conditions. They may be intercalary *(A)*, e.g., between blastoconidia of the pseudohyphae, or terminal on the pseudohyphae *(B)*.

ment. Daughter cells eventually become mother cells in turn. The chlamydospores (Figs. 7.6 and 7.7) produced by *C. albicans* are, in fact, thick-walled vesicles that are simply swollen cells. True chlamydoconidia are asexual reproductive structures with thick walls. Chlamydoconidia are produced directly from the hyphae in response to an unfavorable environment; they are thallic conidia, capable of reproduction if circumstances permit. Chlamydospores and chlamydoconidia are compared in Figure 7.8.

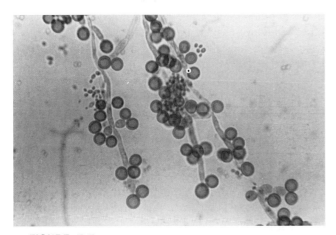

FIGURE 7.7

The many large, round structures with thick walls are chlamydospores. Both terminal and intercalary chlamydospores are evident against the thin-walled elongated cells of the pseudohyphae. The small oval to round structures are simple blastoconidia. (Courtesy of the Centers for Disease Control and Prevention.)

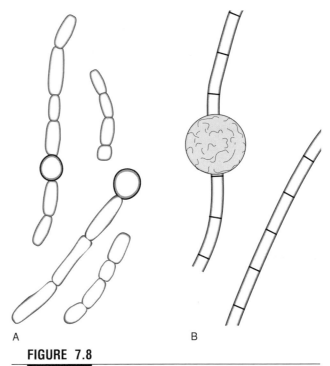

FIGURE 7.8

Chlamydospores and chlamydoconidia look much alike. The differences are that chlamydospores typically have double walls that are more refractile than those of chlamydoconidia and they look empty, while chlamydoconidia usually appear to have some internal contents or structure. Chlamydospores *(A)* are swollen cells found in pseudohyphae; they are storage units rather than reproductive cells. Chlamydoconidia *(B)* are asexual reproductive cells produced directly from true hyphae in thallic conidiogeny.

When colonies appear, a wet prep should be made from the culture. First, wet preps show that the colony is a yeast rather than one of the bacteria with similar colonies. The features noted in direct examination of the specimen—size, shape, number of buds, and how they are connected—should be noted again. The likelihood of determining the way the buds are attached is inversely proportional to the vigor with which the preparation is mixed before it is examined. If the specimen is from a site with normal flora, simply identifying the colony as a yeast may suffice. Colonies from specimens that are normally sterile unless infection is present, such as blood and cerebrospinal fluid, should be further identified.

CMT agar can be inoculated from the primary culture to encourage development of chlamydospores and to see the relationships among hyphae, pseudohyphae, and the other structures. The growth in these clear media can be examined simply by placing the Petri dish on the stage of a brightfield microscope. A composite figure showing all of the organisms in this chapter is included just before the section of laboratory exercises (see Fig. 7.24) because microscopic morphology in wet preps and CMT agar is so important for identification of the yeastlike fungi.

Differential Tests. Most laboratories find it impractical to identify every yeast that is isolated from a clinical specimen since yeast are found in the normal human flora. Those that should always be identified are the isolates from body sites that are normally sterile, yeast recovered as the predominant organism in a culture, and those isolated repeatedly from immunocompromised patients.

A wet prep should always be done first when a yeast-like colony forms. The germ tube test is the second procedure that should be done on each yeast isolated. *Germ tubes* are filamentous outgrowths from the blastoconidium (Fig. 7.9), another form of asexual reproduction. No constriction is seen where the germ tube emerges from the yeast. In contrast, pseudohyphae *are* constricted where they emerge from the blastoconidium. This feature is critical for distinguishing these two structures. More than 90% of the yeasts isolated from clinical specimens that have a positive germ tube test are *C. albicans*. Most laboratories report all germ tube–positive yeasts as *C. albicans* without further testing. More than 90% of the yeasts that produce chlamydospores on CMT agar are *C. albicans*. Laboratories that use both the germ tube and chlamydospore tests have the best assurance of correctly determining whether the yeast is *C. albicans* or another yeast.

When the germ tube test is negative, and the isolate is from a normally sterile body site, additional tests must be done to identify the organism. CMT agar or a similar medium should be inoculated to determine the growth pattern of the organism and the microscopic structures formed. Urease production, nitrate utilization, the phenoloxidase test, and the ability of the organism to assimilate various carbohydrates should also be tested. The ability of the yeast to form a *pellicle* (a film) on the surface of a broth medium is sometimes an important differential fea-

ture; the test should be performed under standard conditions, using Sabouraud's dextrose broth (SDB). Several manufacturers market manual or automated rapid-identification kits featuring the biochemical tests for yeasts in various combinations. Without them many smaller laboratories could not afford to identify yeast because of the expense of maintaining the variety of media required for yeast identification.

Yeast and Yeastlike Organisms

BLASTOMYCETES

CANDIDA ALBICANS (Can-duh-duh or Can-deed'-uh al'[3]-buh-cans)

C. albicans is recognized as the most frequently encountered fungal opportunist and is now regarded as the most common cause of serious fungal disease.

■ **Reservoirs.** *C. albicans* is found worldwide on fruits and vegetables. It is an endogenous inhabitant of the alimentary tract and the mucocutaneous regions of the body. Although it is not usually found in large numbers on normal human skin, it rapidly colonizes the skin after an injury.

■ **Unique Risk Factors.** Any change in hormonal balance can increase the likelihood of infection with *C. albicans*. Depression of the immune response, whether from disease or as a result of various treatments, also increases the probability of a *Candida* infection.

■ **Human Infection.** The clinical diseases caused by *Candida* are collectively called **candidiasis**. *C. albicans* is the most common agent, but other species of *Candida* also cause candidiasis. Minor, self-limiting infections with *C. albicans* are seen in healthy people. *Candida* species, especially *C. albicans*, have been isolated from infections in every area of the human body, causing an enormous diversity of clinical syndromes. They are most often opportunistic pathogens of immunocompromised and debilitated hosts.

■ **Immunology.** Most people normally have low levels of antibody to *C. albicans*. Multiple blood samples should be obtained over time to allow detection of the increasing titers of anti-*Candida* antibodies associated with infection. Most tests for *Candida* antibody in immunosuppressed patients are negative or only weakly positive because antibody production is depressed or abrogated in these patients. The immunologic methods that are most widely used to detect antibodies in patients with func-

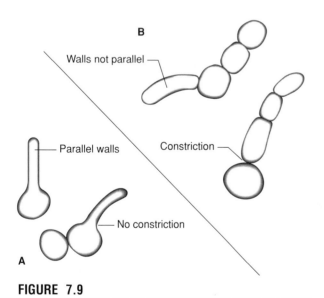

FIGURE 7.9

Germ tubes *(A)* are filamentous outgrowths that emerge from a blastoconidium in the initial stages of asexual reproduction. The sides of the slender tubes are approximately parallel *with no constriction* at the junction between germ tube and blastoconidium. In contrast, the walls of the cells in pseudohyphae *(B)* are not necessarily parallel and *constrictions are present* between cells of pseudohyphae.

[3]"Al" as in al-ligator.

tional immune systems are double immunodiffusion (ID), counterimmunoelectrophoresis (CIE), and latex agglutination (LA). These methods have sensitivity levels of about 80%. CIE and ID tests are the most specific. An enzyme-linked immunoassay (EIA), a test that detects the serum mannan[4] antigen with 80% sensitivity and 98% specificity, is recommended for testing immunocompromised patients suspected of having invasive candidiasis. Using two or more immunologic tests in combination increases the reliability of the diagnosis.

■ **Special Precautions.** None are needed.

■ **Culture Media.** BAP, modified SDA, modified SDA with cycloheximide and antibiotics.

Temperature Considerations. Optimal temperature for growth is 25° to 30°C; Tmax is 42° to 45°C for *C. albicans*.

■ **Macroscopic (Colony) Morphology.** On modified SDA at 25° to 37°C within 1 to 2 days *C. albicans* and most other *Candida* species develop as entire, white, pasty, convex colonies that initially resemble staphylococci. The colonies may produce pseudohyphal fringes around the periphery. Over time, the colonies typically become tan and rough and develop true hyphae that grow into the medium. Colony forms shift and are unstable, particularly when cultures are maintained for any length of time.

---

[4]Mannan is a constituent of the cell wall of *Candida*. It is present in the blood in systemic candidiasis.

■ **Microscopic Morphology** (Fig. 7.10). In a wet prep *C. albicans* demonstrates blastoconidia on pseudohyphae. NOTE that blastoconidia are more prevalent in cultures grown at 37°C than at 25°C. The blastoconidia are approximately the size of a normocytic red blood cell (3×6 μm to 6×10 μm), globose or ovoid, and thin walled. They occur singly or in tight clusters at the constrictions of the pseudohyphae. The pseudohyphae are hyaline, with cells occurring in elongated chains like fat linked sausages. *C. albicans* looks much the same when grown in CMT agar as it does in a wet prep, except for the large number of sessile and terminal chlamydospores that develop.

In *direct examination* (see Figs. 7.2 and 7.3) of specimens *C. albicans* produces the same structures: blastoconidia and pseudohyphae. Rippon says both are significant in infection. The blastoconidium must be present to initiate infection. The pseudohyphae form when the organism is exposed to environmental factors that inhibit the division of the cell wall while allowing growth.

■ **Laboratory Identification of *Candida albicans*.** A positive germ tube test and chlamydospore production on the appropriate media are generally considered adequate for identification of *C. albicans*. Biochemical tests and special methods for examination of the microscopic morphology are recommended for identification of other yeasts and for *Candida* species.

■ **Helpful Features for Identification of *Candida albicans***

Yeast-form colonies and microscopic structures at both 25°C and 37°C

FIGURE 7.10

Blastoconidia, singly and in pairs, are seen in wet preps of *Candida albicans (inset, A)*. Short pseudohyphae may also be present. In cornmeal-Tween 80 agar *(B)* many pseudohyphae are formed by elongated blastoconidia, and smaller oval blastoconidia cluster at the connection between adjacent pseudohyphal cells. Sessile and intercalary chlamydospores may also be seen. The presence of large numbers of terminal chlamydospores in CMT identifies the fungus as *C. albicans.* The 7-μm red blood cells (RBC) (arrow) show the relative sizes of the mycotic elements.

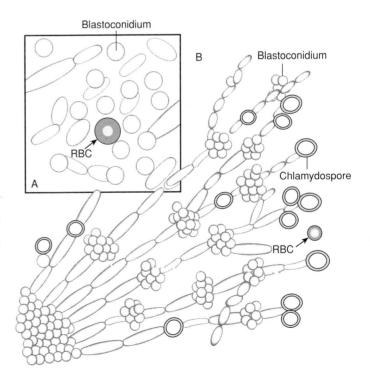

Both blastoconidia and pseudohyphae present
Germ tubes formed within 3 hours at 35°C
Many terminal chlamydospores on carbohydrate-rich agar
Characteristic pattern of carbohydrate utilization
Absence of capsules
General resistance to cycloheximide (a few varieties are sensitive)

■ **Organisms from Which *Candida albicans* Must Be Differentiated** (Tables 7.1 and 7.2; see also Fig. 7.24)

All other *Candida* species and the yeastlike organisms (*Rhodotorula, Saccharomyces, Torulopsis, Hansenula, Cryptococcus*)

Yeast and Yeastlike Organisms

BLASTOMYCETES

CANDIDA SPECIES

Candida species have many features in common with each other and with *Candida albicans*. The properties associated with all species other than *C. albicans* are reviewed here. Only those characteristics that are distinctive are presented in the discussion of individual species.

■ **Reservoirs.** Species of *Candida* are found worldwide as normal endogenous inhabitants of the body.

■ **Unique Risk Factors.** In general *Candida* species other than *C. albicans* are considered opportunistic pathogens, attacking those who are immunocompromised or debilitated.

■ **Human Infection.** *Candida* species are usually isolated as contaminants although various species have been reported as agents of disease. Some species are more prevalent than others as opportunistic pathogens. Almost any site in the body may be attacked by *Candida* species and *C. albicans*.

■ **Immunology.** See the general discussion of immunologic detection of candidiasis in the section for *C. albicans*.

■ **Special Precautions.** None are needed.

■ **Culture Media.** Almost any medium supports the growth of *Candida* for isolation, including media such as sheep blood agar. SDA, SABHI, or BHIA with and without antimicrobials are recommended.

Because *Candida* species vary in their sensitivity to cycloheximide, it is important to use media with and without antimicrobial agents.

CMT agar or another starchy medium may be inoculated to enhance production of characteristic microscopic structures.

Temperature Considerations. Optimal growth temperature for *Candida* species is 25°C, but all species also grow at 37°C.

■ **Laboratory Identification of *Candida* Species.** Special methods for examination of the microscopic morphology, as well as biochemical tests such as carbohydrate utilization, are necessary for distinguishing among *Candida* species. These procedures are discussed in the introduction for this chapter.

Yeast and Yeastlike Organisms

BLASTOMYCETES

CANDIDA GUILLIERMONDII (Can-duh-duh or Can-deed'-uh ghee-ur-mawn'-dee)

■ **Human Infection.** *C. guilliermondii* has been reported as the agent of urinary tract infections, endocarditis, cutaneous candidiasis, mycotic keratitis, and osteomyelitis.

■ **Culture Media.** *C. guilliermondii* is not sensitive to cycloheximide. Some isolates require prolonged incubation before visible colonies are formed.

■ **Macroscopic (Colony) Morphology.** On modified SDA at 25° to 37°C within 3 to 5 days *Candida guilliermondii* is a moist dull-white to cream-colored flat colony that is lacy; it forms wrinkles in a rugose pattern. After 2 to 3 weeks the colony acquires a pale pink color. *C. guilliermondii* occasionally requires a long incubation to form visible colonies.

■ **Microscopic Morphology** (Fig. 7.11). In a wet prep *C. guilliermondii* produces small ovoid blastoconidia in chains and clusters on long, thin, pseudohyphal cells that are slightly curved. The pseudohyphae are slow to develop; they may branch.

On CMT agar *C. guilliermondii* produces long, thin, slightly curved pseudohyphal cells that may be hard to see. Small (2 to 4.5 × 2.5 to 7 μm) blastoconidia form chains or clusters at constrictions of the pseudohyphae.

■ **Helpful Features for Identification of *Candida guilliermondii*** (see Fig. 7.24 and Tables 7.1 and 7.2)

Yeast-form colonies and microscopic structures at both 25°C and 37°C

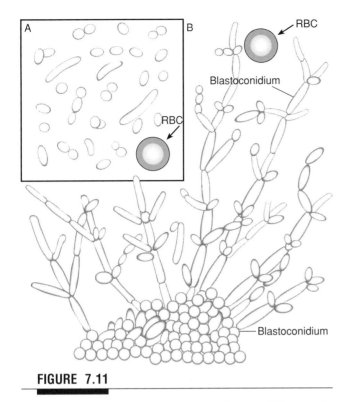

FIGURE 7.11

Wet preps of *Candida guillermondii (inset, A)* show ovoid blastoconidia singly and in pairs and short pseudohyphal chains. In cornmeal-Tween 80 agar *(B) C. guillermondii* develops relatively short, slender pseudohyphal cells that are slightly curved. Groups of blastoconidia form at constrictions between pseudohyphal cells. Chlamydospores are not formed. The 7-μm red blood cells (RBC) (arrow) show the relative sizes of the mycotic elements.

Both pseudohyphae and oval to elongate blastoconidia
Slender, slightly curved pseudohyphal cells
Compact clusters of blastoconidia that soon cover the pseudohyphae
Capsule, germ tube, and chlamydospore negative
Resistance to cycloheximide
No pellicle in broth
Biochemical reactions in urease, nitrate, and carbohydrate assimilation tests

Yeast and Yeastlike Organisms

BLASTOMYCETES

CANDIDA KEFYR[5] (Can-duh-duh or Can-deed'-uh key'-fur)

■ **Human Infection.** *C. kefyr* is one of the four most frequently isolated species of *Candida*. Urinary tract infections, endocarditis, mycotic keratitis, and onychomy-

---

[5]Formerly *Candida pseudotropicalis (sood-oh-trop-uh-callous)*

cosis caused by *C. kefyr* have occasionally been reported in debilitated or immunocompromised hosts.

■ **Culture Media.** *C. kefyr* is not sensitive to cycloheximide.

■ **Macroscopic (Colony) Morphology.** After 2 to 3 days on modified SDA at 25° to 37°C, *C. kefyr* develops smooth, cream-colored colonies. A fringe eventually develops around the periphery of the colony.

■ **Microscopic Morphology** (Fig. 7.12). In a wet prep from a colony *C. kefyr* produces a small number of blastoconidia of varying lengths (2.5 to 5 × 5 to 10 μm), usually with an abundant amount of branching pseudohyphae.

On CMT agar *C. kefyr* produces elongated blastoconidia at the junction of pseudohyphal cells, then separate from the pseudohyphae and lie parallel to it. This characteristic arrangement resembles logs in a river that have "jammed" on an obstruction and is called, logically enough, a "log jam" pattern.

■ **Helpful Features for Identification of *Candida kefyr*** (see Fig. 7.24 and Tables 7.1 and 7.2)

Yeast-form colonies and microscopic structures at both 25°C and 37°C
Both blastoconidia and pseudohyphae
"Log jam" arrangement of blastoconidia and pseudohyphae
Capsule, germ tube, and chlamydospore negative
Resistance to cycloheximide
No pellicle in broth
Biochemical reactions in urease, nitrate, and carbohydrate assimilation tests

Yeast and Yeastlike Organisms

BLASTOMYCETES

CANDIDA KRUSEI (Can-duh-duh or Can-deed'-uh cruise'-ee-eye)

■ **Human Infection.** *C. krusei* has been isolated, rarely, from cases of endocarditis and vaginitis and has been found in bone marrow recipients.

■ **Culture Media.** Some strains of *C. krusei* are sensitive to cycloheximide.

■ **Macroscopic (Colony) Morphology.** Colonies are similar to those of *Candida albicans*, but older colonies are flat and comparatively dull. Very old colonies are greenish yellow and dull, with a mycelial fringe around the colony.

TABLE 7.1 Biochemical Reactions for Yeasts and Yeastlike Fungi

Fungus	Germ Tubes Within 3 Hours at 25°C	Caffeic Acid (Niger Seed) Test	Capsule Present	Pseudohyphae on CMT at 25°C	Arthroconidia on CMT at 25°C	True Hyphae on CMT at 25°C	Urease Production	Nitrate Assimilation	Growth at 37°C on SDA	Growth at 42–45°C on SDA	Ascospores on Special Media
Candida albicans	Positive	Negative	No	Yes	No	Rare	No	Negative	Yes	Yes	No
*Candida stellatoidea**	Positive	Negative	No	Yes	No	No	No	Negative	Yes	—	No
Candida parapsilosis	Negative	Negative	No	Yes	No	No	No	Negative	Yes	—	No
Candida tropicalis	Negative	Negative	No	Yes	No	No	No	Negative	Yes	—	No
Candida kefyr†	Negative	Negative	No	Yes	No	No	No	Negative	Yes	—	No
Candida krusei	Negative	Negative	No	Yes	No	No	Yes‖	Negative	Yes	—	No
Candida guillermondii	Negative	Negative	No	Yes	No	No	No	Negative	Yes	—	No
Saccharomyces	Negative	Negative	No	Yes‖	No	No	No	Negative	Yes	—	Yes
Cryptococcus neoformans	Negative	Positive	Yes‡	Rare	No	No	Yes	Negative	Yes	No	No
Cryptococcus species	Negative	Variable	Yes‖	Rare	No	No	Yes	Negative‖	Variable	No	No
Geotrichum candidum	Negative	Negative	No	No	Yes	Yes	No	Negative	No‖	—	No
Hansenula anomala	Negative	Negative	No	No	No	No	No	Positive	Variable	—	Yes
Rhodotorula species	Negative‖	Negative	No‖	Rare	No	No	Yes‖	Positive‖	Yes	No	No
Prototheca species	Negative	Negative	No	No	No	No	No§	Negative	Yes	—	No
Torulopsis (Candida) glabrata	Negative	Negative	No	Rare	No	No	No	Negative	Yes	No	No
Trichosporon beigelii	Negative	Negative	No	Yes	Yes	Yes	Yes‖	Negative	Variable	—	No

Candida stellatoidea is considered by some mycologists to be a sucrose-negative variant of *Candida albicans*.
†*Candida kefyr* was previously named *Candida pseudotropicalis*.
‡In specimens from patients with a good immune response.
§Some variation in reactions among different strains of this species.
Positive,‖ Yes,‖ or +‖ means more varieties positive.
Negative,‖ No,‖ or 0‖ means more varieties negative.
The growth patterns and biochemical reactions of the yeastlike fungi are essential steps in correct identification.
d, variable (i.e., "differing"); CMT, cornmeal-Tween 80 agar; SDA, Sabouraud's dextrose agar.

■ **Microscopic Morphology** (Fig. 7.13). In a wet prep *C. krusei* produces elongated blastoconidia (3 to 5 × 6 to 20 μm) that chain and form pseudohyphae with treelike branching. On CMT agar *C. krusei* produces long branching pseudohyphae. Chains of blastoconidia develop at the junc-

tion of the pseudohyphal cells, creating a characteristic appearance that has been described as "crossed matchsticks."

Direct Examination. The structures seen in specimens resemble those seen in wet preps from colonies.

Assimilations													Fermentations					
Dextrose	Maltose	Sucrose	Lactose	Galactose	Melibiose	Cellobiose	Inositol	Xylose	Raffinose	Trehalose	Dulcitol	Starch	Dextrose	Maltose	Sucrose	Lactose	Galactose	Trehalose
+	+	+	0	+	0	0	0	+	0	+	0	+	+	+	0	0	+	+
+	+	0	0	+	0	0	0	+§	0	+§	0	+	+	+	0	0	0	0
+	+	+	0	+	0	0	0	+	0	+	0	0	+	0	0	0	0	0
+	+	+	0	+	0	+	0	+	0	+	0	+	+§	0	+‖	0	0	0§
+	0	+	+	+	0	+§	0	+‖	+	0‖	0	0	+	0	+	+‖	+	0
+	0	0	0	0	0	0	0	0	0	0	0	0	+	0	0	0	0	0
+	+	+	0	+	+	+	0	+	+	+	+	+‖	+	0	0	0	0	0
+	+	+	0	+	0	0	0	0	+	+‖	0	0	+	+	+	0	+	+
+	+	+	0	+	0	+	+	+	+‖	+‖	+	+‖	0	0	0	0	0	0
+	+	+	0‖	+§	+‖	+	+	+	+§	+‖	+‖	0	0	0	0	0	0	0
+	0	0	0	+	0	0	0	+	0	0	0	—	0	0	0	0	0	0
+	+	+	0	+	0	+	0	+	0	+	0	0	+	+‖	+	0	+	0
+	+	+	0	+‖	0	+‖	0	+	+	+	0	0	0	0	0	0	0	0
+	0	+‖	0	+	0	0	0	0	0	+‖	0	0	0	0	0	0	0	0
0	0	0	0	0	0	0	0	0	0	+	0	+‖	+	0	0	0	0	0
+	+	+	+	+‖	+§	+‖	+	+	+§	+§	+§	+§	0	0	0	0	0	0

■ **Helpful Features for Identification of *C. krusei*** (see Fig. 7.24 and Tables 7.1 and 7.2)

Yeast-form colonies and microscopic structures at both 25°C and 37°C

Both blastoconidia and pseudohyphae, with blastoconidia at junctions in pseudohyphae

Lo-o-ng pseudohyphal cells

Crossed matchsticks

Capsule, germ tube, and chlamydospore negative

Sensitivity to cycloheximide

Appearance of pellicle; in SDB the pellicle grows up the sides of the test tube

Biochemical reactions in urease, nitrate, and carbohydrate assimilation tests

TABLE 7.2 Morphology of Yeast and Yeastlike Fungi

Fungus	Size of Conidia (μm)	Shape of Conidia	Pseudohyphae (CMT)	Appearance in CMT	Germ Tube Test	Colony Morphology	Growth Rate	Other Helpful Features
Candida albicans	4 × 6	Oval, elliptical, or round blastoconidia	Yes	Elongate pseudohyphal cells with large clusters of blastoconidia at junctures between cells. Sessile, intercalary, and many terminal chlamydospores	Positive	Slightly dry white or cream bacteria-like colony	Growth in 1–2 days	Yeast most frequently isolated from clinical specimens
Candida guillermondii	3 × 5	Oval or elliptical blastoconidia	Yes	Long, slender, slightly curved cells with pairs and small clusters of blastoconidia at junctures between cells. No terminal chlamydospores	Negative	Moist, dull white to creamy flat lacy colony that becomes wrinkled or rugose	Growth in 3–5 days	Pale pink color may develop in colonies after 2–3 weeks
Candida kefyr	3 × 8	Elongate, slender, oval blastoconidia	Yes	Elongate, slender pseudohyphal cells with adjacent free blastoconidia, resembling logs in a stream	Negative	Smooth, cream-colored colonies	Growth in 2–3 days	Older colonies acquire a peripheral fringe
Candida krusei	4 × 12	Spheres, ellipses, and elongate oval blastoconidia of varying sizes	Yes	Long, slender, straight cells with treelike branching and chains of blastoconidia from the juncture between cells resemble "crossed matchsticks"	Negative	Similar to *Candida albicans* but duller	Growth in 2–3 days	Very old colonies become greenish yellow and dull, with a peripheral fringe
Candida parapsilosis	3 × 6	Spherical and elliptical blastoconidia	Yes	Short, thin cells with pronounced curve, and occasional giant cells. Blastoconidia develop singly, in clusters and short chains on the pseudohyphae	Negative	Compact, moist shiny white or cream colonies that may be lacy	Growth in 2–3 days	Old colonies become wrinkled and the periphery turns brown
Candida tropicalis	6 × 8	Ovoid or elongate blastoconidia	Yes	Long branching pseudohyphae with blastoconidia anywhere along the pseudohyphae. Chlamydoconidia and true hyphae occasionally form	Negative	White to cream colonies	Growth in 2–3 days	Peripheral fringe may be submerged in the agar
Cryptococcus species	4–20	Globose blastoconidia	None	Globose cells in varying sizes that do not touch	Negative	Mucoid or moist white colonies that become dull and tan	2–4 days	Colonies become dull and tan as they age

Organism	Size (µm)	Conidia	Pseudohyphae	Microscopic morphology	CMT	Colony morphology	Growth rate	Comments
Geotrichum candidum	4 × 12	Rectangular arthroconidia	None	Hyphae, often fragmented into arthroconidia	Negative	Spreading white yeastlike colonies	2–3 days	Mature colonies are dry and powdery with a submerged hyphal fringe. Germinating arthroconidia resemble hockey sticks
Hansenula anomala	3.5 × 4.2	Globose or ellipical blastoconidia	None	Yeast cells with multilateral budding	Negative	Resembling colonies of *Candida* or *Cryptococcus*	2–3 days	Globose to elliptical blastoconidia with multilateral budding
Malassezia furfur	4.5 × 2.5	Oval blastoconidia (bowling pins)	None	NA	Negative	Black yeast	6–10 days	Requires lipids in media for growth
Pneumocystis carinii	5–12	Globose to ovoid "cysts"	NA	NA	NA	Unknown	NA	Consult a parasitology text for details of cellular morphology†
Rhodotorula species	2–14	Globose blastoconidia	Rare	Globose cells with multilateral budding	Negative	Spectrum of pigment from coral red to yellow, moist to mucoid	3–4 days	Sometimes a faint capsule is produced
Saccharomyces	6 × 12	Oval or ellipsoidal to globose blastoconidia	None	Oval to ellipsoidal yeast with multilateral budding and occasional short chains of blastoconidia	Negative	Flat, moist, shiny or dull white colonies	3 days	Asci and ascospores are produced on special media
Torulopsis (Candida) glabrata	2–4	Globose or oval blastoconidia	None	Globose or oval cells with occasional short branched chains	Negative	Moist, smooth, and shiny white colonies that darken and wrinkle with age	3 days	May be found intracellularly in tissue samples
Trichosporon beigelii	3 × 6	Ovoid or pyriform blastoconidia	Yes	Blastoconidia on pseudohyphae; true hyphae break into arthroconidia	Negative	Moist at first, becoming wrinkled cream to gray	5 days	Growth inhibited by cycloheximide

*Some variation among species or strains within a species.
†May resemble conidia or nonbudding yeast forms.
The yeast and yeastlike fungi that produce pseudohyphae and true hyphae can often be distinguished by details of the walls and shapes of the microscopic structures. Colony morphology, growth patterns, and biochemical reactions are also useful.
NA, not available CMT, cornmeal-Tween 80 agar.

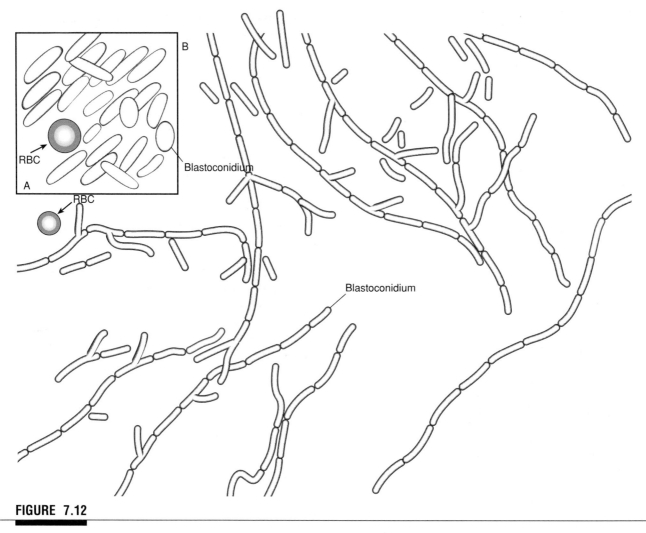

FIGURE 7.12

Wet preps of *Candida kefyr (inset, A)* show relatively long, thin, oval blastoconidia that somewhat resemble frankfurters. Pseudohyphae develop on cornmeal-Tween 80 agar *(B)*. Individual blastoconidia of *C. kefyr* readily separate from the pseudohyphae, then come to rest parallel to the pseudohyphae, resembling a log jam—look in the upper right corner for a hint of this. The 7-μm red blood cells (RBC) (arrow) show the relative sizes of the mycotic elements.

Yeast and Yeastlike Organisms

BLASTOMYCETES

CANDIDA PARAPSILOSIS (Can-duh-duh or Candeed'-uh pair-ap'-sill-o-sis')

■ **Human Infection.** *C. parapsilosis* has been isolated with increasing frequency from urinary tract infections and pyelonephritis, endocarditis, cutaneous candidiasis, paronychia, otitis externa, mycotic keratitis, fungemia, vaginitis, and endophthalmitis. It has also been isolated as the agent of nosocomial infections following cardiovascular surgery or the use of indwelling catheters.

■ **Culture Media.** *C. parapsilosis* is sensitive to cycloheximide.

■ **Macroscopic (Colony) Morphology.** On modified SDA at 25°C after 2 to 3 days, *C. parapsilosis* develops compact, moist colonies that are shiny white to cream colored; they have a smooth or lacy topography. Colonies become wrinkled with age, and the periphery of the colony turns brown in 3 to 4 weeks.

C. parapsilosis forms spider-like colonies in CMT agar, with satellite "fingers" extending outward from the line of the inoculation streak. These fingers can be seen under low-power magnification.

■ **Microscopic Morphology** (Fig. 7.14). In a wet prep *C. parapsilosis* produces small elongate blastoconidia in chains and clusters, together with branching pseudohyphae.

On CMT agar *C. parapsilosis* produces short, thin, markedly curved pseudohyphal cells that sometimes develop into large "giant" pseudohyphal cells. Ovoid or elongate blastoconidia (2.5 to 4 × 2.5 to 9 μm) form

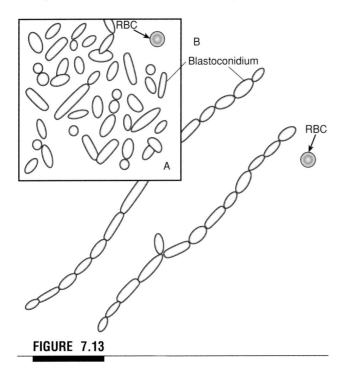

FIGURE 7.13

In wet preps *(inset, A) Candida krusei* has blastoconidia of varying sizes and shapes, including long, slender forms. When *C. krusei* grows in cornmeal-Tween 80 agar *(B)* pseudohyphae branch like trees. Chains of blastoconidia extend from the junctions of the pseudohyphal cells. The 7-μm red blood cells (RBC) (arrow) show the relative sizes of the mycotic elements.

singly or in short chains or clusters along and between the junctions of the pseudohyphae.

- **Helpful Features for Identification of *C. parapsilosis*** (see Fig. 7.24 and Tables 7.1 and 7.2)

    Yeast-form colonies and microscopic structures at both 25°C and 37°C
    Both blastoconidia and pseudohyphae
    Short, curved pseudohyphal cells that may develop into "giant" cells
    Capsule, germ tube, and chlamydospore negative
    Sensitivity to cycloheximide
    No pellicle in broth (a light surface film does develop)
    Biochemical reactions in urease, nitrate, and carbohydrate assimilation tests

Yeast and Yeastlike Organisms

BLASTOMYCETES

CANDIDA TROPICALIS   Can-duh-duh or Candeed'-uh trop[6]-uh-callous)

- **Human Infection.** *C. tropicalis* is presently second only to *Candida albicans* as the cause of serious candidiasis

[6]"Trop" rhymes with drop.

in immunocompromised patients. Vaginitis, intestinal disease, and bronchopulmonary and systemic infections due to *C. tropicalis* are increasing in frequency. The yeast has also been isolated from cases of meningitis, thrush, endophthalmitis, endocarditis, and fungemia.

- **Culture Media.** Some strains of *C. tropicalis* are sensitive to cycloheximide.

- **Macroscopic (Colony) Morphology.** After 2 to 3 days on modified SDA at 25° to 37°C, *C. tropicalis* develops white to cream-colored colonies. They may be smooth, moist, and shiny or heaped, rough, and waxy. A fringe around the periphery of the colony may become submerged into the agar.

- **Microscopic Morphology** (Fig. 7.15). In a wet prep *C. tropicalis* produces ovoid or elongate (4 to 8 × 5 to 11 μm) blastoconidia. They typically occur singly along the hyphae and at the junctions in the pseudohyphae. Rarely, blastoconidia develop on true hyphae growing in the medium.

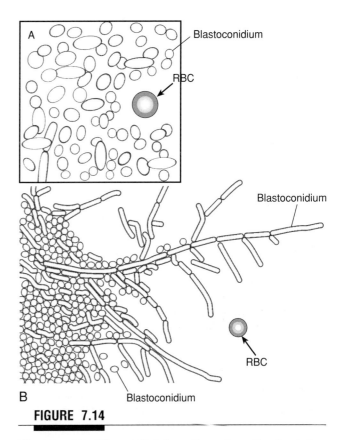

FIGURE 7.14

Wet preps of *Candida parapsilosis (inset, A)* contain small oval and elongate blastoconidia singly and in pairs and chains, with occasional long pseudohyphal cells. In cornmeal-Tween 80 *(B) C. parapsilosis* produces pseudohyphae in which the predominant cell is short and thin with a pronounced curve. Blastoconidia occur singly, in clusters, or in short chains along the pseudohyphae. Under low-power magnification "fingers" of the colony in CMT extend outward from the line of inoculation. The 7-μm red blood cells (RBC) (arrow) show the relative sizes of the mycotic elements.

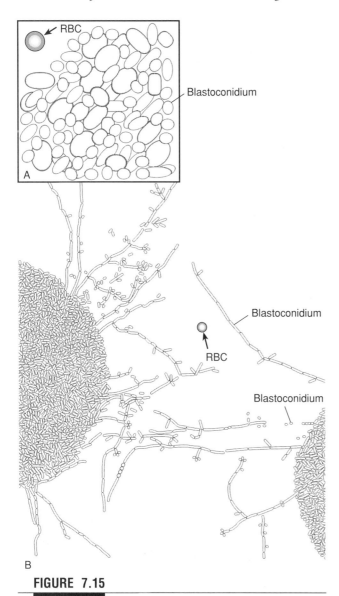

FIGURE 7.15

In wet preps *(inset, A) Candida tropicalis* produces oval or elongate blastoconidia, with occasional pseudohyphae. *C. tropicalis* produces abundant long branching pseudohyphae on cornmeal-Tween 80 agar *(B)*, with blastoconidia formed randomly along the pseudohyphal cells and occasional small chlamydoconidia (that disappear after subculture). True hyphae occasionally develop. The 7-μm red blood cells (RBC) (arrow) show the relative sizes of the mycotic elements.

On CMT agar *C. tropicalis* produces abundant long, branching pseudohyphae. Ovoid or elongate (4 to 8 × 5 to 11 μm) blastoconidia are found anywhere along the pseudohyphae, including adjacent to the junctions. True hyphae may also be present. Small terminal thin-walled oval to tear-shaped chlamydoconidia are produced occasionally in initial culture by some strains but disappear in subcultures. Chlamydoconidia production can be enhanced by first incubating a freshly inoculated CMT agar at 25°C for 2 to 3 days, then refrigerating it for 3 to 6 days.

■ **Helpful Features for Identification of *C. tropicalis*** (see Fig. 7.24 and Tables 7.1 and 7.2)

Yeast-form colonies and microscopic structures at both 25°C and 37°C
Both blastoconidia and pseudohyphae
True hyphae may be formed
Capsule and germ tube[7] negative
Surface film, with bubbles, in SDB
Biochemical reactions in urease, nitrate, and carbohydrate assimilation tests

Yeast and Yeastlike Organisms

BLASTOMYCETES

CRYPTOCOCCUS NEOFORMANS   (Crip-toe-cock'-us knee-oh-for'-munz)

■ **Teleomorph.** *Filobasidiella neoformans.*

■ **Reservoirs.** *C. neoformans* is found worldwide, wherever pigeons roost. Its chief vector is the pigeon *Columbia livia.* The yeast is able to survive passage through the pigeon's gut. It remains viable for 2 years or longer in the excreta deposited around the nesting area, although it typically loses its capsule during this period. When the small (2 μm) virulent nonencapsulated organisms found in environmental dust are inhaled, they enter the alveolar spaces of the host's lung. Here they establish colonies, produce a capsule, and (sometimes) cause disease. *C. neoformans* has also been isolated from dairy products, fruits and vegetables, and the excreta of birds other than pigeons. Kwon-Chung and Bennett postulate that *C. neoformans* in pigeon droppings could be due to eating food contaminated with the yeast.

■ **Unique Risk Factors.** Despite its long history as an agent of meningitis *C. neoformans* is considered an opportunistic pathogen. Exposure to soil contaminated with pigeon excrement is potentially hazardous to those who are immunosuppressed.

■ **Human Infection.** The incidence of *C. neoformans* infection has greatly increased with the spread of AIDS and the increased occurrence of other immunosuppressed conditions. *Cryptococcosis* initially is a chronic or subacute pulmonary infection, but the yeast has a predilection for the central nervous system and the brain. In those who are immunosuppressed *C. neoformans* rapidly spreads to cause a fulminant systemic or central nervous system infection; meningitis (meningoencephalitis) is the most common form of cryptococcosis. Cutaneous cryptococcosis is regu-

---

[7]Some isolates look germ tube positive, but the ability is rapidly lost after repeated subculture.

larly encountered in immunosuppressed patients; the bone is involved in as many as 10% of reported cases. Eye infections may lead to blindness.

■ **Specimen Sources.** *C. neoformans* may be found in almost any tissue. The usual specimens are cerebrospinal fluid, blood, urine, and respiratory secretions, and pus or biopsied tissue from skin lesions.

Direct examination of specimens should follow standard procedures, *except that* care should be taken to concentrate specimens by filtration or centrifugation to increase the likelihood of recovering any *Cryptococcus* present. Filtration is preferred because centrifugation may collapse the yeast cells, making them inviable. If enough specimen is available, an India ink preparation can be run in conjunction with the cryptococcal LA test. The India ink preparation isn't sensitive, but it's fast.

■ **Immunology.** Four serotypes (A, B, C, and D) have been described for *C. neoformans*; Serotype A is the one most often isolated from human infections. Serotype B, once isolated primarily from patients on the U.S. West Coast, since the advent of AIDS, rarely been isolated. Serotype C is prevalent in tropical areas, and Serotype D is prevalent in Europe.

No one has developed a useful skin test for diagnosis of cryptococcosis because of the low antibody response by the host, but several immunologic tests are available for measuring antibody titers in patient serum. Several fluorescent antibody tests are recognized, both for tissue studies and for serotyping cultures. A whole yeast cell tube agglutination test and an EIA procedure are available for detecting Cryptococcus in patient serum. These tests are valuable for early diagnosis of the infection, which improves the prognosis for the patient because the appropriate treatment can be started.

Antigen tests are more specific than tests for antibody. A simple, rapid LA test is commercially available to detect the polysaccharide capsular antigen of *C. neoformans* in serum and cerebrospinal fluid. Methods are reportedly both sensitive and specific, but false-negative results do occur. Serum from patients with rheumatoid factor or disseminated *Trichosporon beigelii* infections may contain a component that reacts with the cryptococcal antigen. The cross-reaction can be eliminated by boiling the specimen with Na^2EDTA or by treating the serum with 5 mg of pronase per milliliter of serum. Titers greater than 1:2 in the LA test indicate active cryptococcosis.

The LA method developed for *C. neoformans* may detect other species of *Cryptococcus*. If the organisms can be isolated, carbohydrate assimilation tests should be done to identify the species. Of course any organism isolated from the cerebrospinal fluid is considered pathogenic.

■ **Culture Media.** Almost any medium can be used, with and without antibacterial antibiotics. *C. neoformans* is sensitive to cycloheximide.

Capsule production can be enhanced by inoculating a plate of standard chocolate agar and incubating it at 35°C in the presence of 5% to 10% CO_2 or by growing the culture in a 1% peptone solution.

Temperature Considerations. *C. neoformans* can grow at temperatures from 25° to 37°C. Most species of *Cryptococcus* other than *C. neoformans* cannot grow at temperatures of 37°C, but *Cryptococcus terreus* does. *Cryptococcus laurentii* varies in its ability to grow at 37°C.

■ **Laboratory Identification of *Cryptococcus neoformans.*** Biochemical tests as well as special methods for examination of the microscopic morphology are useful for distinguishing *C. neoformans* from related organisms. The tests include carbohydrate and nitrate utilization, urease production, and the phenoloxidase test or caffeic acid/bird seed/thistle/niger seed agar.

■ **Macroscopic (Colony) Morphology.** On modified SDA at 25° to 37°C within 2 to 4 days, *C. neoformans* colonies typically are dome shaped and shiny white to tan, but they may be yellow to light pink or light brown. If the organism has a capsule, colonies will be mucoid; they become dry and dull as they age.

■ **Microscopic Morphology** (Figs. 7.16 and 7.17). *Cryptococcus neoformans* is a thin-walled globose or oval-shaped yeast that varies greatly in size. Cells may occur

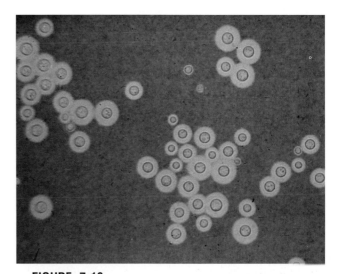

FIGURE 7.16

Positive India ink preps for *Cryptococcus neoformans* show large colorless or white circles against a black background. The cryptococcal cells form the center of the circles. The walls are refractile and the interior generally shows disorganized granules and blobs of material. A featureless amorphous "halo"—the capsule—surrounds the yeast cell. The width of the capsule varies from yeast to yeast and patient to patient. White blood cells can be mistaken for *Cryptococcus*. The differences are that white blood cells have an organized central mass—the nucleus—the walls are less refractile, and the rim of the halo is fuzzy rather than defined. (Courtesy of the Centers for Disease Control and Prevention.)

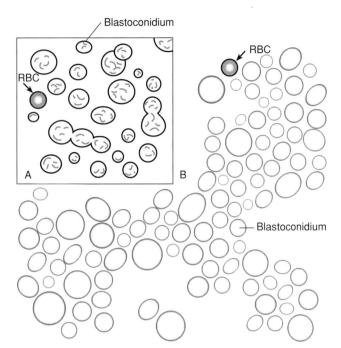

FIGURE 7.17

In a wet prep *(inset, A) Cryptococcus neoformans* typically appears as large globose forms of varying sizes. Pairs and short chains of cells may be seen, but these appear much less frequently than they do with *Candida* species. In densely packed fields of a wet prep most cells of *Cryptococcus* appear not to be in contact because the capsules hold them apart. The appearance of *C. neoformans* in cornmeal-Tween 80 medium *(B)* is not much different than the wet prep, except that the cells are stationary. Globose cells of varying sizes, separated by the invisible capsule, predominate. Pseudohyphae are not formed, and true hyphae rarely develop. The 7-μm red blood cells (RBC) (arrow) show the relative sizes of the mycotic elements.

singly or in pairs; neither pseudohyphae nor true hyphae occur, but very rare strains do produce rudimentary hyphae on CMT agar and in tissue. Budding may be single or double, with narrow points of attachment between the mother and the daughter cells. The cells are usually surrounded by refractile mucopolysaccharide capsules of varying width, especially in preparations made directly from the specimen. The appearance of a capsule is related in some degree to the strength of the host's immune response. Capsules form to protect the organism from the host, remember?

The India ink preparation for detection of *C. neoformans* in cerebrospinal fluid has been replaced by latex agglutination (LA) tests for the capsular antigen in most laboratories because of LA's greater speed and sensitivity. Nonetheless, the India ink prep remains a good technique for viewing encapsulated yeasts in culture.

■ Helpful Features for Identification of *Cryptococcus neoformans*

Yeast-form colonies and microscopic structures at both 25°C and 37°C

Large yeast cells (typically without pseudohyphae or true hyphae)

Capsule positive; germ tube and chlamydospore negative

Sensitivity to cycloheximide

Rapid production of phenoloxidase, and formation of brown colonies on caffeic acid (birdseed) agar

Biochemical reactions in urease, nitrate, and carbohydrate assimilation tests

■ Organisms from Which *Cryptococcus neoformans* Must Be Differentiated (see Fig. 7.24 and Tables 7.1 and 7.2)

Rhodotorula species
Other *Cryptococcus* species

Yeast and Yeastlike Organisms

BLASTOMYCETES

CRYPTOCOCCUS SPECIES (Crip-toe-cock'-us species)

Nineteen species of *Cryptococcus* other than *C. neoformans* are presently recognized. Six species that are most often recovered from clinical specimens as contaminants or, occasionally, as agents of infection, are the following:

Cryptococcus albidus var. *albidus* (al[8]-buh-diss)
Cryptococcus albidus var. *diffluens* (dih-flue-ens)
Cryptococcus luteolus (lute-ee-ohl-us)
Cryptococcus laurentii (law-rent-ee)
Cryptococcus terreus (tear-us)
Cryptococcus gastricus (gas-truh-cuss)

No sexual reproductive method has yet been discovered for these species of *Cryptococcus*. Because of the many

[8]"Al" as in al-ligator.

similarities among these species, biochemical tests must be done to distinguish them from *C. neoformans* and other yeasts and to differentiate among species of *Cryptococcus* (see Tables 7.1 and 7.2). These methods for examination of the microscopic morphology, as well as biochemical tests, are discussed with *C. neoformans*.

Yeast and Yeastlike Organisms

MONILIACEAE

GEOTRICHUM CANDIDUM (Gee'-oh-trick-um can'-deed'-um)

■ **Reservoirs.** *G. candidum* is thought to be normal flora on human skin and in the gastrointestinal tract. It is often isolated from milk and dairy products, vegetables, and fruit.

■ **Human Infection.** *G. candidum* and other species of *Geotrichum* have been isolated from infections in debilitated and immunocompromised patients in cases of vaginitis, thrush, bronchitis, and cutaneous infections. The general term for these infections is *geotrichosis*.

■ **Unique Risk Factors.** None.

■ **Culture Media.** *G. candidum* is sensitive to cycloheximide.

■ **Macroscopic (Colony) Morphology.** After 2 to 3 days on modified SDA at 25°C, *G. candidum* is seen as spreading white yeastlike colonies. As the culture matures it becomes mouldlike with short fuzzy aerial mycelia, acquiring a dry, powdery texture. The pigment becomes more cream colored, and a hyphal fringe of subsurface growth develops around the periphery of the colony.

At 37°C surface growth is sparse, with slow subsurface growth of hyphae predominating, giving a "ground glass" appearance to the colony.

■ **Microscopic Morphology** (Figs. 7.18 and 7.19). In a wet prep *G. candidum* demonstrates wide (3 to 4 × 4 to 12 μm) septate, hyaline true hyphae with lateral branching. Abundant arthroconidia form from the cells of the hyphae by splitting the double septa between the hyphal cells; eventually the hyphae fragment, releasing the arthroconidia. Arthroconidia vary markedly in size and shape but characteristically are rectangular or barrel shaped with thin walls. The ends of the arthroconidia are typically rounded, although they may be square. Arthroconidia that have been liberated germinate by sending out a germ tube from one corner of the cell, creating an arrangement resembling a hockey stick. Neither blastoconidia nor pseudohyphae are formed.

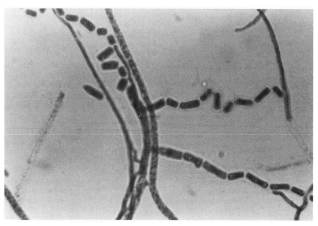

FIGURE 7.18

The "corners" on the rectangular arthroconidia of *Geotrichum candidum* are very square, in contrast with the rounded ends and irregular width of the pseudohyphal cells formed by *Candida* species. The trail of arthroconidia running through this photomicrograph from upper left to lower right shows the typical arrangement of arthroconidia; they seem to "snap," and some cells turn at approximately right angles to the original structure, as if to make room for adjacent cells. (Courtesy of the Centers for Disease Control and Prevention.)

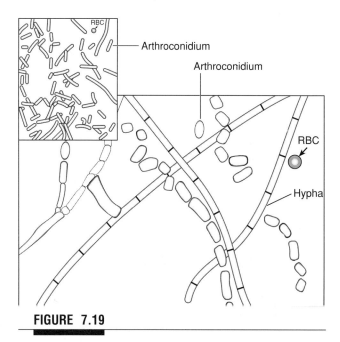

FIGURE 7.19

Wet preps of *Geotrichum candidum (inset)* contain true hyphae with septa and short, broad arthroconidia with rounded ends. Arthroconidia may remain attached, creating a structure resembling pseudohyphae. In cornmeal-Tween 80 agar *G. candidum* has essentially the same structures, except that true hyphae predominate. The arthroconidia are longer, tend to remain in the pattern of the original hyphae, and are more likely to have square—not rounded—corners. Germ tubes emerge from one corner of germinating arthroconidia of *G. candidum*, creating a structure that resembles a hockey stick. The 7-μm red blood cells (RBC) (arrow) show the relative sizes of the mycotic elements.

On CMT agar *Geotrichum* species produce structures similar to its microscopic morphology on modified SDA.

■ Helpful Features for Identification of *Geotrichum candidum*

Yeast-form colonies initially at 25°C, becoming mouldlike as the colony ages
Arthroconidia germinating in a "hockey stick" arrangement
Neither blastoconidia nor pseudohyphae
True hyphae formed
Sensitivity to cycloheximide

Pellicle in broth
Biochemical reactions in urease, nitrate, and carbohydrate assimilation tests

■ Organisms from Which *G. candidum* Must Be Differentiated (Fig. 7.20; see also Figs. 7.24 and 8.7; see also Tables 7.1, 7.2, and 8.3)

Trichosporon species
Coccidioides immitis

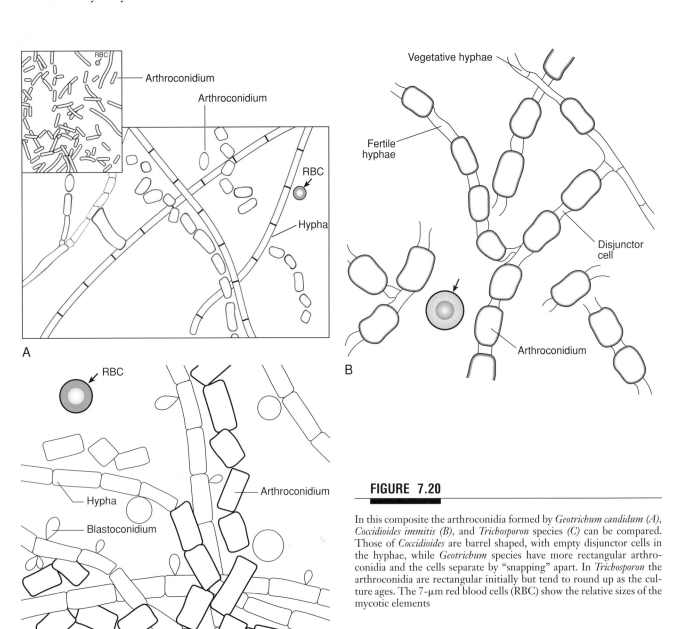

FIGURE 7.20

In this composite the arthroconidia formed by *Geotrichum candidum (A)*, *Coccidioides immitis (B)*, and *Trichosporon* species *(C)* can be compared. Those of *Coccidioides* are barrel shaped, with empty disjunctor cells in the hyphae, while *Geotrichum* species have more rectangular arthroconidia and the cells separate by "snapping" apart. In *Trichosporon* the arthroconidia are rectangular initially but tend to round up as the culture ages. The 7-μm red blood cells (RBC) show the relative sizes of the mycotic elements

Ascomycetous Yeasts

ASCOMYCETES

HANSENULA SPECIES (Hans-en-oooh'-la species)

Two species, *Hansenula anomala* and *Hansenula polymorpha*, are presently included in this genus as opportunistic pathogens of humans. The anamorph of *H. anomala* is *Candida pelliculosa*.

■ **Reservoirs.** *Hansenula* species may occasionally be found as part of the normal endogenous flora of the human throat and alimentary tract. They are frequently found in soil and on various fruits and vegetables.

■ **Unique Risk Factors.** None.

■ **Human Infection.** *Hansenula* species have been isolated from infections in a very small number of debilitated and immunocompromised patients. In 1980 McGinnis reported a case involving *Hansenula* in a child with granulomatous disease. Subsequently, in 1986, Murphy reported colonization and infection in 52 neonates. In the same year Klein reported a case of catheter-related infection due to *Hansenula* in an adult. Although the incidence of infection has rarely been reported to date, it is considered to be rising in association with increasing numbers of compromised and debilitated patients. Increasing awareness of this organism and improved techniques are factors contributing to the (apparent) increase in *Hansenula* infections.

■ **Culture Media.** In addition to the standard media, V-8 ascospore medium is helpful for demonstration of the characteristic features of sexual reproduction of *Hansenula*.

Temperature Considerations. Optimal growth temperature is 25°C. Growth of *Hansenula* at 37°C is variable.

■ **Macroscopic (Colony) Morphology.** Colonies of *Hansenula* appear on modified SDA at 25°C after 2 to 3 days. While the culture typically is recognizable as a colony of yeast, there are several variations of colony morphology. Colonies of *Hansenula* may be confused with colonies of either *Candida* or *Cryptococcus*. The colonies are described as moist, glistening, white to cream to tan, with a smooth to wrinkled topography.

■ **Microscopic Morphology.** On CMT agar at 25°C some species of *Hansenula* produce both pseudohyphae and true hyphae, but this has not been reported for *H. anomala* and *H. polymorpha*. These two species produce many blastoconidia budding from the yeast cells at different sites. The multilateral blastoconidia are globose to elliptical.

H. anomala is an ascosporogenous yeast. To detect the teleomorph phase growth from V-8 agar should be stained with Kinyoun's modified acid-fast stain. ***Asci (sing. ascus)*** are produced that contain up to four ***ascospores*** that have turned-down "brims." The cells resemble derby hats, the typical British "bowler" the actor-mime Charlie Chaplin and comedians Laurel and Hardy wore. The vegetative cells of *Hansenula* species are approximately 1 to 5 × 2 to 5 μm in size.

■ **Helpful Features for Identification of *Hansenula* Species**

> Yeast-form colonies at 25°C (and at 37°C if they can grow at the higher temperature)
> Blastoconidia
> Capsule, germ tube, and chlamydospore negative
> True hyphae or pseudohyphae in some species
> Biochemical reactions in urease, nitrate, and carbohydrate assimilation tests

Yeast and Yeastlike Organisms

ASCOMYCETES

PNEUMOCYSTIS CARINII (New-moe-cyst-iss kuh-wren-ee)

Until recently *P. carinii* was considered a parasite. It was reclassified in 1988 and placed in the Class Ascomycetes because of similarities with *Saccharomyces cerevisiae*. The two fungi have similar structures, RNA patterns, and ribosomal sequences.

Because *P. carinii* has only recently been included with the fungi, some of the characteristics presented for other organisms in this text are not yet known. For additional information, especially about infections, consult a parasitology rather than a mycology text.

■ **Reservoirs.** Human tissue is one reservoir for *P. carinii*. The fungus may be acquired in infancy and remain dormant in tissues until some weakness of the individual's immune system provides it an opportunity for infection. Related strains of the fungus are widespread in nature and in rodents and other mammals. It is believed to be transmitted by airborne routes.

■ **Unique Risk Factors.** Infections are found in debilitated and immunocompromised hosts, especially those

invades MØ

with malignancies, leukemia, and AIDS. They also occur in malnourished babies and children.

■ Human Infection.

Inhaled

P. carinii pneumonia (PCP) is often the first opportunistic infection to develop in patients positive for human immunodeficiency virus. The yeast has been isolated from lung tissue and from aspirates from the lungs and related structures.

The infection is a diffuse interstitial plasma cell pneumonia that at first resembles *Mycoplasma* pneumonias. The yeast multiples in the alveolar spaces of the lung, causing distention of the alveoli from the copious secretions produced. The bronchial secretions contain macrophages that have ingested the *Pneumocystis*. As the infection progresses fibrosis develops in the alveoli. Dissemination of *Pneumocystis* from the lungs to other organs is rare.

■ Specimen Sources.

Specimens most likely to be submitted for culture are lung tissue, bronchial brushings, and respiratory secretions.

■ Specimen Collection and Handling.

Specimens should be collected according to the standard protocol for the type of specimen. If necessary, sputa may be induced by administering an aerosolized spray of sodium chloride and glycerin. Rapid transport to the laboratory is imperative.

Direct examination of specimens of tissue should include *impression smears*, that is, smears made by impressing (touching) the slide with the tissue. Tissues should be prepared for staining by the histology laboratory. Two kinds of stains should be used: Gomori's methenamine silver (GMS) stain or toluidine blue is preferred for the "cyst" form of the fungus; Giemsa or Wright-Giemsa stain is recommended for the "trophozoite" forms.[9]

Direct smears of sputum and other respiratory secretions are likely to be negative even when PCP is present.

■ Immunology.

An immunofluorescence method using a monoclonal antibody is commercially available for detecting *P. carinii* in specimens.

Serologic tests are of little value because a large percentage of the population has antibodies from colonization and asymptomatic infections.

■ Special Precautions.

None are needed, but specimens should be handled within a biologic safety cabinet.

■ Culture Media.

P. carinii has not yet been isolated in culture.

---

[9]The terms "cyst," "sporozoite," and "trophozoite" were used to describe the stages of the life cycle of *P. carinii* when it was considered a parasite. New labels, more appropriate for a fungus, have not yet been attached to these stages.

■ Laboratory Identification of *P. carinii*.

Identification rests on linking the characteristic microscopic structures of the organism found in tissue specimens to the symptoms of the infection. As noted earlier, this requires use of special stains.

■ Macroscopic (Colony) Morphology.

Unknown.

■ Microscopic Morphology.

Pneumocystis species are unicellular organisms that may appear in either of two forms. The "cyst" is the stage in the life cycle of some parasites where the organism is enclosed in a protective wall. The thick-walled cyst ranges from 5 to 12 µm in diameter; cysts may contain up to eight oval "sporozoites"[9] that mature into *trophozoites*. Sporozoites develop within a cyst; trophozoites develop immediately after sporozoites are released from the cyst.

Free trophozoites of *Pneumocystis* are ameboid in shape, and average 5 µm in diameter. They have a visible nucleus in stained preparations. The surface of trophozoites is covered with tiny projections that are thought to be used for attachment to alveolar surfaces.

Direct Examination. Toluidine blue stains the cysts reddish blue or purple against a blue background. This staining method is faster than the GMS stain but results are less definitive. When GMS stain is used the pattern of staining is similar to that of other fungi; organisms are outlined in blue-black against a light green background.

Cysts do not stain with Giemsa stain but are seen as clear areas containing up to eight dots (the sporozoites). Staining trophozoites is more difficult than staining cysts.

■ Helpful Features for Identification of *Pneumocystis*

Characteristic appearance of the organism in stained tissue preparations

■ Related Organisms from Which *Pneumocystis* Must Be Differentiated

Blastomyces
Saccharomyces and other yeasts

Yeast and Yeastlike Organisms

BLASTOMYCETES

RHODOTORULA SPECIES (Row-dough-tore'-you-lah)

The genus *Rhodotorula* contains multiple species. The one of greatest interest in terms of human disease is *Rhodotorula rubra*.

■ **Reservoirs.** *Rhodotorula* species is found worldwide in soil and water and is transmitted by airborne routes. It is also found in dairy products and fruit juice and is part of the normal flora of the human skin, especially the genital area and throat. When urine specimens are collected improperly, *Rhodotorula* may be found in the urine as a contaminant if it is part of the normal genital flora of the host. *Rhodotorula* has been cultured from sputa, throat swabs, and feces of hospitalized patients.

■ **Unique Risk Factors.** *Rhodotorula* is usually nonpathogenic, but infections are occasionally found in debilitated and immunocompromised hosts. Infections are especially likely when the normal protective mechanical barriers to infection are breached or following *iatrogenic* procedures, that is, procedures used by physicians to treat the patient.

■ **Human Infection.** *Rhodotorula* infections are increasing somewhat because of the increased numbers of susceptible people. The yeast has been isolated from lung and urinary tract infections, endocarditis, meningitis, fungemia, mycotic keratitis, and peritonitis.

■ **Specimen Sources.** Specimens are cerebrospinal fluid, blood, urine, respiratory secretions, gastric washings, vaginal secretions, and scrapings from the skin or cornea.

■ **Specimen Collection and Handling.** Specimens should be collected according to the standard protocol for the type of specimen. Rapid transport to the laboratory is imperative.

Direct examination of specimens can usually be done by wet mounts or gram-stained smears. An India ink preparation can be run in conjunction with the cryptococcal LA test. Tenacious or opaque specimens may need to be cleared with KOH before they are examined.

■ **Immunology.** No tests are available commercially for the specific diagnosis of *Rhodotorula* infections.

■ **Special Precautions.** None are needed.

■ **Culture Media.** Almost any medium can be used with and without antibacterial antibiotics, including sheep blood agar. *Rhodotorula* is variably sensitive to cycloheximide.

Temperature Considerations. *R. rubra* can grow at temperatures between 25° and 38°C.

■ **Laboratory Identification of *Rhodotorula*.** Biochemical tests such as carbohydrate utilization, the phenoloxidase test or caffeic acid/birdseed agar, and special methods for examination of the microscopic morphology are useful for distinguishing *Rhodotorula* species from related organisms.

■ **Macroscopic (Colony) Morphology.** On modified SDA at 25°C after 3 to 4 days, well-behaved *Rhodotorula* colonies are typically coral red or orange to golden yellow, but variations among species occur. Rare strains may be white or cream colored. The texture of the colonies is smooth and moist; isolates with capsules may be mucoid. Older cultures become waxy and wrinkled.

■ **Microscopic Morphology** (Fig. 7.21). *Rhodotorula* species are globose or oval yeast cells varying in size from 2.5 to 14 μm, with thin walls. They reproduce by multilateral budding. Cells are usually found singly but may form short chains or clusters.

Pseudohyphae are not produced on ordinary media; rudimentary pseudohyphae are produced, rarely, on CMT agar. Faint capsules may be seen. Neither germ tubes nor chlamydospores are formed.

■ **Helpful Features for Identification of *Rhodotorula* Species**

> Coral red, orange, or golden yellow pigment in colony
> Capsule is faint or absent
> Germ tube and chlamydospore negative
> Production of blastoconidia and rare rudimentary pseudohyphae on CMT agar
> Sensitivity to cycloheximide variable

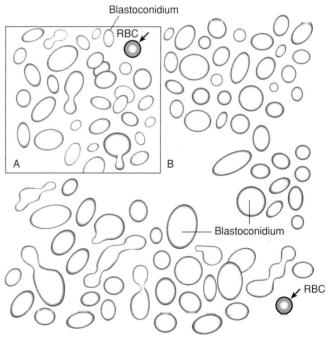

FIGURE 7.21

In wet preps *Rhodotorula* (inset, A) resembles *Cryptococcus*: large globose (or oval) structures that may have buds attached. In cornmeal-Tween 80 medium (B) *Rhodotorula* also resembles *Cryptococcus*, but budding is more common and may be multilateral, and oval cells are frequently seen. The 7-μm red blood cells (RBC) (arrow) show the relative sizes of the mycotic elements.

Negative phenoloxidase

Biochemical reactions in urease, nitrate, and carbohydrate assimilation tests

■ **Organisms from Which *Rhodotorula* Species Must Be Differentiated** (see Fig. 7.24 and Tables 7.1 and 7.2)

Cryptococcus species
Other yeast and yeastlike organisms

Ascomycetous Yeasts

ASCOMYCETES

SACCHAROMYCES CEREVISIAE (Sack'-uh-row-mice'-ees sir-vase'-ee-ay)

S. cerevisiae is a "working yeast." Various strains are used in industry to make bread, beer, wine, and industrial alcohol. This genus is the teleomorph of *Candida robusta.*

■ **Reservoirs.** *S. cerevisiae* may occasionally be found as part of the normal endogenous flora of the human throat and alimentary tract.

■ **Unique Risk Factors.** None.

■ **Human Infection.** *S. cerevisiae* is being isolated with increasing frequency from infections in debilitated and immunocompromised patients. It has been isolated from pulmonary, gastrointestinal, and genitourinary infections, as well as from cases of fungemia, endocarditis, paronychia, and oral thrush.

■ **Culture Media.** Almost any medium with and without chloramphenicol, but without cycloheximide or gentamicin, is recommended. *S. cerevisiae* is inhibited by cycloheximide.

V-8 ascospore medium or Fowell acetate agar is helpful for demonstration of the characteristic features of sexual reproduction.

■ **Macroscopic (Colony) Morphology.** After 2 to 3 days on modified SDA at 25° to 30°C, *S. cerevisiae* produces a flat colony that is moist, with a shiny or dull surface. Pigment ranges from white to cream to tan.

■ **Microscopic Morphology** (Fig. 7.22). In wet preps *Saccharomyces* species are unicellular forms with occasional budding; they vary somewhat in shape from oval to globose.

On CMT agar at 25°C *Saccharomyces* organisms may produce short pseudohyphae or rudimentary hyphae.

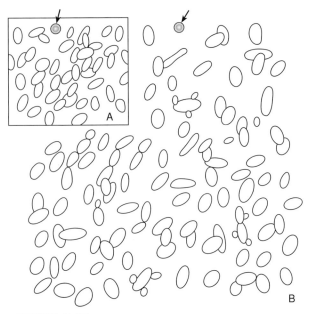

FIGURE 7.22

Wet preps of *Saccharomyces (inset, A)* show predominantly oval yeast cells and occasional round ones, with budding. *Saccharomyces* has the same appearance in cornmeal-Tween 80 medium *(B)*; typically neither pseudohyphae nor true hyphae develop. The 7-μm red blood cells (arrow) show the relative sizes of the mycotic elements.

Single multilateral budding yeast (3 to 9 × 5 to 20 μm) are seen. They vary from oval-ellipsoidal to globose, and they may form short chains.

In the teleomorph phase, after 3 to 4 days on an ascospore medium, suspected *Saccharomyces* should be stained with Kinyoun's modified acid-fast stain. The yeast does not form ascocarps but produces free asci containing one to four globose ascospores. With Kinyoun's stain the asci and ascospores are bright pink against the background of blue vegetative cells.

Direct examination of specimens containing *S. cerevisiae* shows oval to globose to ellipsoidal blastoconidia and rudimentary pseudohyphae. In gram-stained specimens asci are gram negative but the vegetative blastoconidia are gram positive.

■ **Helpful Features for Identification of *Saccharomyces cerevisiae*** (see Fig. 7.24 and Tables 7.1 and 7.2)

Yeast-form colonies at 25°C and 37°C
Blastoconidia, but neither germ tubes nor chlamydospores
Sensitivity to cycloheximide
Biochemical reactions in urease, nitrate, and carbohydrate assimilation tests
No pellicle in broth
Free asci with one to four globose ascospores in teleomorph state, on ascospore agar

Yeast and Yeastlike Organisms

BLASTOMYCETE

TORULOPSIS GLABRATA (Tore-you-lop′-sis glah-brah′-tuh)

References continue to waffle on whether this organism belongs in its own genus, *Torulopsis*, or whether it should be placed in the genus *Candida*. Confusion can be alleviated by recognizing it by its species name, *glabrata*. The taxonomic scheme accepted by McGinnis—*Torulopsis glabrata*—has been adopted for this book.

■ **Reservoirs.** *T. glabrata* is found worldwide, as a saprophyte in soil and dairy products and as part of the normal endogenous flora of the human skin, oral cavity, gastrointestinal tract, and urogenital tract.

■ **Unique Risk Factors.** None.

■ **Human Infection.** The most common infection caused by *T. glabrata* is fungemia. It has been found in lung infections, endocarditis, meningitis, urinary tract infections, and vaginitis, as well as in various tissue infections following iatrogenic procedures.

■ **Immunology.** LA and ID tests are available. Cross-reactions with *Candida* antigens can make interpretation of reactions difficult.

■ **Culture Media.** Media with and without antibacterial antibiotics are recommended. *T. glabrata* is sensitive to cycloheximide

Temperature Considerations. Optimal growth temperature for *T. glabrata* is 25°C. *T. glabrata* grows at 25° to 37°C.

■ **Macroscopic (Colony) Morphology.** On modified SDA at 25° to 37°C after 3 to 4 days, *T. glabrata* colonies are white to cream colored; later they become grayish white or brown. The colonies are moist, smooth, and shiny initially. Older cultures may become wrinkled.

■ **Microscopic Morphology** (Fig. 7.23). In a wet prep *T. glabrata* demonstrates unicellular globose to oval multilateral budding yeasts that are thin walled and smaller (2.5 to 4.5 μm) than other yeasts that cause infections.

In CMT agar the cells form in tight clusters along the line of the streak. Occasionally short branched chains appear. Pseudohyphae are not produced, but rudimentary hyphae are occasionally formed.

In *direct examination* of tissue specimens *T. glabrata* is seen as unicellular oval to globose yeast cells. In a tissue specimen, an occasional cell may be up to 8.5 μm in length, somewhat reminiscent of the budding "cigar-shaped" tissue form of *Sporothrix schenckii*. *Torulopsis* may be found intracellularly in macrophages in tissue samples; in such cases it must be distinguished from *Histoplasma capsulatum*.

■ **Helpful Features for Identification of *Torulopsis glabrata***

Yeast-form colonies and microscopic structures at both 25°C and 37°C
Slow growth and smaller colonies at 37°C
Tiny yeast cells with no pseudohyphae
Capsule, germ tube, and chlamydospore negative
Sensitivity to cycloheximide

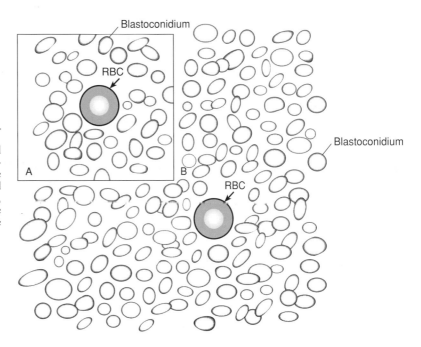

FIGURE 7.23

A wet prep of *Torulopsis glabrata* (*inset, A*) contains small oval or globose cells with occasional budding. In cornmeal-Tween 80 medium (*B*) *T. glabrata* looks the same way, with the addition of occasional short, branched chains of blastoconidia. Pseudohyphae are not produced, but occasionally rudimentary true hyphae develop. The 7-μm red blood cells (RBC) (arrow) show the relative sizes of the mycotic elements.

Thin pellicle in broth
Biochemical reactions in urease, nitrate, and carbohydrate assimilation tests

■ **Related Organisms from Which *T. glabrata* Must Be Differentiated** (Fig. 7.24; see also Tables 7.1, 7.2, and 8.4)

All other unicellular *Candida* species
Sporothrix schenckii
Histoplasma capsulatum

Yeast and Yeastlike Organisms

BLASTOMYCETE

TRICHOSPORON BEIGELII

T. beigelii is an agent of the superficial mycotic infection white piedra. It is discussed in Chapter 4. The organism is listed here because other yeast and yeastlike fungi may be confused with it.

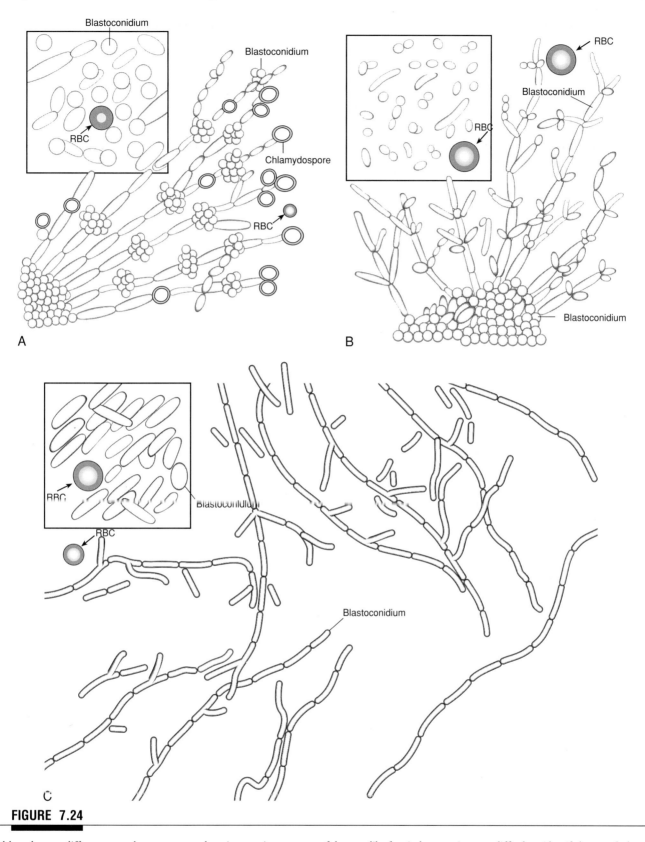

FIGURE 7.24

Although some differences can be seen among the microscopic structures of the yeastlike fungi, the organisms are difficult to identify by morphology alone. Compare the structures produced by *Candida albicans (A)*, *Candida guillermondii (B)*, *Candida kefyr (C)*, *Candida krusei (D)*, *Candida parapsilosis (E)*, *Candida tropicalis (F)*, *Cryptococcus neoformans (G)*, *Rhodotorula (H)*, *Saccharomyces (I)*, and *Torulopsis (J)*. Growth patterns and biochemical tests are needed for definite identification.

Illustrations continued on following page

FIGURE 7.24   CONTINUED

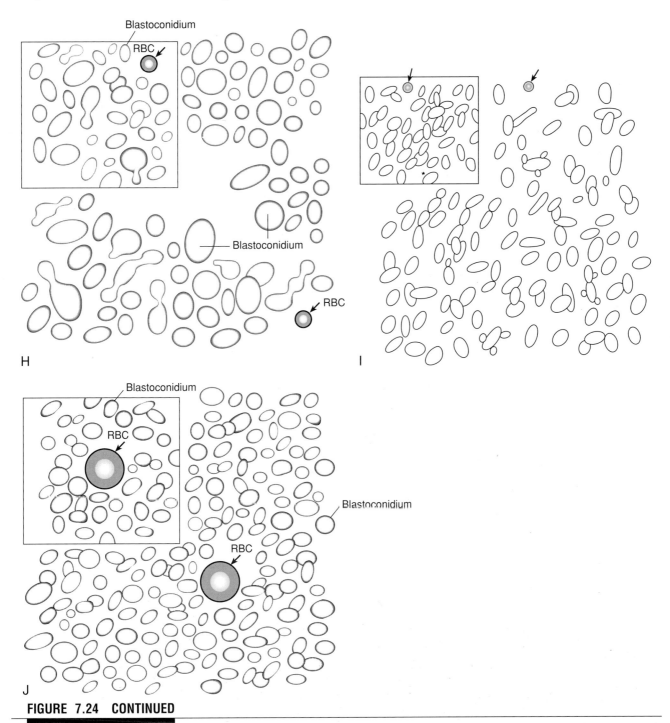

FIGURE 7.24 CONTINUED

SUGGESTED EXERCISES FOR CHAPTER 7

(Yeasts and Yeastlike Organisms)

Exercise 11 (1st Session)

Purpose. To practice the procedures and (again) to set up the cultures needed for the next laboratory. Yeasts are the group of fungi most often isolated from clinical specimens.

Suggested Fungus Cultures

Set 1   *Candida albicans*
Set 2   *Cryptococcus neoformans*
Set 3   *Geotrichum candidum, Trichosporon beigelii*[10]
Set 4   *Candida* species *(Candida parapsilosis, Candida kefyr, Candida tropicalis, Candida guilliermondii, Candida krusei), Rhodotorula rubra, Saccharomyces cerevisiae*

Initial Process. Pick up five plates of Emmon's modified SDA and at least one plate of modified SDA with cycloheximide and chloramphenicol (C&C) from the supply table. At the same time, pick up the new cultures you are working with today. If you have selected *Candida krusei* as one of your cultures, you will need a second plate of SDA with C&C.

You are to study a total of five of the yeastlike fungi. One of the four *must* be *Candida albicans* and one of the four *must* be *Cryptococcus neoformans*. Select the remaining three yeast from the last two sets listed, one organism from Set 3 and two from Set 4. Again, if you have a lab partner, coordinate your choices so that you are working with different organisms (see Tables 7.1 and 7.2). NOTE that the LABORATORY REPORT SHEET for yeasts differs from the one you have been using for moulds; prepare one for each of the cultures you are studying.

Yeast colonies can be transferred just as you would transfer a bacterial culture, with a standard bacterial loop. Use a light inoculum and streak the plate for isolation. Remember to streak *Candida albicans* and *Candida krusei* to both SDA and SDA with C&C.

Exercise 11 (2nd Session)

Procedures to Be Completed

germ tube test on all organisms
CMT plate on all organisms
India ink prep on all organisms
caffeic acid test on encapsulated yeasts
urea, nitrate, and carbohydrate assimilation tests on all germ tube–negative organisms

---

[10]Yes, you have seen *Trichosporon beigelii* before, but you didn't do biochemical tests on the culture. *Trichosporon cutaneum* can be substituted for *Trichosporon beigelii*; using *Trichosporon beigelii* again saves the expense and hassle of obtaining the *Trichosporon cutaneum* culture.

Additional Supplies Needed

rabbit plasma or accepted substitute for germ tube test
small (10 × 75 mm) disposable test tubes
heat block for incubation of germ tube tests (37°C)
method for nitrate assimilation
urea utilization procedures
India ink
caffeic acid substrate
CMT agar plates, one per organism
materials to determine assimilation of carbohydrates

The Process

Get the yeast cultures out of the incubator, and pick up the materials you need from the supply table. Supplies are not listed here in detail because they will vary with the identification system being used. Some methods are provided in Appendix D.

Begin, as usual, by describing the colonies of the organisms and recording the information on the LABORATORY WORK SHEET for yeasts—one sheet per organism. Compare the growth of *Candida albicans* on SDA without antibiotics to its growth when C&C was present in the SDA. Make the same comparison for *Candida krusei* if this is one of the yeasts you selected. Then use a *tiny* amount of the colony to make a wet prep of each yeast; either saline or water can be used for these. Add the drawings of each yeast, uninspiring though they might be, to the appropriate report forms.

Set up a germ tube test on each of the five yeasts so that results can be read before the end of the laboratory session today. The directions are in Appendix D and the procedure has been demonstrated for you. NOTE that these tests are incubated at 37°C.

Inoculate the rapid tests for nitrate assimilation and urea if you are using these methods so that you can read them today.

Make an India ink prep of the *Cryptococcus*, and one of the *Candida albicans* (or another *Candida* species) to serve as a negative control. Read these and record the results; you may wish to make a drawing of the *Cryptococcus*.

Set up the caffeic acid test on the *Cryptococcus*, following the directions for the method you are using.

Prepare morphology studies of the organisms on CMT agar, one organism per plate. The procedure is provided in Appendix D.

To determine the pattern of assimilation of carbohydrates set up the remaining tests.

NOTE that use of commercial kits such as the Uni-Yeast-Tek or API 20C Clinical Yeast System streamlines the process and makes many of the individual steps listed earlier unnecessary. Commercial kits are more expensive, which often prevents their use in student laboratories, but they can be set up by the instructor as demonstrations.

You will need to arrange your schedule so that you can pop into the laboratory several times before the next session to read the results of certain tests. The authors suggest that you might work with your lab partner or another student so that you can alternate visits to the laboratory. You should, however, do your own study of the morphology of the yeasts on CMT agar.

Exercise 11   (3rd Session—for courses longer than 8 weeks)

Read the results of any remaining tests and record the information on the LABORATORY WORK SHEET for yeasts.

Compare the colony morphology of the older yeast cultures to the descriptions you recorded originally and note any differences on the work sheet.

Look at the pattern of reactions for each yeast and, as much as possible, treat the culture as if it were an unknown. Compare the pattern of reactions to the tables in the text to see whether or not the isolates reacted according to type.

ASSESS WHAT YOU HAVE LEARNED

Responses to the questions below are located in Appendix A.

1. Define assimilation, fermentation, iatrogenic, ascospore, pellicle.
2. How does an impression smear differ from a wet prep?
3. What is a micrometer? How is it used in mycology?
4. Compare the following pairs of terms: (A) colonization and infection, (B) fungemia and fungoma, (C) yeast and yeastlike, (D) pseudohyphae and germ tube, (E) chlamydospore and chlamydoconidium.
5. List at least three factors that suggest that the yeast in a clinical specimen is the etiologic agent of the infection.
6. Name the two tests that should be done first on yeastlike organisms isolated in primary culture, and explain why these should be completed before other procedures are initiated.
7. List at least three additional procedures that are useful for identification of yeast and yeastlike organisms.

For questions 8 through 15 **MATCH** the characteristic **(numbered)** with the name of the organism **(lettered)** with which the characteristic is associated. NOTE that responses will be used more than once.

8. agent of thrush
9. causes paronychia
10. forms brown colonies on birdseed agar
11. generally resistant to cycloheximide
12. has a large polysaccharide capsule
13. infection is usually from endogenous organisms
14. infects the central nervous system and brain
15. pseudohyphae and/or true hyphae develop

  a. *Candida albicans*
  b. *Cryptococcus neoformans*

16. Name the substrate or medium, and describe positive and negative reactions for the (A) germ tube test, (B) phenoloxidase method, (C) nitrate and (D) carbon assimilation methods, (E) pellicle formation.

For questions 17 through 24 **NAME** the organism described in each of the items below. NOTE that if a carbohydrate is not listed with the assimilation reactions, it should be assumed to be negative.

17. **Lesion:** colonization and inflammation of the heart valve
    Colony: smooth, creamy colony after 2 days on Sabouraud's dextrose agar
    Microscopic: oval blastoconidia of varying sizes with many branching pseudohyphae in the wet prep. "Log jam" arrangement of pseudohyphae and blastoconidia in cornmeal-Tween 80 agar.
    Other: germ tube negative. Nitrate and urease negative. Cellobiose, dextrose, lactose, raffinose, and sucrose are assimilated.

18. **Lesion:** bronchitis
    Colony: colony is white and spreading after 3 days on Sabouraud's dextrose agar
    Microscopic: septate, hyaline branching hyphae, with arthroconidia, in a wet prep. The cornmeal-Tween 80 agar shows septate branching hyphae, and free arthroconidia, some with germ tubes emerging from one corner of the conidium
    Other: germ tube negative. Nitrate and urease negative. Dextrose and galactose assimilated

19. **Lesion:** vaginitis in a pregnant teenager
    Colony: smooth, creamy colony after 3 days on Sabouraud's dextrose agar
    Microscopic: chains and clusters of small blastoconidia in a wet prep, with branching pseudohyphae. Short, thin, curved pseudohyphal cells with elongate blastoconidia clustered at the septa of the pseudohyphae in cornmeal-Tween 80 agar. Occasional giant pseudohyphae
    Other: germ tube negative. Nitrate and urease negative. Dextrose, galactose, maltose, sucrose, trehalose, and xylose assimilated

20. **Lesion:** keratitis
    Colony: orange-red smooth colony on Sabouraud's dextrose agar after 3 days
    Microscopic: large, thin-walled globose yeast cells with occasional buds in wet prep. In cornmeal-Tween 80 agar cells are large and globose with thin walls; some multilateral budding is seen.
    Other: germ tube negative. Nitrate and urease positive. Cellobiose, dextrose, maltose, raffinose, sucrose, trehalose, and xylose assimilated

21. **Lesion:** fungemia
    Colony: white, moist, smooth and shiny colony on Sabouraud's dextrose agar after 3 days
    Microscopic: tiny round unicellular blastoconidia in the wet prep. In cornmeal-Tween 80 agar some multilateral budding is seen, and a few short branched chains of blastoconidia. Clusters of blastoconidia are grouped along the line of the streak
    Other: germ tube negative. Nitrate and urease negative. Dextrose and trehalose fermented

22. **Lesion:** pulmonary infection in an AIDS patient
    Colony: heaped, rough waxy colony on Sabouraud's dextrose agar after 2 days
    Microscopic: elongate blastoconidia dispersed along the pseudohyphae in the wet prep. In cornmeal-Tween 80 agar the same picture is seen, with occasional chlamydoconidia.
    Other: germ tube negative. Nitrate and urease negative. Dextrose, galactose, maltose, sucrose, trehalose, and xylose assimilated

23. **Lesion:** cutaneous lesion in a patient with leukemia
    Colony: dome-shaped beige mucoid colony
    Microscopic: large globose thin-walled cells, singly and in pairs, in a wet prep. In cornmeal-Tween 80 agar, well-separated large globose thin-walled yeasts with thick capsules
    Other: germ tube negative. Nitrate negative, urease positive. Cellobiose, dextrose, dulcitol, galactose, inositol, maltose, sucrose, raffinose, trehalose, and xylose assimilated

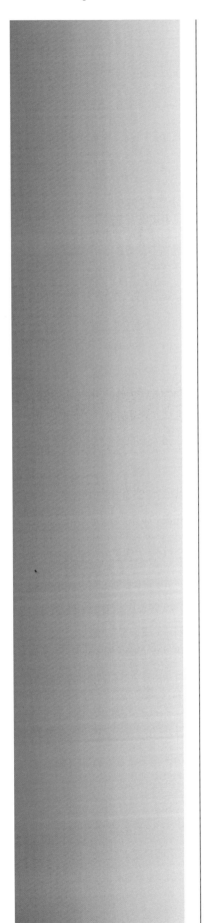

24. **Lesion:** urinary tract infection in a quadriplegic
    Colony: moist, glistening, beige colony with slightly wrinkled topography
    after 3 days on Sabouraud's dextrose agar
    Microscopic: globose blastoconidia with multilateral budding from blasto-
    conidia, in both wet prep and cornmeal-Tween 80 agar
    Other: pseudohyphae and true hyphae seen. On V-8 agar asci containing
    four "derby hats" present

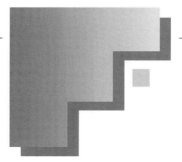

CHAPTER 8

Systemic Fungi

Upon completion of this chapter the reader should be able to:

1. Define the following terms: blastomycin, coccidioidin, histoplasmin, paracoccidioidin, spherulin, Darling's disease, desert rheumatism, mariner's wheels, Valley fever, spelunker's disease.

2. Outline the procedure for converting any dimorphic fungus from one growth form to another.

3. Recognize or describe the distinguishing characteristics of the gross and microscopic morphologies of both yeast and mould forms of *Blastomyces dermatitidis*, *Coccidioides immitis*, *Histoplasma capsulatum*, and *Paracoccidioides brasiliensis*.

4. Correctly identify the systemic fungi studied, given pertinent background information such as patient history and microscopic and colony morphology.

5. Describe the symptoms of primary pulmonary infections caused by the systemic fungi, and name additional tissues typically affected by each of the systemic pathogens.

6. Describe the antigens associated with each systemic pathogen, and list the relative value of each of the immunologic procedures used for each of the fungi.

INTRODUCTION

Systemic mycoses are infections that involve major body systems or that involve more than one kind of tissue or organ. Rippon separates the systemic mycoses into those caused by the dimorphic pathogens and those caused by opportunistic fungi, including yeast. However, in considering the distinction between the groups, Rippon strongly suggests that opportunism is involved in any symptomatic mycotic infection. All fungi are opportunists—but some need less help from opportunity than do others—these he calls "true pathogens." Rippon also suggests that many biologic groups demonstrate some type of dimorphism. In so-called thermal dimorphism, conversion from one form to another is controlled primarily by temperature, although other factors sometimes influence conversion. Among fungi infecting humans, thermal dimorphism is found almost exclusively in the pathogenic fungi—the systemic organisms *Blastomyces dermatitidis*, *Coccidioides immitis*, *Histoplasma capsulatum*, *Paracoccidioides immitis*, plus the subcutaneous agent *Sporothrix schenckii*. The yeasts and the opportunistic moulds that cause systemic infections (Zygomycetes and *Aspergillus*) share certain characteristics that distinguish them from the systemic fungi. They are monomorphic. Each is found throughout the world, in a variety of habitats. Some are part of the normal flora of humans. Primary infection may occur at almost any body site. The fungi are of relatively low virulence so that, for infection to develop, the host's defenses must be compromised in some way. Infections are symptomatic. Typically these opportunists grow rather rapidly. The yeast and yeastlike organisms, *Candida* and *Cryptococcus*, can also cause systemic infections. Table 8.1 highlights the differences between opportunistic and true pathogens.

The systemic dimorphic pathogens described in this chapter also share some common features. The parasitic yeast form is found in tissues and in culture at 37°C. At 25° to 30°C the saprobic mycelial phase is found. To convert a dimorphic fungus from one form to another, the culture is transferred to a fresh container of media and incubated at the "opposite" temperature. The "opposite" temperature means that if it was isolated at 25° to 30°C, the new culture is incubated at 37°C. Conversely, if the yeast form was isolated initially, the mycelial form would be obtained by culture at room temperature. A specific protocol for conversion of dimorphic fungi is found in Appendix D.

The systemic pathogens all are able to adapt to the reduced oxidation-reduction environment within the host and to survive the normal lytic action of the body's cellular defenses. Each is endemic to a specific geographic area. Evidence strongly suggests that each is a saprobe in the soil, although this hasn't been proven for all of them. They are not part of the normal flora of humans. The patient's history is valuable if the laboratory is to isolate and identify a dimorphic fungus in a timely

TABLE 8.1 Comparative Features of Opportunistic and True Pathogens		
Characteristic*	Opportunistic Fungi	"True" Pathogens
Colony morphology	Monomorphic	Thermal dimorphs
Habitat	Worldwide	Endemic zones
Occurrence in humans	Normal flora	Linked to infection or disease
Primary infection	Any body site	Pulmonary
Virulence	Low—requires compromised host	Can infect normal host
Growth rate in culture	Rapid	Intermediate to slow

*Exceptions occur.

fashion. *Paracoccidioides* is endemic to Central and South America, but the remaining three systemic pathogens are endemic in different locations of the United States. The occupation and avocation of the patient can also provide helpful clues about the identity of the fungus.

All systemic fungi are capable of causing multiple kinds of infections, of varying severities. The primary infection for all four of them is pulmonary, contracted through inhalation of the conidia, and the incidence of benign infection is far greater than the incidence of disseminated fatal infection. In most cases in the immunocompetent person the primary infection is asymptomatic and resolves spontaneously. Those who do develop symptoms appear to have a common cold, or the "flu."

The primary infection sometimes progresses to acute or chronic pulmonary disease, characterized by granulomatous lesions in the lungs. A *granuloma* is a collection of macrophages, giant cells and other cells, and proteinaceous substances produced by the host's immune system to surround the infecting organism in an attempt to "wall it off." Rarely, the yeasts are ingested by macrophages in the lung and carried to the lymph nodes, then released into the bloodstream. When this occurs infection develops in other organs, including the lymph nodes, central nervous system, and musculoskeletal system. Disseminated fatal infections are so fast moving, so dramatic, and so frightening that the existence of benign infections is often forgotten.

Each of the dimorphic pathogens is also capable of causing secondary infections of the skin and/or mucous membranes; the tissues attacked and the characteristics of the infection vary with the fungus.

LABORATORY METHODS FOR SYSTEMIC FUNGI

Tissue specimens should be minced or ground, under aseptic conditions, before they are inoculated to media. When possible, materials such as pleural fluid and cerebrospinal fluid should be concentrated by centrifugation or filtration before media is inoculated. Thick or *tenacious* (adhesive; tough) materials such as mucus or pus should be treated with a mucolytic agent such as N-acetyl-L-cysteine before the culture or microscopic preparation is done. The method for digesting specimens is included in most comprehensive microbiology texts, such as the American Society for Microbiology's *Manual of Clinical Microbiology.*

When a dimorphic fungus is suspected, the specimen should be transported and plated as quickly as possible. Specimens should never be held at room temperature and should be stored only briefly in the refrigerator. *H. capsulatum* in particular may be inhibited by bacteria and yeasts that multiply rapidly at room temperature and by enzymes present in many specimens.

Microscopic Examination. The easiest method for direct examination of specimens is a simple 10% potassium hydroxide (KOH) preparation. Blue-black ink can be added to the KOH to make it easier to see the fungal elements, or the calcofluor white method can be used. Papanicolaou staining methods have been used successfully to detect these organisms, especially in tissue. Staining methods specifically developed for tissue sections, such as the hematoxylin and eosin (H&E) method, the periodic acid–Schiff (PAS) stain and Gomori's methenamine silver (GMS) stain may also be helpful for examination of tissue sections.

Culture Media. Emmon's modification of Sabouraud's dextrose agar (modified SDA) without antimicrobials should be used for primary isolation of the systemic pathogens because of its approximately neutral pH and lower glucose content. A second tube of SDA with cycloheximide and/or chloramphenicol may also be inoculated from the specimen if it is likely to contain bacteria or saprophytic fungi. Both tubes should be incubated at approximately 30°C. At 35° to 37°C the use of selective media alone is undesirable because the tissue (yeast) form of most systemic dimorphic pathogens is sensitive to cycloheximide.

Brain-heart infusion agar (BHIA) with added blood or a combination of SDA and BHI (SABHI) is strongly recommended for primary culture of specimens for the dimorphic pathogens; the additional nutrients provided by the blood enhance recovery of the fungus and speed up the rate of growth. If a liquid medium is needed brain-heart infusion broth (BHIB) should be used. Yeast extract phosphate medium or potato agars (potato flake [PFA] or potato dextrose [PDA]) may be used for subcultures of the initial growth to encourage conidiation and speed identification of the fungus.

Within the laboratory, following isolation of the fungus, identification is accomplished by examining the gross and microscopic morphology of the culture. *C. immitis* does not produce yeast-form colonies unless it is grown in a special medium in an environment of increased CO_2. The other three dimorphic pathogens that cause systemic infection (*Blastomyces*, *Histoplasma*, and *Paracoccidioides*) produce yeast-form colonies at body temperature (37°C) on standard solid laboratory media. The yeast-form colonies of these dimorphic fungi are similar initially, resembling colonies of bacteria or of ordinary yeastlike organisms such as *Candida*.

On standard media at 25° to 30°C *and* at 35° to 37°C typical colonies of *C. immitis* are floccose and white to grayish. They become powdery as they develop, with a great variety of pigments, predominantly tan to brown. *Blastomyces*, *Histoplasma*, and *Paracoccidioides* produce similar mould-form colonies on solid agar at room temperature. Initially colonies are flat, with a glabrous texture and white pigment. As they mature they acquire a tan or brownish tinge and become folded or heaped with a woolly or velvety texture. In microscopic preparations the mould-form conidia, or the yeast cell, or both, are usually distinctive enough for definitive identification of the organisms.

Risk Factors. Systemic pathogens are dangerous organisms capable of causing laboratory-acquired infections. *Great care and strict laboratory precautions MUST be taken when working with specimens or cultures believed to contain these organisms!*

Remember that the dimorphic pathogens are all transmitted by the airborne route and are pathogens of the lungs. Colonies that resemble the dimorphic pathogens should *only* be handled within a biologic safety cabinet. Strict safety precautions should be used. *Slide cultures should never be done.*

Immunology. Immunologic methods have been developed for detection of the systemic pathogens for at least two reasons. First, the infections are potentially life threatening. Second, when immunologic methods are not available, invasive procedures such as a lung biopsy are often necessary to obtain appropriate specimens for examination. Moreover, the fungus may be present in the specimen in such small quantities that it may not be recovered in culture.

Development of immunologic methods is hampered by the fact that the fungi are not strong antigens and generally stimulate cellular rather than humoral antibody responses. Cross-reactions occur among the fungi, and standardization of antigens is difficult. In all immunologic testing standardized controls must be used and test protocols should be followed.

Skin tests are useful epidemiologic tools for detection of three of the systemic pathogens (*Coccidioides, Histoplasma,* and *Paracoccidioides*). Skin tests are usually the first immunologic tests to be positive. An attenuated extract of the fungus is injected intradermally. A positive reaction simply means that the patient has been exposed to the fungus; this does not, of course, mean that the patient is necessarily infected. Skin tests should not be done until serum for other immunologic tests has been obtained or false-positive results may occur in the other tests. Skin testing for *Coccidioides* is an exception to this rule. Many people—especially those who have lived in the endemic area—have low titers of antibody to the dimorphic fungi. For this reason accurate diagnosis of an infection by immunologic methods is most likely to result from testing several serum samples drawn over a short period so that any significant change in the titer of antibodies can be seen. A negative skin test in a person who was previously positive indicates the anergy of a disseminated infection, that is, the person's immune system is unable to respond to the antigen with antibody production. Most immunosuppressed patients and patients with acquired immunodeficiency syndrome (AIDS) are seronegative in immunologic tests even when infection is present because they are incapable of producing antibody.

The first antifungal antibodies to be produced are usually precipitins, followed by complement-fixing antibodies. The titer of complement-fixing antibodies usually begins to decrease as the patient recovers, serving as an indicator of the patient's prognosis. Complement fixation (CF) methods are not widely used except in reference laboratories because they are tedious to perform, even for experienced technologists.

Immunodiffusion (ID) methods, which use an agar gel substrate to detect the precipitin antibodies, are available commercially. They are generally more sensitive than the CF methods, are easier to do, and parallel the CF tests in terms of timing of antibody detection. The enzyme-linked immunosorbent assay (ELISA) method has been applied to detection of *B. dermatitidis* and can be expected to be extended to detection of the other three systemic pathogens. A latex particle agglutination (LA) test and a tube precipitin (TP) test have been developed for diagnosis of coccidioidomycosis. The LA test is reported to be more accurate and easier to perform than the CF test, with sensitivity that matches the CF method. LA methods should be used for screening and confirmed by another method, because a false-positive rate of 6% to 10% has been reported for them. The TP method, on the other hand, is complicated, costly, and time consuming. Despite its high specificity it is unlikely to be developed for widespread use in detection of *Coccidioides, Histoplasma,* and *Paracoccidioides*.

An exoantigen test that detects cell-free antigens of a fungus has been used for the identification of cultures of *Blastomyces, Coccidioides, Histoplasma,* and *Paracoccidioides*.

Material is extracted from the mould-form colony and reacted with known antisera for the suspected organism under controlled conditions. The advantage of the exoantigen test is that a culture can be identified much faster than when morphology alone is used. The soluble antigen can be extracted from the culture despite contamination with other fungi or with bacteria, whether the colony of interest is viable or not. Commercially available DNA probes are reported to be faster, more sensitive, and more specific than exoantigen tests but are too expensive to use unless the laboratory does a large volume of tests. *DNA probes* use single strands of DNA isolated from a known organism to "probe" for the complementary DNA sequence in a culture or specimen. The culture or specimen of interest is treated to release the DNA from the organism and fix it to a solid matrix. After the known "reagent" DNA strand and the DNA in the specimen have been allowed to bond the reaction is detected with a dye, a radioisotope, or an enzymatic reaction.

Immunologic tests for diagnosis of systemic mycoses and identification of the fungi are most likely to be performed in reference laboratories or in clinical laboratories of relatively large institutions where many fungus cultures are done annually. Some immunologic testing methods are currently commercially available, and the number and availability are likely to increase. Table 8.2 presents the immunologic tests currently available for detecting the systemic mycoses. The application of immunology is the newest and fastest growing area of clinical mycology, changing so rapidly that the latest information should be sought from journal articles, manufacturers, and researchers rather than texts such as this one.

Systemic Dimorphic Pathogens

HYALINE HYPHOMYCETES

BLASTOMYCES DERMATITIDIS (Blast-oh-mice-ees derm-uh-tih-duh-dis)

■ **Teleomorph.** *Ajellomyces dermatitidis.*

B. dermatitidis is endemic in North America in areas surrounding the Mississippi, Missouri, and Ohio Rivers and their tributaries. The zone extends east into Kentucky and the Carolinas, including the Appalachian region, north into Canada and into Wisconsin. Gilchrist's disease is a synonym for blastomycosis, honoring the first man to publish reports of the infection.

■ **Reservoirs.** The exact ecologic niche of *B. dermatitidis* has not been determined, but the fungus has been

TABLE 8.2 Immunologic Tests to Detect Systemic Mycoses

Systemic Mycosis	Complement Fixation	Counterimmunoelectrophoresis	Enzyme Immunoassay	Exoantigen	Fluorescent Antibody	Immunodiffusion	Latex Agglutination	Nucleic Acid (DNA) Probe	Radioimmunoassay	Skin Test	Tube Agglutination	Tube Precipitation
Aspergillosis	X	X	X		X	X			X	X		
Blastomycosis	X		X	X	X	X		X	X	X		
Candidiasis	X	X	X		X	X	X					
Coccidioidomycosis	X			X	X	X	X	X		X		X
Cryptococcosis			X		X	X	X				X	
Histoplasmosis	X	X		X	X	X	X	X	X	X		
Paracoccidioidomycosis	X	X	X	X	X	X				X		
Sporotrichosis	X		X	X	X	X	X			X	X	

found in moist environments in wood, tree bark, and rotting vegetation, as well as in animal habitats, manure, and wet acid soil from the banks of rivers.

■ **Risk Factors.** The fungus is most often transmitted by airborne routes but is only rarely infectious. *B. dermatitidis* is a relatively small threat to people with competent immune systems, although it can cause fatal infections. Kwon-Chung and Bennett say laboratory-acquired infections are rare; fewer than a dozen cases have been reported.

■ **Human Infection.** *B. dermatitidis* is the etiologic agent of *blastomycosis*, a chronic granulomatous and suppurative disease that may affect the lungs, skin, and mucous membranes, or other organ systems. Pulmonary infections have been described in the Introduction to this chapter.

Chronic cutaneous blastomycosis, with or without lung involvement, is verrucose and ulcerated, with small abscesses that suppurate and weep. They occur more often on exposed skin or mucocutaneous tissue than in other tissues. Without successful treatment the cutaneous blastomycosis disseminates. Systemic blastomycosis may involve any organ of the body or a combination of organs. Bone lesions and painful debilitating arthritis or osteomyelitis are often encountered, as are urogenital infections in males.

■ **Specimen Sources.** Sputum or other pulmonary specimens, aspirated pus from lymph nodes and subcutaneous abscesses, skin scrapings or biopsied tissue from the edges of ulcers, biopsied lung tissue, crusts from skin lesions, oropharyngeal scrapings, bone, blood, prostate secretions, urine, and cerebrospinal fluid are most likely to be submitted for culture.

■ **Specimen Collection and Handling.** Specimens should be collected aseptically according to the standard protocol for the type of specimen, transported to the laboratory without delay, and plated promptly.

Direct examination of pus aspirated from draining sinuses can be done with simple wet mounts, with or without added stains. If necessary, 10% KOH can be added to the mounting fluid to clear the specimen before it is examined. Tissue specimens are best examined as sections that have been fixed and stained with GMS stain by the histology laboratory. Mucus and other thick substances should be treated with N-acetyl-L-cysteine before the wet mount is done. Specific fluorescent antibody (FA) tests are also available to detect the yeast in tissue or other clinical specimens. Special stains such as the Papanicolaou stain, H&E, or Giemsa stain may be helpful, especially for tissue specimens.

■ **Immunology.** *B. dermatitidis* has two antigens, A and B, that have been used in immunologic tests; A is reported to be the more useful of the two. *Blastomycin,* an extract of the yeast form, has been used for skin testing, but Rippon says that "skin testing with this reagent is a useless procedure" (p. 497). Currently no skin test for blastomycosis is commercially available because of the lack of purified antigens.

Kaufman and associates have reported development of purified specific A and B antigens of *B. dermatitidis* that have greatly improved the serologic diagnosis of this mycosis. In a limited study using the purified yeast cell A antigen the sensitivity ranged from 52% to 100%, depending on the method used. Specificity ranges from 84% to 100%. The A antigen has been incorporated into all available tests because it offers the best sensitivity and specificity.

An FA test that uses specific yeast-form conjugates is now available to identify tissue forms of *B. dermatitidis* in culture and in most types of clinical specimens. The advantage of FA tests, like exoantigen tests, is that mixed cultures and colonies that are not viable can be tested.

ID tests using the purified A antigen, reference sera, and sera from cases of *Blastomyces* proven by culture, has a specificity of 84% to 100% and a sensitivity of 57% to 62%. The identification of A precipitin bands that are continuous or identical with the reference antisera indicate a recent or current infection. The identification of *Blastomyces* in a yeast-form culture filtrate is specific using the A antigen with the ID method. Any serum that forms a precipitin band is considered diagnostic of blastomycosis. Negative tests should be repeated at 3-week intervals, if the infection with *B. dermatitidis* is strongly indicated by the symptoms and history of the patient.

A more sensitive and specific serologic test for blastomycosis is the enzyme immunoassay (EIA), which has a sensitivity of 80% and a specificity of 98%. Some cross-reactivity occurs with sera from patients with *H. capsulatum* antibodies; titers greater than 1:16 are considered suspicious of *B. dermatitidis* and titers of 1:32 or greater are considered diagnostic. The optimum protocol is to use the EIA test with the ID test to improve the sensitivity and specificity. A single set of negative tests does not rule out blastomycosis; the procedures should be repeated after 2 to 3 weeks.

Other serologic tests for diagnosis of blastomycosis include a specific A band exoantigen test that is now available commercially for confirmation of the identity of both yeast and mycelial forms of *B. dermatitidis*; titers of 1:16 and greater are considered positive. A CF method is available but it is relatively insensitive and is difficult to perform. Recently Stockman and associates reported a chemiluminescent DNA probe method that allows identification as soon as growth occurs, making it the most rapid diagnostic technique.

In the past, immunologic tests have not been proven valuable in the diagnosis or management of blastomycosis, but the method of antigen preparation developed by Kaufman and associates is likely to change this.

■ **Special Precautions.** Laboratory personnel who are working with *any* fluffy white colony should take special precautions and adhere stringently to laboratory procedures. *As a minimum, cultures should always be studied within a biologic Class II safety cabinet. Slide cultures should never be made.*

■ **Culture Media.** Modified SDA or BHIA with antibiotics at temperatures from 25° to 30°C, SDA without antimicrobials at temperatures above 30°C. Use BHIA containing blood for culture of specimens from body sites that are normally sterile.

Biphasic culture bottles containing both BHI broth and BHI agar are recommended for blood cultures. The agar is layered along one side of the bottle and, after the agar has solidified, the broth is added. Yeast extract phosphate agar can be inoculated directly from the specimen to encourage conidiation and inhibit *Candida* species. PDA or PFA may be used for subculture to encourage conidia production.

Temperature Considerations. Optimal temperature for growth is 25° to 30°C for the mould form on routine media. A temperature of 37°C is needed to induce the yeast phase.

Primary cultures for B. dermatitidis should be held for 4 to 8 weeks before being discarded as "no growth."

■ **Macroscopic (Colony) Morphology**

At 25°C, mould-form colonies of *B. dermatitidis* on modified SDA grow slowly; mature colonies typically grow in 6 to 21 days. The colonies show great variety in form, texture, and pigment. Generally they are white or beige to brown at first with a waxy or glabrous texture, although some isolates may be fluffy. Some are prickly in the center. Later, colonies tend to become fluffy or woolly, and some develop concentric rings. Reverse pigment of the colonies is tan to brown.

At 37°C, colonies of yeast appear after 10 to 15 days on enriched media such as BHIA with blood. They are white to light tan, with a wrinkled or folded topography and a waxy texture.

■ **Microscopic Morphology**

At 25° to 30°C (Figs. 8.1 through 8.3) the mould form of *Blastomyces* produces very fine (1 to 2 μm) hyphae that are septate and hyaline; they may form ropelike strands. Conidia are borne directly on the hyphae or on lateral conidiophores of varying lengths, resembling lollipops. The conidia are hyaline with pyriform or globose shapes. The average diameter is 6 μm. The thick, smooth walls of the conidia are doubly *refractile*; that is, they have a double image. Thick-walled chlamydoconidia approximately 7 μm in diameter may be seen.

At 37°C (Figs. 8.4 and 8.5) *B. dermatitidis* is a yeast. The cells are hyaline, large (up to 20 μm), and spherical to pyriform, with thick walls. They reproduce by forming buds that are typically attached to the mother cell by broad (4 to 5 μm) necks. The buds are often as large as

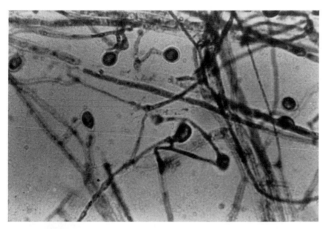

FIGURE 8.1

In typical preparations the mould form of *Blastomyces dermatitidis* is undistinguished looking. Very fine septate hyphae are seen, with oval or globose conidia at the tips of conidiophores and borne directly on the hyphae. (Courtesy of the Centers for Disease Control and Prevention.)

the parent cell before they detach, which causes the "figure eight," or hourglass, configuration of the parent-daughter combination. Rarely the daughter cell buds without separating from the parent, creating a "threesome."

Direct Examination of Specimens. In tissue specimens and body fluids *B. dermatitidis* produces spherical, thick-

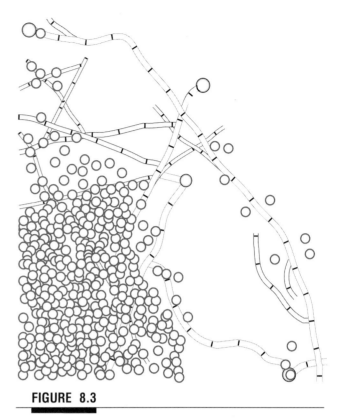

FIGURE 8.3

In bad preparations *Blastomyces dermatitidis* is difficult to identify because it does not have unique structures. The round conidia, septate, hyaline hyphae, and sticklike conidiophores make it resemble a number of other fungi. Tests for thermal dimorphism are helpful to distinguish it from *Trichophyton* species and the anamorphs of *Pseudallescheria boydii.*

walled, doubly refractile budding yeast cells with broad bases (4 to 5 μm or greater) of attachment to the mother cell. Hyphae are rarely present in tissue preparations. Histologic study of tissue specimens using GMS stain are of great diagnostic value when they are positive.

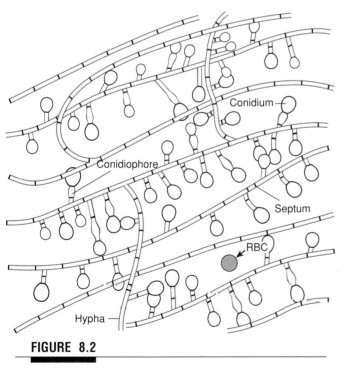

FIGURE 8.2

Blastomyces dermatitidis in the mould form does not have a dramatic look. Small round or pear-shaped conidia grow directly on the septate hyphae or at the tips of conidiophores. Conidiophores are of varying lengths; the central portion of the conidiophore may be slightly swollen. Conidia typically have thick refractile walls. The 7-μm red blood cell (RBC) (arrow) shows the relative sizes of the mycotic elements.

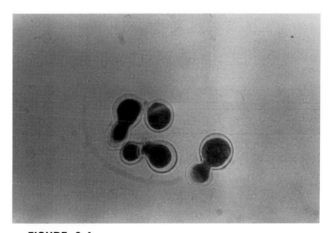

FIGURE 8.4

Blastomyces dermatitidis yeast forms are large and spherical, or pyriform, with thick refractile walls. The thick wall, or retraction of the cell contents from the wall, often makes the yeast appear to be encased in a bubble. Broad connections between budding cells cause it to resemble an hourglass or figure eight. (Courtesy of the Centers for Disease Control and Prevention.)

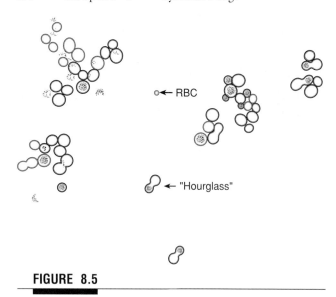

← RBC

← "Hourglass"

FIGURE 8.5

Characteristic preparations of the yeast form of *Blastomyces dermatitidis* contain large globose cells with thick refractile walls. Another notable feature is the thick "neck" that connects the mother and daughter cells. The 7-μm red blood cell (RBC) (arrow) shows the relative sizes of the mycotic elements.

■ **Laboratory Identification of *Blastomyces dermatitidis*.** *B. dermatitidis* is a thermally dimorphic organism. It can be converted from the mould form to the yeast form (using enriched media at 37°C) to confirm identification. During conversion swollen hyphal cells and elements of rudimentary hyphae develop in cultures; cytoplasmic granulation is often seen in mycotic cells during conversion. Alternatively, *Blastomyces* can be identified more safely by the specific exoantigen test or DNA probe.

■ **Helpful Features for Identification of *Blastomyces dermatitidis***

  Colonies with slow to intermediate growth rates at 25°C
  Globose to pyriform "lollipops" on conidiophores of varying lengths at 25° to 30°C
  Waxy, wrinkled, light brown colony of yeast cells at 37°C
  Large, thick-walled budding yeast with thick necks in pairs (figure eights) at 37°C
  Appearance in tissue stained with GMS method

■ **Organisms from Which *Blastomyces dermatitidis* Must Be Differentiated** (Tables 8.3 and 8.4; Figs. 8.6 and 8.7)

  Nonencapsulated forms of *Cryptococcus neoformans*
  Paracoccidioides brasiliensis mould form
  Pseudallescheria boydii/Scedosporium apiospermum
  Detached buds of *P. brasiliensis* yeast form
  Endospores or young spherules of *Coccidioides immitis*

Systemic Dimorphic Pathogens

HYALINE HYPHOMYCETES

COCCIDIOIDES IMMITIS (Cock-sih-dee-oy'-dees imm-ih-tiss)

C. immitis is endemic where the climate is hot and semi-arid, in the Lower Sonoran Life Zone in the southwestern United States and in the littoral zones of northern Mexico and the Pacific Coast of the United States. It is also found, in a lesser degree, in Central and South America. The pulmonary infection caused by the organism is sometimes called *Valley fever* because of its association with the San Joaquin Valley in California.

■ **Teleomorph.** None has been identified.

■ **Reservoirs.** In the saprobic mould form *C. immitis* is found primarily in alkaline desert soil where winters are mild and summers are hot and where rainfall often averages less than 15 inches a year. The infectious conidia become airborne in dust storms. Animals, especially desert rodents, have also been shown to be vectors.

■ **Unique Risk Factors.** Although *C. immitis* can cause fatal infections, it is a relatively small threat to people with a competent immune system. When infection does occur, it is likely to be more severe in dark-skinned people and during pregnancy. Infection is an occupational hazard for people such as construction workers and farmers who are exposed to soil and dust. Person-to-person transmission is rare.

 C. immitis is the dimorphic fungus that most often causes laboratory-acquired infections. *Great care and strict laboratory precautions MUST be taken when working with specimens or cultures believed to contain this organism!*

■ **Human Infection.** *C. immitis* is probably the most virulent of all the agents of human mycoses, according to Rippon. In an immunocompetent host inhalation of a few conidia causes an infection and antibodies may develop, but such people generally do not require treatment for the mild infection.

 C. immitis can cause several different kinds of infections. The most common, primary pulmonary *coccidioidomycosis*, is asymptomatic and *self-limiting* (resolving without treatment) 60% of the time in immunocompetent people. Skin eruptions characterized by *erythema nodosum* or *erythema multiforme* may develop; a third of those with erythema nodosum develop **desert rheumatism,** an arthralgia in one or more joints. Primary coccidioidomycosis with erythema nodosum is more common in women than in men. However, the dissemination rate is four times as high in adult males as it is in women.

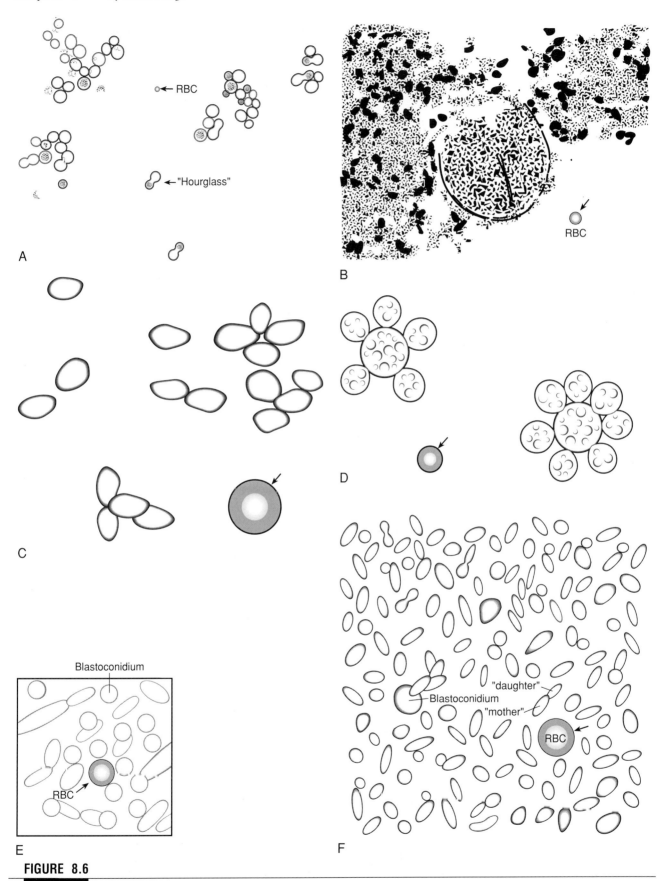

FIGURE 8.6

The yeast (tissue) forms of *Blastomyces dermatitidis (A)*, *Coccidioides immitis (B)*, and *Paracoccidioides brasiliensis (D)* are very distinctive. However, the yeast (tissue) forms of *Histoplasma capsulatum (C)* and *Sporothrix schenckii (F)* are very similar to *Candida (E)* and other yeastlike fungi. Notice the differences in size. The 7-μm red blood cell (RBC) (arrow) shows the relative sizes of the mycotic elements.

TABLE 8.3 Yeast Forms of Dimorphic Fungi and Similar Monomorphic Fungi

Fungus	Size of (Blasto) Conidia (μm)	Shape of (Blasto) Conidia	Pseudohyphae (CMT)	Appearance in CMT	Germ Tube Test	Caffeic Acid (Niger Seed) Test	Capsule Present	Urease Production	Colony Morphology	Growth Rate	Other Helpful Features
Blastomyces dermatitidis	≦20	Spherical to pyriform	No	NA	NA	NA	NA	NA	White to light tan with wrinkled- or folded topography and waxy texture	10–15 days	Thick connection between mother and daughter cells
Candida albicans	4 × 6	Oval, elliptical, or round	Yes	Elongate pseudo-hyphal cells with large clusters of blastoconidia at junctures between cells. Sessile, intercalary, and many terminal chlamydospores	Positive	Negative	None	Negative	Slightly dry, white or cream bacteria-like colony	1–2 days	Grown in 1–2 days at room temperature *or* at 37°C; monomorphic
Coccidioides immitis	None	NA	NA	True hyphae with rectangular or barrel-shaped arthroconidia with thick walls	NA	NA	NA	NA	No yeast form colony	5–15 days	No yeast form in culture on standard media
Cryptococcus species	4–20	Globose	None	Globose cells in varying sizes that do not touch	Negatiave	Variable	Yes	Variable	Mucoid or moist white colonies that become dull and tan	2–4 days	Colonies become dull and tan as they age; monomorphic if encapsulated

240

Organism	Size	Morphology						Colony morphology	Incubation	Comments
Histoplasma capsulatum	4 × 6	Oval, elliptical, or round	NA	Yes	NA	NA	NA	White to pale tan, slightly dry colony that darkens with age	5–15 days	Found intracellularly in reticuloendothelial cells; mould form colony at 25°C
Paracoccidioides brasiliensis	10–30	Oval or elongate cells budding from central cell	NA	NA	NA	NA	NA	Cream or white, dry colony that becomes darker and more wrinkled with age	5–15 days	Yeast cells resemble a ship's wheel; mould form colony at 25°C
Sporothrix schenckii	4–6	Oval or elongate	NA	None	NA	NA	NA	Creamy, dry colonies that may contain black or dark brown striations	5–15 days	Very fine connector between mother and daughter cells. Dematiaceous mould colonies at 25°C
Torulopsis glabrata	3–5	Oval	Small oval or rounded blastoconidia	None	Negative	Negative	Negative	Very small dry, creamy or white colonies	2–3 days	May be found intracellularly in specimens; both cells and colonies are smaller than those of other yeastlike fungi; monomorphic

NA, not applicable; CMT, cornmeal–Tween 80 agar.

TABLE 8.4 Mould Forms of Dimorphic Fungi and Similar Monomorphic Fungi

Fungus	Size of Microconidia (μm)	Shape of Microconidia	Arrangement of Microconidia	Width of Hyphae (μm)	Length of Conidiophore (μm)	Shape of Conidiophore	Arrangement of Conidiophores	Colony Morphology	Growth Rate	Other Helpful Features
Blastomyces dermatitidis species	6	Pyriform or globose	Singly	1–2	4–10	Sticklike	Solitary	Varied. typically waxy white or beige becoming fluffy; reverse tan to brown	Slow	Colony may develop concentric rings or become prickly in the center
Chrysosporium species	5 × 8	Club shaped	Solitary and intercalary	3	3–10	Sticklike	Solitary	Moniliaceous (variations in pigment)	Rapid	Monomorphic. Arthroconidia may be present. Conidia may be intercalary
Coccidioides immitis	NA	Many barrel-shaped arthroconidia	NA	2–6	NA	NA	NA	Initially white and fluffy, becoming membranous later	Rapid	Many barrel-shaped arthroconidia, with disjunctors
Graphium species	8 × 6	Pyriform with truncate base	Single	1–4	Variable	Sticklike with occasional branches	Solitary	Woolly brownish surface with gray to black reverse	Intermediate	Monomorphic mould; synnemata
Histoplasma capsulatum	2–5	Oval or globose	Single	1–2	3–6	Short sticks	Solitary	Fluffy white, becoming woolly and tan	Slow	8–14 μm tuberculate "chlamydospores"; dimorphic
Paracoccidioides brasiliensis	2–3	Oval to pyriform and truncate	Single	1–2	2–3	Short sticks	Solitary	Varied: initially downy white, becoming creamy and membranous or folded	S-l-o-o-ow	Dimorphism
Pseudallescheria boydii	*Pseudallescheria boydii* is a teleomorph. Colonies are mixtures of *P. boydii* and one of its synanamorphs, *Scedosporium apiospermum* or *Graphium* species. Details of conidia, hyphae, and other characteristics can be found in the discussion of those fungi.							Woolly brownish surface with gray to black reverse	Intermediate	Cleistothecia containing asci and ascospores
Scedosporium apiospermum	8 × 6	Pyriform with truncate base	Single	1–3	Variable	Sticklike with occasional branches	Solitary	Woolly brownish surface with gray to black reverse	Intermediate	Monomorphic mould
Sepedonium species	7–19	Round and rough or tuberculate	Single or in clusters	2–3	5–20	Straight or branching	Solitary	White and cottony	Intermediate	Mould at 25°C and 37°C

NA, not applicable.

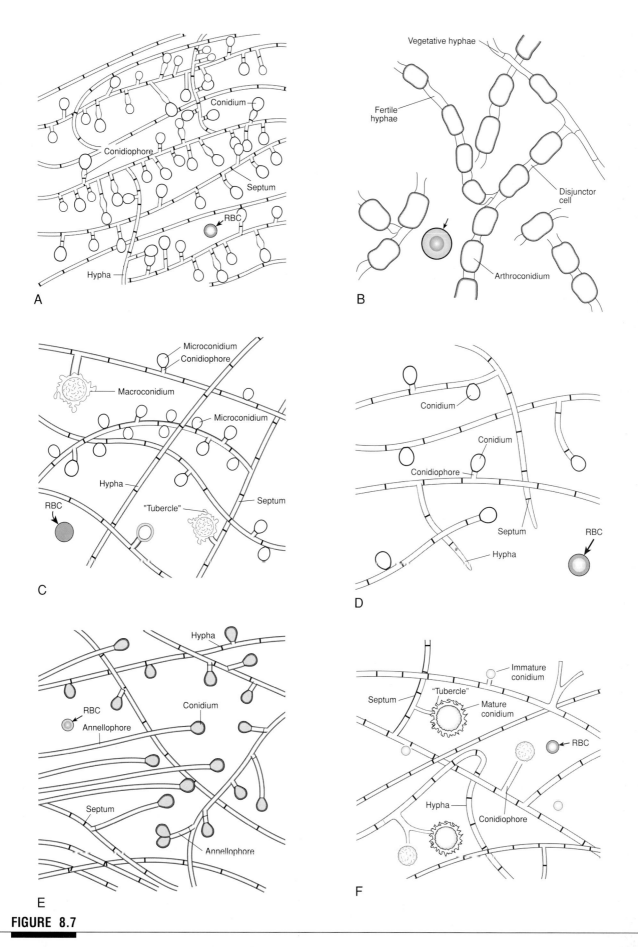

FIGURE 8.7

The mould forms of *Blastomyces dermatitidis* (A), *Paracoccidioides brasiliensis* (D), and *Scedosporium apiospermum* (E) as well as some of the saprobic fungi are very similar. *Histoplasma capsulatum* (C) also resembles these moulds unless macroconidia are present. When macroconidia are present, *Histoplasma* must be distinguised from *Sepedonium* species (F). The thick-walled arthroconidia of *Coccidioides immitis* (B) make it look very different from the other dimorphic pathogens. The 7-μm red blood cells (RBCs) (arrows) show the relative sizes of the mycotic elements.

High serum levels of estradiol and progesterone in pregnant women are thought to account for an increased risk of infection during pregnancy. Rarely, primary cutaneous disease results from inoculation of *C. immitis* into an open lesion on the skin.

Adult males with dark skin, especially African Americans and Filipinos, are most likely to develop severe primary disease with dissemination. Secondary symptomatic infections of the lungs or other organ systems follow primary infections in less than 2% of the cases. Meningitis is one of the commonest causes of death. Fewer than 0.5% of secondary infections are fatal.

■ **Specimen Sources.** Sputum or other pulmonary specimens, aspirated pus, skin scrapings or biopsied tissue, cerebrospinal fluid, blood, or urine are most likely to be submitted for culture when *C. immitis* is suspected.

■ **Specimen Collection and Handling.** Specimens should be collected aseptically according to the standard protocol for the type of specimen and transported to the laboratory without delay. *Because of the potential consequences of infection, the person collecting the specimen should take special precautions.*

Direct examination of pus aspirated from draining sinuses can be done with simple wet mounts, with or without added stains. If necessary, KOH can be added to the mounting fluid to clear debris from the specimen. Tissue specimens are best examined as sections that have been fixed and stained by the histology laboratory. Mucus and other thick substances should be treated with *N*-acetyl-L-cysteine before the wet mount is done. Specific FA tests are also available to detect the spherules in tissue or wet preparations of clinical specimens. Special stains such as the Papanicolaou stain, H&E, or Giemsa stain may be helpful, especially for tissue specimens.

■ **Immunology.** The individual antigens of *C. immitis* have not yet been characterized. The two substances used as antigens are mixtures. *Coccidioidin* is a filtrate prepared from mould cultures; *spherulin* is an extract from a tissue culture of the yeast form. Skin tests using intradermal injections of coccidioidin are primarily useful as epidemiologic tools. The conversion from a negative to a positive skin test is diagnostic of infection with *C. immitis.* When there is no history of a negative test, a positive skin test does not differentiate between past exposure to *C. immitis* and the current condition. When the skin test is positive, other serologic tests should be done; results of other serologic tests are not compromised if skin testing for *Coccidioides* is done first.

Either coccidioidin or spherulin is used as the antigen for CF tests. Complement-fixing IgG antibodies are present within 3 months in 90% of patients infected with *C. immitis.* Although they are the last to appear, they are of the greatest prognostic value. Typically CF titers parallel the severity of the disease, remaining high until the

patient begins to recover, at which time the titer begins to drop. CF antibodies in cerebrospinal fluid are indicative of *Coccidioides* meningitis. Hemolysis of less than 30% in the test and control tubes is considered a positive test; control sera must have titers of 1:32 or greater for results to be considered valid. Detection of antibodies of the IgG class at any titer, within 2 to 6 weeks of the onset of symptoms, is presumptive evidence of coccidioidomycosis when symptoms are present. Titers greater than 1:16 that increase gradually and persist despite treatment are indicative of disseminated infection. CF is quite specific, but a few cross-reactions to coccidioidin occur in patients with acute disseminated histoplasmosis. Their anti-*Coccidioides* CF titers are higher than their anti-*Histoplasma* CF titers when the tests are done simultaneously on the same serum.

In about 90% of those patients who have symptoms of infection precipitins appear within the first weeks of infection before CF tests become positive and disappear within a short period, even if the infection disseminates. The advantage of the TP test is that, as a test for an IgM antibody, it is an early indication of recent infection. The test is highly specific; very few cross-reactions occur with other mycoses. The TP is helpful for diagnosis, but it has no prognostic value. Both CF and TP tests are too complicated, costly, and time consuming to be used for routine screening of patients. They are usually reserved for confirmation of results obtained with simpler, less expensive tests.

ID tests are the most popular screening tests for the detection of both IgG and IgM antibodies to *C. immitis.* With agar gels as the substrate, ID tests are as sensitive as CF tests and more specific, and anticomplementary serum does not interfere with the test. The ID methods roughly parallel CF tests in terms of timing of antibody detection. The identification of one band that is continuous or identical with the reference antisera indicates chronic infection. Two or more bands usually indicate active infection.

In the recent past the LA test was considered to yield results compatible with CF and TP tests but, according to the *Manual of Microbiology* the LA test is being reevaluated because of reports of up to 10% false-positive results with cerebrospinal fluid and diluted sera. Latex particles coated with heat-treated coccidioidin are combined with patient serum. Although the LA test is an excellent screening process, a positive LA test should always be confirmed by another more specific method.

DNA probes, FA, and exoantigen tests are also available to detect *Coccidioides* antigen. The exoantigen test for *C. immitis* detects cell-free F, HL, and HS antigens in mould colonies using an ID method. FA tests can be applied directly to specimens, and cross-reactions with other fungi are rare, making this an excellent screening test for coccidioidomycosis.

■ **Special Precautions.** Laboratory personnel who are working with *any* fluffy white mould colony should take special precautions. *As a minimum, cultures should always be studied within a biologic Class II safety cabinet.* Another excellent practice when *C. immitis* is suspected is to wet the colony with a small amount of sterile saline before removing any portion of the colony for microscopic examination or transfer to new media. An alternative, if the culture does not need to be kept viable, is to flood the colonies with 1% formaldehyde and allow it to stand for 2 to 3 hours before making the microscopic preparations.

■ **Culture Media.** Modified SDA, SDA with antimicrobials, BHIA, and BHIB. *Note:* If *C. immitis* is suspected, initial cultures and subcultures should be done in test tubes or culture bottles rather than Petri dishes. Converse medium and increased CO_2 must be used to convert the mould form to the tissue phase of *Coccidioides*—a practice that is NOT recommended. Levine's modification of Converse medium is an agar containing ammonium acetate, phosphates, sodium and calcium carbonate, glucose, zinc sulfate, and tamol.

Temperature Considerations. Optimal temperature for growth is 25° to 35°C for the mould form on routine media. Temperatures of 37° to 40°C and increased CO_2 are needed to induce the tissue phase in culture (with special media such as Converse medium). Tmax for *C. immitis* is 54°C.

■ **Macroscopic (Colony) Morphology.** Colonies of *C. immitis* on modified SDA at 25°C usually mature in 3 to 5 days—within 48 hours if abundant conidia are present in the specimen. Arthroconidia form in 7 to 10 days. The colonies are white and floccose at first; they develop great varieties of color and form as they mature. Typical mature colonies are membranous or glabrous with hyphae that are adherent to the agar; the surface is partially or completely covered with a cottony aerial mycelium that resembles cobwebs. Mature colonies of *C. immitis* typically become white to gray, but strains with lavender, buff, cinnamon, yellow, or brown obverse pigment may be found. The reverse pigment can range from white through tan to dark brown or orange. Some variants produce a brown pigment that diffuses into the agar around the colony. The powdery texture is caused by the production of many arthroconidia. *C. immitis* does not produce a yeast form in culture on routine media, although it grows in tissue as a spherule. Conversion of the culture to the spherule form is not necessary for identification and is not recommended.

■ **Microscopic Morphology** (Figs. 8.8 and 8.9). In a lactophenol–cotton blue prep, septate hyaline hyphae of varying widths are seen; fertile arthroconidiating hyphae are wider (3 to 6 μm) than the vegetative hyphae. The arthroconidia are usually single celled and barrel shaped or rectangular. Interspersed in the hyphae between the

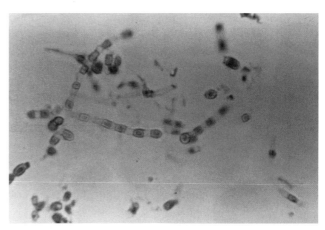

FIGURE 8.8

In typical preparations of the mould form *Coccidioides immitis* is seen as septate, hyaline hyphae containing arthroconidia that are broader than other hyphal cells. Here two hyphae filled with arthroconidia form a Y with the base at the center of the left margin. The typical thick-walled, barrel-shaped arthroconidia are separated from one another by empty thin-walled disjunctor cells. Free arthroconidia are present here, and one hypha without arthroconidia runs between the arms of the Y, parallel to its lower arm. (Courtesy of the Centers for Disease Control and Prevention.)

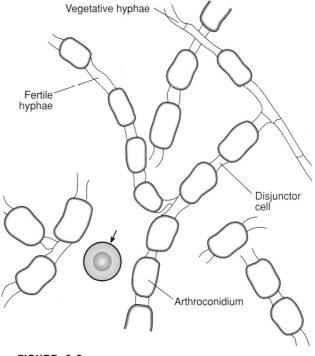

FIGURE 8.9

Coccidioides immitis in the mould form consists of septate, hyaline hyphae of varying widths and arthroconidia. The conidia are typically barrel shaped, although they may be rectangular and have thick walls. Thin-walled disjunctor cells, which appear to be empty, are interspersed between arthroconidia in the hyphae. Disarticulated arthroconidia eventually "round up" into roughly spherical forms. Mould colonies that could be *C. immitis* should not be manipulated *except* in a biologic safety cabinet. The 7-μm red blood cell (RBC) shows the relative sizes of the mycotic elements.

arthroconidia are empty thin-walled "disjunctors" (disjuncture cells) that fragment when they are mature, freeing the arthroconidia to disperse. Remnants of the walls of the disjunctors initially remain attached to the ends of the arthroconidia, where they can be seen with the brightfield microscope, but the remnants may dissolve shortly after fragmentation of the hyphae. Cultures of *C. immitis* are extremely hazardous because enormous numbers of the infectious arthroconidia can be released from the culture when the fungus is manipulated in any way. The arthroconidia "round up" and become spherules in tissue, develop mould colonies in routine culture, or rest quietly in the soil until a likely host comes along. Racquet hyphae may also be observed in culture.

Direct Examination of Specimens (Figs. 8.10 and 8.11). *C. immitis* produces endosporulating spherules in the host's tissue. The spherules are round and refractive and usually have thick (2 μm) walls. They range in size from 10 μm for young forms up to 80 μm at maturity. When they are mature, the spherules contain numerous thin-walled nonbudding endospores (2 to 4 μm in diameter) formed by progressive cleavage of the protoplasm of the spherules. The *endospores* ("endo," within) are freed when the mature spherule ruptures, spilling them into the surrounding tissue. Endospores can be seen in intact or rupturing spherules in tissue sections and other specimens or free in the tissue. Occasionally hyphal fragments may be found in pulmonary lesions located near air passages in the lung.

If spherules are identified and clinical symptoms are evident, the fungus can be definitively identified as *C. immitis*; culture is not required.

■ **Laboratory Identification of *Coccidioides immitis*.** Exoantigen tests can be used to speed identification of

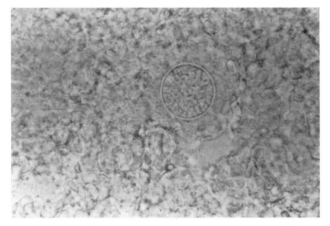

FIGURE 8.10

In tissue and other specimens such as sputum, *Coccidioides immitis* forms spherules, very large spherical structures with thick walls. The cluttered background in this photomicrograph is the tissue cells in which the spherule is lodged. Endospores are present within the spherule, waiting to be liberated to start new sites of infection. (Courtesy of the Centers for Disease Control and Prevention.)

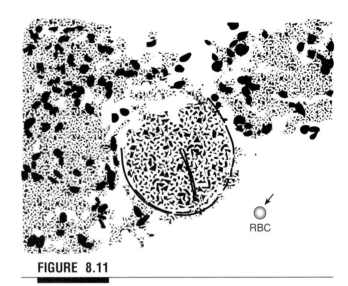

FIGURE 8.11

Coccidioides immitis produces spherules in host tissues but *not* in routine cultures. These large, round, thick-walled structures contain infectious endospores that form by division of the spherule's protoplasm and are released when the mature spherule ruptures. A break in the spherule's wall can be seen in the center of this field. The 7-μm red blood cell (RBC) (arrow) shows the relative sizes of the mycotic elements.

the fungus. Indirect FA tests and a nucleic acid probe for culture confirmation are also available for *C. immitis*.

■ **Helpful Features for Identification of *Coccidioides immitis***

Rapidly growing colonies with early appearance of white cottony aerial mycelium and areas of adherent surface hyphae

Barrel-shaped arthroconidia alternating with disjuncture cells at 25° to 35 °C

Spherules containing endospores in tissue or at 40°C in special media

■ **Organisms from Which *Coccidioides immitis* Must Be Differentiated** (see Tables 8.3 and 8.4 and Figs. 8.6 and 8.7)

Gymnoascus
Malbranchea
Nonbudding yeast forms of *Blastomyces dermatitidis* and *Candida* species
Nonencapsulated forms of *Cryptococcus neoformans*
Geotrichum species
Trichosporon species

Systemic Dimorphic Pathogens

HYALINE HYPHOMYCETES

HISTOPLASMA CAPSULATUM   (Hiss-toe-plaz-muh cap-suh-lot-um)

H. capsulatum is found worldwide and is endemic in central North America in areas surrounding the Mississippi, Missouri, and Ohio Rivers. *H. capsulatum* var. *duboisii* is primarily found in Africa. It is identical to *H. capsulatum* var. *capsulatum* except that it develops larger, thick-walled yeast cells.

The pulmonary infection is sometimes called **Darling's disease,** in honor of the pathologist who first recognized it in a patient in the Ancon Canal Zone Hospital in Panama. Darling believed the organism to be a parasite because of its size and staining characteristics and its presence within histiocytes.

■ **Teleomorph.** *Ajellomyces capsulatus.*

■ **Reservoirs.** The ecologic niche with which *H. capsulatum* is most often associated is soil with a high nitrogen content resulting from deposits of the excreta of starlings, chickens, and bats. Histoplasmosis has been nicknamed **spelunker's disease,** or caver's disease, because of its occurrence in those who explore caves, which are often inhabited by bats.

■ **Unique Risk Factors.** The fungus is transmitted by airborne routes and is considered highly infectious. Epidemics of histoplasmosis have occurred, usually in groups of people who are exposed to large numbers of conidia through some common activity such as tearing down an old chicken house or cleaning up a site invaded by starlings. Although *H. capsulatum* can cause fatal infections, it is a relatively small threat to people with a competent immune system.

■ **Human Infection.** *H. capsulatum* is the etiologic agent of *histoplasmosis,* a chronic granulomatous and suppurative disease that primarily involves the lungs and the reticuloendothelial (RE) system. In approximately 5% of patients with primary pulmonary histoplasmosis the infection progresses to chronic disease or "an acute fulminating, rapidly fatal disease. The latter form is particularly common in children" (Rippon, p. 381). Fibrosis around the cavities in the lung creates dense, round, flattened areas that are described as "coin lesions." In untreated infections the macrophages begin hematogenous spread of the *Histoplasma* to other tissues and organs early in the disease.

The yeast form of *H. capsulatum* was first discovered in *histiocytes,* that is, connective tissue macrophages, in the RE system, where Darling described a capsule in the stained tissue sections. The apparent capsule has been proven to be an artifact, caused by the protoplasm of *Histoplasma* shrinking away from the cell wall during the staining process, leaving an unstained area (Fig. 8.12). In specimens the yeast cells resemble *Candida*, and two parasites, *Toxoplasma gondii* and *Leishmania*; the fungi can be differentiated from the parasites by the GMS stain that is specific for fungi.

H. capsulatum has been found in various clinical conditions in increasing numbers of immunocompromised patients. Patients with AIDS are at particular risk of developing cutaneous lesions and disseminated infections.

■ **Specimen Sources.** Sputum or other pulmonary specimens, aspirated pus from lymph nodes and subcutaneous abscesses, skin scrapings or biopsied tissue from the edges of ulcers, biopsied lung tissue, crusts from skin lesions, oropharyngeal scrapings, bone marrow, blood, cerebrospinal fluid, and urine are most likely to be submitted for culture.

■ **Specimen Collection and Handling.** Specimens should be collected aseptically according to the standard protocol for the type of specimen and transported to the laboratory without delay. The tissue phase of *H. capsulatum* is sensitive to enzymes that are present in specimens and is injured by the metabolites of yeasts that may also be present. Specimens should be inoculated to culture media as rapidly as possible when histoplasmosis is suspected.

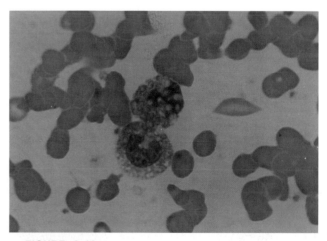

FIGURE 8.12

Tissue forms of *Histoplasma capsulatum* have invaded the leukocytes in this blood film; the pale oval forms are most easily seen in the nucleus of the upper cell, although they are also scattered through the cytoplasm. A free yeast cell lies just to the left of the lower white blood cell, at approximately 9 o'clock. A second free cell can be seen adjacent to the red blood cell in the lower left, and other free cells are scattered through the field.

Direct Examination. *H. capsulatum* is a pathogen of the RE system and is most likely to be found within cells instead of free in fluids. Bone marrow, or a preparation of the buffy coat of a blood sample, should be examined. The materials should be stained by Wright's method, the Giemsa stain, or the combined Wright-Giemsa stain and examined under oil immersion. A KOH preparation is not useful in this situation.

Direct examination of pus aspirated from draining sinuses can be done with simple wet mounts, with added stains. Tissue specimens are best examined as sections that have been fixed and stained by the histology laboratory. Mucus and other thick substances should be treated with *N*-acetyl-L-cysteine before the wet mount is done. Specific FA tests are also available to detect the yeast forms in tissue or other clinical specimens. Special stains such as the Papanicolaou stain or H&E stain may be helpful, especially for tissue specimens.

■ **Immunology.** One of the antigens used to detect *H. capsulatum* and histoplasmosis is ***histoplasmin,*** a mixture of H and M antigens and other materials. A yeast antigen, extracted from yeast cultures of *H. capsulatum*, is more sensitive than the histoplasmin antigen.

Skin tests with intradermal injections of histoplasmin, a filtrate of the mycelial phase of growth, are useful as epidemiologic tools. Because a positive skin test indicates *either* past or present exposure to *H. capsulatum*, and because the skin test procedure causes production of antibodies to *Histoplasma* and some related fungi, Kwon-Chung and Bennett consider that it has little diagnostic value and should not be used. Serologic tests can be done on serum, plasma, peritoneal fluid, cerebrospinal fluid, and urine. Specimens for other tests should be obtained first if skin testing is done.

The CF test is the most widely used procedure for the diagnosis of all stages of histoplasmosis, including meningeal infections, despite problems with the method. Although it is very sensitive, the CF test is less specific than other methods, and positive tests do not occur with anticomplementary sera. The antigen for the CF test may be histoplasmin or the yeast extract. CF tests are used for diagnosis and for following the response to treatment. Titers between 1:8 and 1:32 are generally considered presumptive evidence of histoplasmosis. A decreasing titer with both antigens is indicative of the patient's improvement; titers to the yeast antigen fall more slowly than titers to histoplasmin. CF titers generally appear within 2 to 3 weeks of exposure or by the time symptoms appear, if the yeast extract is used. A titer that remains high is usually considered to be indicative of active or progressive disease. A fourfold change in the titer in either direction, of course, signifies progression or regression of the disease. Cross-reactions may occur in patients with blastomycosis or paracoccidioidomycosis when histoplasmin is the antigen. Cross-reactions with leishmaniasis also occur when the yeast antigen is used. A negative CF test does not exclude the possibility of histoplasmosis. The test should be repeated with fresh serum after a 2- to 3-week interval.

ID and counterimmunoelectrophoresis tests, using histoplasmin as the antigen, are useful screening procedures. The formation of two precipitating bands representing specific reactions to the H and M antigens are diagnostic of histoplasmosis, although additional bands representing other antigens may form. The H band may be present in active infection, while the M band appears early and persists even after recovery; it is often found without the H band. Either or both bands are also found in meningeal histoplasmosis. ID and CF tests are often used in combination to assess the patient's progress after treatment. Reagents for both methods are available commercially.

Other immunologic methods developed for diagnosis or identification of *H. capsulatum* include an LA test that uses latex particles coated with histoplasmin as the antigen. Many false-positive tests have been reported; this screening test should always be confirmed with another method. The radioimmunoassay (RIA) test, performed in reference laboratories, is highly sensitive but not very specific. It tests for the *Histoplasma* polysaccharide antigen and has been useful for the diagnosis of histoplasmosis in patients with AIDS. The RIA can be used with serum, urine, and cerebrospinal fluid. The antigen cross-reacts with *Coccidioides immitis* and *Blastomyces dermatitidis*. Because of the low specificity, results of the RIA test should be confirmed by another method.

An exoantigen test for detection of the H or M antigens of *H. capsulatum* is now available commercially to confirm the identity of an isolate. Antiserum is tested against an extract of mould colonies of the unknown fungus. Bands that are continuous with or identical to the reference bands indicate that the unknown is *H. capsulatum*. The exoantigen test is faster than conventional methods of identification and can be applied to contaminated and nonviable cultures. A commercially available FA test can be used for identification of yeast cells.

■ **Special Precautions.** Laboratory personnel who are working with *any* fluffy white mould-form colony should take special precautions and adhere stringently to laboratory procedures. *As a minimum, cultures should always be studied within a biologic Class II safety cabinet. Slide cultures should never be made.*

■ **Culture Media.** Blood agar plate (BAP) or modified SDA, BAP or modified SDA with antimicrobials at temperatures from 25° to 30°C. SDA without antimicrobials at temperatures above 30°C. Media must be moist for successful growth!

SABHI or BHIA containing blood are strongly recommended for specimens from sites that are ordinarily sterile. Biphasic culture bottles containing BHIA and

BHIB are recommended for blood cultures. Yeast extract phosphate agar with ammonium hydroxide can be inoculated from the specimen to encourage conidiation and inhibit *Candida species.*

Use PDA or PFA for subculture from colonies to encourage conidia production.

Temperature Considerations. Optimal temperature for growth is 25° to 30°C for the mould form on routine media. Temperature of 37°C is needed to induce the yeast phase.

Primary cultures for H. capsulatum should be held for 10 to 12 weeks before being discarded as "no growth."

■ Macroscopic (Colony) Morphology

At 25°C, mould-form colonies of *H. capsulatum* develop slowly on modified SDA; mature colonies are usually produced in 15 to 25 days. The colonies show great variety in form, texture, and pigment. They may be white or beige to brown at first with a fluffy or glabrous texture. Later they become woolly, as aerial hyphae develop. Typical colonies have a tan pigment, but albino- and brown-type colonies also occur. On BHI or SABHI containing blood, colonies of *H. capsulatum* are cream colored, tan, or pink, with heaped or wrinkled topography and moist or prickly texture. The reverse pigment of the colonies is white or yellow to yellow-orange.

At 37°C H. capsulatum is a yeast. Colonies typically appear after 10 to 15 days on an enriched medium, such as BHIA with blood. They are white to light tan and mucoid, with a rough membranous texture.

■ Microscopic Morphology

At 25° to 30°C (Figs. 8.13 through 8.15), *Histoplasma* produces very fine (1 to 2 μm) hyphae that are septate and hyaline; they may form ropelike strands on media containing blood. Microconidia are produced in some isolates. They are borne directly on the hyphae or on short conidiophores; the small (2 to 5 μm) conidia are unicellular and hyaline and may be smooth or echinulate.

Macroconidia are also produced by *H. capsulatum.* They develop directly on the hyphae or on short, slender conidiophores that develop at right angles to the vegetative hyphae. The macroconidia are hyaline, unicellular, and relatively large (8 to 14 μm), with spherical to pyriform shapes. As the macroconidia age (or in subculture) they become *tuberculate;* that is, they form finger-like extensions of the thick wall of the conidium. Mature macroconidia are sometimes described as resembling sunflowers in bloom.

At 37°C (Figs. 8.16 and 8.17), *H. capsulatum* resembles cells of *Candida.* The blastoconidia are small (2 to 5 μm) and globose to ovoid. When buds are produced, they form at the smaller end of the mother cell, with narrow necks of attachment.

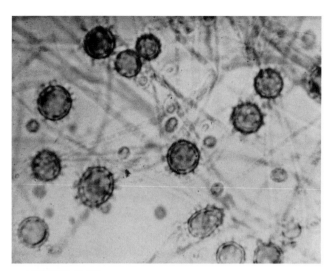

FIGURE 8.13

Typical preparations of mould form colonies of *Histoplasma capsulatum* are frequently unremarkable in young cultures. The delicate hyphae in the background of this photomicrograph are not distinctive; the small oval microconidia and matchstick-like conidiophores such as the one at 6 o'clock add no real clues to the identity of this isolate. The presence of large macroconidia with thick walls extending into finger-like tubercles strongly suggests *H. capsulatum.* This must be confirmed by immunologic tests or by proving the isolate is thermally dimorphic. (Courtesy of the Centers for Disease Control and Prevention.)

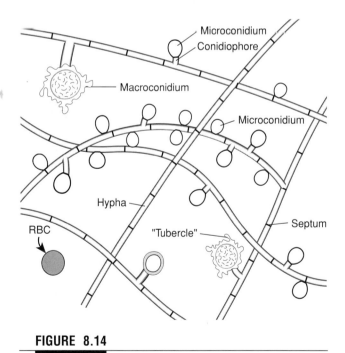

FIGURE 8.14

Histoplasma capsulatum mould colonies contain hyaline, septate hyphae and round conidia borne directly on the hyphae and at the tips of short, sticklike conidiophores. Large, thick-walled macroconidia, with the exterior walls of the macroconidium extended into finger-like projections, are also seen in older cultures. The 7-μm red blood cell (RBC) (arrow) shows the relative sizes of the mycotic elements.

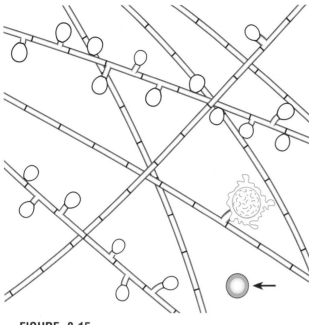

FIGURE 8.15

In bad preparations the mould form of *Histoplasma capsulatum* is difficult to identify, especially if tuberculate macroconidia are not seen. The dimorphic fungus must be distinguished from *Trichophyton* species, the monomorphic opportunist *Sepedonium*, and anamorphs of *Pseudallescheria boydii*. The 7-μm red blood cell (arrow) shows the relative sizes of the mycotic elements.

Direct Examination of Specimens. In tissue specimens and body fluids *H. capsulatum* produces small (2 to 5 μm), round to oval yeast cells that may show budding from the parent cell by a narrow neck. The yeast are often clustered within histiocytes. Histologic study of tissue specimens using GMS, PAS, and H&E stains are of great diagnostic value when they are positive.

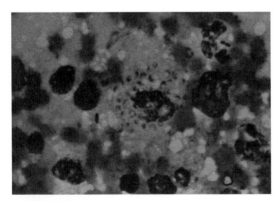

FIGURE 8.16

In tissue specimens and body fluids *Histoplasma capsulatum* is seen as small round to oval yeast cells resembling species of *Candida*. The leukocyte in the center of this section of liver tissue is filled with the dark oval cells of *Histoplasma*. Other *Histoplasma* cells are free in the intercellular spaces. (From Rippon JW: Medical Mycology: The Pathogenic Fungi and the Actinomycetes, 3rd ed. Philadelphia, WB Saunders, 1988, p 403.)

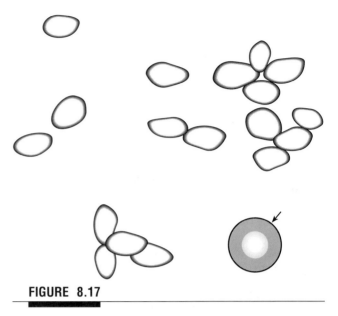

FIGURE 8.17

Histoplasma capsulatum in its tissue phase forms oval or round yeast cells that resemble other yeasts such as *Candida*. The only significant differences is the smaller size of *Histoplasma*, a feature that may be missed unless a micrometer is used to examine the preparation.

■ **Laboratory Identification of *Histoplasma capsulatum.*** Exoantigen tests are available for identification of cultures.

H. capsulatum is a thermally dimorphic organism. It must be converted from the mould form to the yeast form (using enriched media at 37°C) or identified by the exoantigen test or by nucleic acid hybridization to confirm identification. During thermal conversion swollen hyphal cells, pseudohyphae, and blastoconidia develop in cultures.

■ **Helpful Features for Identification of *Histoplasma capsulatum***

> Colonies with slow to intermediate growth rates at 25°
> Thick-walled tuberculate macroconidia ("sunflowers") at room temperature
> Waxy, wrinkled, light brown colony of yeast at 37°C
> Small blastoconidia, 2 to 5 μm in diameter, with narrow necks of attachment, at 37°C
> Intracellular yeast in tissue sections and white blood cells

■ **Organisms from Which *Histoplasma capsulatum* Must Be Differentiated** (see Tables 8.3 and 8.4 and Figs. 8.6 and 8.7)

> Nonbudding yeast forms of *Blastomyces dermatitidis*
> Nonencapsulated forms of *Cryptococcus neoformans*
> Detached buds of *Paracoccidioides brasiliensis*
> Endospores or young spherules of *Coccidioides immitis*
> *Candida* species, especially *Torulopsis (Candida) glabrata*

Chrysosporium species
Scedosporium species
Sepedonium species

Systemic Dimorphic Pathogens

HYALINE HYPHOMYCETES

PARACOCCIDIOIDES BRASILIENSIS (Pair-uh-cock-sih-dee-oy'-dees bruh-zill-ee-en-sis)

P. brasiliensis is endemic in the Holdridge Life Zones (on both sides of the equator and the Tropic of Capricorn) in northwestern, central, and southeastern South America, Central America, and southern Mexico.

■ **Teleomorph.** None has been identified.

■ **Reservoirs.** In the saprobic mould form *P. brasiliensis* is found primarily in acid soil in the humid areas in which it is endemic. The exact ecologic niche of the fungus has not been determined, but the infectious conidia are believed to be found in the soil and on plants. Armadillos may be carriers of *P. brasiliensis*. Paracoccidioidomycosis is also called *South American blastomycosis*.

■ **Unique Risk Factors.** *P. brasiliensis* is transmitted by airborne routes or by contact with contaminated plants and is considered highly infectious. Although mild subclinical infection occurs, fatal infection is a relatively minor threat to people with a competent immune system. Paracoccidioidomycosis occurs most often in adult males; this may be the combined effect of their hormonal makeup and their occupations. Malnutrition and immunocompetence are important factors influencing susceptibility to this organism.

■ **Human Infection.** *P. brasiliensis* may cause multiple kinds of infections of varying severities. The most common, primary pulmonary *paracoccidioidomycosis,* is usually asymptomatic or subclinical and self-limiting. People who do develop symptoms in subacute primary pulmonary disease may have only mild changes in the lungs and a positive skin test.

Secondary symptomatic infections, involving either pulmonary disease or dissemination to other organs and adjacent tissues, follow primary infections in a small number of cases. The skin of the face is the most common site of infection; mucous membranes of the nose, mouth, throat, and intestine are frequently involved. In disseminated disease any organ of the body can be involved. Pyogenic abscesses and ulcers that become granulomatous may also develop. Lymphadenitis is common.

■ **Specimen Sources.** Sputum or other pulmonary specimens, pus aspirated from lymph nodes, skin scrapings or biopsied tissue from the edges of ulcers, biopsied lung tissue, and crusts from skin lesions are most likely to be cultured.

■ **Specimen Collection and Handling.** Specimens should be collected aseptically according to the standard protocol for the type of specimen and transported to the laboratory without delay.

Direct examination of pus aspirated from draining sinuses can be done with simple wet mounts, with added stains. KOH may be added to the mounting fluid to clear debris from the specimen. Tissue specimens are best examined as sections that have been fixed and stained by the histology laboratory. Mucus and other thick substances should be treated with *N*-acetyl-L-cysteine before the wet mount is done. Special stains such as the Papanicolaou stain, H&E, or Giemsa stain may be helpful, especially for tissue specimens. Specific FA tests are also available to detect the yeast forms in tissue.

■ **Immunology.** The antigens for immunologic tests for paracoccidioidomycosis and *P. brasiliensis* have not been purified enough yet to be separated and designated by individual names. The extract of moulds is **paracoccidioidin**; an E2 antigen extracted from the yeast phase is also used. In precipitin tests the antigens are referred to by the band number (the position of the band relative to the well containing the antigen) and "band 1" is apparently identical to the E2 antigen extracted from yeast.

Skin tests with intradermal injections of paracoccidioidin are primarily useful as epidemiologic tools. They are usually the first serologic tests to be positive in patients, but they do not differentiate between past exposure to *P. brasiliensis* and the current condition. A negative skin test in a person who was previously positive indicates the anergy of disseminated infection.

The CF test, using yeast filtrate antigens, is recommended for the serologic detection of *P. brasiliensis.* One study showed positive CF tests in 97% of patients with paracoccidioidomycosis. CF titers appear late and remain detectable for several months after the patient is considered cured. They are reportedly useful in following the response to treatment. Cross-reactions may occur at low titers in patients with acute histoplasmosis and blastomycosis.

ID tests using concentrated yeast antigens and reference sera are available. The reported sensitivity is 94%; when ID tests are done using reference sera as controls, the method is highly specific. The identification of one to three precipitin bands that are continuous or identical with the reference antisera is indicative of infection. The number of bands is apparently correlated with the CF titer. Low titers are usually indicative of localized infection, while high titers indicate acute infection or dissemination. Band 1 is the first to disappear during treatment. When symptoms are present a combination of ID and CF tests is 98% specific for diagnosis of paracoccidioidomycosis.

Exoantigen methods are useful for speeding up the identification of cultures of *P. brasiliensis*. Direct FA tests to detect *P. brasiliensis* cells in smears of clinical materials are especially useful because most specimens contain few cells of the fungus and those that are present may not have the morphology typical of the fungus.

■ **Special Precautions.** Laboratory personnel who are working with *any* fluffy white mould-form colony should take special precautions. *As a minimum, cultures should always be studied within a biologic Class II safety cabinet. Slide cultures should never be made.*

■ **Culture Media.** Modified SDA with antimicrobials can be used at temperatures from 25° to 30°C. SDA (or any other medium, such as BHIA with blood) without cycloheximide should be used at temperatures above 30°C. Media containing antibacterial antibiotics, but without cycloheximide, may be necessary for primary inoculation of specimens that are thought to be contaminated with bacteria, but this initially slows the growth of the fungus.

Use SABHI or BHIA containing blood for specimens from body sites that are expected to be sterile. Yeast extract agar can be used for primary culture to encourage initial growth and conidiation. PDA or PDA can also be used for subculture of colonies to encourage co-nidia production.

Temperature Considerations. Optimal temperature for growth is 25° to 30°C for the mould form on routine media. Temperatures of 35° to 37°C are needed to induce the yeast phase.

■ **Macroscopic (Colony) Morphology**

At 25°C, mould-form colonies of *P. brasiliensis* on modified SDA mature slowly—they are approximately 2 cm in diameter after 2 to 3 weeks' incubation. Colonies show great variety in form, texture, and pigment. Typically they are white to cream colored at first, with short, downy aerial mycelia and elevated centers. Later they become flat, with a membranous or velvety texture and cerebriform or folded topography. The pigment becomes beige or brown, with a yellow-brown reverse, in mature colonies.

At 37°C, the yeast form of *P. brasiliensis* is produced. On enriched media, and media containing blood, pasty yeastlike colonies appear in 10 to 15 days. They are white to light tan or gray, with a wrinkled or folded topography.

■ **Microscopic Morphology**

At 25° to 30°C (Fig. 8.18), the mould form of *Paracoccidioides* produces very fine (1 to 2 μm) hyphae that are sep-

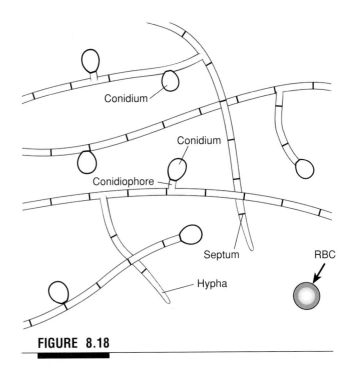

FIGURE 8.18

Paracoccidioides brasiliensis mould forms are oval to pyriform conidia with truncate bases; they develop directly on the hyphae and on sticklike conidiophores. Miscellaneous vegetative hyphal structures such as chlamydoconidia and racquet hyphae may also be present. The 7-μm red blood cell (RBC) (arrow) shows the relative sizes of the mycotic elements.

tate and hyaline. Conidiation may be absent on modified SDA, or a few small (2 to 3 μm) oval to pyriform truncate conidia may be found on short conidiophores or sessile on the hyphae. Usually only chlamydoconidia, both terminal and intercalary, racquet hyphae, and coiled hyphae are seen on modified SDA. When yeast extract agar without glucose—or any medium deficient in glucose—is used, the oval to pyriform conidia are seen in larger numbers, with thick-walled arthroconidia that develop in an alternating pattern.

At 37°C (Figs. 8.19 and 8.20), *P. brasiliensis* grows in the yeast form. The cells are large (up to 30 μm; average

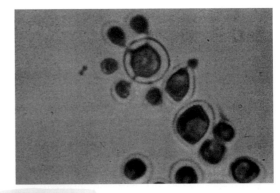

FIGURE 8.19

Characteristically the tissue form of *Paracoccidioides brasiliensis* consists of large round or pyriform cells. These are surrounded by multiple buds that may cover the entire surface of the parent cell, creating the "mariner's wheel." (Courtesy of A. Restrepo.)

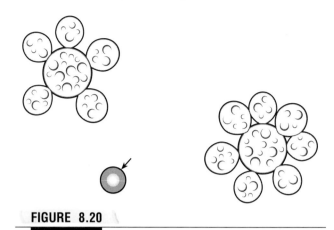

FIGURE 8.20

Paracoccidioides brasiliensis yeast forms are large cells with thick walls from which multiple buds form, creating an arrangement resembling the wheel used to steer sailing ships. Free buds resemble the yeast cells of *Candida* and *Histoplasma*. The 7-μm red blood cell (arrow) shows the relative sizes of the mycotic elements.

diameter, 15 μm) and spherical to pyriform, with thick (0.2 to 1 μm) walls. *Paracoccidioides* reproduces by forming multiple buds that are up to 10 μm in diameter; buds may cover the entire surface of the parent cell. The buds are typically attached by relatively thin necks and are easily dislodged; free buds resemble *Candida* and the yeast phase of *Histoplasma*. The mature cells with the buds attached have been described as resembling a *mariner's wheel*—the pilot wheel found on sailing ships.

Direct Examination of Specimens. *P. brasiliensis* produces *mariner's wheels*, the refractile multiple budding yeast forms, in tissue. The buds may elongate or form short chains while they are still attached to the parent cell, or they may break off in the surrounding tissue when they are mature and begin budding.

■ **Laboratory Identification of *Paracoccidioides brasiliensis*.** *P. brasiliensis* is a thermally dimorphic organism. It must be converted from the mould form to the yeast form (using enriched media at 37°C) to confirm identification. During conversion, swollen hyphal cells and elements of rudimentary hyphae develop in cultures; cytoplasmic granulation is often seen in mycotic cells during conversion.

Exoantigen tests and DNA probes can detect the presence of cell-free antigens produced from the mould-form colonies.

■ **Helpful Features for Identification of *Paracoccidioides brasiliensis***

   Slow-growing colonies with early appearance of white cottony aerial mycelium and heaped-up topography with membranous or velvety texture at 25°C
   Chlamydoconidia and coiled hyphae
   Arthroconidia, especially on media without glucose at 25°C
   Folded colony of yeast cells at 37°C
   Large, thick-walled, multiple budding yeast cells ("mariner's wheels") at 37°C
   Histologic studies of tissue with GMS, PAS, and H&E stains

■ **Organisms from Which *Paracoccidioides brasiliensis* Must Be Differentiated** (see Tables 8.3 and 8.4 and Figs. 8.6 and 8.7)

   Nonbudding yeast forms of *Blastomyces dermatitidis*
   Nonencapsulated forms of *Cryptococcus neoformans*
   Chrysosporium species
   Scedosporium apiospermum
   Blastomyces dermatitidis mould form

SUGGESTED EXERCISES FOR CHAPTER 8

(S y s t e m i c   F u n g i)

Exercise 12   (Single Session)

Purpose. To study the gross and microscopic morphologies of the systemic pathogens without risk, using demonstration materials provided by the instructor.

Suggested Fungus Cultures

Blastomyces dermatitidis
Coccidioides immitis
Histoplasma capsulatum
Paracoccidioides brasiliensis

Process. WORK WITH ONE ORGANISM AT A TIME. Describe the colony morphology of each of the fungi grown at 25–30°C and at 35–37°C. Record the information, as usual.

Then examine the permanent mounts of the organism from cultures grown at the different temperatures. Make drawings on the LABORATORY WORK SHEET for dimorphic fungi.

Bonus. You need not scrub your desk with disinfectant today, and you certainly should not discard the cultures or permanent slides!

ASSESS WHAT YOU HAVE LEARNED

Responses to the questions below are located in Appendix A.

1. Define endospore, mariner's wheel, spherule, tuberculate, coin lesion, granuloma.
2. List at least three characteristics that distinguish true pathogens from the opportunistic moulds, yeasts, and yeastlike organisms.
3. Name four media that may be inoculated for primary culture or subculture when a dimorphic pathogen is suspected.
4. Describe safety precautions that should be implemented when the mould form of a potential systemic pathogen is to be subcultured.

For questions 5 through 14 **MATCH** the name of the organism **(lettered)** with the related disease state(s). NOTE that responses will be used more than once

5. chronic cutaneous infection with ulcers and abscesses
6. Darling's disease
7. desert rheumatism
8. erythema nodosum
9. Gilchrist's disease
10. infects mucous membranes of mouth, nose, and throat
11. intracellular parasite of the reticuloendothelial system
12. South American blastomycosis
13. spelunker's disease
14. Valley fever

a. *Blastomyces dermatitidis*
b. *Coccidioides immitis*
c. *Histoplasma capsulatum*
d. *Paracoccidioides brasiliensis*

For questions 15 through 19 **MATCH** the name of the fungus **(lettered)** with the endemic zone and the reservoir **(numbered)**. NOTE that responses may be used more than once.

15. alkaline desert soil
16. Appalachian region
17. Central and South America
18. bat guano
19. wet acid soil and rotting vegetation

a. *Blastomyces dermatitidis*
b. *Coccidioides immitis*
c. *Histoplasma capsulatum*
d. *Paracoccidioides brasiliensis*

For questions 20 through 25 **MATCH** the name of the fungus **(lettered)** with the characteristics of the organism **(numbered)**. NOTE that responses may be used more than once.

20. large budding yeasts with broad bases of attachment and thick walls
21. mould-form colony is produced at 25°C and at 37°C
22. mould form consists of septate hyphae and barrel-shaped arthroconidia with disjuncture cells
23. thick-walled yeast cells covered with multiple buds attached by narrow necks
24. tuberculate macroconidia resemble a sunflower
25. yeast forms resemble *Leishmania* and *Toxoplasma gondii*

a. *Blastomyces dermatitidis*
b. *Coccidioides immitis*
c. *Histoplasma capsulatum*
d. *Paracoccidioides brasiliensis*

For questions 26 through 30 **MATCH** the fungus **(lettered)** with serodiagnostic properties **(numbered)**. NOTE that responses may be used more than once.

26. a chemiluminescent DNA probe has recently been designed to identify this fungus as soon as the colony appears
27. complement fixation tests are relatively insensitive for this fungus
28. complement fixation tests in combination with immunodiffusion is 98% specific for diagnosis of infection with this fungus
29. exoantigen tests detect free H and M antigens of the mould form of this fungus
30. immunodiffusion is the most popular screening method for both IgG and IgM antibodies to this fungus

a. *Blastomyces dermatitidis*
b. *Coccidioides immitis*
c. *Histoplasma capsulatum*
d. *Paracoccidioides brasiliensis*

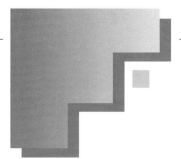

APPENDIX **A**

Answer Key for "Assess What You Have Learned"

CHAPTER

1. Fungi are eukaryotic, devoid of chlorophyll, parasitic, heterothallic, lacking leaves or true roots, and chemosynthetic, and they reproduce by formation of conidia and/or spores. *At least three* of these characteristics should be included in your answer.

2. The two important routes of infection with fungi are inhalation of conidia or spores and accidental traumatic inoculation of conidia or spores into tissues of the host.

3. The factors that predispose a person to a mycosis include exposure to an overwhelming dose of the infecting fungus; a dysfunctional immune system; prolonged use of antibiotics, steroids, or immunosuppressive drugs; iatrogenic procedures; or debilitating disease. *At least three* of these elements should be included in your answer.

4. (a) -mycota, (b) -mycetes, (c) -ales, (d) -aceae, (e) none, (f) none

5. *Superficial mycoses* affect the outer "dead" layer of the skin and hair, while *cutaneous mycoses* involve the deeper layers of the hair, skin, and nails. *Subcutaneous mycoses* infect the connective tissues, bones, muscles, and lymphatic system. *Systemic mycoses* can occur in any part of the body, especially the organ systems and deep tissues. *Opportunistic mycoses* are "wild card" infections of virtually any tissue that occur when the person becomes debilitated or immunocompromised.

6. (i) without cross walls

7. (a) cell from which conidia are produced

8. (c) fungus causing the infection

9. (g) tubular structures comprising mould-form growth of fungi

10. (d) mass of hyphae

11. (b) fungal infection

12. (f) reproductive structures produced sexually. (asexual propagules of Zygomycetes are also called spores)

13. The *aerial* hyphae are the visible portion of the colony growing above the surface of the medium. The *vegetative* hyphae grow on or in the medium and absorb nutrients from the medium. Conidia and/or spores develop from the *reproductive* hyphae.

14. *Anamorphs* are asexual states of fungi; *teleomorphs* are the sexual states. When a teleomorph has more than one anamorph, the group of anamorphs are *synanamorphs*, i.e., siblings. The combination of anamorphs (syn-anamorphs) and teleomorphs for a fungus is the *holomorph*. The Classes Ascomycetes, Basidiomycetes, and Zygomycetes have both teleomorphic states and anamorphic (synanamorphic) states and are holomorphs. The Class Deuteromycetes is composed of anamorphs.

15. True pathogens are consistently able to cause infection, even at relatively low doses of conidia/spores, while opportunistic pathogens must be present in overwhelming numbers and/or find a debilitated or immunocompromised host.

16. When both sexual and asexual forms of a fungus are known, the teleomorphic form is placed in the correct taxonomic position in a class of "perfect" fungi, while the anamorphic form remains in the Class Deuteromycetes (Fungi Imperfecti). The anamorph is maintained as if it were a separate organism because it has a history that should be preserved and

because the asexual form is the one isolated from infections in patients.

17. Normocytic red blood cells, with a normal diameter of 7 μm, are used in the drawings.

CHAPTER

1. The general requirements that must be met to ensure the quality of a specimen to be cultured for fungi include (a) take the specimen with as little contamination as possible; (b) take it from the area most likely to yield a positive culture; (c) obtain the specimen at the appropriate stage of the infection; (d) take an adequate amount of the specimen. *Any three of the four* requirements comprise a correct response.

2. The response has several essential elements. The area should be cleansed as thoroughly as possible before the specimen is collected; this includes discarding loose debris from under the nail before the specimen is shaved off. Specimens of skin should be scraped from inside the rim of the lesion. Hairs should be plucked, not clipped, and the hair root should be included. All specimens should be kept dry until they can be treated with KOH (or KOH plus stain) and examined. NOTE that the desirable concentration of KOH varies for hair, skin, and nail specimens.

3. All specimens (except those to be cultured for dermatophytes/cutaneous fungi) should be placed in sterile containers and delivered to the laboratory immediately.

4. Deep cough sputa, respiratory secretions, cerebrospinal fluid, tissue biopsies, urine, and/or blood should be collected to diagnose systemic mycoses and cryptococcoses. Your procedure manual should include the following information: *Sputa* and other tenacious respiratory secretions should be digested with a mucolytic agent such as *N*-acetyl-L-cysteine; bloody flecks should be studied with particular care because they often contain fungal elements. *Tissue* biopsies are minced or ground[1] with sterile sand before the tissue is placed on culture media. *Clear fluids* (cerebrospinal fluid, urine) should be filtered or centrifuged so that the sediment can be cultured and examined microscopically. *Blood* is cultured in blood culture bottles containing the appropriate medium; thin blood smears (like differentials) can be stained with Wright's stain and examined.

5. Procedures designed to keep the laboratory clean and prevent cross-contamination are (a) follow uni-

versal precautions; (b) follow procedures in the microbiology safety manual; (c) keep open wounds bandaged; (d) do not smoke, drink, eat, or apply make-up in the laboratory; (e) wear goggles over contact lenses and do not clean contact lenses in the laboratory; (f) manipulate cultures within a biologic safety cabinet; (g) avoid creating aerosols; (h) disinfect work areas daily; (i) dispose of contaminated materials in appropriate containers. *Any five* of these procedures could have been included in your response.

6. The advantages of Petri dishes are the larger surface area, a better oxygen supply, and the relative ease with which mixed cultures can be detected. These advantages are offset by the faster rate of drying of the agar, the insecurity of the lid, and the relatively high probability of disseminating fungal elements from the culture.

    Test tubes have the advantages of a slower rate of drying, a secure closure, and the relatively small probability that fungal elements will be disseminated if good technique is used. These advantages are counterbalanced by a smaller surface area for growth, the more limited access to oxygen, and the difficulty of detecting mixed cultures.

7. Primary cultures may need to be subcultured to determine thermotolerance of the fungus, enhance pigmentation, determine nutritional requirements of the organism, encourage conidiation/sporulation, and determine resistance of the fungus to an antimycotic agent such as cycloheximide. *Any two* of these reasons constitute a correct response.

8. Macroscopic (colony), microscopic

9. The (a) symptoms, (b) travel history, (c) hobbies, (d) place of residence, and (e) occupation of the patient all may provide clues to the identity of the etiologic agent. *Any four elements* of patient history should have been included in your response.

10. Direct microscopic examination of specimens for fungus culture is always important to (a) help select media for the primary culture; (b) generate a preliminary report to the physician; (c) contribute to appropriate therapy if the mycotic elements are distinctive; (d) detect mycotic elements that are not viable. *Any two* of these reasons should be included in your response.

11. (e) resembling the surface of the brain

12. (c) long, thin, tangled aerial hyphae

13. (g) volcano-like

14. (b) possessing a large number of conidia/spores

15. (f) short aerial hyphae of approximately equal length

16. (a) featuring many warts and rough knobs

17. Wet preps are simple suspensions of a culture or specimen in sterile water or saline. Place 1 or 2 drops of fluid on a clean glass slide. Add a small amount of the material to be examined, and stir it into the fluid

---

[1]Remember that grinding sometimes destroys the mycotic elements if they are large.

until the fluid becomes barely cloudy. Lower a coverslip into position on the mixture carefully, to reduce air bubbles in the final preparation. Let the wet prep stand for a few minutes to allow the particles in it to settle, then examine the prep with a brightfield microscope, using the high-power lens and reduced light. Do *NOT* use oil immersion—it is unnecessary and can be dangerous.

18. Lactophenol–cotton blue is the most frequently used mounting fluid. It is composed of lactic acid (to fix fungal elements), phenol (to kill the cellular elements), and cotton blue (staining agent).

19. *KOH preps* are used to detect mycotic elements in specimens. *India ink preps* are negative stains, most useful for detecting encapsulated yeasts in liquid specimens. *Tease mounts/LPCB preps* are used to examine reproductive structures of mould-form colonies. *Scotch tape preps* are also used to examine reproductive structures of moulds. *Slide cultures* are useful for examining reproductive structures of moulds; they are best used to study fungi that could not be identified by using a tease mount or Scotch tape prep and to create permanent mounts of fungi.

20. Emmon's modification of Sabouraud's dextrose agar (SDA), SDA with antimicrobial agents, brain-heart infusion agar (BHIA) with or without blood, SABHI medium.

21. Antimicrobial agents are added to media to prevent overgrowth of the etiologic agent by bacteria or saprobic fungi. The two that are most often used are the antimycotic agent cycloheximide and the antibiotics chloramphenicol and gentamicin.

22. Potato dextrose agar (PDA), potato flake agar (PFA), and cornmeal agar (CMA) all can be used to enhance pigment production and conidiation/sporulation.

23. Texture, topography, and pigmentation of the colony should always be recorded along with the colony's age and rate of growth, temperature of incubation, and medium on which the fungus is growing.

24. **Dematiaceous:** darkly pigmented; colonies with dark green, brown, or black pigment on the obverse and reverse of the colony; microscopic structures with brown to black pigment in unstained specimens.
Moniliaceous: having white, light brown, or pastel pigment on the reverse of the colony; microscopic structures are clear and colorless.
Hyaline: having clear and colorless microscopic structures
Anergy: diminished reactivity to antigen, either immediate or delayed. The person's immune system is unable to respond to antigen by producing antibody.

25. Immunologic tests that can be used for the detection and/or identification of fungal antibodies are (*include four* in your answer): immunodiffusion (ID), indirect immunofluorescence (IFA), complement fixation (CF), latex agglutination (LA), counterimmunoelec-trophoresis (CIE), and tube agglutination (TA). Fungal antigens can be detected and/or identified by (*include two):* enzyme-linked immunosorbent assay (ELISA), enzyme immunoassay (EIA), fluorescent antibody (FA), and exoantigen methods.

CHAPTER

1. Opportunistic fungi are those that can cause infection only when the opportunity is created by the debilitated condition of the host or when the infecting dose of spores or conidia is massive. Opportunistic fungi are becoming increasingly important because they are being seen more frequently in clinical microbiology laboratories as the result of medicine's improved ability to keep people with massive injuries or severe disease alive.

2. A *contaminant* is an organism that is present without causing infection (although it may be infectious in other circumstances). A *commensal* is a microorganism that lives on or in the host without either injuring or benefitting the host.

3. *Hyalohyphomycosis* and *phaeohyphomycosis* are both infections caused by opportunistic fungi that (at least so far) only occasionally cause infections. *Hyalohyphomycoses* are, as you would expect, caused by hyaline moulds, while *phaeohyphomycoses* are caused by dematiaceous moulds.

4. (b) conidiogenous cell that continues to lengthen after producing the first conidium

5. (a) conidium produced by an annellide

6. (d) hyphal cell that supports an annellide

7. (e) production of or genesis of conidia

8. (c) conidiogenous cell that stops elongating after production of the first conidium

9. If the fungus isolated is to be recognized as the agent of the infection the patient's symptoms must be consistent with a fungal infection, fungal elements should be seen in material from the infected site, the fungus should be isolated from cultures of the infected area, the fungus isolated should be capable of causing the patient's symptoms, and the fungus must be identified correctly. Your response should include *four of the five* elements.

10. The opportunistic fungi are divided into dematiaceous fungi, hyaline fungi, and Zygomycetes by colony morphology and the presence or absence of septa in the hyphae.

11. **Clavate:** club shaped
Elliptical: shaped like an ellipse—approximately like an egg with both ends of equal size
Phialide: a macronematous conidiogenous cell that is determinate and typically resembles a vase
Pyriform: pear shaped

Sporodochia: a tight mat or patch of conidiating conidiophores within the mycelium

Tuberculate: having wartlike protuberances

Vesicle: a swelling; specifically, the swollen terminal end of the conidiophore typical of the aspergilli

12. *Macronematous,* or complex, conidiophores are distinctively shaped or produce branching structures so that the conidiophores are easily differentiated from the vegetative hyphae. *Micronematous* conidiophores cannot be distinguished from the vegetative hyphae unless conidia are attached.

13. *Aspergillus* species all have septate hyphae that branch at an angle of approximately 45 degrees, especially in tissue. The free end of the long conidiophore terminates in a vesicle; a "foot cell" anchors the conidiophore in the hyphae. A series of phialides (uniseriate or biseriate) support compact columns of chaining conidia.

Zygomycetes have hyphae that are aseptate or sparsely septate, and broader than the hyphae of other fungi that infect humans. They sporulate by producing asexual sporangiospores within sacklike sporangia formed around swollen columellae at the ends of sporangiophores. Some Zygomycetes produce rhizoids.

14. (c) youngest conidium is produced at the tip of the chain of conidia

15. (h) youngest conidium is found at the base of the chain of conidia

16. (e) phialides arising from the vesicle in two series

17. (f) rhizoids are formed between the sporangiophores

18. (a) conidia produced through openings in the wall of the conidiophore

19. (b) conidia produced together at the same time

20. *Absidia* species have branching internodal sporangiophores, rhizoids, columellae shaped like Hershey's Kisses and an apophysis with collarette; it grows at temperatures from 25°C to 42°C.

Mucor has branching sporangiophores and collarettes on the columellae but no apophyses or rhizoids; it does not grow at 50°C.

Rhizomucor has short branching internodal sporangiophores with globose columellae and collarettes but not apophyses; primitive rhizoids are present. *Rhizomucor* grows at temperatures up to 55°C.

Rhizopus has well-developed rhizoids and branching sporangiophores with hemispherical columellae; the sporangiophores are nodal. Some species of *Rhizopus* grow at temperatures up to 50°C.

Syncephalastrum produces tubular merosporangia from globose vesicles supported by branching sporangiophores.

21. (e) *Mucor*

22. (g) *Penicillium*

23. (b) *Curvularia*

24. (i) *Scopulariopsis*

25. (a) *Aspergillus*

26. (c) granular colony with pastel surface pigment and a white or cream reverse pigment

27. (a) dark brown velvety surface with a black reverse pigment

28. (c) granular colony with pastel surface pigment and white or cream reverse pigment

29. (a) dark brown velvety surface with a black reverse pigment

30. (b) gray woolly colony with a cream reverse pigment

CHAPTER 4

1. In *black piedra* the hard dark nodules form primarily on scalp hair, eyebrows, eye lashes, and pubic hair. Asci and spores are found in the nodules. The fungus is *Piedraia hortae.*

In *white piedra* the nodules are soft and pale. The hair of the mustache, axilla, and groin are most often affected. *Trichosporon beigelii* is the etiologic agent.

2. **Piedra:** literally, "stone." Piedras are superficial infections of the hair

Tinea: superficial infections of the skin, and cutaneous infections of the hair, skin, and nails

Wood's lamp: a lamp with an ultraviolet bulb that is used to detect fluorescent substances in the hair and skin

Lipophilic: lipid loving

Glabrous: resembling pressed felt, with tightly woven vegetative hyphae and few or no aerial hyphae or spores

Cerebriform: resembling the brain

Rugose: topography featuring radial grooves from the center of the colony toward the rim

Fusiform: having pointed ends

Ascus: a saclike cell in which ascospores develop

Ascospore: sexual spore formed within an ascus following karyogamy and meiosis

Arthroconidia: asexual conidia produced directly from the hyphae by modification of hyphal cells

Annellation: A scar, formed when the conidium is released from the annellide

Collarette: ring of fragments of the sporangium that remains attached to the sporangiophore at the base of the columella when the sporangium ruptures or disintegrates

3. Colonies of *Piedraia hortae* are dematiaceous velvety moulds. Microscopically brown hyphae are seen, with arthroconidia and chlamydospores.

Trichosporon beigelii forms creamy yeastlike colonies that become wrinkled and folded as they age. In microscopic preparations hyphae are seen with arthroconidia and blastoconidia.

4. **Tinea nigra** (tinea nigra palmaris) is caused by *Exophiala werneckii.* Dark macular lesions resembling silver nitrate stains develop on the palms of the hands

and, less commonly, on the soles of the feet. The lesions are flat and are not scaly. It is generally considered a tropical disease, occurring most often in people younger than 19 years of age.

A lipophilic yeast, *Malassezia furfur*, causes tinea versicolor (pityriasis versicolor). This is a transient furfuraceous infection of the stratum corneum on the upper chest, back, arms, and neck. The melanosomes are apparently affected, so that the normal skin color changes from light to dark, or dark to light, in the affected areas. It is found primarily in young adults.

5. Colonies of *Malassezia furfur* resemble colonies of bacteria; they are white initially and become a dull beige in older cultures. Hyphae are rarely seen in microscopic preparations. The predominant cells are unicellular yeasts with distinct collarettes that make them resemble medicine capsules or bowling pins. In *tissue preparations* the round conidia and remnants of hyphae have caused *M. furfur* to be described as "spaghetti and meatballs."

Young colonies of *Exophiala werneckii* are yeast-like, with off-white to dark gray pigment. The cells of young cultures are hyaline to olive-black ellipses that are typically two celled. In 2- to 3-week-old cultures *E. werneckii* colonies are velvety dematiaceous moulds. Septate hyphae are seen microscopically, with annellophores bearing annellides. The unicellular annelloconidia accumulate in clusters around the apices of the annellides and slide down onto the hyphae. Microscopic structures of the mould are dematiaceous, with the hyphae more intensely pigmented than the annellophores.

6. (c) *Piedraia hortae*
7. (b) *Malassezia furfur*
8. (b) *Malassezia furfur*
9. (d) *Trichosporon beigelii*
10. (a) *Exophiala werneckii*

C H A P T E R

1. A dermato*phytosis* is any infection caused by dermatophytes, while a dermato*mycosis* is an infection of the cutaneous tissues due to fungi other than dermatophytes.
2. In *gray-patch* tinea capitis the hair becomes grayish, dull, and brittle due to ectothrix invasion of the hair, and hairs break off near the base of the shafts. In *black-dot* tinea capitis endothrix invasion of the hair occurs and arthroconidia accumulate within the hair shaft. When the hair breaks off, the remaining stub is a "black dot" because of the conidia in the stub.
3. **Folliculitis:** inflammation of the hair follicles
Kerion: a "boggy tumefaction," i.e., a spongy swelling
Alopecia: hair loss, which may be permanent

Sebum: fatty secretions of the sebaceous glands, believed related to the differential ability of some dermatophytes to cause tinea capitis in children and adults
Scutula: yellowish cup-shaped crusts composed of mycelium, sebum, and other debris; they are found in tinea favosa
Echinulate: spiney; prickly; rough

4. *Microsporum* species infect the hair and skin but rarely the nails. Macroconidia are characteristically fusiform or spindle shaped with relatively thick echinulate walls; microconidia are produced but are less abundant than the macroconidia.

Epidermophyton floccosum infects the skin and nails but not the hair. Macroconidia are shaped like snowshoes or beaver's tails, with thin, smooth walls; microconidia are not produced.

Trichosporon species invade the hair, skin, and nails. Macroconidia are typically pencil- or cigar-shaped with relatively thin, smooth walls; microconidia are more abundant than the macroconidia.

5. (a) tinea barbae
6. (e) tinea manum
7. (c) tinea corporis
8. (f) tinea pedis
9. (d) tinea cruris
10. (b) tinea capitis
11. The *ectothrix* pattern of invasion involves development of the fungus outside the hair shaft, with fragmentation of the hyphae into arthroconidia that accumulate around the hair shaft or just beneath the cuticle. In *endothrix* invasion of hair the fungus penetrates into the hair shaft and arthroconidia accumulate in it. *Favic-type* invasion is characterized by development of filaments of fungi in the hair where they degenerate to leave tunnels containing oil deposits and air.
12. Figure 5.5 shows most of the vegetative structures associated with dermatophytes (and which may occur in other fungi). *Pectinate hyphae* resemble a comb, with multiple irregular "teeth" extending from one side of the hyphae. *Racquet hyphae* are composed of a series of club-shaped structures in which the walls of successive cells swell to form the "heads" of the racquets. *Spiral hyphae* are hyphae that seem to have been twisted around a rod or pencil and released, creating hyphae that resemble corkscrews. *Nodular bodies* are roundish masses formed when two or more hyphae become entangled into a knot. *Favic chandeliers* (Fig. 5.28) resemble the branches of trees or the antlers of reindeer.
13. Figure 5.4 demonstrates the principle groupings of microconidia of dermatophytes. Microconidia *en grappe* are arranged in groups that resemble clusters of grapes. Microconidia *en thryses* develop in an arrangement resembling a sleeve.
14. A Wood's lamp, containing a bulb that emits ultraviolet rays, is used to detect the yellow-green fluores-

cence in hair and skin infected with some species of *Microsporum*. Some medications and some hair oils cause false-positive reactions.

15. (g) large sac or blister filled with a clear fluid
16. (e) inanimate objects that harbor microorganisms and transmit infection
17. (a) allergic reaction to a dermatophyte
18. (b) between the folds of the skin
19. (c) general term for a nail infection
20. (f) itching
21. DTM is an acidic medium containing basic nutrients and the antimicrobial agents cyclohexamide, chlortetracycline, and gentamicin. Phenol red indicator is included, so that the freshly prepared medium is yellow. This color changes to red if a dermatophyte, *or any organism that is not susceptible to the antimicrobials*, grows on the medium and produces alkaline by-products.
22. *Trichophyton verrucosum*
23. *Microsporum gypseum*
24. *Trichophyton mentagrophytes*
25. *Epidermophyton floccosum*
26. *Trichophyton tonsurans*
27. *Microsporum audouinii*
28. *Trichophyton rubrum*
29. *Trichophyton schoenleinii*
30. *Microsporum canis*

CHAPTER 6

1. **Autoinoculation:** transfer of the organism (and the infection) from one area of the body to another
   Primary conidiation: formation of the first "set" of conidia on the conidiophore or conidiogenous cell
   Secondary infection: infection due to a second microorganism that takes advantage of favorable conditions created by the first disease or infection
   Shield cells: blastoconidium that is approximately triangular with three thickened disjuncture scars where it was attached to other conidia
   Sclerotic bodies: also known as copper pennies. Pleomorphic spherical brown forms divided by muriform septa into two or four cells
   Synnemata: bundles or tufts of conidiophores
   Verrucoid: rough and raised; wartlike
2. Subcutaneous mycoses typically result from "traumatic inoculation," i.e., minor injuries caused by a thorn or splinter, which introduce the fungus into the tissues. They occur most frequently in tropical and subtropical areas to those who work outdoors as farmers and laborers. Working conditions, poor nutrition, scanty clothing, and going barefooted increase the risk of infection.
3. A *mycetoma* is a tumorlike swelling, with draining sinus tracts and "granules" in the exudate from the si-

nuses. Mycetomas usually appear on the hands and feet. Infections tend to remain localized in the subcutaneous tissues; the lymphatic system is not involved. *Pseudallescheria boydii* is the most common agent of eumycotic mycetoma in the United States and Europe. Other mycotic agents of mycetoma are *Cladosporium carrionii*, *Xylohypha bantianum*, *Exophiala jeanselmei*, *Wangiella dermatitidis*, *Phialophora verrucosa*, and *Fonsecaea* species. Some bacteria cause actinomycotic mycetomas.

Sporotrichosis ("rose gardener's disease") is a chronic mycotic infection. Five different types of infection may be seen. In the most common type the infection is on an extremity and ascends the lymph vessels from the site of inoculation, causing characteristic ulcers at successive lymph nodes along the route. Usually the bone is not involved but the infection may disseminate. The causative organism is *Sporothrix schenckii*.

Chromoblastomycosis is characterized by crusted verrucoid nodules on the skin, usually on the lower limbs. Untreated lesions eventually become elevated and may resemble a cauliflower. Microabscesses resembling cayenne pepper may develop on the surface. The bone and subcutaneous tissues, as well as the lymphatic system, may be involved. Sclerotic bodies may form in the tissue. Chromoblastomycosis is caused by *Cladosporium carrionii*, *Exophiala jeanselmei*, *Fonsecaea* species, *Phialophora verrucosa*, *Wangiella dermatitidis*, and *Xylohypha bantianum*.

4. The subcutaneous fungi—*except Pseudallescheria boydii*—are dematiaceous organisms that are found as saprobes in soil, plants, wood, and rotting vegetation. All are slow growing, except *Sporothrix schenckii* and *P. boydii*. Generally they remain dormant in tissue until a second injury, after the fungus has acclimated to the tissue environment, occurs.

Colonies are usually flat or heaped, with a velvety texture, dark gray-green or olive-green obverse pigment and jet black reverse—except (again) for *P. boydii*.

Three types of anamorphic conidiation are found in the subcutaneous fungi, plus the production of annelloconidia.

5. *Cladosporium-type* conidiation is associated with conidiophores of various lengths, long branching chains of blastoconidia, and ovoid to elliptical conidia. In *phialophora*-type conidiation phialides are produced; they may or may not have collarettes. Conidia cluster in balls at the tip of the phialide and may slide down the phialide to rest on the hypha. In *rhinocladiella*-type conidiation the conidia are produced sympodially on short denticles around the swollen tip of the conidiophore. Secondary and tertiary conidia may form from the primary conidia.

For Matching Questions 6–13:

6, 11, 12   (a) *Cladosporium carrionii*
7, 8, 9, 10, 13 (b) *Xylohypha bantianum*

For Matching Questions 14–18:

14, 15   (a) *Exophiala jeanselmei*
16, 17, 18   (b) *Wangiella dermatitidis*

For Matching Questions 19–22:

20   (a) *Exophiala jeanselmei*
19, 22   (b) *Pseudallescheria boydii*
21   (c) *Wangiella dermatitidis*

For Matching Questions 23–28:

24, 26, 27   (a) *Pseudallescheria boydii*
23, 25, 28   (b) *Sporothrix schenckii*

29. *Sporothrix schenckii*
30. *Exophiala jeanselmei*
31. *Pseudallescheria boydii*
32. *Cladosporium carrionii*
33. *Fonsecaea pedrosoi* or *Fonsecaea compacta*
34. *Phialophora verrucosa*
35. *Wangiella dermatitidis*

CHAPTER 7

1. **Assimilation:** oxidative metabolism of a substrate, used for speciation of yeasts and other microorganisms
   Fermentation: fermentative metabolism of a substrate, used for speciation of microorganisms, including yeasts
   Iatrogenic: resulting from procedures used by a physician in treatment of a patient
   Ascospore: sexual spore formed in a sac followed by karyogamy and meiosis
   Pellicle: a film or "scum" formed on the surface of a liquid
2. An *impression smear* is made by pressing a segment of infected tissue against a clean glass slide, which is subsequently stained and examined microscopically. A *wet prep* (like most of the other preparations for identification of fungi) is done by suspending a portion of the colony in a fluid and examining it; stain may or may not be used.
3. A micrometer is a calibrated device that is placed in one of the oculars of the microscope. This allows the microscopist to measure the size of objects seen through the ocular. Micrometers are most often used

in mycology to determine the size of yeasts. Micrometers are also used in parasitology, especially for the protozoa.

4. (A) *Colonization* means that microorganisms are present in host tissues without causing infection. All animals, including humans, are colonized by microorganisms that comprise the normal flora of the host. *Infection*, on the other hand, means that the microorganisms have an active presence in the host, invading healthy tissue and damaging it.
   (B) The presence of fungi in the blood is a *fungemia*; usually it is associated with infection, although the fungi may simply be present for a brief period. A tumor caused by (and containing) mycotic elements is a *fungoma*.
   (C) *Yeast* are true fungi with both a sexual and an asexual form of reproduction, while *yeastlike* organisms do not have a sexual mode of reproduction. In practice yeast and yeastlike are often used interchangeably to indicate predominantly unicellular fungi that reproduce, in the asexual phase, by budding.
   (D) *Pseudohyphae* ("false" hyphae) resemble a string of sausages. They are chains of blastoconidia that remained attached. True septa are not present, but there is a *constriction* where the newest blastoconidium is produced by the older one. *Germ tubes* are "sprouts," filamentous extensions from blastoconidia. Septa are not present. *No constriction* is present between the germ tube and the blastoconidium.
   (E) *Chlamydoconidia* are thick-walled asexual reproductive cells produced blastically from the hyphae in response to an unfavorable environment. *Chlamydospores* are thick-walled vesicles—swollen cells—that serve as storage units for the yeast in an unfavorable environment; they are not reproductive cells.
5. First, the yeast should be recovered in significant numbers and, second, it should be recovered from multiple specimens from the same site. Third, the microscopic morphology of the yeast should suggest infection rather than colonization. The symptoms of the infection should be consistent with the identity of the yeast. The specimen must, of course, be fresh if the number of organisms and the microscopic morphology is to be assessed accurately. Note that the "rules" change for the yeast form of dimorphic fungi, when *any* isolate is important.
6. The first two tests that should be done from colonies resembling yeast are the wet prep and the germ tube test. The wet prep confirms that the organism is a yeast rather than a bacterium. The germ tube test identifies most *Candida albicans*—the yeast most often isolated from clinical specimens—without further testing, which reduces the workload (and the cost) of identifying yeast significantly.
7. Cornmeal-Tween 80 (CMT) agar should be inoculated to determine the microscopic morphology in this medium. Urease production and utilization of

nitrate and various carbohydrates should also be tested. Phenoloxidase production and the ability to form a pellicle in broth should also be determined when the morphology of the yeast in CMT suggests this will be helpful. The biochemical tests can be done with conventional procedures or as rapid tests.

For Matching Questions 8–15:

8, 9, 11, 13, 15   (a) *Candida albicans*
10, 12, 14   (b) *Cryptococcus neoformans*

16. (A) **Germ tube test**
    Substrate: rabbit plasma; sheep serum; fetal bovine serum
    Positive: filamentous outgrowths from blastoconidia without a constriction between the sprout and the blastoconidium, developing within 3 hours at 37°C
    Negative: any other morphology
    (B) **Phenoloxidase**
    Substrate: caffeic acid
    Medium: birdseed agar, thistle medium, niger seed agar
    Positive: brown to black pigment in the colonies
    Negative: no color development
    (C) **Nitrate assimilation**
    Substrate: a nutritionally complete agar or broth devoid of nitrates except for measured quantities of potassium nitrate
    Positive: growth (cloudiness)
    Negative: lack of growth (no cloudiness)
    (D) **Carbohydrate assimilation**
    Substrate: a nutritionally complete agar or broth that contains no carbohydrate other than a measured amount of the carbohydrate being tested
    Positive: growth (cloudiness)[2]
    Negative: lack of growth (no cloudiness)
    (E) **Pellicle formation**
    Medium: Sabouraud's dextrose broth
    Positive: formation of a film or plug on the surface of the broth
    Negative: no growth on the broth's surface
17. *Candida kefyr (Candida pseudotropicalis)*
18. *Geotrichum candidum*
19. *Candida parapsilosis.* Although the pattern of carbohydrate assimilations is suggestive of *Candida tropicalis*, the morphology clearly indicates this isolate is *Candida parapsilosis.* A negative test for pellicle formation would confirm the identity of this isolate as *C. parapsilosis.*
20. *Rhodotorula rubra*
21. *Torulopsis (Candida) glabrata*

---

22. *Candida tropicalis.* Although the pattern of carbohydrate assimilations is suggestive of *Candida parapsilosis*, the morphology clearly indicates that this isolate is *C. tropicalis.* A positive test for pellicle formation would confirm the identity of this isolate as *C. tropicalis.*
23. *Cryptococcus neoformans*
24. *Hansenula* species

CHAPTER 8

1. **Endospores:** literally, spores formed within. Endospores are formed within the spherules produced by *Coccidioides immitis*, by cleavage of the protoplasm.
    Mariner's wheel: nickname for tissue forms of *Paracoccidioides brasiliensis*, which resemble the mariner's wheel because of their large size and many knobby projections from the cell wall
    Spherule: the tissue form of *Coccidioides immitis*, which does not develop a yeast form colony at 37°C on standard media
    Tuberculate: having wartlike protuberances
    Coin lesion: dense, round, flattened area in the lungs created by the deposition of fibrin around a cavity resulting from *Histoplasma capsulatum* infection
    Granuloma: a collection of macrophages, giant cells, and other cells, mixed with the proteinaceous materials formed by the host's immune system to fight the infection. The host attempts to surround the invader and "wall it off," creating the tumor-like mass.
2. True pathogens generally differ from opportunistic pathogens in their habitats, number of morphotypes, existence as normal flora, site of the primary infection, virulence, growth rate, and nutrient requirements. See Table 8.1 to review the characteristics of each group of pathogens.
3. Sabouraud's dextrose agar with and without antimicrobials, SABHI or brain-heart infusion (BHIA) agar with blood, BHI broth, yeast extract phosphate medium, potato dextrose or potato flake agar, Converse medium (for suspected *Coccidioides immitis* only).
4. Protective garments should be worn. All work should be done within a biologic safety cabinet. If *Coccidioides immitis* is suspected, the mould-form colony should be flooded with sterile saline before subculture is attempted and before microscopic preparations are done.

For Matching Questions 5–14:

5, 9   (a) *Blastomyces dermatitidis*
7, 8, 14   (b) *Coccidioides immitis*
6, 11, 13   (c) *Histoplasma capsulatum*
10, 12   (d) *Paracoccidioides brasiliensis*

For Matching Questions 15–19:

16, 19	(a)	*Blastomyces dermatitidis*
15	(b)	*Coccidioides immitis*
18	(c)	*Histoplasma capsulatum*
17	(d)	*Paracoccidioides brasiliensis*

For Matching Questions 20–25:

20	(a)	*Blastomyces dermatitidis*
21, 22	(b)	*Coccidioides immitis*
24, 25	(c)	*Histoplasma capsulatum*
23	(d)	*Paracoccidioides brasiliensis*

For Matching Questions 26–30:

26	(a), (b), and (c)	
27	(a)	*Blastomyces dermatitidis*
30	(b)	*Coccidioides immitis*
29	(c)	*Histoplasma capsulatum*
28	(d)	*Paracoccidioides brasiliensis*

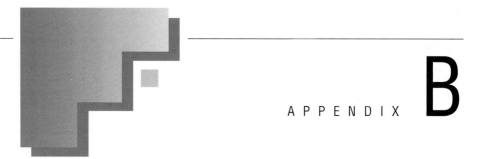

Glossary of Terms with Pronunciations

Term	Pronunciation	Definition
Absidia species	Ab-syd´-ee-uh ("ab" as in absent)	
Acremonium species	Ack-ruh-moan´-ee-um	
acropetal	ack-row-pet-ul	Conidiogeny in which the youngest conidium is at the tip of the chain of conidia
acrotheca-type conidiation	ack-row-thee-kuh (pronounce the "th" as you do in "thin")	Term used formerly for rhinocladiella-type conidiation
Acti-Dione	ack-tuh-dye-own (rhymes with "spin")	Brand name for cycloheximide, an antimycotic agent used in media to suppress fungi
actinomycotic	ack-tin-oh-my-cot-ick	Related to ray ("actino") fungi—the Actinomyces, which are now considered bacteria, not fungi
adiaspiromycosis	uh-dee-oh-spir-oh-my-koh-sus	Condition that occurs in tissue when elevated temperatures are present. The conidia of some fungi enlarge in size without replication
adiaspore	uh-dee-oh-spore (rhymes with "dough")	Conidium produced by some fungi in response to elevated temperatures. Instead of forming a new conidium the conidium enlarges, without replication, to create a vesicle. Despite use of the term -*spore*, this is an asexual process
aerial hyphae		Hyphae growing above the surface of the medium or substrate; the visible colony
aleuric	uh-lure-ick	"Fractured"; released from the conidiophore by fracture of the conidiophore
alopecia	al-oh-peesh-ee-uh	Hair loss
Alternaria species	All-tur-nair´-ee-uh ("al" as in alligator)	
anamorph	ann-uh-morff	Asexual (imperfect) form of a fungus that is related to a sexual teleomorph (perfect) form
anergy		Diminished reactivity to antigen. Either delayed or immediate hypersensitivity may be diminished. The person's immune system is unable to respond to the antigen by producing antibody
annellation	ann-L-aye-shun	Scar on the tip of the annellide formed by material from the outer layer of cell wall of the conidium as each conidium is released
annellide	ann-L-lid	Conidiogenous cell that is indeterminate and that produces annelloconidia that leave a ringlike "collar" of cell wall material on the annellide as they are released
annelloconidium (pl. annelloconidia)	ann-L-oh-koh-nid-ee-um & ann-L-oh-koh-nid-ee-uh	Conidium produced from an annellide
annellophore	ann-L-oh-four	Conidiophore that bears annellides
annular frill	ann-you-lure frill	Ring of fragments of the conidiophore or hypha that remains attached to the conidium when the conidium is released

Table continued on following page

Term	Pronunciation	Definition
anthropophilic	ann-throw-poe-fill-ick	People loving; dermatophytes whose primary reservoir is people
antibiotic	ann-tuh-by-ott-ick	Agent that inhibits bacteria. Gentamicin, chloramphenicol, penicillin, and streptomycin are antibiotics commonly used in media
antigenemia	ann-tuh-jhuh-neem-ee-uh	Antigens in the blood
antimicrobial agent	ann-tuh-my-crow-be-ull agent	General term for chemicals and dyes that inhibit bacteria or fungi
antimycotic agent	ann-tuh-my-kot-ick	Agent that inhibits fungi. Cycloheximide (Acti-Dione) is used to inhibit the saprophytic fungi
apex (pl. apices)	aye-pex & aye-puh-sees	The tip or end of a structure
apiculate	aye-pick-you-late	Having a short projection at one or both ends
apophysis	aye-poff-oh-sis	Swelling at the base of the columella
apothecium	ap-oh-thee-key-um	Cup-shaped ascocarp; asci form on the inside of the cup
arthroconidia	are-throw-koh-nid-ee-uh	Asexual conidium produced directly from the hyphae by modification of hyphal cells; they are released from the hypha by fragmentation of the hypha
ascocarp	ask-oh-carp	Fruiting body within which asci form
ascospore	ask-oh-spore	Sexual spore formed within an ascus following karyogamy and meiosis
ascostroma (pl. ascostromata)	ass-koh-strome-uh & ass-koh-strome-ah-tuh	Ascocarp composed of hard masses of hyphae (stroma) in which asci are produced
ascus (pl. asci)	ask-us & ass-key	Saclike cell in which ascospores develop
aseptate		without cross walls
asexual reproduction		Reproduction of the daughter cell or conidium from a single parent
aspergilloma	ass-purr-jill-ome-uh	Fungus ball (literally, fungus tumor) caused by a species of *Aspergillus*
aspergillosis	ass-purr-jill-oh-sus	Any infection caused by a species of *Aspergillus*
Aspergillus flavus	Ass-per-jill-us flay-vus	
Aspergillus fumigatus	Ass-per-jill-us fume-uh-got´-us	
Aspergillus niger	Ass-per-jill-us nigh-jhur	
Aspergillus terreus	Ass-per-jill-us tare-us	
assimilation		Oxidative metabolism of a carbohydrate
asteroid body		Basophilic staining yeast cell in tissue that is surrounded by an eosinophilic covering of a precipitated antigen-antibody complex. Associated with *Sporothrix schenckii*
athlete's foot		Ringworm of the feet
Aureobasidium pullulans	Are-ee-oh-buh-syd´-ee-um pull´-yo-u-lans	
autoinoculation		Inoculation of the organisms from one area of the body to another

rhymes with "map"

rhymes with "home"

rhymes with "home"

"us" rhymes with "fuss"

rhymes with "pan(s)"

Term	Pronunciation	Notes	Definition
balanitis	bahl-uh-night-us		Candidiasis of the penis
barbae	bar-bay		Beard, or bearded area
barber's itch			Ringworm of the bearded areas of the face and neck
basidiospore	buh-cyd-ee-oh-spore		Sexual spore formed on a basidium following karyogamy and meiosis
basidium	buh-cyd-ee-um		Club-shaped reproductive structure
basipetal	base-uh-pet-ul		Pattern of conidiation where the newest conidium is at the base and the oldest one at the tip of the chain of conidia
battery			An array of similar materials such as antigens, antibodies or test methods
beaked			Having a long tapered end; the arrangement of certain conidia in which the tapered end of one conidium is attached to the broader, rounded, blunt end of the next conidium in the chain
biologic safety cabinet			Enclosed area with a system to remove particles from the air before the air is returned to general circulation. Designed to prevent the spread of microbes to the laboratory environment and to protect personnel from pathogenic organisms
biphasic bottle	buy-fays-ick bottle		Culture bottle containing both liquid and solid media
Bipolaris species	By-pole-air'-us		
biseriate	buy-sear-ee-utt		Pattern in *Aspergillus* species where secondary phialides arise from primary phialides, creating two series of phialides
black-dot tinea capitis	teen-ee-uh cap-uh-tiss		Endothrix pattern of hair invasion so that the stub remaining after the hair breaks off is a "black dot"
black piedra	pee-aye-druh		Superficial hair infection characterized by hard black nodules of mycotic elements surrounding the hair shaft; the etiologic agent is *Piedraia hortae*
blastic conidiogeny	blast-ick koh-nid-ee-oj-uh-knee	"koh" rhymes with "dough"; "oj" rhymes with "dodge"	Conidiogeny in which the new conidium begins to enlarge and then is differentiated from the parent cell by development of a septum
blastoccnidium (pl. blastoconidia)	blast-oh-koh-nid-ee-um & blast-oh-koh-nid-ee-uh	rhymes with "dough"	Asexual conidium produced blastically from the parent cell; typically it is released by fission. Blastoconidia can be produced singly or synchronously in chains
blastogenesis	blast-oh-jenn-uh-sis		Budding process of asexual reproduction
Blastomyces dermatitidis	Blast-oh-mice-ees derm-uh-tih-duh-dis	"uh" rhymes with "puh" as in puddle	
blastoycin	blas-toe-my-sun		Extract of the yeast form of *Blastomyces dermatitidis*
blastorycosis	blas-toe-my-koh-sus	rhymes with "dough"	Infections caused by *Blastomyces dermatitidis*
boggy			Spongy
budding			Initial stage of production of some conidia; small protuberances or buds "push out" from the parent cell

Table continued on following page

	Pronunciation	Term	Definition
		buffy coat	The layer of leukocytes and platelets formed at the interface between the erythrocyte mass and the plasma when blood is centrifuged or allowed to settle
	bull-uh & bull-aye	bulla (pl. bullae)	Large bulbous sac or blister filled with clear fluid
		C-reactive protein	Protein that is increased in the serum of patients with severe injury or inflammation. Because it is nonspecific it cross-reacts with the antigen in some immunologic tests. Also known as CRP
"kah" as in "calf"	kah-fay-ick	caffeic acid	Substrate that is converted to melanin by action of the enzyme phenoloxidase produced by some species of *Cryptococcus*
"cal" as in California	cal-coe-flure white	calcofluor white	Colorless dye that binds to chitin and cellulose and that fluoresces when exposed to ultraviolet light
"can" rhymes with "pan"; "duh"/"buh" rhyme with "puh" as in puddle	Can-duh-duh/Can-deed′-uh al′-buh-cans	*Candida albicans*	
rhymes with "pan"	Can-duh-duh/Can-deed′-uh ghee-ur-mawn′-dee	*Candida guillermondii*	
rhymes with "pan"	Can-duh-duh/Can-deed′-uh key′-fur	*Candida kefyr*	
rhymes with "pan"	Can-duh-duh/Can-deed′-uh cruise′ee-eye	*Candida krusei*	
"can" rhymes with "pan"; "ap" rhymes with "map"	Can-duh-duh/Can-deed′-uh pair-ap′-sill-oh-sus′	*Candida parapsilosis*	
"can" rhymes with pan; "trop" rhymes with "hop"	Can-duh-duh/Can-deed′-uh trop-uh-callous	*Candida tropicalis*	
	can-duh-dye-uh-sus	candidiasis	Infections caused by *Candida* species, including *Candida albicans*
	cap-uh-tiss	capitis	Related to the head
		Carmen Miranda	1950s performer who wore a hat or turban consisting of an arrangement of bananas and other fruits
		cask shaped	Shaped like a barrel but smaller
		caver's disease	Nickname for histoplasmosis. The presence of the yeast form of *Histoplasma* in the waste products of cave bats can result in infection of the spelunker, i.e., the person who goes "caving"
	suh-reeb-ruh-form	cerebriform	Topography resembling the surface of the brain, heaped with shallow folds and convolutions
rhymes with "dough"	cluh-me-dough-koh-nid-ee-um & cluh-me-dough-koh-nid-ee-uh	chlamydoconidium (pl. chlamydoconidia)	Asexual conidia produced directly from the hyphae and larger than the surrounding hyphal cells. Chlamydoconidia usually have thickened walls.
	cluh-me-dough-spores	chlamydospores	Swollen, thick-walled vesicles that do not reproduce

Term	Pronunciation	Definition
chromoblastomycosis	chrome-oh-blass-toe-my-koh-sus	Chronic mycotic infection involving subcutaneous and cutaneous tissues that is characterized by crusted, cauliflower-like lesions on the skin and sclerotic bodies in the exudate (formerly chromomycosis)
chromomycosis	chrome-oh-my-koh-sus	Chronic mycotic infection involving subcutaneous and cutaneous tissues that is characterized by crusted, cauliflower-like lesions on the skin and sclerotic bodies in the exudate (now called chromoblastomycosis)
Chrysosporium species	Chris-oh-spore'-ee-um "Chris" as in crystal	
Cladosporium carrionii	Clad-o-spore'-ee-um care-ee-own'-ee "clad" rhymes with "lad"; "oy" rhymes with "boy"	
Cladosporium trichoides	Clad-o-spore'-ee-um trick-oyd'-ease rhymes with "dad"	
cladosporium-type conidiation	clad-oh-spore'-e-um	Pattern of anamorphic conidiation characterized by conidiophores of various sizes from which branching chains of blastoconidia are produced
clavate	clah-vate "clah" as in clavicle	Club shaped
cleistothecium	clice-toe-key-um rhymes with "rice"; "th" as in "thin"	Ascocarp that has no opening; asci are released when the cleistothecium ruptures
clinical mycology	clinical my-koll-oh-gee	Identification of fungi infecting humans
Coccidioides immitis	Cock-sih-dee-oy'-dees imm-uh-tiss "uh" rhymes with "puh" as in puddle; "oy" rhymes with "boy"	
coccidioidin	cock-sid-ee-oy-din	Antigen prepared from mould cultures of *Coccidioides immitis*
coccidioidomycosis	cock-sid-ee-oy-dough-my-koh-sus	Infections caused by *Coccidioides immitis*
coin lesion		Dense, round flattened area in the lungs created by the deposition of fibrin around a cavity resulting from *Histoplasma capsulatum* infection
collarette		Ring of fragments of the sporangium that remains attached to the sporangiophore at the base of the columella when the sporangium ruptures or disintegrates
colonization		Situation in which microorganisms are just "hanging out" in body tissue without causing infection
columella (pl. columellae)	koll-you-mell-uh & koll-you-mell-aye "koll" as in college	Sterile domelike structure at the distal end of a sporangiophore; it extends into and supports the sporangium
columnar	koh-lumm-nar rhymes with "dough"	Arranged in columns
commensal	koh-men-sull rhymes with "dough"	Organisms that live on or in the host without either injuring or benefitting the host
compact		Tightly grouped
complex		Conidiophores that branch or that are markedly different from the vegetative hyphae

Table continued on following page

Term	Pronunciation	Definition
compromised host		Person whose immune system is not functioning normally, for whatever reason
conidiation	koh-nyd-ee-aye-shun	Production of conidia
conidiogenous cell	koh-nid-ee-oj-uh-nuss cell	Cell from which conidia are produced
conidiogeny	koh-nid-ee-oj-uh-knee	Asexual reproduction involving formation of specialized cells; the production or genesis of conidia
conidiophore	koh-nid-ee-oh-four	Structure that supports conidia; it may be conidiogenous or it may support a conidiogenous cell
conidium (pl. conidia)	koh-nid-ee-um & koh-nid-ee-uh	Reproductive structures of fungi produced by asexual means
contaminant		Fungi (or other microorganisms) from the environment that are found in a patient specimen but that are not causing infection. Likewise, organisms found in culture that were not present in the patient's specimen
copper pennies		Pleomorphic spherical brown forms divided by muriform septa into two to four cells; found in the exudate in chromoblastomycosis. More formally known as sclerotic bodies
corporis	core-priss	Related to the body
cottony		Texture produced by large quantities of long aerial hyphae that usually become tangled. Technically, cottony colonies are less densely woven than woolly colonies. Synonym: woolly, floccose
crateriform		Topography resembling a volcano, or mashed potatoes with a "well" for the gravy
crossed matchsticks		Arrangement of elongate or cylindrical blastoconidia in which they lie across one another. Typical of *Candida krusei*
CRP		Protein that is increased in the serum of patients with severe injury or inflammation. Because it is nonspecific, it cross-reacts with the antigen in some immunologic tests. Also known as C-reactive protein
cruris	crurr-us	Related to the groin
cryptococcosis	krip-toe-kah-koh-sus	Infections caused by *Cryptococcus* species, including *Cryptococcus neoformans*
Cryptococcus albidus var. *albidus*	Crip-toe-cock'-us al-buh-diss	
Cryptococcus albidus var. *diffluens*	Crip-toe-cock'-us dih-flew-ens	
Cryptococcus gastricus	Crip-toe-cock'-us gas-truh-cuss	
Cryptococcus laurentii	Crip-toe-cock'-us law-rent-ee-ee	
Cryptococcus luteolus	Crip-toe-cock'-us lute-ee-ohl-us	
Cryptococcus neoformans	Crip-toe-cock'-us knee-oh-for'-munz	

rhymes with "dough"

"koh" rhymes with "dough"; "oj" rhymes with "dodge"

"koh" rhymes with "dough"; "oj" rhymes with "dodge"

rhymes with "dough"

rhymes with "dough"

rhymes with "purr"

rhymes with "dough"

"us" rhymes with "fuss"

Term	Pronunciation	Definition
Cryptococcus terreus	Crip-toe-cock'-us tare-us	
Curvularia species	Curve-you-lair'-ee-uh	
cutaneous mycoses	cue-tain-ee-us my-koh-sees	Mycotic infections of the deeper layers of the hair, skin, and nails
cyst	sisst	Stage in the life cycle of *Pneumocystis carinii* (and protozoan parasites) where they are enclosed with a protective wall; a bag of fluid
daisy-like pattern		Pattern of conidiation in *Sporothrix* moulds, where conidia are produced sympodially at the tip of the conidiophore and attached by delicate denticles
Darling's disease		Pulmonary histoplasmosis
daughter cell		Cells that are formed from a mother cell in mitotic division of cells. Cells that are produced by blastogenesis from a mother cell
debilitated		Weakened—perhaps by poor diet, illness, or stress
dematiaceous	dee-mat-ee-ay-shus	Darkly pigmented; refers to colonies with dark olive-green to dark brown to black pigment on the surface and the reverse of the colony *and* microscopic structures with a brown to black pigment in unstained specimens
denticle	den-tuh-cull	Peg
denticulated	den-tick-you-lay-ted	Toothlike; surface covered by fine serrations
derby hat		Shaped like the hats worn by Charlie Chaplin, and the comedy team of Laurel and Hardy. The crown of the hat is small and the narrow brim is turned up
dermatomycosis	durr-mat-oh-my-koh-sus	Infection of the cutaneous tissues caused by fungi other than dermatophytes
dermatophyte	durr-mat-oh-fight	Fungus that invades the keratinized portions of the hair, skin, and/or nails
dermatophytid reaction	durr-mat-oh-fy-tid	Allergic response to a dermatophytic infection elsewhere in the body
dermatophytosis	durr-mat-oh-fy-toe-sus	Infection caused by dermatophytes
desert rheumatism		Arthralgia in one or more joints resulting from *Coccidioides* infection
desquamation		Shedding of the epidermis
determinate		Conidiogenous cells that stop elongating when the first conidium is produced
dimethylsulfoxide (DMSO)		Penetrating agent, often combined with other chemicals and compounds as a carrier to increase the rate of penetration of the second chemical and/or compound into some structure or tissue
dimorph.c	dye-morff-ick	Having two bodies; fungi with different morphotypes under different conditions of growth
disease		Microorganisms penetrate into tissues and reproduce, causing injury and/or illness in the host
disjunctor	diss-junk-tur	Cell that releases an arthroconidium after fragmentation or lysis of the cell wall

rhymes with "dough"

rhymes with "dough"

rhymes with "purr"

Table continued on following page

Term	Pronunciation	Definition
disjuncture cell	diss-junk-shure cell	Cell that releases a conidium by fragmentation or lysis
distal	diss-tul	Away from the origin or source
DMSO		See dimethylsulfoxide
Drechslera species	Dresh-lair'-uh; rhymes with "mesh"	
echinulate	ee-kine-you-late; rhymes with "wine"	Rough or prickly
ectothrix	ek-toe-thricks; "th" as in "thin"	Pattern of invasion of hair in which the hyphae of the fungus fragments into arthroconidia that accumulate around the hair shaft or just beneath the cuticle
elephantiasis		Condition, related to infection, where blocked lymph vessels cause accumulation of lymph, with swelling of the skin and subcutaneous tissues. The scrotum and legs are most likely to be affected
elliptical		Shaped like an ellipse—approximately like an egg with both ends of equal size
embolus (pl. emboli)		Plug, which may be composed of solid material, liquid, or gases, that is present in the bloodstream or lymphatic channel. The blood or lymph vessel may be occluded, and infarcts may occur
en grappe	enn grah-pay	Arrangement resembling clusters or bunches of grapes
en thyrses	enn thris-us	Sleevelike arrangement around the hypha
endemic		Native to a particular geographic area and benign for immunocompetent natives, i.e., infections occur, but the mortality is low
endophthalmitis	end-opp-thall-mite-us; rhymes with "shall"	Inflammation of the eye
endospore		Spore formed within a spherule by cleavage of the cytoplasm
endothrix	en-doe-thricks; rhymes with "tricks"; pronounce "th" as in "thin"	Pattern of invasion of hair in which the hypha of the fungus fragments into arthroconidia that accumulate within the hair shaft
endotoxin		Toxin that is not released until the structure that contains it dissolves or disintegrates
enteroblastic		Production of conidia that involves only the inner layer of the cell wall of the conidiogenous cell
entire		Unbroken
Epicoccum species	Epp-ee-cock'-um	
Epidermophyton floccosum	Epp-ee-derm-oh-phy-ton flock-oh-some	
erythema multiforme	ear-uh-theme-uh mull-tee-form-ee	Pattern of reactions in the skin and mucous membranes caused by multiple agents. The erythema has a sudden onset. The typical pattern is erythematous papules with concentric rings
erythema nodosum	ear-uh-theme-uh no-dough-sum	Type of panniculitis, characterized by transient inflammatory nonulcerating nodules. Usually a hypersensitivity reaction; multiple agents may elicit the reaction

Term	Pronunciation	Definition
etiologic agent		Organism causing the infection
eukaryote	you-carry-ott	Organism in which the cell nucleus is surrounded by a membrane
eumycotic	you-my-cot-ick	Related to true ("eu-") fungi
exoantigen		Water-soluble cell-free antigens that are released into the medium (or which can be extracted in aqueous solution)
exogenous	X-oj-uh-nus (rhymes with "dodge")	Generated outside—not part of the normal flora of the host
Exophiala dermatitidis	X'-oh-fee-ah'-lah derm-ah-tid'-duh-dis (rhymes with "bah," as in "bah, humbug")	
Exophiala werneckii	X-oh-fee-ah'-luh were-neck-ee	
favic chandelier	fah-vick shan-duh-leer	Hypha that resembles reindeer antlers or branches of trees
favic-type hair invasion	fah-vick type	Characterized by development of filaments of fungi in the hair where they degenerate to leave tunnels containing oil deposits and air
favus	fah-vuss	Special variety of tinea capitis, associated with masses of mycelium and debris that form scutula
fermentation		Anaerobic utilization of carbohydrates
fertile hyphae		Mycelia from which the reproductive structures form
filamentous	fill-a-men-tus	Tubular
fixation		Treating a specimen, especially tissues, with a series of solutions to prevent shrinkage of the specimen and preserve it for further study
floccose	flah-kose	Texture produced by large quantities of long aerial hyphae that usually become tangled. Synonyms: woolly, cottony
fluctuant	fluck-shew-unt	Movable; not attached to adjacent tissues
folded		Topography featuring random folds
folliculitis	foe-lick-you-light-us	Inflammation of the hair follicles
fomite	foe-might	Inanimate object such as a doorknob, towel, or pencil that contains or carries microbial agents and spreads disease
Fonsecaea compacta	Fahn-seek'-uh komm-pack'-ta	
Fonsecaea pedrosoi	Fahn-seek'-uh puh-drow-soy	
foot cell		Specialized cell that forms in aconidium or conidiophore originates. Typically seen in the aspergilli and in *Fusarium*
fulminant	full-muh-nent	Occurring very rapidly
fungemia	fun-jheem-ee-uh (rhymes with "gleam")	Fungi in the bloodstream
fungicidal	fun-jhuh-side-ull ("jhuh" as in "justice")	Able to kill fungi

Table continued on following page

Pronunciation	Term	Definition
fun-gome-uh	fungoma	Fungus tumor; a ball or mass of mycelium
fun-gus & fun-jhy	fungus (pl. fungi)	Nonmotile eukaryotic organisms that have definite cell walls, lack chlorophyll, and reproduce sexually and/or asexually
fur-fur-aye-shus	furfuraceous	Resembling scales or dandruff
Few-sarh-ee-um	*Fusarium* species	
few-suh-form	fusiform	Having pointed ends; spindle shaped
jenn-ick-you-lut	geniculate	Resembling a bent knee
gee-oh-fill-ick	geophilic	Earth loving; dermatophytes whose primary reservoir is the soil
gee-oh-trick-oh-sus	geotrichosis	Infections caused by *Geotrichum candidum*
Gee-ah'-trick-um can-deed'-um	*Geotrichum candidum*	
	germ tube	Initial filamentous outgrowth from a conidium or a spore; an asexual reproductive structure
	germinate	Developing germ tubes; "sprouting"
geem-suh	Giemsa stain	Routine hematology stain, useful for detecting yeast forms of *Histoplasma capsulatum* in specimens
glay-brus	glabrous skin	Defined as smooth by Kwon-Chung and Bennett, and McGinnis. Smooth skin is glabrous skin
glay-brus	glabrous texture	Resembling pressed felt, with tightly woven vegetative hyphae and few or no aerial hyphae or spores. May be brittle and difficult to subculture or examine. The texture is less pronounced than in leathery colonies. Synonym: leathery
Glee-oh-clay'-dee-um	*Gliocladium* species	
glow-bose	globose	Round
	granular	Texture produced by presence of large numbers of conidia or spores. Technically granular colonies are coarser than powdery colonies. Synonym: powdery
	granule	Microcolony in tissue that is composed of an organized mass of hyphae
gran-you-loam-uh	granuloma	Collection of macrophages, giant cells, and other cells, mixed with the proteinaceous substances resulting from the host's immune response to the presence of infecting organisms. The host attempts to surround the invader and "wall it off"
teen-ee-uh cap-uh-tiss	gray-patch tinea capitis	Dermatophytic infections with ectothrix invasion of the hair; hair becomes grayish, dull, discolored, and brittle
jim-know-thee-key-um	gymnothecium	Ascocarp with loosely woven walls that allow asci to escape through them
"th" as in "thin"	H&E stain	Routine histologic stain that is useful for demonstrating the tissue response to mycotic infection; fungi stain pink to pinkish blue

	Pronunciation	Term	Definition
	Hans-en-oooh′-la	*Hansenula* species	
		haploid nuclei	Nuclei with half the number of chromosomes found in mature cells
	Hell-minth′-oh-spore′-ee-um	*Helminthosporium* species	
rhymes with "dodge"	heem-uh-todj-uh-nuss	hematogenous	Pertaining to or originating in the blood
	heem-uh-tocks-uh-linn & ee-oh-sun	hematoxylin and eosin stain	Routine histologic stain that is useful for demonstrating the tissue response to mycotic infection; fungi stain pink to pinkish blue
"thall" rhymes with "shall"	hett-urr-oh-thall-ick	heterothallic	Mating of two compatible thalli
rhymes with "growth"	hett-urr-oh-trowff	heterotroph	Derives energy from oxidation of organic compounds
	high-lum & high-luh	hilum (pl. hila)	Scar
	hiss-tee-oh-sight	histiocyte	Cell in the mononuclear phagocytic system (MPS), also called a connective tissue macrophage
"plaz" rhymes with jazz	Hiss-toe-plaz-muh cap-suh-lot-um	*Histoplasma capsulatum*	
	hiss-toe-plas-men	histoplasmin	Mixture of H and M antigens extracted from mould cultures of *Histoplasma capsulatum*
	hiss-toe-plas-moe-sis	histoplasmosis	Infections caused by *Histoplasma capsulatum*
	whole-oh-blast-ick	holoblastic	Production of conidia that involves all the layers of the cell wall of the conidiogenous cell
	whole-oh-morff	holomorph	The complete fungus—teleomorph and anamorph(s)
"thall" rhymes with "shall"	home-oh-thall-ick	homothallic	Self-fertilization; only one thallus is involved
		host	Organism (animal, vegetable, or mineral) that entertains the bacterium, fungus, or parasite
	hume-or-ull	humoral	Related to body fluids; specifically used to denote fluid-borne products of the immune system, such as antibodies
rhymes with "tin"	high-ah-linn	hyaline	Having white, light brown, or pastel pigment on the reverse of the colony. Microscopic structures are clear and colorless
"al" as in "alligator"	high-al-oh-high-foe-my-koh-sus	hyalohyphomycosis	Any subcutaneous mycotic infection that is not identified as a specific disease state and that is caused by a hyaline fungus
	high-fuh & high-fee	hypha (pl. hyphae)	Filamentous or tubular structure; collectively the hyphae comprise the body of a mould-form fungus
	eye-aye-trow-jenn-ick	iatrogenic	Related to procedures done by a physician in treatment of a patient
		id reaction	Allergic response to a dermatophytic infection elsewhere in the body
		immunocompromised	Person whose immune system is not functioning normally, for whatever reason
		immunofluorescence tests	Tests that use antigen or antibody labeled with a fluorescent dye to detect the specific (antigen or antibody) counterpart in specimens

Table continued on following page

Term	Pronunciation	Definition
imperfect fungi		Fungi that have not been proven to have a sexual method of reproduction
impression smears		Smears made by pressing a segment of biopsied tissue against a glass slide
indeterminate		Conidiogenous cells that continue to grow longer as conidia are produced
India ink preparation	in-dee-turr-min-nut	Wet prep using India ink as the mounting fluid. Primarily used for detecting encapsulated yeasts
infarct	inn-farkt	Area of tissue that becomes necrotic because the blood supply is cut off
infection		Situation in which microorganisms penetrate into tissues and reproduce (disease may or may not be present)
intercalary	in-turr-cow-lure-ee	Formed within the hyphae between the hyphal cells
intermediate grower		Fungus that produces mature colonies in 6–10 days
internodal	in-turr-node-ull	Describes the position of sporangiophores that arise from the hyphae between the rhizoids
intertriginous	in-ter-tridge-uh-nuss	Between the folds of the skin
intralipid therapy	in-truh-lip-id	Use of an intravenous hyperalimentation fat emulsion to correct a deficiency of fatty acids during total parenteral nutrition for those who cannot take adequate amounts of food orally
jock itch		Nickname for ringworm of the groin
karyogamy	care-ee-ogg-oh-me	Fusion of two nuclei in sexual conjugation
keratosis	care-uh-toe-sus	Condition (infection) involving the cornea of the eye
kerion	care-ee-awn	Spongy swelling
KOH preparation		Wet mount that uses an aqueous solution of 10–20% potassium hydroxide (KOH) as the mounting fluid
lactophenol–cotton blue preparation	lack-toe-fee-nol	Wet mount that uses lactophenol–cotton blue (LPCB) as the mounting fluid
leathery		Resembling leather, due to the tightly woven vegetative hyphae and the absence of aerial hyphae. May be difficult to separate a portion for subculture or microscopic preparations. Synonym: glabrous
lid-lifter		Fungus that grows with such enthusiasm and rapidity that the mycelium pushes up the lid of a plastic Petri dish
lipophilic	lye-poe-fill-ick	Lipid loving
locules	lock-yules	Compressions or cavities in an astrostroma
locus	loke-us	Site
log jam		Arrangement of blastoconidia in which they separate from the pseudohyphae but remain lying parallel to it, like logs in a river that have "jammed" on some obstruction

"min" as in minute

"uh" rhymes with "puh" as in puddle

rhymes with "bridge"

rhymes with "dawn"

Term	Pronunciation	Definition
LPCB prep		Wet mount that uses lactophenol–cotton blue (LPCB) as the mounting fluid
lymphocutaneous	limff-oh-cue-tain-ee-us	Related to the lymphatic system and cutaneous tissues
lyophilization	lye-off-uhl-uh-zay-shun	Using ultra-cold temperatures and a vacuum pump to freeze-dry microorganisms or other materials
maceration	mass-ur-aye-shun	Softening of the skin, similar to that which occurs when skin is soaked in water
macroconidium (pl. macroconidia)	mack-row-koh-nid-ee-um & mack-row-koh-nid-ee-uh	The larger of two types of conidia produced in the same manner by a single fungus
macronematous	mack-row-nem-uh-tus	Conidiophores that produce branching structures or that are distinctively shaped, e.g., can be distinguished from the vegetative hyphae
macular patches	mack-you-lurr	Discolored patches or spots that are not raised or sunken into surrounding skin
Malassezia furfur	Mal-uh-see-zee-uh fur-fur	
malt diastase	malt dye-uh-stace	Mixture of autolytic enzymes from malt that convert starch to simple sugars
manuum		Related to the hand
mariner's wheel		Large wheel with multiple knobs used to steer a ship in a body of water. The nickname for tissue forms of *Paracoccidioides brasiliensis*, which resemble mariner's wheels
mature colony		Colony possessing reproductive structures that can be used to identify the fungus
meiosis	my-ose-us	Process of nuclear reduction and division that results in formation of daughter cells with one half the number of chromosomes of the parent cell
melanoma	mell-an-ohm-uh	Pigmented mole or tumor which may be cancerous
melanosome	mell-ann-oh-sohm	Literally, black body; the pigment granules produced by melanocytes
merosporangiospore	"merr" as in merry merr-oh-spoe-ran-gee-oh-spore	Sporangiospore produced in a merosporangium
merosporangium (pl. merosporangia)	"merr" as in merry merr-oh-spoe-ran-gee-um & merr-oh-spoe-ran-gee-uh	Sporangium in which the sporangiospores are arranged in a single row or column within a cylindrical sac
methenamine silver stain	"th" as in "thin" muh-theen-uh-mean	Recommended histologic stain for demonstrating fungi in tissue; mycotic elements are black with paler lavender-gray central areas. Also referred to as MS stain
metula (pl. metulae)	met-you-luh & met-you-lay	Sterile branches within the reproductive system
Meyer's mucicarmine stain	rhymes with "loose" muce-uh-car-men	Stain for demonstrating *Cryptococcus neoformans* in tissue; *Cryptococcus* stains rose to red, nuclear material of tissue cells is black, and the other tissue elements are yellow. Also referred to as MM stain

Table continued on following page

Pronunciation	Term	Definition
rhymes with "dough"	microconidium (pl. microconidia)	Smaller of two conidia produced in the same manner by a single fungus
mick-row-koh-nid-ee-um & mick-row-koh-nid-ee-uh		
rhymes with "hem"	micrometer	Instrument used for measuring objects seen through the microscope
my-krom-uh-ter	micronematous	Condiophores that cannot be distinguished from the vegetative hyphae unless conidia are attached. Straight tubular or sticklike conidiophores without branching
my-crow-nem-uh-tuss		
My-crow-spore-um aw-dough-een-ee/awd-ween-ee	*Microsporum audouinii*	
My-crow-spore-um cane-us	*Microsporum canis*	
My-crow-spore-um cookie-eye	*Microsporum cookei*	
My-crow-spore-um gip-see-um	*Microsporum gypseum*	
My-crow-spore-um nan-um	*Microsporum nanum*	
	mince	To cut a specimen, usually tissue, into tiny bits with a scalpel
my-tose-us	mitosis	Division of nuclear chromosomes between two daughter cells so that each daughter has the same number of chromosomes as the parent cell
	MM stain	Meyer's mucicarmine stain for demonstrating *Cryptococcus neoformans* in tissue; *Cryptococcus* stains rose to red, nuclear material of tissue cells is black, and the other tissue elements are yellow
moan-ill-ee-ay-shus	moniliaceous	Having white, light brown, or pastel pigment on the reverse of the colony. Microscopic structures are clear and colorless
moe-nill-oh-form	moniliform	Colorless or lightly pigmented; not dematiaceous. Synonym: moniliaceous
	monomorph	Fungus that has the same structural form under all growth conditions
	morphology	Study of the body or shape; the macroscopic and microscopic details of fungus colonies
	mosaic sheath	Pattern of arthroconidia around the hair shaft resembling a tile mosaic
	mother cell	Cell from which the bud ("daughter") is produced. A conidiogenous cell. "Mother" and "daughter" are typically used to describe reproduction by budding in yeast and yeastlike fungi
	mold	A plastic, glass or metal container for puddings and gelatins
	mould	Fungal colonies composed of hyphae
	MS stain	Methenamine silver stain, the recommended histologic stain for demonstrating mycotic fungi in tissue; mycotic elements are black with paler lavender-gray central areas
rhymes with "dough"	*Mucor* species	
Mhew'-core		
mhew-core-my-koh-sus & mhew-core-my-koh-sees	mucormycosis (pl. mucormycoses)	Any infection caused by one of the Zygomycetes
	multilateral	Development of blastoconidia on several sides of a parent cell

Pronunciation	Term	Definition
rhymes with "lure"	muriform	Having both transverse and longitudinal septa
my-seal-ee-uh stir-ill-ee-uh	mycelia sterilia	Nonconidiating hyphae; sterile isolates; a colony with hyphae that do not produce reproductive propagules
my-seal-ee-um & my-seal-ee-uh	mycelium (pl. mycelia)	Masses of hyphae that comprise the colony of the mould
rhymes with "home"	mycetoma	Subcutaneous infection caused by fungi or bacteria that is characterized by tumor-like swelling, draining sinus tracts, and granules in the exudate from the infection
my-koll-oh-just	mycologist	One who studies fungi
"koll" as in college	mycology	Study of fungi
"koll" as in college	mycosis (pl. mycoses)	Infection caused by a fungus
rhymes with "dough" my-koh-sus & my-koh-sees	mycotic	Adjective, meaning pertaining to fungi
my-kot-ick	N-acetyl-L-cysteine	Mucolytic agent used to digest tenacious specimens such as sputa, to free the microorganisms so they can be seen in microscopic preparations or grow in culture
N-uh-see-till-L-sis-tuh-een	nail head hypha	Hypha that is swollen at the tip to resemble roofing nails
	negative stain	Staining method that creates a dark background against which structures that are not penetrated by the stain can be seen
nurr-oh-trope-ism	neurotropism	Selective affinity or fondness for (and invasion of) neural tissue
neh-vrus & neh-vee	nevus (pl. nevi)	Congenital discoloration of the skin (a birthmark) or a vascular tumor of the skin that is usually congenital
Nigh-grow-spore-uh	Nigrospora species	
noe-dull	nodal	Describes the position of sporangiophores that arise from the hypha at a point opposite rhizoids
	nodular body	Roundish mass formed when two or more hyphae become twisted together in a knot
non-sin-crow-nus	nonsynchronous	Produced at different times
	normocytic	Erythrocyte (red blood cell) with average diameter of approximately 7 µm
rhymes with "home"	nosocomial	Hospital-acquired
know-sow-comb-ee-ul	nuchal rigidity	Stiff neck. Specifically, the patient is unable to touch his (her) breastbone with his (her) chin
new-cull rigidity	obverse	Surface
	occluded	Blocked
rhymes with "dough" onk-oh-my-koh-sus	onychomycosis	Mycotic infection of the nail
	opportunist	See opportunistic pathogen

Table continued on following page

Term	Pronunciation	Definition
opportunistic fungi		Fungi that infect a great variety of tissues in compromised hosts when the opportunity arises; "wild cards"
opportunistic pathogen		Fungi (or other microorganisms) that have no invasive properties but that are able to cause infection when they are introduced into the host under conditions (such as depression of the immune system) that favor them
otomycosis	oh-toe-my-koh-sus	Mycotic infection of the ear
oval		Shaped like an ellipse—approximately like an egg with both ends of equal size
Paecilomyces species	Pay-sill-oh-my-sees	
Papanicolaou stain	pap-uh-nick-oh-low	Stain for the detection of changes in tissue due to malignancy or infection. George Papanicolaou, a Greek physician, developed the method that is widely used for examination of cervical smears and sputa. It is also known as the "Pap" smear
Paracoccidioides brasiliensis	Pair-uh-cock-sih-dee-oy´-dees bruh-zill-ee-en-sis	
paracoccidioidin	pear-uh-cock-sid-ee-oy-din	Antigen extracted from yeast form cultures of *Paracoccidioides brasiliensis*
paracoccidioidomycosis	pear-uh-cock-sid-ee-oy-dough-my-koh-sis	Infections caused by *Paracoccidioides brasiliensis*
parasite		Organism that grows in or on another organism (the "host") and that derives benefit from the host
paronychia	pear-onch-ee-uh	Infection of the tissues surrounding the nail
PAS stain		Periodic acid–Schiff stain, a histologic stain for demonstrating fungi in tissues; fungi stain deep pink
pathogen		Organism that can initiate infection in people with normal immune systems
pathogenic		Capable of causing infection or disease
pathognomonic	path-oh-no-mon-ick	Characteristic of the infection or disease
pectinate hypha	peck-tuh-nate	Hypha resembling a comb, with multiple "teeth" of varying lengths extending from one side of the hypha
pedis	pedd-us	Related to the foot
pellicle		Thin to thick film that forms on the surface of a broth medium
Penicillium species	Pen-uh-sill´-ee-um	
penicilliosis	pen-uh-sill-ee-oh-sus	Condition, usually an infection, caused by *Penicillium* species
penicillus	pen-uh-sill-us	Brushlike arrangement created by branching of the conidiophores

Pronunciation notes (left margin):

rhymes with "dough"

rhymes with "map"

"uh" rhymes with "puh" as in puddle; "oy" rhymes with "boy"

"uh" rhymes with "puh" as in puddle

"uh" rhymes with "puh" as in puddle

rhymes with "honk"

rhymes with "home"

rhymes with "late"

rhymes with "head"

Term	Pronunciation	Definition
perfect fungi	"shiff" as in shift	Fungi that have been demonstrated to have both sexual and asexual modes of reproduction
periodic acid-Schiff stain	purr-eye-oh-dick acid shiff	Histologic stain for demonstrating fungi in tissues; fungi stain deep pink. Also referred to as the PAS stain
perithecium	"th" as in "thin"; pear-uh-thee-key-um	Flask-shaped ascocarp with an opening through which ascospores escape
Phaeoannellomyces	Fay-oh-ann-ell-oh-my-seas	
Phaeococcomyces	Fay-oh-cock-oh-my-seas	
phaeohyphomycosis	rhymes with "dough"; fay-oh-high-foe-my-koh-sus	Any subcutaneous mycotic infection that is not identified as a specific disease state and that is caused by a dematiaceous fungus
phenoloxidase		Enzyme produced by *Cryptococcus neoformans* (and occasionally other *Cryptococcus* species) that converts caffeic acid to melanin
phialide	fy-ale-id	Macronematous conidiogenous cell that is determinate and typically shaped somewhat like a vase
phialoconidium	fy-ale-oh-koh-nid-ee-um	Conidium produced from a phialide
Phialophora verrucosa	Fy-uh-loff-or-uh verr-uh-kose-uh	
phialophora-type conidiation	fy-uh-loff-or-uh	Pattern of anamorphic conidiation characterized by conidiophores that are more or less vaselike, with clusters of phialoconidia clustered around the tip of the phialide
piedra	pee-aye-druh	Superficial hair infection with nodular masses of fungal elements ("stones") surrounding the hair shaft
Piedraia hortae	Pee-ay-dree-uh harr-tay/hoar-tay	
pityriasis versicolor	pit-uh-rye-uh-sis verse-uh-color	Superficial skin infection characterized by changes in the pigment of the skin, especially on the trunk of the body; the etiologic agent is *Malassezia furfur.*
Pneumocystis carinii	new-moe-sis-tiss care-in-ee	Parasite recently reclassified as a fungus (an Ascomycete). It exists within host cells and is similar to the yeast *Saccharomyces cerevisiae.* Often associated with pneumonia in patients with AIDS
polytridic	rhymes with "doll"; poll-ee-tryd-ick	Conidiogeny in which multiple conidia are produced through tiny pores in the cell walls of the conidiogenous cell
polyvinyl alcohol	rhymes with "doll"; poll-ee-vine-ul alcohol	Mounting fluid useful for examination of cultures; it hardens into a permanent mount. A carcinogenic substance that requires care in handling
polyvinyl alcohol-cotton blue	rhymes with "doll"; poll-ee-vine-ul alcohol-cotton blue	Polyvinyl alcohol combined with cotton blue (Poirrer's blue) dye for use as a mounting fluid
poroconidium (pl. poroconidia)	poor-oh-koh-nid-ee-um	Holoblastic conidia produced through pores in the cell wall of the conidiogenous cell or conidiophore
powdery		Texture associated with production of large numbers of conidia or spores. Technically powdery colonies are less coarse than granular colonies. Synonym: granular

Table continued on following page

Term	Pronunciation	Definition
primary		First level or stage
primary condition		First infection, injury, or disease
primary culture		Set of media inoculated from the specimen
pruritic	prew-it-ick	Itching
Pseudallescheria boydii	Sood-al-ush-shear-ee-uh boy-dee	
pseudohypha	sood-oh-high-fuh	Chain of cells (blastoconidia) that resembles a hypha but that lacks septa (although constrictions between cells are present)
purulent	pure-you-lent	Containing pus
pustule		Small sac or blister containing purulent fluid
PVA		Mounting fluid useful for examination of cultures; it hardens into a permanent mount. A carcinogenic substance that requires care in handling
PVA-CB		Polyvinyl alcohol combined with cotton blue (Poirrier's blue) dye for use as a mounting fluid
pyriform	pie-ruh-form	Pear shaped
racquet hyphae		Series of swollen cells in which the walls of successive cells swell to form the "head" of racquets
radial grooves		Grooves that radiate from the center like spokes from a bicycle wheel. Synonym: rugose
rapid grower		Fungus that produces mature colonies in 5 days or less
rat tail conidium		Macroconidium whose free end is long, thin, and tail like
refractile		Ray of incident light is split into two refractive rays, producing a double image. Refractile structures look sharper and brighter than nonrefractile ones
refraction		Deflection of a ray of light at a certain angle when the ray passes from one transparent medium into another of different density. In double refraction the incident ray is divided into two refracted rays, producing a double image
reproductive hyphae		Mycelia from which the reproductive structures form
reservoir		Place where the fungus is found in nature—soil, water, vegetation, or some combination of these factors
rhinocladiella-type conidiation	rine-oh-clad-ee-L-uh	Pattern of anamorphic conidiation characterized by production of conidia sympodially on short denticles around the tip of the swollen conidiophore. Secondary and tertiary levels of conidia may be produced
rhizoid	rye-zhoid	Rootlike structures for anchoring the fungus to the substrate and absorbing nutrients
Rhizomucor species	Rye'-zo-mhew-core	

rhymes with "drew"

"al" as in alligator; "sood" rhymes with "dude"

"sood" rhymes with "dude"

rhymes with "dad"

rhymes with "annoyed"

rhymes with "dough"

Term	Pronunciation	Definition
Rhizopus species	Rye-zo-puss	
Rhodotorula species	Row-dough-tore´-you-lah	
ringworm		Nickname for tineas, recognizing the circular pattern of typical skin lesions
rose gardener's disease		Sporotrichosis
rosette pattern		Pattern of conidiation in *Sporothrix* mould colonies. Conidia, attached by delicate denticles, are produced sympodially at the tip of the conidiophore
rudimentary		Primitive; poorly developed
rugose	rew-ghose	Topography featuring radial grooves from the center of the colony toward the rim
Saccharomyces cerevisiae	Sack´-uh-row-mice´-ees sir-vase´-ee-ay	
salt and pepper		Colony surface that looks as if it had been sprinkled with these two seasonings due to the presence of dark conidia on the hyaline hyphae
saprobe	sah-probe	Organism that uses dead organic material for nutrition and does not harm the host. These contaminants or commensals may cause infection in immunodeficient hosts, i.e., some are also opportunistic pathogens
Scedosporium apiospermum	Ski-dough-spore-ee-um ape-ee-oh-sperm-um	
sclerotic body	slare-ah-tick	Pleomorphic spherical brown forms divided by muriform septa into two to four cells; found in the exudate in chromoblastomycosis. Sometimes called "copper pennies"
Scopulariopsis species	Scope-you-lair-ee-op´-siss	
Scotch tape prep		Microscopic preparation in which cellophane tape is used to pick up a portion of the colony and transfer it to the mounting fluid
scutula (pl. scutulae)	scoot-you-luh & scoot-you-lee	Yellowish cup-shaped crusts composed of mycelium, scales, sebum, and other debris
sebum	see-bum	General term for fatty secretions of the sebaceous glands
secondary		Second stage or level
secondary infection		Infection of an area by a second microorganism that takes advantage of the conditions created by the first disease or infecting organism
section		Process of cutting tissue into ver-r-r-y thin slices (microns thick) in preparation for staining it. Also, the slice of tissue
selective media		Media containing antimicrobial agents and/or chemicals or dyes to select for some microorganisms and prevent the growth of others
self-limiting		Asymptomatic infection, usually of brief duration, that resolves without treatment

Pronunciation guide notes:
"rew" rhymes with "drew"; "ghose" rhymes with "dose"

rhymes with "dare"

rhymes with "hop"

Table continued on following page

Term	Pronunciation	Definition
sensitivity	"sep" rhymes with "pep"; "doan" rhymes with "moan"	Conditional probability that the antigen or antibody will be detected when it is present
Sepedonium species	Sep-uh-doan´-ee-um	
septate		Having cross-walls
serial testing		Testing of a succession of specimens collected over a period of time. Usually done in immunology to detect changes in the level of the response
sessile	sess-ul	Without a pedicle; attached directly by a broad base
sexual reproduction		Union of nuclei or gametes through meiosis
shield cell		Blastoconidium of certain dematiaceous fungi that is approximately triangular with three thickened disjuncture scars
ship's wheel		*See* mariner's wheel
simple		Conidiophores that cannot be distinguished from the vegetative hyphae unless conidia are attached. Straight tubular or sticklike conidiophores without branching
sleevelike pattern		Pattern of conidiation in which conidia are produced on threadlike denticles along the hyphae, covering it like a "sleeve." Typical of *Sporothrix* moulds
slide culture		Fungi are grown on agar blocks on slides and harvested to make permanent preparations for examination
slow grower		Fungus that needs 11 or more days to produce mature colonies
South American blastomycosis	blas-toe-my-koh-sus	Nickname for paracoccidioidomycosis
spaghetti and meatballs		Arrangement of conidia and hyphae that causes the characteristic appearance of *Malassezia furfur* in tissue
speciation	spee-see-aye-shun	Identifying the organism to species
specificity		Conditional probability that when the test is positive, the patient has the disease or infection
spelunker's disease	spee-lunk-urr	Nickname for histoplasmosis. The presence of *Histoplasma* in the waste products of cave bats can result in infection of the spelunker, i.e., the person who goes "caving"
spherulin	sphere-you-lin	Antigen prepared from the tissue form (spherule) of *Coccidioides immitis*
spicule	spick-yule	Small projection or peg; denticle
spindle shaped		Resembling the spindles used to hold wool or thread. Spindles swell from one end to the center, then taper to the opposite end
spinulose	spin-you-lose	Having spines
spiral hypha	"spin" rhymes with "tin"; "lose" rhymes with "dose"	Hypha that seems to have been twisted around a pencil and released; resembling curly fries

Term	Pronunciation	Definition
sporangiophore	spo-rangh-ee-oh-four (rhymes with "flange")	Structure supporting the sporangium and sporangiospores
sporangiospore	spo-rangh-ee-oh-spore (rhymes with "flange")	Primary asexual reproductive structure formed by the Zygomycetes. It is formed in a sac
sporangium (pl. sporangia)	spo-rangh-ee-um & spo-rangh-ee-uh (rhymes with "flange")	Saclike structure in which sporangiospores are formed by cleavage
spore		Reproductive structure of fungi produced by sexual means. Conventionally the asexual reproductive structures of the Zygomycetes, which are formed by cleavage of the cell wall, are also called spores (sporangiospores)
sporodochium (pl. sporodochia)	spore-oh-doke-ee-um & spore-oh-doke-ee-uh (rhymes with "poke")	Tight mat or patch of conidiating conidiophores within the mycelium; sporodochia may be grossly visible on the surface of the colony
Sporothrix schenckii	Spore-oh-thricks shenk-ee (rhymes with "tricks"; pronounce "th" as in "thin")	
sporotrichin	spore-oh-trick-in	*Sporothrix* antigen made from heat-killed yeast cells of the fungus
sporotrichosis	spore-oh-trick-oh-sis	Chronic mycotic infection, involving the cutaneous and subcutaneous tissues and adjacent lymphatic tissues, characterized by ulcers along the lymph channels
sporozoite	spore-oh-zoe-ight	Stage in the life cycle of *Pneumocystis carinii* (and protozoan parasites). Sporozoites develop within cysts of *P. carinii*
sterile hyphae		Hyphae that do not produce conidia or conidiophores; mycelia sterilia
stolon	stole-un	Runner; a horizontal hypha from which hyphae, rhizoids, or sporangiophores develop
stratum corneum	strat-um corn-ee-um (rhymes with "fat")	Outermost horny layer of the epidermides
striated	stry-ate-ud	Striped
striation	stry-aye-shun	Stripe
stroma	strome-uh (rhymes with "home")	"Mattress"; a hard mass of tightly interwoven hyphae
subculture		Transferring a culture from growth in one culture to another medium
subcutaneous mycoses	sub-cue-tain-ee-us my-koh-sees	Mycotic infections of the bone, muscle, connective tissues, and lymphatic system
subglobose	sub-glow-bose (rhymes with "close")	Irregularly rounded
substrate		Material on which the fungus is growing—medium, tissue, or organic/inorganic compound
subungual	sub-ung-you-ull (rhymes with "hung")	"Beneath the nail," i.e., involving the deep areas of the nail plate
suede		Texture created by short aerial hyphae of approximately equal length and few conidia or spores. Synonym: velvety
superficial mycoses		Mycotic infections of the outer "dead" layers of the skin and hair
suppurative	soup-urr-uh-tive	Producing pus

Table continued on following page

Term	Pronunciation	Definition
sympodial	sim-poe-dee-ul ("rhymes with "dough"")	Indeterminate conidiogeny in which the oldest conidium is found at the tip of the conidiophore and younger conidia are produced successively on either side of and behind the older conidium, creating a repetitive zigzag pattern
synanamorph	sin-ann-uh-morff ("rhymes with "tin"")	Anamorphs associated with a teleomorph
Syncephalastrum species	Sen-seff'-uh-last'-rum ("rhymes with "deaf"")	
synchronous	sin-kruh-nus ("rhymes with "tin"")	Produced at the same time
synnemata	sin-uh-mott-uh ("rhymes with "tin"")	Bundles or tufts of conidiophores
systemic mycoses		Mycotic infections of organ systems and deep tissues of the body
Tmax		Maximum temperature of growth
tease mount		Microscopic preparation that uses two needles to gently separate the hyphal strands so the hyphae and reproductive structures of fungi can be examined
teasing needle		Needle used in mycology to transfer cultures or make slides. The needle is thicker and stronger than the needles and loops used for bacteria
teleomorph	teal-ee-oh-morff	Sexual (perfect) form of a fungus
tenacious	tuh-nay-shus	Adhesive; tough; holding together
terminal		At the end of the chain of conidia—the end of the line
tertiary	turr-shuh-ree ("rhymes with "purr"")	Third level or stage
texture		Refers to the colony surface and describes the way it would feel if you could (yuk!) touch it
thallic conidiogeny	thall-ick koh-nid-ee-oj-uh-knee ("th" as in "thin" "thall" rhymes with "shall" "koh" rhymes with "dough" "oj" rhymes with "dodge")	Conidiogeny in which the septum is formed in the parent cell before the new conidium is produced
thallus (pl. thalli)	thall-us & thall-eye ("th" as in "thin"; rhymes with "shall")	Mass of the colony; all of the hyphae
thermal dimorph		Fungus that has "two bodies," the mould form at room temperature and another form at human body temperature
thermotolerant		Able to grow at temperatures above 37.5°C
thrush		Candidiasis of the mucous membranes of the mouth
tinea	teen-ee-uh	Superficial or cutaneous infection of the hair, skin, or nails
tinea barbae	teen-ee-uh bar-bay	Ringworm of the bearded areas of the face and neck
tinea capitis	teen-ee-uh cap-uh-tiss	Ringworm of the hair, scalp, eyebrows, and eyelashes
tinea corporis	teen-ee-uh car-pore-us	Ringworm of the glabrous skin
tinea cruris	teen-ee-uh crurr-iss ("rhymes with "purr"")	Ringworm of the groin, perineum, and perineal regions

Term	Pronunciation	Definition
tinea favosa	teen-ee-uh fah-voe-suh	Special variety of tinea capitis, associated with masses of mycelium and debris that form scutula
tinea manuum	teen-ee-uh man-um	Ringworm of the palms and interdigital spaces of the hands
tinea nigra (tinea nigra palmaris)	teen-ee-uh nye-grah (pal-mire-us)	Superficial skin infection characterized by development of irregular black or brown macular patches on the palmar surfaces of the hands and fingers; the etiologic agent is *Exophiala werneckii*
tinea pecis	rhymes with "me"	Ringworm of the interdigital spaces and soles of the feet
tinea unguium	teen-ee-uh un-ghwee-um	Ringworm of the nails
tinea versicolor	teen-ee-uh verse-uh-color	Superficial skin infection characterized by changes in the pigment of the skin, especially on the trunk of the body; the etiologic agent is *Malassezia furfur*.
topography	top-og-ruh-fee (rhymes with "frog")	Arrangement of the colony surface—its peaks and valleys
Torulopsis glabrata	Tore-you-lop'-sis glah-brah'-ruh ("lop" rhymes with "hop"; "glah" rhymes with "bah," as in "bah, humbug")	
transverse		Crosswise; lying at right angles to the long axis
traumatic inoculation		Any minor or not so minor injury that breaks the skin; a common route of infection for fungi
Trichoderma species	Trick-oh-derm-uh	
Trichophyton mentagrophytes	Trick-oh-phy-tun/Try-koff'-uh-'tun men-tag-row-phy'-tees	
Trichophyton rubrum	Trick-oh-phy-tun/Try-koff'-uh-'tun rube'-rum	
Trichophyton schoenleinii	Trick-oh-phy-tun/Try-koff'-uh-'tun show-en-leen-ee/shane-line-eye	
Trichophyton tonsurans	Trick-oh-phy-tun/Try-koff'-uh-'tun tohn-sir-anns	
Trichophyton verrucosum	Trick-oh-phy-tun/Try-koff'-uh-'tun verr-uh-kose-um (rhymes with "dose")	
Trichophyton violaceum	Trick-oh-phy-tun/Try-koff'-uh-'tun vi-oh-lay'-see-um	
Trichosporon beigelii	Trick-oh-spore-un bay-jhuh-lee ("jhuh" as in "justice")	
trophozoite	troff-oh-zoe-ight	Developmental stage of *Pneumocystis carinii* (and protozoan parasites). After sporozoites are released from the mature cyst, they develop into ameboid trophozoites
truncate	trun-kate	"Cut off"; ending abruptly; square at the tip

Table continued on following page

Term	Pronunciation	Definition
tuberculate	two-burr-kew-lut	Having wartlike protuberances
tumefaction		Swelling resembling a tumor
unguium	un-ghwee-um (rhymes with "me")	Related to the nail
uniseriate	une-uh-sear-ee-ut (rhymes with "moon")	Single series
Valley fever		Nickname for coccidioidomycosis. It is based on the endemicity of *Coccidioides immitis* to the San Joaquin Valley in California
vegetative hyphae		Mycelia growing in or on the substrate; its role is absorption of nutrients
velvety		Texture created by short aerial hyphae of approximately equal length. Synonym: suede
vermiform		Wormlike; shaped like a worm
verrucoid	vuh-rew-koid	Wartlike; raised and rough
verrucose	vuh-rew-kuss	Topography featuring many warts or rough knobs. Synonym: warty
vesicle		Swelling at the terminal end of the conidiophore, typical of the aspergilli. Also, a small sac or blister on the skin that contains clear fluid
Wangiella dermatitidis	Wang-ee-ell-uh derm-ah-tid-duh-dus (rhymes with "bah", as in "bah, humbug")	
wet preparation (wet mount)		Microscopic preparation made by suspending a small amount of the specimen or culture in mounting fluid and covering it with a coverslip on a slide
white piedra	white pee-aye-druh	Superficial hair infection characterized by soft, white nodules of mycotic elements surrounding the hair shaft; the etiologic agent is *Trichosporon beigelii*
Wood's lamp		Ultraviolet light used to detect fluorescent substances that develop in the hair and skin in certain mycotic infections
woolly		Texture produced by large quantities of long aerial hyphae that usually become tangled. Technically, woolly colonies are more dense than cottony colonies. Synonym: cottony, floccose
Wright-Giemsa stain (Wright's stain)	right gheem-suh stain (rhymes with "gleam")	Routine hematology stain, useful for detecting yeast forms of *Histoplasma capsulatum* in specimens
Xylohypha bantiana	Zy-low-high-fah bann-tee-ann-uh	
yeast		Perfect fungi composed of predominantly unicellular forms that bud
yeastlike		Imperfect fungi composed of predominantly unicellular forms that bud
zoophilic	zoe-oh-fill-ick (rhymes with "dough")	Animal loving; dermatophytes whose primary reservoir is animals
zygomycosis (pl. zygomycoses)	zigh-go-my-koh-sus & zigh-go-my-koh-sees ("sus" rhymes with "fuss")	Any infection caused by one of the Zygomycetes

Term	Pronunciation	Definition
zygosporangium	zigh-go-spo-rangh-ee-um "rangh" rhymes with "flange"	Saclike structure in which a zygospore is formed after the fusion of the tips of two compatible hyphae
zygospore	zigh-go-spore	Round, thick-walled spore formed in a zygosporangium by fusion of the tips of two compatible hyphae

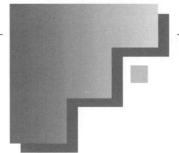

Suggested Student Laboratory Schedules

INTRODUCTION

Laboratory examination of fungi is a critical component of mycology that should be integrated into the broader didactic portion of the course. Without some element of practical experience the identification of unknown fungi in the clinical laboratory is far more difficult, if not impossible.

Every mycology text—including this one—has wonderfully detailed drawings of "perfect" organisms, sometimes with equally explicit photographs showing how the fungi look on a good day. In the real world fungi don't often look perfect or behave perfectly. The two or three characteristics that identify the organism are likely to be lost in a maze of imperfectly "teased" hyphae and free conidia. Only practice helps the laboratorian learn which characteristics are important and which can be ignored.

In designing the laboratory sessions to accompany this text, we have drawn on our combined experience in teaching mycology to generations of students in the medical laboratory sciences. Users of this text who have taught mycology for years, and have their own ways of doing things, will find some hints that will be helpful. By providing detailed instructions and lists of the stock cultures, media, and equipment needed, we have also tried to accommodate the instructor who is teaching a mycology course for the first time.

The three most important tasks in the laboratories are *drawing, drawing, and drawing*. Great artistic ability is not required. Nonetheless, drawing the microscopic structures is important because the process forces the observer to notice *all* the details of the structures and

the manner in which they are connected to one another.[1]

Laboratory exercises have been designed to accompany Chapters 2 through 8 of the text. These are found near the end of each chapter, with all the sessions for each exercise arranged sequentially. This format allows the reader to see how all the parts fit together to achieve the goal—acquiring a good working knowledge of the organisms being studied. Which sessions should be included and the frequency of the sessions are of course left to the instructor, with the caveat that few fungi grow enough to be studied in less than 7 days. Figure C.1 provides a general plan for laboratories, with a brief description of the tasks to be accomplished in each of the recommended sessions for a given laboratory exercise.

One of us (F.F.) regularly taught mycology in a 2-week period, in conjunction with other courses for herself and her students, which made them all think they were going to explode from knowledge overload and fatigue. The other one (N.C.) teaches a more conventional 8-week course, which still creates the sensation of "so many fungi, so little time." The optimum is a course that spans a full 16-week semester. The key differences among the three task outlines are that as the course becomes shorter (1) the instructor must set up more demonstrations, (2) some exercises must be omitted, and (3) students must rely more on memorization and less on assimilation of the information.

---

[1]We agree that, in preparing accurate, realistic illustrations for this text, we have been more completely "tuned in" than ever before and have greatly improved our knowledge and understanding of certain of the fungi.

GENERAL SCHEDULE FOR LABORATORY EXERCISES

	First Session	INTERIM	Second Session	INTERIM	Third Session	INTERIM	Fourth Session
Ex. 1 (Ch. 2)	Set up environmental cultures		Describe colony morphology of isolates from environmental cultures. Do tease mounts and Scotch tape preps on two different colonies and read the results.				
Ex. 2 (Ch. 2)	Describe colony morphology of a saprobe. Do tease mounts of a saprobic fungus and read the results.						
Ex. 3 (Ch. 2)	Do a Scotch tape prep of a saprobic fungus and read the results.						
Ex. 4 (Ch. 2)	Set up a slide culture of a saprobic fungus.	*CHECK CULTURE*	Harvest slide culture if possible.		Read slide culture.		Read slide culture if necessary.
Ex. 5 (Ch. 3)	Transfer 3 organisms to fresh media and set up slide cultures.	*CHECK SLIDE CULTURES*	Describe the colony morphology of each culture. Do tease mounts and Scotch tape preps. Harvest slide cultures if possible.	*CHECK SLIDE CULTURES*	Read slide culture.	*CHECK SLIDE CULTURES*	Read slide culture if necessary.
Ex. 6 (Ch. 4)	Transfer 2 superficial fungi to fresh media and set up slide cultures of each.	*CHECK SLIDE CULTURES*	Describe the colony morphology of each culture. Do tease mounts and Scotch tape preps. Harvest slide cultures if possible.	*CHECK SLIDE CULTURES*	Read slide culture.		Read slide culture if necessary.
Ex. 7 (Ch. 5)	Transfer 3 dermatophytes to fresh media and set up slide cultures of each.	*CHECK SLIDE CULTURES*	Describe the colony morphology of each culture. Do tease mounts and Scotch tape preps. Harvest slide cultures if possible.	*CHECK SLIDE CULTURES*	Read slide cultures.		Read slide culture if necessary.
Ex. 8 (Ch. 5)	Set up differential tests for dermatophytes	*CHECK TESTS*	Read differential tests.		Complete differential tests if necessary.		Finish hair perforation tests.
Ex. 9 (Ch. 6)	Transfer *Sporothrix schenckii* and 2 other subcutaneous fungi to fresh media and set up slide cultures of each.	*CHECK SLIDE CULTURES*	Describe the colony morphology of each culture. Do tease mounts and Scotch tape preps. Harvest slide cultures if possible.	*CHECK SLIDE CULTURES*	Read slide cultures if time permits.	*CHECK SLIDE CULTURES*	Read slide cultures if necessary.
Optional Ex. (Ch. 6)	Set up differential tests on subcutaneous organisms.	*CHECK TEST RESULTS*	Read differential tests and use charts to "key out" the organisms.	*CHECK TEST RESULTS*	Read remaining differential tests, if necessary, and use charts to "key out" the organisms.		
Ex. 10 (Ch. 6)	Describe the colony morphology of the yeast form of *Sporothrix schenckii*. Do a wet prep and examine it.						
Ex. 11 (Ch. 7)	Transfer 5 yeasts to fresh media.		Describe the colony morphology of the 5 yeasts. Do a wet prep of each with saline/water and India ink prep and examine them.				
Ex. 12 (Ch. 7)	Set up a germ tube test and other differential tests on each yeast. Read the germ tube test today.	*CHECK TEST RESULTS*	Read remaining differential tests and use charts to "key out" the organisms. Set up any "rapid" tests.	*CHECK TEST RESULTS*			
Ex. 13 (Ch. 8)	Describe colony morphology of prepared killed cultures of the systemic fungi if these are available. Read prepared slides of systemic fungi.						
Ex. 14 (Ch. 2-8)	*REVIEW FOR PRACTICAL EXAM*						

FIGURE C.1

General schedule for laboratory exercises.

Schedules specific to each of the three courses are proposed (see Figs. C.5, C.9, and C.10). These show the session of each exercise that should be done during a 3-hour laboratory; the final day of each proposed course has been left blank with the assumption that the instructor will use that day for written and practical examinations.

Within each schedule the exercises overlap, of course. The procedures that should be demonstrated and the recommended materials for the demonstrations are provided for each schedule, with an outline of the students' tasks and a list of the exercises/sessions to be included. All these elements can be rearranged to suit individual instructors. We have simply attempted to provide a foundation.

Laboratory Safety

Common sense and good *aseptic technique* should be used.

Students should *wear lab coats and gloves* at all times while working in the laboratory.

No extraneous items (such as purses and backpacks) should be left on the counters during laboratories.

A *"place mat"* moistened with disinfectant should be used at the work area.

Countertops and equipment should be disinfected *before and after* each laboratory.

The *safety* of those working in the laboratory is paramount. We recommend that cultures be transferred and slide cultures be handled within a biologic safety cabinet whenever possible, while acknowledging that this can be a logistical nightmare in a busy student laboratory. Because of the fungi that have been suggested for study, this recommendation is more the result of concern with contamination of the laboratory environment than fear of laboratory-acquired infections.

Each student should have one slide "flat" (a rectangular folder of heavy cardboard containing niches into which microscope slides fit) to hold slides while they dry, and one to house the permanent slide collection. Each student should also keep a notebook containing the notes and drawings from each exercise. A notebook helps maintain continuity throughout the course, should be useful in preparing for examinations, and—who knows?—may be an important part of clinical practice for anyone later employed in a microbiology laboratory.

Three *laboratory work sheets* have been developed: one for monomorphic moulds, one for monomorphic yeasts, and one for dimorphic fungi. Each demonstrates the characteristics that have been emphasized in the text and that we believe should be recorded in the study of a fungus. See

Figures C.2 through C.4 for blank forms. A completed example of each form (see Figs. C.6 through C.8) is given as a guide for those doing the exercises, as a part of the session where they are introduced in the 16-week course.

Students should compile notebooks of their laboratory work sheets, drawings, and notes from laboratory sessions. We feel strongly that drawing the microscopic morphology of the fungi is a critical element of learning. Skilled artistry is not expected or required. Few students (or teachers) reproduce drawings suitable for framing. Nonetheless, *nothing else* is as effective in forcing the observer to carefully examine all the structures and the way they fit together.

Materials You Always Need[2]

glass microscope slides
coverslips (22 × 22 and 22 × 30)
marking pen
labels for permanent slides
pencil
forms for recording information about cultures
electric incinerator[3]
disinfectant (such as Septisol or Amphyll)
place mat (brown paper towels or similar material)
teasing needles with straight and bent tips
microscope
disposable gloves
small (8 × 10 inch) autoclavable "biohazard" bag in a frame
test tube rack
standard incubator(s)—*not* CO_2—calibrated to 25–30°C
laminar-flow biologic safety cabinet(s)
slide flat
lens paper
immersion oil

Recommended Media for Every Session

Emmon's modification of Sabouraud's dextrose agar (SDA)
potato flake agar (PFA) or potato dextrose agar (PDA)

Additional Materials for a Tease Mount

lactophenol–cotton blue (LPCB) or other mounting fluid in a dropper bottle
a culture
patience

---

[2]Listed items in **bold type** should be placed in the individual student's drawer or locker and restocked as needed.

[3]If electric incinerators are not available, a beaker half-filled with sand and disinfectant should be added to the list of *Materials You Always Need*. Hyphae and conidia that remain on the tips of forceps and needles should be "scrubbed off" in the sand before the tips are flamed in a burner.

LABORATORY WORK SHEET FOR MONOMORPHIC MOULDS

Your Name		Date Inoculated	Identity of the Fungus

Macroscopic Characteristics	Obs	Dates of Observations (see footnote*)	Age of Culture and Rate of Growth (Rapid, Intermediate, Slow) Temp, Medium	Colony Size (fills plate or tube, restricted, etc.)	Pigmentation		Topography (convex, rugose, etc.) Texture (velvety, glabrous, etc.)
					Obverse	Reverse	
	1st						
	2nd						
	3rd						

Microscopic Characteristics	Obs	Hyphae: width? Presence of septa?	Describe how conidia are produced (budding? on phialides? etc.)	Microconidia: Size? Shape? Other features?	Macroconidia: Size? Shape? Width & texture of cell wall? Other features?	Describe other structures on or in the hyphae
	1st					
	2nd					
	3rd					

	Obs	Dates of Observations	Confirmatory tests done, if any	Reactions to confirmatory tests
	1st			
	2nd			
	3rd			

Make your drawing(s) in the spaces provided below. Each drawing should include hyphae, micro- and macroconidia, and any miscellaneous vegetative structures you see. Show how the structures are connected to one another. LABEL THE STRUCTURES!

*Indicate the type of procedure/observation in this column, with the date. Use abbreviations. Direct Mount, DM; Scotch Tape Prep, STP; Slide Culture, SC

FIGURE C.2

Blank laboratory work sheet for monomorphic moulds.

LABORATORY WORK SHEET FOR DIMORPHIC FUNGI

| Your Name | | Date Inoculated | | Identity of the Fungus | |

OBS	Dates of Observations	Age of Culture and Rate of Growth (Rapid, Intermediate, Slow) Medium, Temp of growth	Colony Size (fills plate or tube, restricted, etc.)	Pigmentation		Topography (convex, rugose, etc.) Texture (velvety, glabrous, etc.)
				Obverse	Reverse	

	OBS						
MOULD	1st						
	2nd						
	3rd						
YEAST	1st						
	2nd						
	3rd						

OBS	Hyphae: Width? Presence of septa?	Describe how conidia are produced (budding? on phialides? etc.)	Microconidia: Size? Shape? Other features?	Macroconidia: Size? Shape? Width & texture of cell wall? Other features?	Describe other structures on or in the hyphae

	OBS					
MOULD	1st					
	2nd					
	3rd					
YEAST	1st					
	2nd					
	3rd					

for Mould

for Yeast

FIGURE C.3

Blank laboratory work sheet for dimorphic fungi.

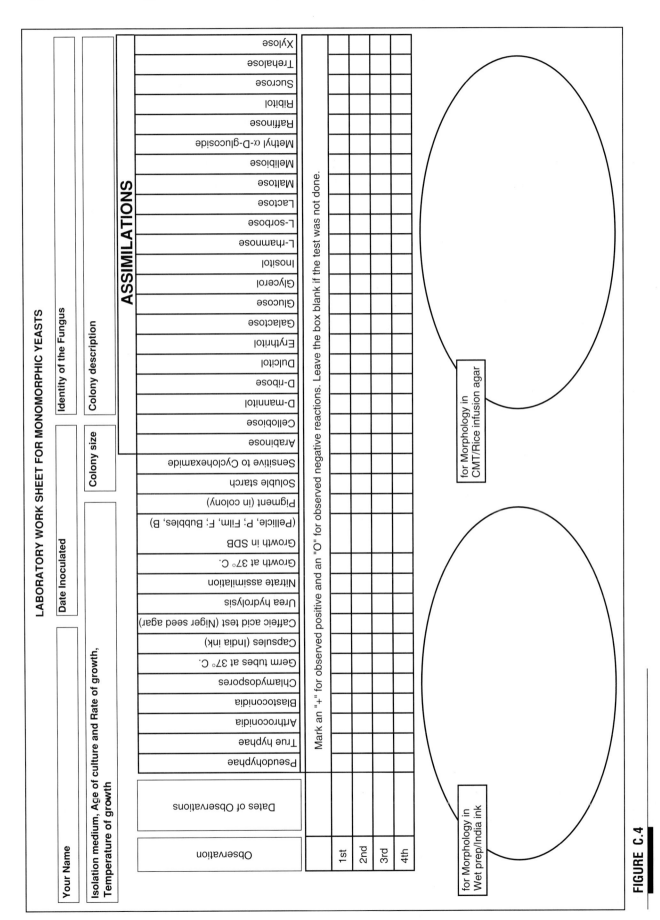

FIGURE C.4

Blank laboratory work sheet for monomorphic yeasts.

Additional Materials for a Scotch Tape Prep

LPCB (or other mounting fluid) in a dropper bottle
clear Scotch tape—*not* the "invisible" variety
tongue blades/tongue depressors
a culture

Additional Materials for a Slide Culture

To set it up

plate of agar (for the agar block)
scalpel (to cut the agar)—Bard-Parker handle and
  #11 blades, or disposable units
forceps with straight or bent points (to handle
  the coverslip)
alcohol bottle with alcohol (to sterilize the scalpel
  and forceps)
sterile slide culture set-up (glass Petri dish containing
  slide, coverslip, filter paper, glass rod, or other "mount")
sterile water
sterile pipette (dropper or transfer)
rubber bulb to use with pipette
a culture

To harvest it

forceps with straight and bent tips
LPCB (or other mounting fluid) in a dropper bottle
beaker of disinfectant (for agar blocks after they are
  removed from the slides)

Additional Materials to Transfer a Fungus Culture

tube or plate of fresh medium
a culture

RECOMMENDED TASK OUTLINE FOR A 16-WEEK COURSE

Detailed instructions for each laboratory exercise are
found in the related chapters and are not repeated here. A
proposed schedule for a 16-week mycology lab course
can be found in Figure C.5.

Laboratory Safety

Common sense and *aseptic technique* should be used.

Students should *wear lab coats and gloves* at all
times while working in the laboratory.

No extraneous items (purses, backpacks, etc.)
should be left on the counters during laboratories.

A *"place mat"* moistened with disinfectant should
be used at the work area.

Countertops and equipment should be disinfected *before and after* each laboratory.

FIRST LABORATORY (Techniques)

Demonstrations by the Instructor

1. Preparation of *direct mounts, Scotch tape preps,* and *slide cultures.*
2. Transfer (subculture) of a fungus culture to fresh medium.
3. Demonstration of various textures, topographies, and pigments.

Demonstration Materials

1. Culture of *Aspergillus fumigatus* to demonstrate preparation of tease mounts, Scotch tape preps, slide cultures, and methods for transfer of cultures.
2. Cultures of fungi showing various pigments, topographies, and textures to demonstrate features of colony
   morphology. Environmental cultures (prepared 3–4 days
   ahead) or a selection of saprobic fungi are good for this.

The Tasks (in the order in which they should be done)

1. Take cultures of airborne contaminants (Exercise 1:
   Environmental Cultures).
2. Examine and describe the morphologic features of a
   colony of a saprobic fungus (Exercise 2: Colony Description). Record the results on the LABORATORY
   WORK SHEET for monomorphic moulds (see Fig.
   C.2). A sample showing how the form can be used is
   provided (Fig. C.6).
3. Describe and draw the microscopic characteristics of
   the saprobe in two different kinds of preparations (Exercise 2: Tease Mount; Exercise 3: Scotch Tape Prep).
   Again, record your work on the LABORATORY
   WORK SHEET.
4. Set up a slide culture (Exercise 4: Slide Culture).

Laboratory Exercises

Exercise 1: Environmental Cultures (1st Session)
Exercise 2: Colony Description (1st Session)
Exercise 3: Scotch Tape Prep (1st Session)
Exercise 4: Slide Culture (1st Session)

Suggested Cultures for Exercises 2–4. 5–7-day
cultures of *Alternaria, Aspergillus, Cladosporium,* and
Penicillium on SDA.

LAB DATE	1	2	3	4	5	6	7	8	9	10	11	12	13	14	15
Exercise 1	1st session	2nd session													
Exercise 2	1st session														
Exercise 3	1st session														
Exercise 4	1st session	2nd session	3rd session												
Exercise 5		1st session	2nd session	3rd session	4th session										
Exercise 6				1st session	2nd session	3rd session									
Exercise 7						1st session	2nd session	3rd session							
Exercise 8							1st session	2nd session	3rd session						
Exercise 9									1st session	2nd session	3rd session				
Exercise 10									1st session	2nd session	3rd session				
Optional										1st session	2nd session	3rd session			
Exercise 11												1st session	2nd session	3rd session	
Exercise 12													1st session	2nd session	3rd session
Exercise 13														1st session	2nd session
Exercise 14															1st session

*The columns indicate the exercises to be done during a laboratory period.
The rows show the session of the exercise to be completed during each laboratory.

FIGURE C.5

Proposed laboratory schedule for a 16-week course.

LABORATORY WORK SHEET FOR MONOMORPHIC MOULDS

Your Name	Mary Edwards	Date Inoculated	4/10	Identity of the Fungus	Scopulariopsis species	4/19

MACROSCOPIC CHARACTERISTICS

Obs	Dates of Observations (see footnote*)	Age of Culture and Rate of Growth (record Rapid, Medium, Slow) Medium, Temp. of growth	Colony Size (fills plate or tube, restricted, etc.)	Pigmentation Obverse	Pigmentation Reverse	Topography (convex, rugose, etc.) Texture (velvety, glabrous, etc.)
1st	4/10	Inoculated on modified SDA–25°C				
2nd STP	4/14	Rapid growth 5 days old Note:–prepared slide culture	Restricted	Off white	Light Tan	Glabrous
3rd SC	4/19	9 days old Note:–Harvested SC	Almost fills the petri dish	Buff brown	Dark tan	Powdery/granular rugose wrinkled

MICROSCOPIC CHARACTERISTICS

Obs	Hyphae: Width? Presence of septa?	Describe how conidia are produced (budding? on phialides? etc.)	Microconidia: Size? Shape? Other features?	Macroconidia: Size? Shape? Width & texture of cell wall? Other features?	Describe other structures on or in the hyphae
1st DM	Hyaline septate 5 µm	NA	Globose 5-6 µm short chains	Only one type of conidia is produced	NA
2nd STP	Hyaline septate 5-6 µm	Conidia are produced by conidiophores that are individual or in penicillii	Globose 5-8 µm	Same	NA
3rd SC	Hyaline septate 5-6 µm	Conidia are produced in chains	Conidia are rough walled globose/pyriform with flattened bases 5-9 µm	Same	Conidiophores are cylindrical

Obs	Dates of Observations	Confirmatory tests done, if any	Reactions to confirmatory tests
1st		-0-	
2nd		-0-	
3rd		-0-	

Make your drawing(s) in the spaces provided below. Each drawing should include hyphae, micro- and macroconidia, and any miscellaneous vegetative structures you see. Show how the structures are connected to one another. LABEL THE STRUCTURES!

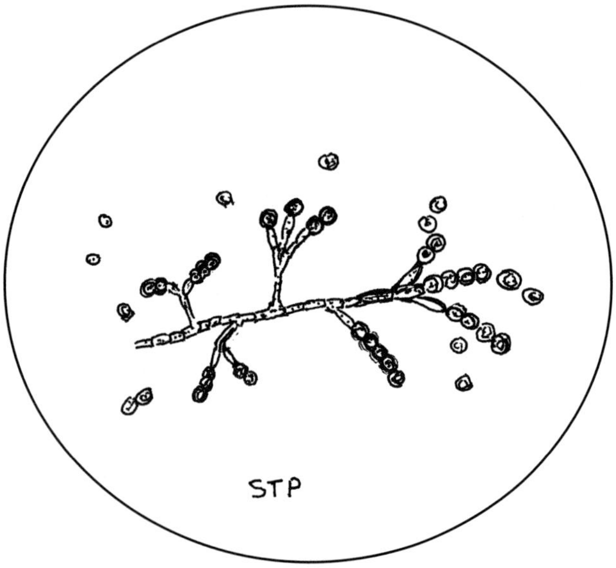

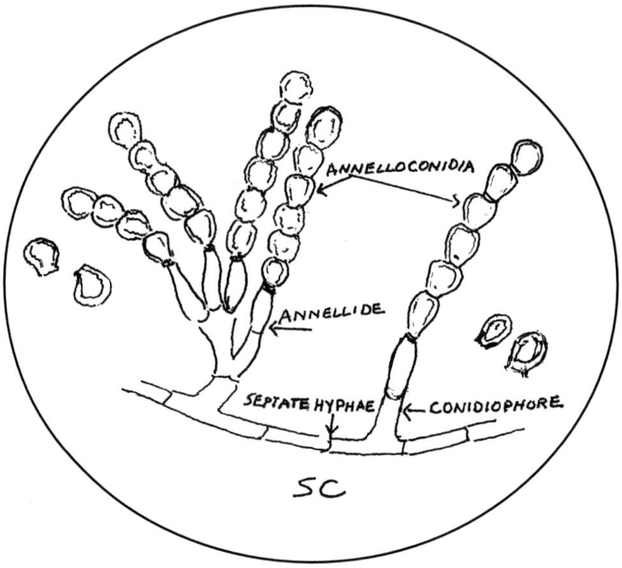

*Indicate the type of procedure/observation in this column, with the date. Use abbreviations. Direct Mount, DM; Scotch tape prep, STP; Slide culture, SC

FIGURE C.6

Sample laboratory work sheet for monomorphic moulds.

Reincubation of Cultures

> We assume that the maturity of a culture is always checked before further study is done. *This will not be stated for every session of every exercise.*
>
> Checking the maturity of a culture is good laboratory practice. Continuous repetition of this should not be necessary and only makes the book longer.
>
> The *consequences* of using an immature culture are that you have to repeat all or part of an exercise or that your conclusions will be based on misinformation.

SECOND LABORATORY (TECHNIQUES)

Demonstration by the Instructor

1. Correct procedure for microscopic examination of an intact slide culture to see whether it is mature ("ripe").

Demonstration Materials

1. Slide cultures of *Aspergillus fumigatus* of varying ages (2, 4, and 7 days) to demonstrate the method for ensuring that the slide culture is "ready" to be harvested and to show how slide cultures are harvested.

The Tasks (in the order in which they should be done)

1. Harvest the slide culture (Exercise 4).
2. Examine the environmental culture (Exercise 1) taken from the laboratory or classroom.
3. Subculture three saprobic fungi (Exercise 5) and set up slide cultures.

Laboratory Exercises

Exercise 1: Environmental Cultures (2nd Session)
Exercise 4: Slide Culture (2nd Session)
Exercise 5: Opportunistic Fungi (1st Session)

Suggested Cultures.[4] 5–7-day cultures of (Set 1) *Alternaria, Aureobasidium, Cladosporium;* (Set 2) *Curvularia, Drechslera, Helminthosporium;* (Set 3) *Fusarium;* (Set 4) *Gliocladium;* (Set 5) *Paecilomyces, Penicillium, Scopulariopsis;* (Set 6) 1 Zygomycetes (*Absidia, Mucor, Rhizopus, Syncephalastrum*); (Set 7) 1 *Aspergillus (A. fumigatus, A. flavus, A. niger, A. terreus).*

---

[4]Organisms in **bold type** were recommended for Exercises 2–4.

THIRD LABORATORY (SAPROBES)

Demonstrations by the Instructor

None

Demonstration Materials

None

The Tasks (in the order in which they should be done)

1. Study the three organisms that were subcultured last week (Exercise 5: Opportunistic Fungi) and harvest the slide cultures.
2. Examine the preparations from the slide culture (Exercise 4) and compare the three methods for examination of microscopic morphology of fungi.
3. Examine as many as possible of the slide preparations made by other students; describe the colonies also.

Laboratory Exercises

Exercise 4: Slide Culture (3rd Session)
Exercise 5: Opportunistic Fungi (2nd Session)

FOURTH LABORATORY (SAPROBES)

Demonstrations by the Instructor

None

Demonstration Materials

None

The Tasks (in the order in which they should be done)

1. Compare the advantages and disadvantages of the three procedures for the identification of microscopic structures (Exercises 2–4).
2. Examine the slide culture preparations of opportunistic fungi (Exercise 5).
3. Subculture the superficial fungi (Exercise 6) and set up slide cultures on them.
4. Study as many as possible of the slide preparations made by other students, including a description of the colonies.

Laboratory Exercises

Exercise 4: Slide Culture (4th Session)
Exercise 5: Opportunistic Fungi (3rd Session)
Exercise 6: Superficial Fungi (1st Session)

Suggested Cultures. *Exophiala werneckii* (2–3 weeks old[5]), *Trichosporon beigelii* on SDA, *Trichosporon beigelii* in malt extract broth.

FIFTH LABORATORY (SUPERFICIAL FUNGI)

Demonstrations by the Instructor

None

Demonstration Materials

1. Stock cultures and permanent mounts of superficial fungi other than *Exophiala werneckii* and *Trichosporon beigelii* for the students to examine are desirable but not essential.
2. Cultures (2–3 days old) of *Trichosporon beigelii* in malt extract broth, one per 3 or 4 students.

The Tasks (in the order in which they should be done)

1. Harvest the slide cultures set up last week (Exercise 6: Superficial Fungi).
2. Complete Exercise 5: Opportunistic Fungi.
3. Study the superficial fungi subcultured last week, including colony descriptions, tease mounts, and Scotch tape preps.
4. Do a wet prep of *Trichosporon beigelii* if a broth culture is available.
5. Compare the colony morphology of the young and the older mature cultures of superficial fungi.

Laboratory Exercises

Exercise 5: Opportunistic Fungi (4th Session)
Exercise 6: Superficial Fungi (2nd Session)

SIXTH LABORATORY (Superficial Fungi)

Demonstrations by the Instructor

None

---

[5]Using *Exophiala* cultures that are 2–3 weeks old allows students to compare the morphology of the young culture that they set up with the morphology of the older culture—a good opportunity to make the point that young cultures are yeastlike and mature colonies are mould forms.

Demonstration Materials

1. Permanent mounts and stock cultures of mature cultures of *Exophiala werneckii* and *Trichosporon beigelii*.
2. Stock cultures and permanent mounts of the other superficial fungi for the students to examine are desirable but not essential.

The Tasks (in the order in which they should be done)

1. Make drawings from the slide cultures of superficial fungi (Exercise 6: Superficial Fungi).
2. Compare the microscopic morphology of the young and mature cultures of the superficial fungi.
3. Subculture three dermatophytes and prepare slide cultures of them (Exercise 7: Dermatophytes).

Laboratory Exercises

Exercise 6: Superficial Fungi (3rd Session)
Exercise 7: Dermatophytes (1st Session)

Suggested Cultures. (Set 1) *Epidermophyton floccosum*; (Set 2) *Microsporum canis, M. gypseum, M. nanum, M. cookei, M. canis*; (Set 3) *Trichophyton mentagrophytes, T. rubrum, T. tonsurans*.

SEVENTH LABORATORY (Dermatophytes)

Demonstrations by the Instructor

1. Inoculation of differential tests for identification of dermatophytes without "carryover" of nutrients from the original culture.
2. Inoculation of urea agar, or "set up" of the rapid urea method (and interpretation of results of the test).
3. Preparation of the hair perforation test.

Demonstration Materials

Stock cultures of dermatophytes for use in demonstrating methods.

The Tasks (in the order in which they should be done)

1. Harvest the slide cultures of the dermatophytes (Exercise 7).
2. Study the organisms that were subcultured last week (Exercise 7), including colony descriptions, tease mounts, and Scotch tape preps.

3. Set up the differential tests for the dermatophytes (Exercise 8).

Additional Materials Needed for Exercise 8

Note that two sets of materials are needed for each medium or method, so that students set up both positive and negative tests. These quantities are the same whether students are working independently or are working in pairs to obtain the complete set of results.

> *Trichophyton* agars #1, #2, #3, and #4
> urea agar, or rapid urea method
> sterile water
> sterile yeast extract (10%$^{w/v}$)
> sterile hair that has not been treated with chemicals such as dyes, hair spray, or permanent wave solution—preferably from a young child
> sterile Petri dishes
> rice grain medium

Laboratory Exercises

> Exercise 7: Dermatophytes (2nd Session)
> Exercise 8: Differential Tests for Dermatophytes (1st Session)

> **Suggested Differential Procedures.** Growth on sterile rice grains; hair perforation test; urea utilization; growth on *Trichophyton* agars.

EIGHTH LABORATORY (DERMATOPHYTES)

Demonstrations by the Instructor

1. Reading "positive" and "negative" results of the hair perforation tests.
2. Colony morphology of dermatophytes and other organisms on dermatophyte test medium (DTM).
3. Interpretation of results of differential tests.

Demonstration Materials

1. Cultures (12–21 days old) of *Trichophyton verrucosum* and *Trichophyton tonsurans* on *Trichophyton* agars (#1, #2, #3, and #4), one set per 3 or 4 students.
2. Sterile rice grains inoculated with *Microsporum audouinii* and *Microsporum canis*, one set per 3 or 4 students.
3. Plates or tubes of DTM inoculated with each of the dermatophytes being studied, as well as a DTM plate/tube of one or two nondermatophytes (one positive, *Acremonium*, and one negative, *Paecilomyces*), one set per 3 or 4 students.
4. Slide preparations of positive and negative hair perforation tests, one set per 3 or 4 students.

5. Positive and negative urea tests (urea agar or rapid method), one set per 3 or 4 students.

The Tasks (in the order in which they should be done)

1. Make drawings from the slide culture preparations harvested last week (Exercise 7: Dermatophytes).
2. Examine the demonstration DTM cultures for the dermatophytes you selected and add the information to your LABORATORY WORK SHEETS.
3. Read the differential tests on the dermatophytes (Exercise 8) and interpret the results.
4. Interpret the hair perforation tests.

Laboratory Exercises

> Exercise 7: Dermatophytes (3rd Session)
> Exercise 8: Differential Tests for Dermatophytes (2nd Session)

NINTH LABORATORY (SUBCUTANEOUS FUNGI)

Demonstrations by the Instructor

> None

Demonstration Materials

> None

The Tasks (in the order in which they should be done)

Note that a different LABORATORY WORK SHEET is suggested for use with dimorphic fungi such as *Sporothrix*. The blank is provided (Fig. C.3). A sample showing how the form can be used is also provided (Fig. C.7).

1. Make a final reading of the differential tests for identification of the dermatophytes (Exercise 8) and interpret the results.
2. Examine as many as possible of the slide preparations made by other students (and the colony morphologies). Add the information *and the drawings* to your notebook.
3. Subculture three subcutaneous fungi and prepare slide cultures of them (Exercise 9: Subcutaneous Moulds; Exercise 10: *Sporothrix*).
4. Read hair perforation (Exercise 8: Differential Tests for Dermatophytes).

LABORATORY WORK SHEET FOR DIMORPHIC FUNGI

our Name	Date Inoculated	Identity of the Fungus
Susan Stanley	5/20	Sporothrix schenckii 5/28

	OBS	Dates of Observations	Age of Culture and Rate of Growth (Rapid, Intermediate, Slow) Medium, Temp of growth	Colony Size (fills plate or tube, restricted, etc.)	Pigmentation Obverse	Pigmentation Reverse	Topography (convex, rugose, etc.) Texture (velvety, glabrous, etc.)
MOULD	1st	5/24	MOD. SDA 30°C–4 days– rapid subcultured to BHIA– 37°C	Restricted	White to cream colored	Cream colored and mottled	Flat Yeast-like glabrous
MOULD	2nd						
MOULD	3rd						
YEAST	1st	5/28	BHIA at 37°C–8 days in 5% CO_2 slow	Restricted	Cream colored	Cream colored	Yeast-like glabrous– moist convex
YEAST	2nd						
YEAST	3rd						

	OBS	Hyphae: Width? Presence of septa?	Describe how conidia are produced (budding? on phialides? etc.)	Microconidia: Size? Shape? Other features?	Macroconidia: Size? Shape? Width & texture of cell wall? Other features?	Describe other structures on or in the hyphae
MOULD	1st	1–2μm septate hyaline	Mould at 30°C: produced on slender conidiophores and occasionally on hyphae	Pyriform 2-5μm arranged around apex of conidiophore	NA	Conidiophores arise at 90° angles and are swollen at their apices
MOULD	2nd					
MOULD	3rd					
YEAST	1st	NA	Yeast on BHIA at 37°C produced by budding	2-3 x 3-8μm	NA	Some typical cigar-shaped yeast forms are present
YEAST	2nd					
YEAST	3rd					

for Mould

for Yeast

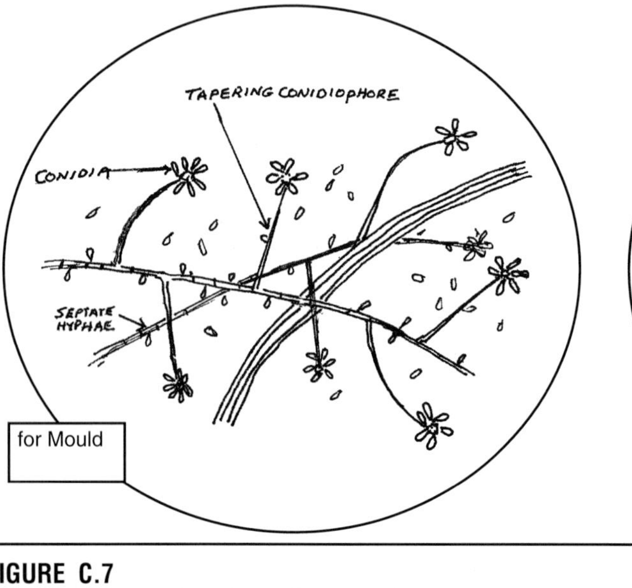

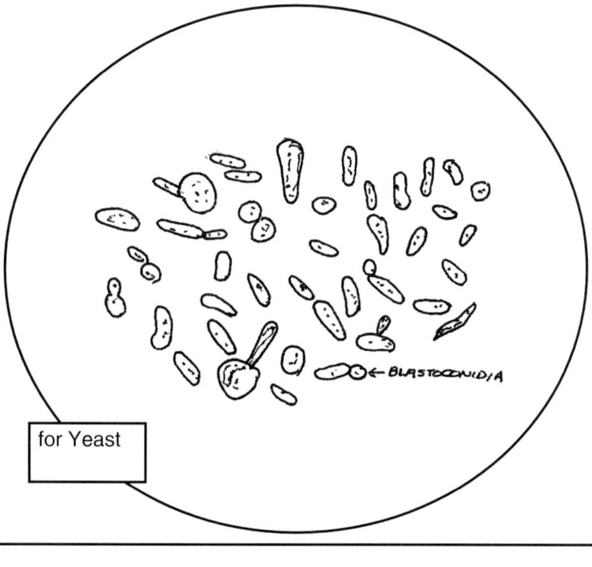

FIGURE C.7

Sample laboratory work sheet for dimorphic fungi.

304

Laboratory Exercises

> Exercise 8: Differential Tests for Dermatophytes (3rd Session)
> Exercise 9: Subcutaneous Moulds (1st Session)

> **Suggested Cultures.** (Set 1) 2–3-week cultures of *Exophiala jeanselmei*, *Wangiella dermatitidis*; (Set 2) *Cladosporium carrionii*, *Fonsecaea pedrosoi*, *Phialophora verrucosa*; (Set 3) *Pseudallescheria boydii*, *Scedosporium apiospernum*.

> Exercise 10: *Sporothrix* (1st Session)

> **Culture Needed.** *Sporothrix schenckii*.

TENTH LABORATORY (SUBCUTANEOUS FUNGI)

Demonstrations by the Instructor

1. Inoculation of differential tests for identification of the subcutaneous fungi.

Demonstration Materials

1. Cultures of *Sporothrix schenckii* in the yeast phase on brain-heart infusion (BHI) agar with blood (or on SDA) and in BHI broth, one set per 3 or 4 students.
2. Mould cultures of several subcutaneous fungi to demonstrate inoculation of differential tests for identification of these organisms.

The Tasks (in the order in which they should be done)

1. Harvest the slide cultures of the subcutaneous organisms (Exercise 9).
2. Study the organisms that were subcultured last week and incubated at 25°C (Exercise 9), including colony descriptions, tease mounts, and Scotch tape preps.
3. Describe the colony of *Sporothrix schenckii* incubated at 37°C (Exercise 10). Make a wet prep of the colony and examine it.
4. Compare the colony morphologies and the microscopic structures of *Sporothrix schenckii* at the two different temperatures of incubation.
5. Set up tests for the differentiation of subcutaneous fungi (Optional Exercise).

Additional Materials Needed for Optional Exercise

Note that two sets of materials are needed for each medium or method, so that students set up both positive and negative tests. These quantities are the same whether students are working independently or in pairs to obtain the complete set of results.

> Gelatin medium
> SDA medium (two tubes per organism)
> Casein medium
> SDA plus cycloheximide
> Nitrate medium *or* rapid nitrate medium

Laboratory Exercises

> Exercise 9: Subcutaneous Moulds (2nd Session)
> Exercise 10: *Sporothrix* (2nd Session)
> Optional Exercise: Differential Tests for Subcutaneous Moulds (1st Session)
>> Growth at 37°C
>> Gelatin liquefaction
>> Rate of growth
>> Casein digestion
>> Nitrate utilization
>> Resistance to cycloheximide

ELEVENTH LABORATORY (SUBCUTANEOUS FUNGI)

Demonstrations by the Instructor

1. Interpretation of results of differential tests for identification of subcutaneous fungi.

Demonstration Materials

1. Differential tests for subcutaneous organisms, showing positive and negative results in each test.

The Tasks (in the order in which they should be done)

1. Read the permanent mounts of your subcutaneous fungi that were prepared from the slide cultures and make your drawings (Exercise 9: Subcutaneous Moulds; Exercise 10: *Sporothrix*).
2. Record the reactions in the differential tests for subcutaneous moulds (Optional Exercise) and interpret the results.
3. Transfer five yeasts to fresh media (Exercise 11: Yeasts and Yeastlike Fungi).

Laboratory Exercises

> Exercise 9: Subcutaneous Moulds (3rd Session)
> Exercise 10: *Sporothrix* (2nd Session)
> Optional Exercise: Differential Tests for Subcutaneous Fungi (2nd Session)
> Exercise 11: Yeasts and Yeastlike Fungi (1st Session)

Suggested Cultures. (Set 1) *Candida albicans;* (Set 2) *Cryptococcus neoformans;* (Set 3) *Geotrichum candidum, Trichosporon beigelii*[6]; (Set 4) *Candida* species (*C. parapsilosis, C. kefyr, C. tropicalis, C. guilliermondii, C. krusei), Rhodotorula rubra, Saccharomyces cerevisiae.*

TWELFTH LABORATORY (YEASTS)

Demonstrations by the Instructor

1. Setting up, reading, and interpreting the germ tube test.
2. "Cut-streak" method for assessing the microscopic morphology of yeasts in CMT or rice infusion agar.
3. Inoculation of differential tests for identification of yeasts.
4. Preparation and interpretation of India ink preps.

Demonstration Materials

1. Stock cultures of yeasts to use in demonstrating differential methods.
2. Germ tube tests demonstrating positive and negative reactions.
3. India ink preps that show "positive" and "negative" reactions.

The Tasks (in the order in which they should be done)

Note that a different LABORATORY WORK SHEET is suggested for identification of yeasts. It is provided (Fig. C.4), with a sample showing how the form can be used (Fig. C.8) following this laboratory.

1. Set up the germ tube tests (Exercise 12).
2. Make and examine wet preps of your yeast cultures, including both simple wet preps and India ink preps (Exercise 11).
3. Read the differential tests for subcutaneous moulds (Optional Exercise).
4. Read the germ tube tests.
5. Set up the cut-streak plates and the other differential tests on your yeast cultures. Wait until the next laboratory to do any "rapid" tests.
6. Examine as many as possible of the slide preparations of subcutaneous fungi done by your classmates. Record colony morphologies and the results of differential tests, as well as the drawings, in your notebook.

---

[6]Yes, you have seen *Trichosporon beigelii* before, but you didn't perform biochemical tests on the culture. *Trichosporon cutaneum* can be substituted for *T. beigelii;* using *T. beigelii* again saves the expense of obtaining the *T. cutaneum* culture.

Laboratory Exercises

Optional Exercise: Differential Tests for Subcutaneous Moulds (3rd Session)
Exercise 11: Yeast and Yeastlike Fungi (2nd Session)
Exercise 12: Differential Tests for Yeast and Yeastlike Fungi (1st Session)

Suggested Differential Procedures. Germ tube test, morphology in CMT/rice infusion agar, India ink prep, caffeic acid test, assimilations (carbohydrates and nitrate), urea hydrolysis, pellicle formation, temperature tolerance.

THIRTEENTH LABORATORY (YEASTS)

Demonstrations by the Instructor

1. Inoculation of rapid methods for differentiation of yeasts, if these were not done during the previous session.
2. Recording and interpreting the results of differential tests for yeasts.
3. Microscopic examination and interpretation of cut-streak plates.

Demonstration Materials

1. Cut-streak plates demonstrating various morphologies of the yeasts, especially chlamydospore production.
2. Sets of differential tests for yeasts, showing positive and negative reactions.
3. Stock cultures of yeasts for inoculation of rapid methods, if these are to be demonstrated.

The Tasks (in the order in which they should be done)

1. Set up rapid methods for yeasts (if any): urea, nitrate, and/or commercial kits.
2. Examine your cut-streak plates and add the drawings to the LABORATORY WORK SHEETS.
3. Read and interpret the results of the differential tests on your yeasts.
4. Examine as many as possible of the yeast cultures and cut-streak plates prepared by your classmates, adding the information and drawings to your notebook (including test results).

Laboratory Exercises

Exercise 11: Yeasts and Yeastlike Fungi (3rd Session)
Exercise 12: Differential Tests for Yeasts and Yeastlike Fungi (2nd Session)

LABORATORY WORK SHEET FOR MONOMORPHIC YEASTS

Your Name	Date Inoculated	Identity of the Fungus
Ron Ferrigno	3/8	Candida guillermondii 3/12

Isolation medium, Age of culture and Rate of growth, Temperature of growth
Mod. SDA–3 days–rapid 25°C

Colony size
small/entire

Colony description
White, pasty, convex with short pseudohyphal fringes

ASSIMILATIONS

Mark an "+" for observed positive and an "O" for observed negative reactions. Leave the box blank if the test was not done.

Observation	Dates of Observations	Pseudohyphae	True hyphae	Arthroconidia	Blastoconidia	Chlamydospores	Germ tubes at 37° C.	Capsules (India ink)	Caffeic acid test (Niger seed agar)	Urea hydrolysis	Nitrate assimilation	Growth at 37° C.	Growth in SDB (Pellicle, P; Film, F; Bubbles, B)	Pigment (in colony)	Soluble starch	Sensitive to Cyclohexamide	Arabinose	Cellobiose	D-mannitol	D-ribose	Dulcitol	Erythritol	Galactose	Glucose	Glycerol	Inositol	L-rhamnose	L-sorbose	Lactose	Maltose	Melibiose	Methyl a-D-glucoside	Raffinose	Ribitol	Sucrose	Trehalose	Xylose
1st	3/10–3/12	+	O	O	+	O	O	O	O	O	O	+	F	O	O	+	+	+		+	+	O	+	+	+	O			O	+	+	+	+	+	+	+	+
2nd																																					
3rd																																					
4th																																					

for Morphology in CMT/Rice infusion agar

(labels: PSEUDOHYPHAE, BLASTOCONIDIA)

for Morphology in Wet prep/India ink

(label: BUDDING BLASTOCONIDIA)

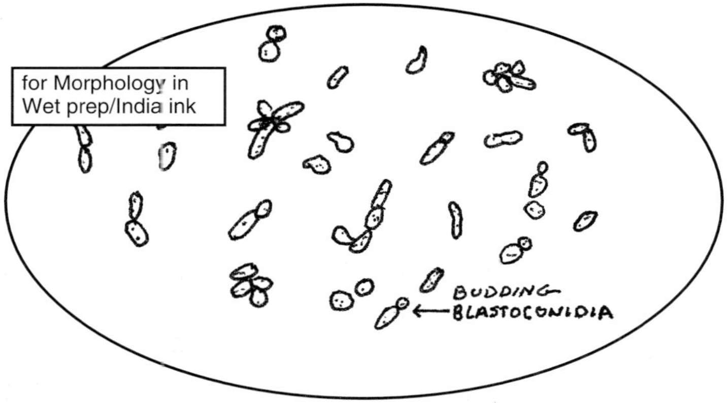

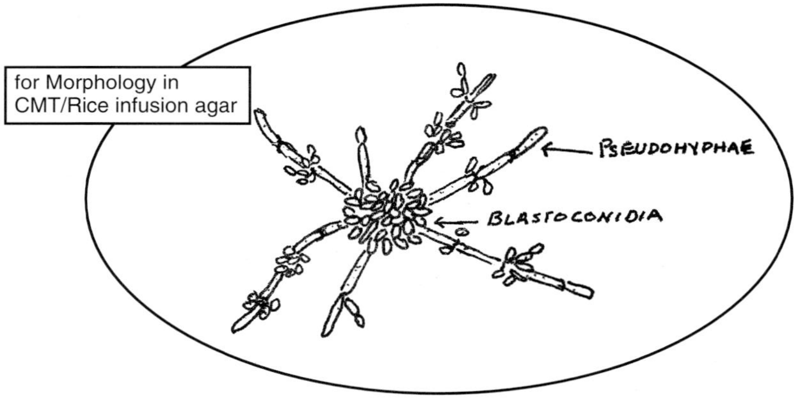

FIGURE C.8

Sample laboratory work sheet for monomorphic yeasts.

FOURTEENTH LABORATORY (SYSTEMIC FUNGI)

Demonstrations by the Instructor

None

Demonstration Materials

1. Stock cultures of nonviable yeast and mould form cultures of as many of the systemic fungi as possible *or* 35-mm slides or other illustrations of the cultures.
2. Permanent slide mounts of yeast/tissue and mould forms of as many of the systemic fungi as possible *or* 35-mm slides or other illustrations of the microscopic structures.

The Tasks (in the order in which they should be done)

1. Complete Exercise 12 (Differential Tests for Yeasts and Yeastlike Fungi).
2. Examine colony morphologies of the systemic fungi (Exercise 13).
3. Examine microscopic morphologies of yeast/tissue and mould forms of the systemic dimorphic fungi, and make drawings in your notebook!

Laboratory Exercises

Exercise 12: Differential Tests for Yeasts and Yeastlike Fungi (3rd Session)
Exercise 13: Systemic Fungi (1st Session)

Suggested Cultures. *Blastomyces dermatitidis, Coccidioides immitis, Histoplasma capsulatum, Paracoccidioides brasiliensis.*

FIFTEENTH LABORATORY (SYSTEMIC FUNGI)

Demonstrations by the Instructor

None

Demonstration Materials

None

The Tasks

REVIEW!   REVIEW!   REVIEW!

1. Complete any exercises that are outstanding.
2. Review your notes and drawings to ensure that they are as complete as possible.
3. Examine as many as possible of the cultures and slide preparations, done by your classmates, that you have not read previously.

4. Clean your work area, discarding any extraneous materials that have been pushed to the back of your drawer or locker and arranging your permanent mounts neatly in a slide flat or box for your instructor to review.

RECOMMENDED TASK OUTLINE FOR AN 8-WEEK COURSE

Detailed instructions for each laboratory exercise are found in the related chapters; they are not repeated here. A proposed schedule for an 8-week mycology lab course can be found in Figure C.9. Teaching the course in 8 rather than 16 weeks means that subcultures and slide cultures are less likely to mature "on schedule" so that some exercises may drag out longer than the suggested plan indicates.

Laboratory Safety

Common sense and *good aseptic technique* should be used at all times.

Students should *wear lab coats and gloves* while working in the laboratory.

Purses and backpacks—*ALL nonessential stuff*—should be removed from the work areas.

A *"place mat"* dampened with disinfectant should be used.

Countertops and equipment should be disinfected *before and after* each laboratory.

Exercise 4 may be omitted since Exercise 5 (Opportunistic Fungi) is scheduled for the same laboratory session. Retaining Exercise 4 is recommended, because it does not lengthen the laboratory significantly *and* because the most complete instructions for the technique are given here. If Exercise 4 is skipped, these instructions should still be used for making the first slide culture.

The Optional Exercise, methods for identification of subcutaneous fungi, is omitted. Exercise 8 (tests for identification of dermatophytes) can also be omitted, but the procedures and results should be demonstrated.

FIRST LABORATORY (TECHNIQUES)

Demonstrations by the Instructor

1. Techniques for the preparation of *direct mounts, Scotch tape preps,* and *slide cultures.*
2. Demonstration of various textures, topographies, and pigments.
3. Transfer of a fungus culture to fresh medium.

LAB DATE	1	2	3	4	5	6	7
Exercise 1	1st session	2nd session					
Exercise 2	1st session						
Exercise 3	1st session						
Exercise 4	1st session	2nd session	3rd session				
Exercise 5	1st session	2nd session	3rd session	4th session			
Exercise 6		1st session	2nd session	3rd session			
Exercise 7			1st session	2nd session	3rd session		
Exercise 8				1st session	2nd session	3rd session	
Exercise 9				1st session	2nd session	3rd session	
Exercise 10				1st session	2nd session	3rd session	
Optional							
Exercise 11					1st session	2nd session	3rd session
Exercise 12						1st session	2nd session
Exercise 13							1st session
Exercise 14							1st session

*The columns indicate the exercises to be done during a laboratory period.
The rows show the session of the exercise to be completed during each laboratory.

FIGURE C.9

Proposed laboratory schedule for an 8-week course.

Demonstration Materials

1. Culture of *Aspergillus fumigatus* to demonstrate methods.
2. Cultures demonstrating a variety of topographies, pigments, and textures. Environmental cultures can be taken in advance for this demonstration, or a selection of saprobic fungi can be used.

The Tasks (in the order in which they should be done)

1. Take cultures of airborne contaminants (Exercise 1: Environmental Cultures).
2. Examine and describe the morphologic features of a colony of a saprobic fungus (Exercise 2: Colony Description). Record the results on the LABORATORY WORK SHEET for monomorphic moulds (see Fig. C.2). A sample showing how the form can be used is provided (see Fig. C.6).
3. Make two different kinds of preparations (Exercise 2: Tease Mount; Exercise 3: Scotch Tape Prep). Examine the preparations and describe and draw the microscopic characteristics of the saprobic fungus. Again, record your work on the LABORATORY WORK SHEET.
4. Compare the advantages and disadvantages of the two procedures for the identification of microscopic structures (Exercises 2 and 3).

5. Prepare four slide cultures (Exercise 4: Slide Culture[7]; Exercise 5: Opportunistic Fungi).
6. Subculture the opportunistic fungi to fresh media (Exercise 5).

Reincubation of Cultures

We assume that the maturity of a culture will always be checked before further study is done. *This will not be stated for every session of every exercise.*

Checking the maturity of a culture is good laboratory practice. Continuous repetition of this should not be necessary and only makes the book longer.

The *consequences* of using an immature culture are that you will have to repeat all or part of an exercise or that your conclusions will be based on misinformation.

---

[7]The additional slide culture done in Exercise 4 may be omitted, but the instructions provided in Exercise 4 should be used for the Exercise 5 slide cultures.

Laboratory Exercises

Exercise 1: Environmental Cultures (1st Session)
Exercise 2: Colony Description (1st Session)
Exercise 3: Scotch Tape Prep (1st Session)
Exercise 4: Slide Culture (1st Session)

Suggested Cultures. 5–7-day cultures of *Alternaria, Aspergillus, Cladosporium, Penicillium* on SDA.

Exercise 5: Opportunistic Fungi (1st Session)

Suggested Cultures.[8] 5–7-day cultures of (Set 1) ***Alternaria,*** *Aureobasidium,* ***Cladosporium;*** (Set 2) *Curvularia, Drechslera, Helminthosporium;* (Set 3) *Fusarium;* (Set 4) *Gliocladium;* (Set 5) *Paecilomyces,* ***Penicillium,*** *Scopulariopsis;* (Set 6) 1 Zygomycetes *(Absidia, Mucor, Rhizopus, Syncephalastrum);* (Set 7) 1 ***Aspergillus*** *(A. fumigatus, A. flavus, A. niger, A. terreus).*

SECOND LABORATORY

Demonstrations by the Instructor

1. Techniques for harvesting slide cultures.
2. Procedure for microscopic examination of an intact slide culture to see whether it is mature ("ripe").

Demonstration Materials

1. Slide cultures of *Aspergillus fumigatus* of varying ages (2, 4, and 7 days) to demonstrate the method for ensuring that the slide culture is "ready" to be harvested and to show how slide cultures are harvested.

The Tasks (in the order in which they should be done)

1. Harvest the slide culture (Exercise 4) and examine the microscopic preparation(s).
2. Harvest the three slide cultures (Exercise 5: Opportunistic Fungi).
3. Examine the environmental cultures (Exercise 1) taken from the laboratory or classroom.
4. Subculture superficial fungi (Exercise 6) and set up a slide culture on each.

---

[8]Organisms in **bold type** were recommended for Exercises 2–4.

Laboratory Exercises

Exercise 1: Environmental Cultures (2nd Session)
Exercise 4: Slide Culture (2nd Session)
Exercise 5: Opportunistic Fungi (2nd Session)
Exercise 6: Superficial Fungi (1st Session)

Suggested Cultures. *Exophiala werneckii* (2–3 weeks old[9]), *Trichosporon beigelii* on SDA, *T. beigelii* in malt extract broth.

THIRD LABORATORY

Demonstrations by the Instructor

None

Demonstration Materials

1. Stock cultures and permanent mounts of superficial fungi other than *Exophiala werneckii* and *Trichosporon beigelii* for the students to examine are desirable but not essential.
2. Cultures (2–3 days old) of *Trichosporon beigelii* in malt extract broth, one per 3 or 4 students.

The Tasks (in the order in which they should be done)

1. Examine the slide cultures (Exercise 5: Opportunistic Fungi) from the previous laboratory.
2. Complete the slide cultures (Exercise 4) that you set up during the first laboratory session.
3. Study the three organisms that were subcultured last week (Exercise 6: Superficial Fungi), including colony descriptions, tease mounts, and Scotch tape preps. Harvest the slide cultures.
4. Compare the tease mount, Scotch tape, and slide culture methods for examining the microscopic morphology of fungi.
5. Do a wet prep of *Trichosporon beigelii.*
6. Compare the colony morphology of young and older mature cultures of superficial fungi.
7. Subculture three dermatophytes and prepare slide cultures of them (Exercise 7).

Laboratory Exercises

Exercise 4: Slide Culture (3rd Session)
Exercise 5: Opportunistic Fungi (3rd Session)
Exercise 6: Superficial Fungi (2nd Session)
Exercise 7: Dermatophytes (1st Session)

---

[9]Using *Exophiala* cultures that are 2–3 weeks old allows students to compare the morphology of the young culture that they set up with the morphology of the older culture—a good opportunity to make the point that young cultures are yeastlike and mature colonies are mould forms.

Suggested Cultures. (Set 1) *Epidermophyton floccosum;* (Set 2) *Microsporum canis, M. gypseum, M. nanum, M. cookei, M. canis;* (Set 3) *Trichophyton mentagrophytes, T. rubrum, T. tonsurans.*

FOURTH LABORATORY

Demonstrations by Instructor

1. Inoculation of differential methods without "carry-over" of nutrients from the original culture medium.
2. Setting up the hair perforation test, and microscopic examination of infected hairs to see the presence and absence of perforations.
3. Interpretation of growth on DTM.

Demonstration Materials

1. Stock cultures of dermatophytes on SDA for inoculation of differential tests for dermatophytes.

The Tasks (in the order in which they should be done)

Note that a different LABORATORY WORK SHEET is suggested for use with dimorphic fungi such as *Sporothrix* (see Fig. C.3). A sample showing how the form can be used (see Fig. C.7) is provided.

1. Harvest the slide cultures of the dermatophytes (Exercise 7), if enough mature conidia have been produced.
2. Complete the slide cultures (Exercise 5: Opportunistic Fungi; Exercise 6: Superficial Fungi) that you harvested last week.
3. Study the organisms that were subcultured last week (Exercise 7: Dermatophytes), including colony descriptions, tease mounts, and Scotch tape preps.
4. Set up the differential tests for the dermatophytes (Exercise 8).
5. Compare the microscopic and colony morphology of cultures of superficial fungi (Exercise 6).
6. Subculture three subcutaneous fungi and prepare slide cultures of them (Exercise 9: Subcutaneous Moulds; Exercise 10: *Sporothrix*).

Additional Materials Needed for Exercise 8

Note that two sets of materials are needed for each medium or method, so that students will set up both positive and negative tests. These quantities are the same whether students are working independently or are working in pairs to obtain a complete set of results. *The demonstration planned for the Fifth Laboratory Session may be substituted for this laboratory exercise.*

Trichophyton agars #1, #2, #3, and #4
urea agar, or rapid urea method

sterile water
sterile yeast extract (10%$^{W/V}$)
sterile hair that has not been treated with chemicals such as dyes, hair spray, or permanent wave solution—preferably from a young child
sterile Petri dishes
rice grain medium

Laboratory Exercises

Exercise 5: Opportunistic Fungi (4th Session)
Exercise 6: Superficial Fungi (3rd Session)
Exercise 7: Dermatophytes (2nd Session)
Exercise 8: Differential Tests for Dermatophytes (1st Session)

Suggested Differential Procedures. Growth on sterile rice grains; hair perforation test; urea utilization; growth on *Trichophyton* agars.

Exercise 9: Subcutaneous Moulds (1st Session)

Suggested Cultures. (Set 1) 2–3-week cultures of *Exophiala jeanselmei*[10], *Wangiella dermatitidis;* (Set 2) *Cladosporium carrionii, Fonsecaea pedrosoi, Phialophora verrucosa;* (Set 3) *Pseudallescheria boydii, Scedosporium apiospernum.*

Exercise 10: *Sporothrix* (1st Session)

Culture Needed. *Sporothrix schenckii.*

FIFTH LABORATORY

Demonstrations by the Instructor

1. Reading and interpreting positive and negative tests for the identification of dermatophytes.

Demonstration Materials

1. Cultures (12–21 days old) of *Trichophyton tonsurans* and *T. verrucosum* on *Trichophyton* agars (#1, #2, #3, and #4), one set per 3 or 4 students.
2. Sterile rice grains inoculated with *Microsporum audouinii* and *M. canis*, one set per 3 or 4 students.
3. Plates or tubes of DTM inoculated with each of the dermatophytes being studied, as well as a DTM plate/tube with 1 or 2 nondermatophytes (1 positive, *Acremonium*, and 1 negative, *Paecilomyces*), one set per 3 or 4 students.
4. Slide preparations of positive and negative hair perforation tests, one set per 3 or 4 students.

---

[10]Using *Exophiala* cultures that are 2–3 weeks old allows students to compare the morphology of the young culture that they set up with the morphology of the older culture—a good opportunity to make the point that young cultures are yeastlike and mature colonies are mould forms.

5. Positive and negative urea tests (urea agar or rapid method), one set per 3 or 4 students.
6. Culture of *Sporothrix schenckii* in the yeast phase on BHI agar and in BHI broth, one set per 3 or 4 students.

The Tasks (in the order in which they should be done)

1. Set up the urea test for dermatophytes *if* this is the method being used and *if* you did not accomplish this during the previous laboratory.
2. Harvest the slide cultures of the subcutaneous organisms (Exercise 9: Subcutaneous Moulds; Exercise 10: *Sporothrix*).
3. If necessary, complete the slide cultures (Exercise 7: Dermatophytes) that you harvested last week.
4. Study the organisms that were subcultured last week (Exercise 9: Subcutaneous Moulds; Exercise 10: *Sporothrix*), including colony descriptions, tease mounts, and Scotch tape preps.
5. Make a wet prep of the culture of *Sporothrix schenckii* that was incubated at 35–37°C. Examine it and make the drawing.
6. Compare the colony morphologies and the microscopic structures of *Sporothrix schenckii* at the two different temperatures of incubation.
7. Transfer five yeasts to fresh media (Exercise 11: Yeasts and Yeastlike Fungi).

Laboratory Exercises

> Exercise 7: Dermatophytes (3rd Session)
> Exercise 8: Differential Tests for Dermatophytes (2nd Session)
> Exercise 9: Subcutaneous Moulds (2nd Session)
> Exercise 10: *Sporothrix* (2nd Session)
> Exercise 11: Yeasts and Yeastlike Fungi (1st Session)

> **Suggested Cultures.** (Set 1) *Candida albicans;* (Set 2) *Cryptococcus neoformans;* (Set 3) *Geotrichum candidum, Trichosporon beigelii*[11]; (Set 4) *Candida* species (*C. parapsilosis, C. kefyr, C. tropicalis, C. guilliermondii, C. krusei*), *Rhodotorula rubra, Saccharomyces cerevisiae.*

SIXTH LABORATORY

Demonstrations by the Instructor

1. Setting up and reading a germ tube test.
2. Reading an India ink prep—identification of capsule.
3. Inoculation of differential methods for identification of yeasts.

4. "Cut-streak" method for determining microscopic morphology of yeasts in CMT or rice infusion agar.

Demonstration Materials

1. Stock cultures of yeasts to use in demonstrating differential methods.
2. Germ tube tests demonstrating positive and negative reactions.
3. India ink preps that show "positive" and "negative" reactions.

The Tasks (in the order in which they should be done)

Note that a different LABORATORY WORK SHEET is recommended for identification of yeasts. The blank form is provided (see Fig. C.4). A sample showing how the form can be used is provided (see Fig. C.8).

1. Describe the colony morphologies of the yeast cultures. Make and examine wet preps of the cultures, including both simple and India ink preps (Exercise 11).
2. Set up the germ tube test and any other "rapid" differential tests you are using for identification of yeasts (Exercise 12).
3. Harvest the slide cultures of the subcutaneous organisms, if growth is sufficient, or reincubate them (Exercise 9: Subcutaneous Moulds; Exercise 10: *Sporothrix*).
4. Complete the slide cultures (Exercise 7: Dermatophytes) that you harvested last week.
5. Describe the colony of *Sporothrix schenckii* incubated at 37°C (Exercise 10). Make a wet prep of the colony and examine it.
6. Compare the colony morphologies and the microscopic structures of *Sporothrix schenckii* at the two different temperatures of incubation.
7. Set up the remaining tests for differentiation of yeasts (Exercise 12).

Laboratory Exercises

> Exercise 8: Differential Tests for Dermatophytes (3rd Session)
> Exercise 9: Subcutaneous Moulds (3rd Session)
> Exercise 10: *Sporothrix* (3rd Session)
> Exercise 11: Yeasts and Yeastlike Fungi (2nd Session)
> Exercise 12: Differential Tests for Yeasts and Yeastlike Fungi (1st Session)

> **Suggested Differential Procedures.** Germ tube test, morphology in CMT/rice infusion agar, India ink prep, caffeic acid test, assimilations (carbohydrates and nitrate), urea hydrolysis, pellicle formation, temperature patterns.

---

[11]Yes, you have seen *Trichosporon beigelii* before, but you didn't perform biochemical tests on the culture. *Trichosporon cutaneum* can be substituted for *T. beigelii;* using *T. beigelii* again saves the expense of obtaining the *T. cutaneum* culture.

SEVENTH LABORATORY

Demonstrations by the Instructor

None

Demonstration Materials

1. Positive and negative reactions in the germ tube and India ink tests and in other tests for the identification of yeast.
2. Nonviable representative cultures of the systemic pathogens in both the tissue/yeast and mould forms *or* 35-mm slides (or other illustrations) of colony morphology of these fungi.
3. Permanent slides of the systemic pathogens in culture and/or in tissue *or* 35-mm slides (or other illustrations) of the microscopic morphology of the systemic pathogens in both the tissue/yeast and mould forms.

The Tasks (in the order in which they should be done)

Use the correct LABORATORY WORK SHEET (Fig. C.3) for the dimorphic fungi (presented in the Fourth Laboratory) and for the yeasts (Fig. C.4).

1. Complete Exercises 11 and 12 (Yeasts and Yeastlike Fungi).
2. Examine colony morphologies of the systemic fungi (Exercise 13).
3. Examine microscopic morphologies of yeast/tissue and mould forms of the systemic dimorphic fungi, and make drawings in your notebook!
4. Complete any exercises that are outstanding.

REVIEW!   REVIEW!   REVIEW!

5. Review your notes and drawings to ensure that they are as complete as possible.
6. Examine as many as possible of the cultures and slide preparations, done by your classmates, that you have not read previously.
7. Clean your work area, discarding any extraneous materials that have been pushed to the back of your drawer or locker and arranging your permanent mounts neatly in a slide flat or box for your instructor to review.

Laboratory Exercises

Exercises 11 and 12: Yeasts and Yeastlike Fungi
Exercise 13: Systemic Fungi

Suggested Cultures. *Blastomyces dermatitidis, Coccidioides immitis, Histoplasma capsulatum, Paracoccidioides brasiliensis.*

RECOMMENDED TASK OUTLINE FOR A 10-DAY COURSE

The suggested plan for a 10-day mycology laboratory is somewhat like a jigsaw puzzle in which some of the pieces are warped. Laboratory sessions for selected exercises are ignored, and the sessions for other exercises are widely separated to allow time for cultures to mature. The instructor must also use ingenuity in configuring the instructions in the chapters so they will fit the abbreviated time frame. A 10-day course is certainly not ideal, or even optimal, but it can be done. Continuing increases in the incidence of mycotic infections have raised the demand for clinical mycologists; a 10-day lab course is infinitely better than no lab course at all.

Laboratory Safety

Common sense and *good aseptic technique* should be used at all times.

Students should *wear lab coats and gloves* while working in the laboratory.

Purses and backpacks—*ALL nonessential stuff*—should be removed from the work areas.

A *"place mat"* dampened with disinfectant should be used.

Countertops and equipment should be disinfected *before and after* each laboratory.

A proposed schedule for the 10-day mycology lab course can be found following this introductory section (Fig. C.10). *Note* that two exercises (Exercise 8 and the Optional Exercise) that involve setting up differential tests are omitted. Demonstrations can be substituted but, frankly, in such a short course, the value is negligible because students are already staggered by the amount of material to be studied.

The brief time frame also means that subcultures and slide cultures have no time to develop. For this reason the first session is omitted for most exercises. Sessions for Chapter 3 (Opportunistic Fungi) and Chapter 7 (Yeasts and Yeastlike Fungi) are interspersed with those for other chapters. We propose this schedule because, although it is potentially confusing, students have the opportunity to do the basic techniques at least once.

One potential advantage of the 10-day course is that the time saved from preparing slide cultures and LPCB preps, and transferring the organisms to be studied, is available for more thorough examination of prepared cultures and slides. Students also have time for the examination of a larger group of organisms.

The instructor has the burden of ensuring that an adequate number of mature cultures and slide preparations (preferably from slide cultures) are available for the students. No effort has been made to lay out a schedule for inoculating the cultures and slide preparations in a timely manner. Instructors should be warned that preparation must begin 3–4 weeks before the first scheduled laboratory session. The growth rates of the fungi, provided in the text, can guide the instructor in scheduling preparation of materials for the laboratories.

FIRST LABORATORY

Demonstrations by the Instructor

1. Preparation of *direct mounts*, *Scotch tape preps*, and *slide cultures.*
2. Transfer of a fungus culture to fresh medium.
3. Demonstration of various textures, topographies, and pigments of colonies.

Demonstration Materials

1. Culture of *Aspergillus fumigatus* to demonstrate preparation of tease mounts, Scotch tape preps, slide cultures, and methods for transfer of cultures.
2. Cultures of fungi demonstrating a variety of pigments, topographies, and textures. A selection of saprobic fungi can be used, or environmental cultures can be taken in advance and used for this demonstration.

The Tasks (in the order in which they should be done)

1. Take cultures of airborne contaminants (Exercise 1: Environmental Cultures).
2. Examine and describe the morphologic features of a colony of a saprobic fungus (Exercise 2: Colony Description). Record the results on the LABORATORY WORK SHEET for monomorphic moulds (see Fig. C.2). A sample showing how the form can be used (see Fig. C.6) is also provided.

Reincubation of Cultures

We assume that the maturity of a culture will always be checked before further study is done. *This will not be stated for every session of every exercise.*

Checking the maturity of a culture is good laboratory practice. Continuous repetition of this should not be necessary and will only make the book longer.

The *consequences* of using an immature culture are that you will have to repeat all or part of an exercise or that your conclusions will be based on misinformation.

Note that in this "short course" you can expect more of a problem with immature cultures than you would have in the 8-week or 16-week courses. You will need to be patient and ever so careful to do the procedures right the first time.

3. Describe and draw the microscopic characteristics of the saprobe in two different kinds of preparations (Exercise 2: Tease Mount; Exercise 3: Scotch Tape Prep). Again, record your work on the LABORATORY WORK SHEET.
4. Compare the advantages and disadvantages of the two procedures for the identification of microscopic structures (Exercises 2 and 3).
5. Set up a slide culture (Exercise 4: Slide Culture).
6. Subculture 3 saprobic fungi (Exercise 5) and set up slide cultures.

Laboratory Exercises

Exercise 1: Environmental Cultures (1st Session)
Exercise 2: Colony Description (1st Session)
Exercise 3: Scotch Tape Prep (1st Session)
Exercise 4: Slide Culture (1st Session)

Suggested Cultures for Exercises 2–4. 5–7-day cultures of *Alternaria, Aspergillus, Cladosporium, and Penicillium* on SDA.

Exercise 5: Opportunistic Fungi (1st session)

Suggested Cultures.[12] 5–7-day cultures of (Set 1) *Alternaria, Aureobasidium, Cladosporium;* (Set 2) *Curvularia, Drechslera, Helminthosporium;* (Set 3) *Fusarium;* (Set 4) *Gliocladium;* (Set 5) *Paecilomyces, Penicillium, Scopulariopsis;* (Set 6) 1 Zygomycetes (*Absidia, Mucor, Rhizopus, Syncephalastrum*); (Set 7) 1 *Aspergillus* (*A. fumigatus, A. flavus, A. niger, A. terreus*).

SECOND LABORATORY

Demonstrations by the Instructor

None

Demonstration Materials

None

---

[12]Organisms in **bold type** were recommended for Exercises 2–4.

LAB DATE	1	2	3	4	5	6	7	8	9
Exercise 1	1st session		2nd session						
Exercise 2	1st session								
Exercise 3	1st session								
Exercise 4	1st session					2nd session	3rd session		
Exercise 5	1st session			2nd session		3rd session		4th session	
Exercise 6				2nd session					
Exercise 7					2nd session				
Exercise 8									
Exercise 9						2nd session			
Exercise 10						1st session			
Optional									
Exercise 11							1st session	2nd session	3rd session
Exercise 12								1st session	2nd session
Exercise 13									1st session
Exercise 14									1st session

*The columns indicate the exercises to be done during a laboratory period.
The rows show the session of the exercise to be completed during each laboratory.

FIGURE C.10

Proposed laboratory schedule for a 10-day course.

The Tasks (in the order in which they should be done)

1. Begin examination of colony morphology of prepared cultures of saprobic fungi.
2. Examine prepared slides of saprobic fungi.

Remember to Alternate These Tasks. First, examine the colony, then follow this with examination of the slide preparation of the same organism. And, DRAW! DRAW! DRAW!

Laboratory Exercise

Exercise 5: Opportunistic Fungi (2nd Session)

THIRD LABORATORY

Demonstrations by the Instructor

1. Preparation of wet prep of *Trichosporon beigelii*.

Demonstration Materials

1. Permanent mounts and stock cultures of mature cultures of *Exophiala werneckii* and *Trichosporon beigelii*.
2. Stock cultures and permanent mounts of other superficial fungi for the students to examine are desirable but not essential.
3. Cultures (2–3 days old) of *Trichosporon beigelii* in malt extract broth, one per 3 or 4 students.

The Tasks (in the order in which they should be done)

1. Complete the examination of prepared cultures of saprobic fungi (Exercise 5).
2. Study the superficial fungi, including colony descriptions and prepared slides (Exercise 6).
3. Do a wet prep of *Trichosporon beigelii* if a broth culture is available (Exercise 6).
4. Compare the colony morphology of the young and the older mature cultures of superficial fungi, if possible (Exercise 6).

Laboratory Exercises

Exercise 5: Opportunistic Fungi (2nd Session)
Exercise 6: Superficial Fungi (2nd Session)

Suggested Cultures. *Exophiala werneckii* (2–3 weeks old[13]), *Trichosporon beigelii* on SDA, *T. beigelii* in malt extract broth.

---

[13]Using *Exophiala* cultures that are 2–3 weeks old allows students to compare the morphology of the young culture that they set up with the morphology of the older culture—a good opportunity to make the point that young cultures are yeastlike and mature colonies are mould forms.

FOURTH LABORATORY

Demonstrations by the Instructor

1. Techniques for *harvesting slide cultures*.
2. Procedure for microscopic examination of an intact slide culture to see whether it is mature ("ripe").
3. Preparation of the hair perforation test.

Demonstration Materials

1. Slide cultures of *Aspergillus fumigatus* of varying ages (2, 4, and 7 days) to demonstrate the method for ensuring that the culture is "ready" to be harvested and to show how slide cultures are harvested.

The Tasks (in the order in which they should be done)

1. Harvest the slide culture (Exercise 4) and examine the microscopic preparation(s).
2. Harvest the three slide cultures (Exercise 5: Opportunistic Fungi).
3. Examine the environmental culture (Exercise 1) taken from the laboratory or classroom.
4. Study the prepared slides and cultures of the dermatophytes (Exercise 7). Record colony morphologies and drawings of microscopic structures on the LABORATORY WORK SHEETS.

Laboratory Exercises

Exercise 1: Environmental Cultures (2nd Session)
Exercise 4: Slide Culture (2nd Session)
Exercise 5: Opportunistic Fungi (2nd Session)
Exercise 7: Dermatophytes (2nd Session)

Suggested Cultures. (Set 1) *Epidermophyton floccosum*; (Set 2) *Microsporum canis, M. gypseum, M. nanum, M. cookei*; (Set 3) *Trichophyton mentagrophytes, T. rubrum, T. tonsurans*.

FIFTH LABORATORY

Demonstrations by the Instructor

None

Demonstration Materials

1. Culture of *Sporothrix schenckii* in the yeast phase on BHI agar and in BHI broth, one set per 3 or 4 students.

The Tasks (in the order in which they should be done)

Note that a different LABORATORY WORK SHEET (see Fig. C.3) is suggested for use with dimorphic fungi such as *Sporothrix*. An example showing how the form can be used is provided (see Fig. C.7).

1. Describe the colony of *Sporothrix schenckii* incubated at 37°C (Exercise 10). Make a wet prep of the colony and examine it.
2. Make a wet prep of the broth culture of *Sporothrix schenckii* that was incubated at 35–37°C. Examine it and make the drawing.
3. Compare the colony morphologies and the microscopic structures of *Sporothrix schenckii* at the two different temperatures of incubation.
4. Study the monomorphic subcutaneous fungi, both the colony morphology and the microscopic structures.
5. Transfer five yeasts to fresh media (Exercise 11: Yeasts and Yeastlike Fungi).

Laboratory Exercises

Exercise 9: Subcutaneous Moulds (1st Session)

Suggested Cultures. (Set 1) 2–3-week-old cultures of *Exophiala jeanselmei, Wangiella dermatitidis;* (Set 2) *Cladosporium carrioinii, Fonsecaea pedrosoi, Phialophora verrucosa;* (Set 3) *Pseudallescheria boydii, Scedosporium apiospernum.*

Exercise 10: *Sporothrix* (1st Session)

Culture Needed. *Sporothrix schenckii.*

Exercise 11: Yeasts and Yeastlike Fungi (1st Session)

Suggested Cultures. (Set 1) *Candida albicans;* (Set 2) *Cryptococcus neoformans;* (Set 3) *Geotrichum candidum, Trichosporon beigelii*[14]; (Set 4) *Candida* species (*C. parapsilosis, C. kefyr, C. tropicalis, C. guilliermondii, C. krusei*), *Rhodotorula rubra, Saccharomyces cerevisiae.*

SIXTH LABORATORY

Demonstrations by the Instructor

None

Demonstration Materials

None

---

[14]Yes, you have seen *Trichosporon beigelii* before, but you didn't perform biochemical tests on the culture. *Trichosporon cutaneum* can be substituted for *T. beigelii;* using *T. beigelii* again saves the expense of obtaining the *T. cutaneum* culture.

The Tasks (in the order in which they should be done)

1. Finish Exercises 4 and 5 by sealing the coverslips on the slide culture preparations, if necessary.
2. Complete the examination of colony morphologies and microscopic structures of the superficial fungi, dermatophytes, and subcutaneous fungi.

Laboratory Exercises

Exercise 4: Slide Culture (3rd Session)
Exercise 5: Opportunistic Fungi (3rd Session)
Exercise 6: Superficial Fungi (3rd Session)
Exercise 7: Dermatophytes (3rd Session)
Exercise 9: Subcutaneous Moulds (3rd Session)
Exercise 10: *Sporothrix* (3rd Session)

SEVENTH LABORATORY

Demonstrations by the Instructor

1. Setting up, reading, and interpreting a germ tube test.
2. Preparing and reading an India ink prep.
3. Inoculation and interpretation of methods for identification of yeasts.
4. "Cut-streak" method for determining microscopic morphology of yeasts in CMT or rice infusion agar.

Demonstration Materials

1. Stock cultures of yeasts to use in demonstrating differential methods.
2. Germ tube tests demonstrating positive and negative results.
3. India ink preps that show "positive" and "negative" reactions.

The Tasks (in the order in which they should be done)

Note that a different LABORATORY WORK SHEET is suggested for identification of yeasts (see Fig. C.4). An example is provided (see Fig. C.8) to show how the form can be used.

1. Set up the germ tube tests (Exercise 12).
2. Make and examine wet preps of your yeast cultures, including both simple wet preps and India ink preps (Exercise 11).
3. Read the germ tube tests.
4. Set up the cut-streak plates and the other differential tests on your yeast cultures. Wait until the next laboratory to do any "rapid" tests.

Laboratory Exercises

Exercise 11: Yeasts and Yeastlike Fungi (2nd Session)
Exercise 12: Differential Tests for Yeasts and Yeastlike Fungi (1st Session)

EIGHTH LABORATORY

Demonstrations by the Instructor

1. Assessment of the microscopic morphology of yeasts in CMT or rice infusion agar.
2. Interpretation of differential tests for identification of yeasts.

Demonstration Materials

1. Stock cultures of yeasts to use in demonstrating differential methods.
2. CMTs of various yeasts and yeastlike fungi.

The Tasks (in the order in which they should be done)

1. Finish microscopic examination of yeasts in cut-streak plates and germ tube tests.
2. Record results of differential tests for yeasts in the appropriate sections of the work sheet, then identify them by reference to the appropriate chart.

Laboratory Exercises

Exercise 11: Yeast and Yeastlike Fungi (3rd Session)
Exercise 12: Differential Tests for Yeast and Yeastlike Fungi (2nd Session)

Suggested Differential Procedures. Germ tube test, morphology in CMT/rice infusion agar, India ink prep, caffeic acid test, assimilations (carbohydrates and nitrate), urea hydrolysis, pellicle formation, temperature tolerance.

NINTH LABORATORY

Demonstrations by the Instructor

None

Demonstration Materials

1. Stock cultures of nonviable yeast and mould forms of as many of the systemic fungi as possible *or* 35-mm slides or other illustrations of the cultures.

2. Permanent slide mounts of yeast/tissue and mould forms of as many of the systemic fungi as possible *or* 35-mm slides or other illustrations of the microscopic structures.

The Tasks (in the order in which they should be done)

1. Complete Exercise 12 (Differential Tests for Yeasts and Yeastlike Fungi).
2. Examine colony morphologies of the systemic fungi (Exercise 13).
3. Examine microscopic morphologies of yeast/tissue and mould forms of the systemic dimorphic fungi, and make drawings in your notebook!

REVIEW!   REVIEW!   REVIEW!

4. Complete any exercises that are outstanding.
5. Review your notes and drawings to ensure that they are as complete as possible.
6. Examine as many as possible of the cultures and slide preparations, done by your classmates, that you have not read previously.
7. Clean your work area, discarding any extraneous materials that have been pushed to the back of your drawer or locker and arranging your permanent mounts neatly in a slide flat or box for your instructor to review.

Laboratory Exercises

Exercise 12: Differential Tests for Yeasts and Yeastlike Fungi (3rd Session)
Exercise 13: Systemic Fungi (1st Session)

Suggested Cultures. *Blastomyces dermatitidis, Coccidioides immitis, Histoplasma capsulatum, Paracoccidioides brasiliensis.*

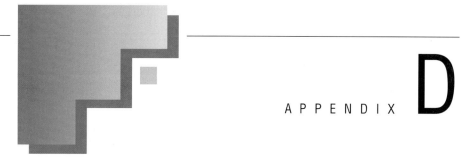

Reagents, Stains, Media, and Methods

INTRODUCTION

The appendix dealing with reagents, stains, media, and methods is perhaps the least interesting section of any text *until you need the information*. We have tried, without being too tedious, to provide enough information for each reagent, stain, medium, and method in this appendix to show its value and to indicate when it is best used. Our expectation is that the user knows the basic principles of aseptic technique and applies them and waits for media to reach room temperature before beginning to use them. We also expect the user to know that cultures and differential tests must be labeled with enough information to link them to the unknown organism being identified.

General methods that are widely used with a variety of media and fungi are presented in the first portion of this appendix. Formulas and methods for specific reagents, stains, and media used exclusively in mycology are given in alphabetical order in the remainder of the appendix. We hope that you will find this different approach less annoying than the customary use of separate appendices with numerous cross-references among them.

For the experienced mycologist the steps for a procedure may seem agonizingly detailed. We have chosen this approach rather than writing the procedures in "shorthand," which is only useful if you've the experience to fill in the blanks. Those blanks can be treacherous for the novice. This appendix shows one way, not The Way, to do things. Individual instructors and practitioners can, and should, modify procedures to fit their circumstances.

Lists of materials for methods include those that are important for that method. These are needed in addition to those listed as "Materials You Always Need" in the in-troduction to the laboratory. For example, a method list may include sterile Pasteur pipettes and assume that the user will know a rubber bulb is also needed to use the pipettes. Specific methods essential for mycology are presented, especially if they are unlikely to be found in all-purpose bacteriology-mycology-parasitology-virology texts.

Most reagents needed for mycology should probably be purchased prepared from laboratory supply houses if the budget allows it, because this removes the burden of most of the quality control procedure from the working laboratory. If the reagents are to be made "in house," they should be prepared according to the instructions, using volumetric glassware when this is specified. They should be stored in glass bottles with screw caps, with a label bearing the reagent name, its formula,[1] the date of preparation, the expiration date (usually 6–12 months), and the initials of the person preparing it. Most reagents are stored at room temperature; variations should be included with directions for preparation and noted on the bottle's label. Reagents are not included in this appendix except when they are necessary for an included medium or method; the others can be found in any standard text.

We believe that if only one item can be purchased already prepared, stains should be that item. The problem is not that stains are especially hard to make; the problem is that they can be so *messy*. The very fine dry particles of dye are carried easily on air currents so that a moment's lack of attention can leave the most astonishing things, and people, wearing tiny specks of purple or magenta. Purchasing prepared stains also reduces the amount of quality control the

---

[1]This does not mean all the exhausting detail of how many grams and milliliters of each ingredient. This is more like citing the reference, e.g., Schlumpfl's modification of mercuric chloride.

working laboratory must do. As with reagents, if stains are to be made in house, they should be prepared according to the instructions, using volumetric glassware when this is specified. They should be stored in glass bottles with screw caps, with a label bearing the name of the stain, the formula,[2] the date it was made, the expiration date (usually 6–12 months), and the initials of the person who made it. Most stains are stored at room temperature; the correct temperature for storage is specified with the instructions for preparation. Mark the storage temperature on the label also. Stains and mounting fluids essential for examining cultures are included in this appendix, with our comments and prejudices.

Most mycology media can be purchased as the basal medium, and many can be purchased from reputable laboratory suppliers as prepared plates or tubes. Purchasing media already prepared has some clear advantages for the teaching laboratory and the clinical laboratory. One obvious advantage is the time saved by the laboratory. Another is that most of the quality control is done by the manufacturer, although the purchaser must ensure that the medium was handled properly in transit and verify the sterility of the product.

Whether you are purchasing prepared media or making it in house from a commercial base, remember that the composition varies even for common media; Sabouraud's agar and potato-based media are two examples in which this occurs. *No formulation is entirely good or entirely bad. To interpret the results, however, you should know which formula you are using and what you can expect from it.* Some tips for "Preparation of Media" are included in the "General Methods" section of this appendix.

Only special media that are not commercially available and are unlikely to be found in a standard text are presented here. Most of these, such as hay infusion agar, are rarely if ever needed routinely. On the other hand, when you need a special medium, you are more likely to make it and use it if the formula is in hand—and some of these "recipes" were very difficult to locate.

GENERAL METHODS

CHLAMYDOSPORE PLATES

The general methods discussed in this section can be used with any "chlamydospore agar" to enhance chlamydospore production by reducing the oxygen available to the yeast or yeastlike fungus. Other characteristic microscopic features are also encouraged by the reduced oxygen tension and the nutrient characteristics of the media. The specific choice of medium is dictated by what is

available in the laboratory, which is in turn determined by the prejudices of the mycologist.

Tween 80 in the medium encourages the formation of microscopic structures by reducing surface tension and thus increasing the rate at which the nutrients can be absorbed by the fungus, which speeds the rate of chlamydospore production as well as the development of other structures. False positives may result if the culture plate is incubated more than 72 hours before it is examined. Control cultures should always be used, especially by the inexperienced mycologist.

Chlamydospore agar with trypan blue, cornmeal agar, cornmeal-Tween 80 agar, rice infusion/rice extract agar, rice infusion/rice extract agar with Tween 80 and/or trypan blue, and Tween 80–oxgall–caffeic acid (TOC) medium all can be used to detect chlamydospore production.

Cut-Streak (Coverslip) Method

1. Touch the tip of a bacteriology needle to several isolated colonies of the organism to be identified. Suspicious colonies typically are 1–2 mm in diameter and creamy or white with a dry texture.
2. Make two parallel streaks about ½ inch apart on one half of the chosen medium. Scarify the agar, i.e., scratch it but do not cut deeply into it.
3. *Flame the loop.* Streak across the parallel "scars" with the flamed loop to form the letter **W** in the center of the parallel lines.
4. Cover the streaked area with a sterile[3] coverslip.

"Scratch" Method for Chlamydospore Plates

1. Touch the tip of a *bent* mycology needle to several isolated colonies of the organism to be identified. Suspicious colonies typically are 1–2 mm in diameter and creamy or white with a dry texture.
2. Use the tip of the needle to cut through the agar to the bottom, then rotate the needle so that the bent tip is parallel to the bottom of the plate. Drag the tip of the needle along the bottom of the plate for the length of the cut.
3. *Without flaming the needle*, repeat the inoculation in a second cut parallel to the first one.

Interpretation

After the plate has incubated at room temperature for 24–48 hours, examine the growth to look for chlamy-

---

[2]As with reagents this means to indicate whose formula is used rather than listing all the ingredients with their amounts on the label.

[3]If sterile coverslips are not available, one can be sterilized by holding it *briefly* in the flame of a Bunsen burner. If the coverslip is held in the flame too long, it will crack or shatter and scatter over the work area. A reasonable alternative, if incinerators are used instead of Bunsen burners, is to flood the coverslip with alcohol, drain it, and ignite the alcohol to sterilize the coverslip.

dospores (see "Procedure for Microscopic Examination of Colonies"). Note whether pseudohyphae and true hyphae are present. Also record the size, shape, and arrangement of the blastoconidia and any other structures that may be present. If trypan blue is present in the medium, the chlamydospores will be dark blue owing to absorption of the dye (see Fig. 7.7).

For controls use *Candida albicans* (positive) and *Candida krusei* (negative).

Positive: numerous terminal chlamydospores
Negative: good growth, but few or no chlamydospores

MEDIA PREPARATION

Making media is no more difficult than making pudding. You must measure the ingredients correctly, add them in the correct order, and ensure that everything is mixed thoroughly. We believe that every laboratorian should know the basic steps in media preparation. One reason is that some media needed occasionally in mycology cannot be purchased prepared or even as a prepared base. Another reason is that if you have to make a medium in an emergency or for a special purpose, you will be able to do so.

The method of sterilization varies with the medium. The recommended method for sterilization of each medium is provided in the directions for the medium. Most can be sterilized by applying steam under pressure. The plug or cap should be seated loosely during sterilization so that steam can enter the container and effect sterilization. When the medium is completely cool, the caps should be tightened to delay dehydration and to make sure they will not be knocked off accidentally. When any of the constituents are sensitive to heat, two choices are available. If the medium is an agar, the heat-sensitive component is filter sterilized separately and added to the agar after it has cooled to approximately 50°C. If the medium is broth, all of it can be filter sterilized.

The desired pH (±0.2) is for the completed medium at room temperature; it is usually stated as part of the formula. In a few instances specific instructions are given for adjusting the pH of the medium or of components during preparation. Generally if the water used for media preparation has a neutral pH, the resulting medium will have the desired pH. Checking and adjusting the pH are not likely to be necessary *except* for those media in which adjusting the pH is emphasized as part of preparing the medium. Media must, of course, be labeled with its identity and the date it was prepared.

Formulas are usually given for 1 L of medium, as they are here. This makes it easier to compare similar media; larger or smaller amounts can, of course, be prepared. The questions that usually determine the volume to prepare are

How much is needed?
How much storage space is there?

How much medium will be dispensed per tube or plate?
What is the shelf life of the medium?

Instructions for preparation are given with each medium and provided with every unit of commercially prepared base. When commercially prepared base is being used, the manufacturer's directions for preparation should be consulted, if only to determine how many grams of base to use. Some tips that we have used in media preparation will help smooth the process when you are doing it.

#1. Be Safety Conscious.

Molten agar is too thick to cool rapidly on contact, and when it is spilled it tends to stick to a surface rather than run off. Use protective autoclave gloves to handle containers of media while you are heating them and as you transfer them into and out of the autoclave. If the gloves get wet, swap them for another pair—the moisture helps conduct heat rather than protect against it.

If you aren't sure you can snatch a flask of medium off the heat source before it boils over, don't try. *Remember that cleaning up a mess is always preferable to a trip to the emergency room or infirmary.*

#2. Select the Container for Making the Medium Carefully.

The container must be clean and dry. The volume of the container should be at least twice the volume you are preparing, e.g., use a 2-L container to make 1 L of agar. You must be able to cap the container securely to autoclave it, and you must be able to remove the cap and manage it safely if you are pouring the medium into plates.

Erlenmeyer flasks work best because they have a large bottom surface for cooking and most people can grasp the top in one hand to move the container or snatch it off the heat. Several layers of aluminum foil or paper towel secured by tape or a rubber band can be used to cap the flask, or a wad of cotton wrapped in gauze can be used as a plug.

Beakers are poor containers for anything that must be autoclaved before it is dispensed, but they make good containers for broths and other media that are dispensed into tubes before they are autoclaved.

#3. Don't Heat It if You Don't Have to, and Don't Heat It Any Longer than You Must.[4]

Media contain various combinations of proteins and amino acids, carbohydrates, vitamins, and minerals.

---

[4]One author takes this one step further. Agar to be poured into plates is added to the water, allowed to stand until it is wet and sinks to the bottom, then autoclaved directly with a magnet in the container. All mixing occurs after the medium is autoclaved.

Sometimes antimicrobial agents are added. All of these constituents are affected somewhat by heat; some are more heat sensitive than others.

In practical terms this means that if the base will go into solution without being heated, as most broths will, don't heat it. This reduces breakdown of the constituents due to heat. It saves energy. Cool medium is handled more easily, and more safely, than hot medium.

#4. Use a Wetting Agent in Agars.

One or two drops of a wetting agent such as Tween 80 or another detergent has no effect on the way the medium works, but it makes a major difference in the number of bubbles that form while the medium is being dispensed. Some media are more likely than others to form annoying bubbles. Media that contain blood are worse than most.

Add the wetting agent to the water before the agar is added, and swirl the container to disperse the wetting agent. Alternatively, add the wetting agent after the agar base is in solution. NOTE that if you fail to disperse the agent in the cold water before the agar base is added, you are likely to end up with a lump in the medium that is difficult to break up.

#5. Add Agar to Water, Not Vice Versa.

When the agar base is added first, and the water poured in on top, you create a sticky mass against the floor of the container—an ideal place for the material to stick and burn.

When water is poured in first, and the agar base added on top, the base gradually wets itself and sinks toward the bottom of the flask. The sticky part is at the top, where it won't burn, and it can eventually be swirled off and mixed in as the medium heats and dissolves.

#6. Use a Hot Plate That Contains a Motor-Driven Magnetic Stirrer.

Stirring the agar-water mixture manually is difficult to do without leaving a burned patch. Swirling the flask to stir it is a good way to prevent the burned patch on the bottom but gets some of the wet agar on the sides so that it has to be mixed back in. A stir-heat plate keeps the bottom from burning, and the magnetic stir bar creates enough of a "swirl" that as the medium gets hot the swirling motion also washes off the wet agar clinging to the sides.

#7. Never Turn Your Back on a Container of Medium that Is Beginning to Boil.

When the cooking medium begins to clear, and tiny bubbles begin to appear, put on your asbestos glove and give the container your complete attention. You want the medium to come to a full boil so that all the agar will be in solution, but once it starts to boil, it will boil over in no time if the container is not lifted off the heat source.

You want to keep the medium from boiling over because, first, you may not salvage enough to make the number of tubes or plates needed. Second, when media burns onto the hot surface, it makes a terrible mess that has to be scrubbed off. Third, burned medium smells worse than the mess it makes.

MICROSCOPIC EXAMINATION OF CULTURES

Subsurface growth in media must be examined microscopically to learn what kinds of structures are present. Growth beneath the coverslip on chlamydospore plates is checked for the production of chlamydospores. Slide cultures are read before they are harvested to see if they are mature and have reproductive structures. A brightfield microscope can be used to do all these things.

1. When you are checking growth in Petri dishes, the first step is always to loosen the screws or clips that attach the slide clamp to the stage of the microscope. When you can, lift off the clamp with the screws attached (so you won't lose the screws) and set the clamp aside. Turn on the microscope lamp.
2. Next, place the object you are examining on the stage of the microscope.

   Examination of Subsurface Growth. If necessary, dry the lid of the Petri dish you wish to examine so that the condensed moisture will not interfere with your examination. Invert the Petri dish on the stage of the microscope, centering the edge of the inoculum over the light source.

   Examination of Coverslipped Growth in Agar. Remove the lid of the Petri dish you wish to examine and place the Petri dish on the stage of the microscope, centering the edge of the inoculum over the light source.

   Checking Slide Cultures. Carefully get a grip on both ends of the slide culture and remove it from the incubation chamber, i.e., Petri dish.[5] Wipe the bottom of the slide with dry gauze so that the slide will not stick to the microscope stage. Place the slide in the clamps on the microscope stage.
3. Carefully move the ocular into place, raising the lens if necessary so that the lens doesn't crash into the cov-

---

[5]Your instructor may prefer to have the slide culture examined without removing it from the Petri dish. This reduces the likelihood of aerosols somewhat, but makes it more difficult to see the structures. If *in situ* examination is preferred, follow the instructor's directions, of course.

erslip or the agar. While you look at the slide culture and the lens from the side, use the coarse adjustment to move the low-power lens as close to the surface as possible.

4. Look through the oculars and use the fine adjustment to *raise the lens only, never lower it*—until the growth beneath the coverslip is in focus. If you lower the lens, you may crack the coverslip or "tip" it. This makes it more difficult to see the results, creates a mess, and means the lens must be decontaminated before you can continue. When you have the field in view with the low-power lens, try to change to the high-power lens; NOTE that this isn't always possible, especially if the slide is sitting in the Petri dish.

5. Find an area of good growth, where the structures are not too crowded, and decide whether the culture is ready to be harvested or whether it should be reincubated. This means that if you have removed the clamp from the microscope, you must wiggle the Petri dish or slide it around on the stage. You may need to increase the amount of light because of the amount of agar between the lens and the light source.

6. If necessary, reincubate the culture. If it is a slide culture, return it to its Petri dish. Add sterile water, if necessary, cover the dish, and let it incubate at room temperature. To harvest the culture, see "Slide Cultures."

PRESERVATION OF CHARACTERISTIC MOULD COLONIES

When the budget is too tight to allow each student to cultivate his or her own fungi, or when the time is too short for the fungi to grow in culture, preserved cultures can be prepared and shared among students. Preserved cultures are also useful for other kinds of training and can serve as good reference materials.

Cultures must obviously be labeled with an identifying number or the name of the fungus. Each label should also show the type of medium used, the temperature of incubation, and the age of the culture when it was preserved.

Materials

cotton balls or square cotton pledgets
formaldehyde (40%) in a dropper bottle
cultures to be preserved
paraffin[6]
rubber gloves

For Method #2, add a large wide-mouth jar such as a Brewer jar, with a tight seal.

---

[6]The paraffin can be obtained at the local grocery store, from among the supplies for canning and preserving foods. Cooks have used it for years to seal jars of jelly.

Methods

The *first* step is always to transfer the fungus to a fresh screw-cap tube of the desired medium, following the usual procedure for "Subculture of Moulds." Allow the subculture to incubate at the appropriate temperature until characteristic colony morphology develops.

To introduce the formaldehyde to the culture, work in a fume hood; the fumes of formaldehyde can be very annoying and should not be inhaled. Wear rubber gloves to soak the cotton with formaldehyde.

Method #1

2. Moisten a cotton pledget or cotton ball with 10 drops of formaldehyde. Remove the cap from the culture and insert the formaldehyde-soaked cotton. Allow the tube to stand at room temperature in the fume hood.

3. After 24 hours trim the cotton so that it is even with the top of the tube. Replace the screw cap, catching a few cotton strands between the cap and the top of the tube to hold the cotton plug in place, and tighten the cap. Seal the top of the tube by dipping the top into melted paraffin to prevent drying of the agar and subsequent deterioration of the colony.

Method #2

2. Remove the cap from the tube and set it aside to be decontaminated. Stand the culture(s) in a beaker or rack in the wide-mouth jar.

3. Moisten several cotton pledgets or cotton balls with formaldehyde. Drop the formaldehyde-soaked cotton into the jar around the culture tubes. Close the jar and tighten the lid.

4. After 48 hours open the jar and remove the cultures. Wrap the mouth of each tube with Parafilm and cover it with a clean screw cap. Tighten the cap. Seal the top of the tube with melted paraffin to prevent drying of the agar and subsequent deterioration of the colony.

PURIFICATION OF FUNGUS CULTURES

Mixed cultures of yeast and bacteria or mould and bacteria inevitably occur sometimes because a bacterial flora is normally present in many kinds of specimens that are cultured for fungi. Sputum is a good example of a specimen that is likely to produce a mixed culture. The likelihood of a mixed culture can, of course, be reduced by using selective as well as nonselective media for primary isolation.

Mould Colonies

Bacterial contamination of mould cultures is usually much less of a problem than bacterial contamination of yeasts because the identification of most moulds relies heavily on the gross and microscopic morphology rather than on biochemical reactions. These morphologic characteristics can usually be distinguished in all but the worst cases of contamination. If necessary, hyphae and conidia/spores from the least contaminated part of the culture can be subcultured to selective media again to eliminate the bacteria.

Yeast Colonies

Unlike moulds, yeast and yeastlike fungi are usually identified by biochemical reactions and growth patterns as well as by the gross and microscopic morphology. Contamination with bacteria rudely interferes with the reactions and growth patterns. A pure culture must be obtained before identification can progress. To determine the presence of bacteria look closely at the colonies on the plate to see if more than one kind of organism is present. A Gram's stain of growth on the primary plates also helps determine if bacteria are present.

The Easy Way to Purify a Yeast Culture. If the contaminated culture is a broth, use a bacteriology loop to streak it for isolation to a variety of media, including blood agar or brain-heart infusion agar (BHIA) as well as at least one selective medium. If it isn't a broth, make a suspension of the yeast, then streak it for isolation.

The Hard Way to Get a Pure Culture of Yeast

1. Obtain four tubes containing 10 ml of Sabouraud's dextrose broth and label them #1 through #4.
2. Add increasing amounts of 1 N HCl to each tube: 1 drop to tube #1, 2 drops to tube #2, and so forth.
3. Make a suspension of the contaminated yeast in sterile water or broth. Add 1 drop of the suspension to each tube. Incubate all tubes at 25–30°C for 24 hours. The lower incubation temperature favors the yeast over bacteria, which tend to grow better at 37°C.
4. After 24 hours, streak from each of the acidified broths to a plate of blood agar. Incubate the blood agar plates for 48 hours at 37°C, then examine them.
5. Look carefully to determine whether more than one kind of colony is present. Do wet preps or Gram's stains from each colony type to find the yeast.
6. *If a pure culture of yeast has been obtained*, streak the yeast to another blood agar plate for isolation before attempting differential tests.
7. If the plates from all four tubes still contain mixed cultures, you should *first* take inoculum from tube #4 and start over again at step 1 above. *Second*, streak from tube #4 to additional media such as cornmeal agar. Consider also streaking isolation plates of selective media such as mycotic medium and Emmon's modification of Sabouraud's dextrose agar (SDA) with chloramphenicol.

SCOTCH TAPE PREPARATIONS[7]

Scotch tape preps are a kind of direct smear made from a mould form colony. This is a substitute for the tease mount. The advantage is that Scotch tape preps usually produce good results quickly, showing the conidia attached to the conidiophores, without requiring the same skill and patience as tease mounts. The disadvantages are that the Scotch tape prep cannot be preserved for long periods, that carelessness can cause widespread dispersion of conidia from the culture, and that Scotch tape isn't sterile (nor can it be handled aseptically) so the mould can be contaminated. This procedure should *always* be done in a biologic safety cabinet.

The traditional mounting fluid, lactophenol–cotton blue (LPCB), creates a good temporary preparation. Using LPCB with polyvinyl alcohol (PVA) is equally good, but the resulting preparation is still not permanent as a tease mount. Both mounting fluids are discussed elsewhere in this appendix. *Tease mounts* and *slide cultures* are alternative methods for examining the microscopic structures of a mould. The procedures for both are described in this appendix.

Do *not* attempt these preparations with *any* mould that could possibly be *Coccidioides immitis*.

Materials

clear cellophane ("Scotch") tape[8]
mould to be examined
microscope slides
mounting fluid in a dropper bottle (LPCB *or* LPCB with PVA)

Procedure (see Fig. 2.3)

1. Place a drop of mounting fluid in the center of a clean microscope slide.
2. Touch the surface of the colony firmly with the adhesive side of the Scotch tape and move it gently sideways. You don't want to punch a dent in the agar, but you do want to ensure that hyphae as well as conidia and conidiophores are picked up on the tape.

   One way to do this is to pull off a strip of tape about 8 inches long and fold it, sticky side out, over a pencil eraser or the end of a tongue blade. The tape must be long enough for you to keep a grip on the ends without getting your fingers into the culture.

   Another way to do this is to pull off a strip of tape about 8 inches long and fold the ends back so the tape

---

[7]We are divided on the value of Scotch tape preps. One feels that the advantage of a good quick preparation outweighs the disadvantages. The other feels that the risks of contamination more than offset the advantages.

[8]*Not* the invisible kind of tape for wrapping gifts; it should be as broad as possible.

can be held without sticking to your glove. Hold both ends with one hand. Place one gloved finger of the other hand within the loop and press the sticky side of the tape firmly onto the colony about midway between the center and the rim.

3. Stick one end of the tape to the top of the slide so the "mould-y" section is centered over the LPCB. Stretch the tape across the stain and stick the remaining end to the slide. The excess tape at either end can be torn off against the edge of the slide. Avoid, as much as possible, creating air bubbles or a crease in the tape.

4. If necessary, use a paper towel to remove excess mounting fluid. Wipe the slide very carefully so that the tape isn't moved, or simply lay the paper towel on the slide and allow it to absorb the LPCB.

5. To examine the slide place it on the stage of a bright-field microscope and examine it under low power and high power. Adjust the light, if necessary, by lowering the condenser. Record what you see, and use the information as a springboard for deciding what to do next. Scotch tape preparations can, if necessary, be kept 1–2 days for further examination, but permanent mounts cannot be created.

SLIDE CULTURE (MICROCULTURE) TECHNIQUE

Slide cultures are microcultures that show the microscopic morphology of a fungus, especially the way the structures are connected, better than either a tease mount or a Scotch tape prep can. Some moulds, such as *Fusarium* and *Sporothrix*, have such delicate linkages between conidium and conidiophore that attached conidia are rarely seen in either tease mounts or Scotch tape preps. Slide cultures are most useful in preparing permanent mounts for teaching. They are used less often in the clinical laboratory, even though they show the morphology best, because of the time the culture needs to develop.

For these microcultures an agar block is placed on a glass slide and inoculated, then covered with a coverslip; two permanent mounts can be prepared from each slide culture. The microculture is incubated in its own chamber—a glass Petri dish—and water is added to provide the necessary moisture. Water on the slide or the agar block spoils the culture, so something (a glass rod or applicator sticks) must be placed under the slide to hold it above the surface of the water.

The materials used for the slide culture must be sterile to prevent contamination of the mould and confusion of the mycologist. Long coverslips are recommended because they provide more surface for growth of the mould. The agar used is poured as thick plates to reduce the chance that it will dry out during incubation. Filter paper is placed in the incubation chamber, e.g., the glass Petri dish, to "hold" the water that is added; this helps prevent drying and keep the water from sloshing over the slide and agar.

Slide culture setups can be prepared in batches and stored until they are needed. Place the components for one culture (except the agar and water, of course) in the glass Petri dish and wrap the dish in paper towel, securing the paper with autoclave indicator tape. Sterilize the setups with dry heat in an oven or the autoclave.

Materials

For setting up the culture

> mycology needle—preferably a bent one
> mould to be examined
> scalpel
> forceps
> sterile water
> sterile Pasteur pipette
> plate of suitable agar (usually potato flake [PFA] or potato dextrose [PDA]) *poured to a depth of 4 mm— a THICK plate*
> sterile glass Petri dish containing 1 sterile microscope slide with frosted end
> 1 sterile (20 × 30 mm or 20 × 50 mm) coverslip
> 1 piece sterile filter paper (Whatman #1 or #2)
> 1 sterile glass rod or tube bent into a V shape *or* 2 pieces sterile applicator stick, broken to fit into the Petri dish

For harvesting the culture

> forceps
> slide flat
> microscope slide
> coverslips (20 × 30 mm or 20 × 50 mm)
> dropper bottle with LPCB or LPCB with PVA

Procedure for Setting Up Microcultures (see Fig. 2.4 A–E)

A special plea for good aseptic technique is in order here, without reiterating all of the necessary moves in every step. Keep the plate of agar and the slide culture setup covered as much as possible. This means holding the lid in one hand while you use sterile tweezers to shift the pieces inside around with the other hand.

---

1. Use a heavy marking pen to draw a grid of 12 × 20 mm or 12 × 40 mm rectangles to fit the bottom of the Petri dish so that the same agar plate can be used efficiently for multiple agar blocks.

2. Position the Petri dish of agar over the grid. Sterilize the blade of the scalpel by dipping it in alcohol

and flaming it. Hold the blade of the scalpel perpendicular to the surface of the agar and cut through
the agar to the bottom along the grid's lines. To
make it easier to remove the blocks you will use, lift
out one of the odd-shaped blocks along the rim of
the dish and discard it.

3. Label the lid of the Petri dish/incubation chamber.
You can't label the slide until you harvest the culture
without contaminating it and the culture.

4. Flame the forceps by dipping them in alcohol and
flaming them. Using aseptic technique, center the
filter paper in the dish. Then position the bent glass
rod in the center of the filter paper (or place the
pieces of applicator stick parallel to each other on the
paper, far enough apart that each piece supports one
end of the microscope slide).

5. Use the forceps to lay the microscope slide on the
supporting rod or sticks so that the frosted side of the
slide is facing up. Put the forceps aside. Sterilize the
scalpel blade again and pick up a rectangular block of
agar. Place it on the microscope slide so that the bottom of the agar is against the slide and so that the
long axis of the agar is aligned with the long axis of
the slide.

6. Sterilize the mycology needle and pick up some
conidia and hyphae from the mould being studied.
Inoculate all four sides of the agar block by gently
scraping the agar near the center of each side of the
block. You can probably do this with a single "pick"
from the original culture, but you can go back to the
culture two, three, or even four separate times if you
wish.

7. Use sterile forceps to seat the sterile coverslip on the
top of the agar block, aligning its sides with those of
the agar. Gently warming the coverslip first ensures
that it seals to the agar surface.

8. Add a small amount of sterile water (3–5 ml) to the incubation chamber. Using the sterile Pasteur pipette is
better than pouring the water in because you have
better control over the rate of flow and where the water lands. Replace the lid of the chamber.

9. Incubate the microculture at room temperature until
growth appears; the time varies with the mould.
Check the culture every 2–3 days to ensure that it
does not dry out.

10. When the culture seems mature,[9] you may wish to
examine it microscopically. The procedure is provided in "Microscopic Examination of Cultures."
When conidia are present, harvest the culture.

Procedure for Harvesting Microcultures[10] (see Fig.
2.4*F* and *G*)

Work inside a biologic safety cabinet. The culture you are harvesting is beyond contamination,
but the process of harvesting inevitably creates
aerosols containing conidia that can—and probably will—contaminate lots of other cultures unless the aerosols are controlled.

---

1. If water has condensed on the slide or coverslip of
the slide culture, you should dry it out first. The best
way is to let the chamber stand several hours or
overnight in the biologic safety cabinet with the lid
cracked open slightly. If it is very wet, you may want
to carefully remove the wet filter paper without damaging the slide culture before you set the culture
aside to dry. Discard the filter paper into a biohazard
container.

2. Place a paper towel on the work surface and moisten it
with disinfectant. Lay a clean glass slide on the towel.
Label it with the necessary information about the culture and add 1–2 drops of mounting fluid to the center
of the slide.

3. Remove the lid of the incubation chamber and set it
aside. Hold the glass slide down by placing one finger
on the frosted end. Gently but firmly grasp the ends of
the coverslip and twist it off the agar block. Cover the
chamber again.

4. Lower the coverslip carefully onto the mounting fluid
so that the rectangle of growth left hollow by the agar
block is centered over the mounting fluid. You want to
seat the coverslip with as few air bubbles as possible.
Avoiding bubbles is sometimes impossible because of
air trapped in the mould colony. Set the slide preparation aside in a slide flat to dry completely. NOTE that
you can stop at this point and examine the slide preparation. If it is satisfactory, i.e., conidia are present and
attached in their natural pattern, continue with the
harvest. If it is not satisfactory, the slide with the attached agar block can be reincubated and harvested
later. If you reincubate the slide and agar block, do remember to add water.

5. Take the lid off the chamber again and pick up the
slide. Invert it over a biohazard container or a beaker
of disinfectant. With your other hand place the tip of
a mycology needle at the base of the agar block and
use the needle as a lever to flick the agar into the biohazard container/beaker.

6. Lay the slide on the disinfectant-soaked paper towel
with the hollow rectangle of growth left by removing

---

[9]You will see hyphae—"fuzz"—first. The colony is approaching
maturity when you also see conidia—"dust" or specks.

[10]Two slide mounts are created from one slide culture. Mounting
the cultures in LPCB with PVA is the best choice if the slide preparations are intended to be used "permanently."

the agar block facing up. Place 1–2 drops of mounting fluid in the hollow rectangle left by the agar block.

7. Lower a clean coverslip carefully onto the mounting fluid, seating it with as few air bubbles as possible. Label the slide with the necessary information about the culture, and set the slide preparation aside in a slide flat to dry completely.

STORAGE TECHNIQUES FOR MAINTAINING FUNGI

Cultures of known organisms are important for teaching students, maintaining the mycologist's skills, and doing quality control. All of the storage methods operate by reducing the metabolism of the fungus, generally by decreasing the oxygen available to the organism and cutting the supply of nutrients. None of the available procedures maintain a culture indefinitely, and none of them completely prevent changes in the fungus. The methods for maintaining viable fungal cultures for future use vary in how hard they are to do and how good the results are. "Good" in this case means large numbers of viable spores are available after storage *and* the characteristics of the fungus are affected very little by the experience.

The method you use depends on how much time you have to fiddle with the cultures and the space and equipment you have available. No method works equally well for all fungi. Some organisms, such as *Epidermophyton floccosum*, are extremely difficult to maintain as stock cultures, no matter what method is used. The most complex method, lyophilization, is least likely to cause changes in the fungus; it is not available in most clinical laboratories. If a lyophilizer is available, follow instructions for its use. The other methods are detailed later, with instructions for subculturing the stored organism.

The starting point for *all* storage techniques is growing a fresh culture of the fungus; the usual medium is PDA or PFA. *Step 1* is to transfer the fungus to a screw-cap tube of fresh PDA or PFA medium and incubate it at the appropriate temperature until good growth is obtained.

Growth in Culture

The easiest method, keeping the fungus on agar with periodic transfers, is also the one most likely to cause changes in the fungus over time.

2. Screw the cap of the tube down very tightly when the culture is mature and/or seal the tube with Parafilm or paraffin. Reducing access to oxygen stops growth of the organism and causes it to, in effect, hibernate. Store the cultures at room temperature.

3. Cultures must be transferred at intervals of 6–12 months to maintain them in culture. The repeated transfers result in morphologic changes in most fungi.

To subculture remove the seal and transfer an agar plug to a fresh plate or tube of medium in the usual fashion. Incubate the subculture at 25–30°C until growth appears.

Storage of Culture Under Oil

One refinement to keeping the fungus on agar in a sealed tube is to cover the mycelium with sterile mineral oil. This makes a big mess whenever you remove some of the growth from the tube, but most organisms survive better for a longer period so that fewer subcultures are needed.

2. When you have good growth, cover the colony *and the agar slant* entirely with sterile mineral oil. If the tip of the agar is exposed, it will begin to dry out.

3. Screw the cap of the tube down tightly and seal the tube, as you do for maintaining a fungus on the growth medium. Store the cultures at room temperature.

4. Cultures must be transferred at intervals of 24 months to maintain them in culture. The repeated transfers result in morphologic changes in most fungi and the oil is messy.

To subculture remove the seal. Wipe the lip of the tube with alcohol and transfer an agar plug to a fresh plate or tube of medium in the usual fashion. Oil is inevitably transferred with the mycelium, creating a slimy sort of subculture. *Mineral oil is flammable.* Be careful when sterilizing the mycology needle[11]; usually lots of spattering occurs, creating fungus-laden aerosols, even if you don't have a small fire. Incubate the subculture at 25–30°C until growth appears.

Frozen Storage of Cultures

Another relatively simple refinement of storing the fungus at room temperature in a sealed tube is to freeze the fungus on the agar. Again, most organisms survive better for a longer period so that fewer subcultures are needed. Eliminating the mess caused by the sterile oil is the bonus for freezing the cultures.

2. When the colony has matured screw the cap of the tube down very tightly and store the cultures in the freezer at −20° to −70°C.

3. Cultures must be transferred at intervals of 1–2 years (sometimes longer) to maintain them. The repeated transfers result in morphologic changes in most fungi.

To subculture remove the cap and "chip off" a piece of the frozen mycelium with a sterile mycology needle. Transfer the inoculum to a fresh plate of PDA or PFA. Quickly recap the frozen culture tightly and return it to the freezer before it begins to thaw. Incubate the subculture at 25–30°C until growth appears.

Storage in Sterile Water

Storage in sterile water is the optimum "low-tech" method for maintaining stock cultures of fungi. Most or-

---

[11]An incinerator is recommended rather than a Bunsen burner, but incinerators are not always available, especially in student laboratories.

ganisms survive with few changes for long periods, there is no mess, and freezer space is not tied up in storing them.

2. Add 2 ml of sterile distilled water to the culture tube when the colony has matured. Use a sterile cotton applicator to rub the conidia and hyphae off the slant into the water. A stiff long-handled needle can also be used but it tends to scrape up bits of agar as well.

3. Transfer the water and the suspended fungal elements to one or more small screw cap tubes or vials.[12] Tighten the caps and seal the tops with Parafilm or a similar material. Store the vials/tubes at room temperature.

4. Cultures can be maintained in sterile water for varying intervals

> 2 weeks: *Alternaria* and *Cladosporium*
> 4 weeks: *Acremonium, Aspergillus fumigatus, Curvularia, Drechslera, Epicoccum, Epidermophyton floccosum, Exophiala jeanselmei, Exophia werneckii, Fonsecaea pedrosoi, Microsporum canis, Microsporum cookei, Microsporum gypseum, Microsporum nanum, Mucor, Nigrospora, Phialophora verrucosa, Piedraia hortae, Rhizopus, Sepedonium, Syncephalastrum*
> 6 months: All others—when in doubt, hold one set for 6 months while transferring a second set at 4-week intervals during the 6 months until you ensure that 6 months is appropriate

To subculture shake the vial or tube to resuspend the particles. Flame the mouth of the vial/tube or wipe the lip with alcohol. Remove 1–2 drops of the suspension with a sterile Pasteur pipette and transfer it to a fresh plate or tube of PDA or PFA. Incubate the subculture at 25–30°C until growth appears.

SUBCULTURE OF FUNGI

Fungi may require subculture to fresh media to obtain more inoculum or to get a young culture for tests, to test their ability to grow or to use certain substrates, or to encourage development of specific characteristics such as pigmentation or conidiation/sporulation. They may be subcultured in an attempt to determine if they are biphasic or to learn if they can grow at different temperatures. For any subculture, for any reason, the same rules apply.

1. Use good aseptic technique, to protect yourself and your coworkers as well as to prevent contamination of the work area and other cultures.

2. Use fresh sterile media.

3. Label plates and tubes properly, including as a minimum the date the transfer is done and the identification number or name of the culture. The medium used and the temperature of incubation are also helpful notes.

Materials

> bacteriologic loop for yeast *or* mycology needles for moulds
> initial culture to be transferred
> any control organisms that are needed
> appropriate medium/media for subculture
> for moulds, alcohol (optional)[13] and a beaker of sterile sand overlaid with disinfectant[14] are also desirable

Procedure

NOTE that these are the required steps for standard subcultures. Consult the specific procedure if you are doing a differential test; in some instances it is important to transfer the fungus without transferring any of the agar.

Moulds

1. Sterilize the mycology needle and use it to cut a small plug of the mycelium from the colony. Choose a section midway between the center and the periphery of the colony. If the initial culture is in a Petri dish rather than a tube, you may find it convenient to use two mycology needles in tandem to make the cut.

2. Scratch the surface of the new agar slightly with a needle to roughen it, or make a small slit or gouge in the surface. The base of the transferred material must be seated firmly against the new surface so that nutrients can be absorbed and so that the transferred plug doesn't slide around or fall off.

3. Impale the agar plug on one needle and transfer it to the fresh plate or tube of medium. Press the *base* of the plug firmly onto the new medium—if you slap the plug in there upside down, the fungus will find it difficult, if not impossible, to grow.

4. Incubate the plate or tube at the appropriate temperature (generally 25–30°C) until growth appears or until the maximum incubation time for the test has expired.

---

[12]One of the authors used vials and Whatman Vial Files for the cultures. The files are easily stored in a small space, and an index is easily maintained on the lid of the file.

[13]Dipping the needle into the alcohol and flaming it effects sterilization of the needle faster and is easier on the metal than holding the thick mycology needle in the flame or incinerator until it is red hot.

[14]A beaker of sterile sand with a layer of disinfectant is desirable when desktop incinerators are not available for cleansing and sterilizing needles and loops. Rubbing the needle in the sand scrubs the mycelial fragments and conidia from the needle, and the disinfectant kills or inactivates the fungus.

Yeasts and yeastlike fungi

1. Sterilize the bacteriology loop. Touch it to the colony to be subcultured, then streak in your usual pattern as if you were streaking bacteria for isolation.
2. Incubate the plate or tube at the appropriate temperature (generally 25–30°C) until growth appears or until the maximum incubation time for the test has expired.

TEASE MOUNTS

A tease mount is a kind of direct smear made from a mould-form colony. Two mycology needles are used to gently pull at ("tease") the fungus. The idea is to separate the hyphae into individual strands so that they, and the conidia, can be examined. The trick is to spread the parts out without disconnecting them so you can see the hyphae and the conidia *and the way they are connected to each other*. Free-floating conidia and remnants of hyphae are not very helpful.

A tease mount is the original method for examining moulds. It takes time and requires patience. The quality of the preparation is directly related to the skill and patience of the mycologist. With some fungi even great skill and great patience cannot make a "good preparation," i.e., one in which the conidia are attached to the conidiophores. *Scotch tape preps* and *slide cultures* are good alternatives to tease mounts; these procedures are also included in this appendix. The traditional mounting fluid is LPCB, which creates a good temporary preparation; using LPCB with PVA means that the slide prep can be saved for future study. Both mounting fluids are discussed elsewhere in this appendix.

Materials

  2 mycology needles
     patience
  mould to be examined
     patience
  microscope slides
     patience
  coverslips
     patience
  slide flat
  mounting fluid in a dropper bottle (LPCB *or* LPCB with PVA)
  Permount or nail polish (if LPCB with PVA is not used)

Procedure

1. Place a drop of mounting fluid on a clean microscope slide. Sterilize the mycology needles by holding them in a flame or incinerator or by dipping them in alcohol and flaming them.

2. Use the two needles to remove a sliver of the colony from an area halfway between the center and the rim of the colony. Do *not* scrape the mycelium from the agar—cut out a tiny plug of the colony with the agar attached.
3. Place the colony plug in the LPCB on the slide. With one mycology needle in each hand *gently* pluck at the fungus, teasing it into separate strands that will lay flat under the coverslip (see Fig. 2.2). If you do this too quickly or too roughly, your final preparation will be useless and you will have to begin again.
4. When the teasing is done, place a coverslip over the suspended cells. Be careful in lowering the coverslip so that you don't trap a lot of air, which creates bubbles, which makes the preparation hard to read. Coverslipping the suspension without getting air bubbles is difficult because the mixture of agar and fungus tends to be lumpy and uneven. Tapping the coverslip gently with the handle of the needle tends to help seat the coverslip and remove trapped air; it can also knock the conidia free of the conidiophores.

   Large bits of agar can be melted by holding the slide *briefly* over the Bunsen burner flame or at the mouth of the incinerator. Be careful—heating the preparation too long or too intensely will spoil it and you will have to begin again at step 1.
5. If necessary, use a paper towel to remove excess mounting fluid. Wipe the slide very carefully so that the coverslip isn't moved, or simply lay the paper towel on the slide and allow it to absorb the LPCB.
6. To examine the slide place it on the stage of a bright-field microscope and examine it under low power and high power. Adjust the light, if necessary, by lowering the condenser.
7. Record what you see, and use the information as a springboard for deciding what to do next.
8. *To preserve the slide* label it with the age of the culture, temperature of incubation and medium used (as well as the mould's name or number, of course). Seal the edges of the coverslip with Permount or nail polish after it is dry when LPCB is the mounting fluid. When LPCB with PVA is the mounting fluid, no seal is needed. Hardening of the PVA keeps the coverslip in place and protects the fungus. A seal can be added, as insurance, if desired. *In either case*, set the preparations aside in a slide flat until the fluid has dried—accidentally touching the microscope lens to the wet sealer or LPCB-PVA will make a mess of the lens.

WET PREPARATIONS (WET PREPS AND WET MOUNTS)

Wet preparations, also called wet preps and wet mounts, may be done to examine a clinical specimen before it is placed on culture media or to examine a colony. The purpose is the same in either case—to see what is present, mycologically speaking, so that you know what needs to be done next. Various mounting fluids are used for wet preps. Water or saline is most often used for wet mounts from colonies. For specimens the fluid almost always contains potassium hydroxide (KOH), usually in combination with other components. Calcofluor white stain can also be used for wet preps.

The slides, coverslips, and mounting fluid do not need to be sterile but it is important that you don't contaminate the "source," i.e., the culture or specimen, in the process of making the wet preparation.

Wet Preps from Yeast Colonies

This procedure is appropriate for colonies resembling bacteria, i.e., colonies that you suspect are one of the yeast or yeastlike fungi. For fuzzy mould colonies do a *tease mount;* that procedure is presented just above.

Materials

bacteriology loop
initial culture to be examined
microscope slides
coverslips
mounting fluid—usually water or saline, sometimes
    LPCB with or without PVA

Procedure

1. Place a drop of water or saline on a slide.
2. Sterilize the bacteriology loop so that you can touch the colony without contaminating it. Remove a SMALL amount of material. Touch the loop to the drop of fluid on the slide and scrub the organisms off in the drop of fluid with a circular motion. NOTE that you do not want to transfer a lot of material and make a thick film. *Look at the drop of water as you scrub and STOP just when the drop begins to look cloudy.*
3. Flame the loop, and place a coverslip over the suspension of cells. Be careful in lowering the coverslip so that you don't trap a lot of air, which creates bubbles, which makes the preparation hard to read.
4. Allow the preparation to stand for 3–5 minutes until streaming (the random movement of cells in the fluid) has stopped. Place the slide on the stage of a brightfield microscope and examine it under low power and high power. Because the suspending fluid is colorless you may need to reduce the light, by lowering the condenser, to see the cells.
5. Record what you see, and use the information as a springboard for deciding what to do next.

Wet Preps from Specimens Using KOH

This procedure is appropriate for specimens that are thick or tenacious, making it difficult to see the mycotic elements against the background material. Consider the type of specimen and choose the mounting fluid accordingly. Ten percent KOH is a relatively mild agent for clearing cellular debris from skin scrapings, hair, mucus, and purulent materials. Twenty percent KOH is a stronger clearing agent that is useful for nail scrapings or clippings. KOH plus ink or dye makes it easier to see the mycotic elements. Dye or ink may be added to both 10% and 20% KOH. KOH plus dimethyl sulfoxide (DMSO) penetrates the cells faster than straight KOH. DMSO may be added to either concentration of KOH, but KOH with DMSO should not be used with hair, thin scales of skin, or materials such as mucus and pus.

Other materials

bacteriology loop or mycology needle
the specimen
microscope slides
coverslips
mounting fluid

Procedure

1. Place a drop of mounting fluid on a slide.
2. Sterilize the bacteriology loop or mycology needle so that you can touch the specimen without contaminating it. Remove a SMALL amount of material; if blood or pus is present, select the material from those areas. Touch the loop to the drop of fluid on the slide and scrub the specimen off in the drop of fluid with a circular motion. Most specimens "scrub off" fairly easily, but you may sometimes need to use two needles to tease the specimen apart and flatten it so that it can be examined.

NOTE that this is a balancing act—you want to transfer enough material to find any mycotic elements that are present, but you do *not* want to make the preparation too thick. Experience helps. It's better to make two or three good thin preps than one bad thick prep.

---

3. Flame the loop/needle, and place a coverslip over the suspension. Be careful in lowering the coverslip so that you don't trap a lot of air, which creates bubbles, which makes the preparation hard to read.
4. To help the KOH do its job of clearing cellular debris from the specimen

    (a) lay the coverslipped specimen in a Petri dish at room temperature and wait 15–20 minutes (or longer, if it is very thick) for the specimen to clear before you examine it *or*

    (b) *gently* heat the slide over a flame. Be very, very careful not to boil it; boiling crystallizes the mounting fluid and distorts the fungus.

> *Do not heat the specimen if the mounting fluid contains DMSO.* The DMSO already hastens the clearing process. When heat is added, you are at serious risk for dissolving any mycotic elements as well as the debris.

5. Monitor the slide while it is standing or after briefly heating it. Eventually the KOH begins to dissolve fungal elements as well as the cellular debris. You can always let the slide stand longer to clear, but you can't go back if it stands too long[15]—except by making another preparation.

6. To examine the slide place it on the stage of a bright-field microscope and examine it under low power and high power. Because the suspending fluid is colorless, you may need to reduce the light (by lowering the condenser) to see the cells.

7. Record what you see, and use the information as a springboard for deciding what to do next.

SPECIFIC REAGENTS, STAINS, MEDIA, AND METHODS

CONVERSE LIQUID MEDIUM

Converse liquid medium was developed by J. L. Converse for converting *Coccidioides immitis* from the mould phase to the yeast form. Mycologists have used media such as BHIA with blood in plates for years to convert the other dimorphic pathogens from the mould phase to the yeast form, but until Converse medium was formulated the dimorphism of *C. immitis* could be demonstrated only by animal inoculation. This was not only hard on the animals but it also placed personnel at significant risk for infection.

The relatively low concentration of agar means that the medium is semisolid rather than either agar or liquid. Because of the high potential for infection, we recommend that the medium be used in test tubes rather than Petri dishes. This medium can be prepared from the components but may be available commercially. To prepare the medium "from scratch," follow the instructions for "Preparation of Media" in the "General Methods" section of this appendix. If commercially prepared base is used, determine the amount of basal medium to use from the manufacturer's directions for preparation.

Converse medium has been further modified by Brosbe, and subsequently by Sun, to create a solid variant. When this is used at 40°C with 20% CO_2, the development of spherules is reported to be much faster.

Media Components (desired final pH 6.6)

Ammonium acetate	1.23 g
Dextrose	4 g
Dipotassium phosphate	0.5 g
Calcium chloride	2 mg
Potassium phosphate	0.4 g
Magnesium sulfate	0.4 g
Sodium carbonate	12 mg
Sodium chloride	14 mg
Tamol	0.5 g
Zinc sulfate	2 mg
Purified agar or Ionagar #2	10 g
Distilled water	1000 ml

Media Preparation

Mix ingredients and boil for 1 minute to dissolve the agar. Tubed Converse medium has a shelf life of 30 days. *Before sterilization* dispense approximately 8 ml per 16 × 125 mm screw-cap tube for slants. Sterilize the medium by autoclaving it at 121°C (15 pounds pressure) for 15 minutes. After the medium has cooled, store it in the refrigerator (4–6°C) with the usual precautions to prevent drying.

Use and Interpretation

> ALL work with suspected dimorphic pathogens should be done within a laminar-flow biologic safety cabinet. This means that *all work* done with cottony white colonies—especially isolates from sputum and other respiratory specimens—should be done in a laminar-flow biologic safety cabinet.

1. Flood the surface of the unknown colony with sterile saline to counter, as much as possible, the tendency of the conidia to become airborne when they are disturbed. Use a sterile mycology needle to remove a small portion of the mycelium and conidia. Aseptically transfer the growth to a fresh tube of Converse medium.

2. Incubate the inoculated tube at 40°C in a 20% CO_2 incubator for 4–5 days. Place the tube in a cup or small rack so that it remains upright. Examine the tube every 24–36 hours.

3. When growth appears in the tube, go to the biologic safety cabinet and make a wet mount from the culture, using LPCB as the mounting fluid. The "Procedure for Wet Preparations" is provided with the other general mycology techniques in another section of this appendix. *Be very careful about making, transporting,*

---

[15]Honesty compels us to say that, of course, you will probably never know if the mycotic elements were digested along with the debris unless you report "No organisms or mycotic elements seen" and a magnificent fungus colony later appears in culture.

and *examining this slide preparation!* Do *not* allow it to dry out. Carefully dispose of the slide and all other materials so that neither you nor anyone else is exposed to arthroconidia. Laboratory accidents *do* happen, but many can be prevented by using common sense and attending to standard safety precautions.

COTTONSEED CONVERSION MEDIUM

Cottonseed conversion medium was recommended by the Centers for Disease Control and Prevention as the medium of choice for conversion of *Blastomyces dermatitidis* from the mould phase to the yeast form. Reportedly most isolates of the fungus grow within 2–3 days after subculture. This medium must be prepared from scratch. The Traders Oil Mill Company in Fort Worth, Texas, was given as the source for the key ingredient *Pharmamedia*, which presumably is a processed form of cottonseed[16]; other sources may be available.

Media Composition (desired final pH 6.0)

Pharmamedia	20 g
Dextrose	20 g
Agar	20 g
Distilled water	1000 ml

Media Preparation

Add all ingredients to the distilled water. Bring the suspension to a boil and boil for 1 minute to bring the agar into solution. *Before sterilization* dispense approximately 8 ml per 16 × 125 mm screw-cap tube for slants. Sterilize the medium by autoclaving it at 121°C (15 pounds pressure) for 15 minutes. After the medium has cooled, store it in the refrigerator (4–6°C) with the usual precautions to prevent drying.

Use and Interpretation

See the "*In Vitro* Conversion of Dimorphic Fungi" in this appendix for the method.

GERM TUBE TEST

Production of germ tubes is an important characteristic in rapid economical identification of *Candida albicans*. In most clinical laboratories a positive germ tube test is considered definitive, although some mycologists insist that the yeast must also be tested for chlamydospore production and sucrose assimilation to positively eliminate *Candida stellatoidea*.

All yeast and yeastlike fungi produce germ tubes eventually. Because of this the incubation time of 3 hours maximum must be strictly observed. Several substrates can be used for the germ tube test, including bovine serum, rabbit serum or plasma, fetal calf serum, and sheep serum. The substrate is usually purchased in the lyophilized state and reconstituted as needed. The substrate does not need to be kept sterile since it is used for a brief (3-hour) test rather than a culture, but it should be protected from gross contamination. Pooled human serum or plasma *can* be used, but this is not wise. Either may contain the hepatitis or human immunodeficiency viruses or other infectious agents. Human serum or plasma may also contain antibodies or other agents that can interfere with the growth of *Candida* or the development of germ tubes, although this threat is mitigated somewhat by using pooled serum or plasma.

Materials

small (10 × 75 mm) tubes
plasma substrate
organisms for positive and negative controls
plastic film to cover tubes
disposable Pasteur pipettes
glass slides and coverslips
heat block (optional—a 37°C incubator will do, or a test tube rack in a 37°C water bath, but the heat block is convenient)

Procedure

1. Inspect the working container of substrate for clots or gross contamination before using it. Label small (10 × 75 mm) test tubes[17]: positive control, negative control, and number(s) of the culture(s) being tested. Use *Candida albicans* as the positive control and *Candida krusei* as the negative control. Dispense approximately 0.3 ml of substrate into each tube.
2. Touch the colony to be tested with the tip of a sterile Pasteur pipette. Introduce the tip of the pipette into the tube of substrate and twirl the pipette gently to transfer yeast cells from the pipette into suspension. *Leave the pipette in the tube!* Prepare positive and negative controls in the same manner.
3. Wrap plastic film around the pipette and the mouth of the tubes, and incubate them in a heat block or the incubator at 37°C for 2 to 3 hours. *Incubation for more than 3 hours can cause false-positive results.*
4. After incubation, use the Pasteur pipette to transfer 1 or 2 drops from the "unknown" to a labeled glass slide. Coverslip the mixture and set it aside for a few minutes until

---

[16]According to the third (1973) edition of *Laboratory Methods in Medical Mycology*, published by the U.S. Department of Health, Education, and Welfare.

[17]A "batch" of serum or plasma can be dispensed into tubes when the material is reconstituted. The tubes should be sealed with Parafilm or a similar material and frozen until they are needed.

brownian movement has stopped. Return the pipette to the tube. Repeat the transfer process with the control tubes.

5. Examine the slides with the low- and high-power lenses of a brightfield microscope, as you would any wet prep. Look for germ tubes on all three slides. Do *not* fall into the trap of seeing germ tubes in the positive control because they are supposed to be there *or* of missing germ tubes in the negative control because they should be absent. Accidents happen. Mistakes are made. Controls have no value if you assume you know the results and use the controls incorrectly.

Interpretation

Germ tubes, blastoconidia, and pseudohyphae all may form in the substrate during the period of incubation. *Germ tubes* are longer than the parent cell and approximately half as wide, with parallel sides. They are *not* constricted where they emerge from the parent cell. *Pseudohyphae* are blastoconidia that have not (yet) separated from the parent cell. The sides of pseudohyphae are not parallel, and pseudohyphae *are* constricted where they emerge from the parent cell (see Fig. 7.9). Results cannot be quantitated, but you should see numerous germ tubes in the preparation before you call the organism *Candida albicans*. If only one or two cells have germ tubes, consider repeating the test or confirming the results by chlamydospore production or assimilation tests.

HAIR PERFORATION TEST

The *in vitro* hair perforation test is used for identification of the dermatophytes, especially to differentiate *Trichophyton mentagrophytes* and *Trichophyton rubrum*. Sterile hair is presented for the mould, with yeast extract as the source of nutrition. The hair used should be from a young child (<5 years old). This is logical if you consider who is most likely to have tinea capitis. Using a child's hair also means that the hair has probably not been exposed to dyes or permanent wave solutions or other chemicals likely to make the hair resistant to penetration or interfere with the growth of the fungus. Dermatophytes do not prefer blondes, but using light-colored hair makes it easier to see the results of the test.

Materials

sterile Petri dish
sterile filter paper
sterilized human hair
sterile 10% yeast extract
sterile distilled water, 10 ml
sterile Pasteur pipette
forceps and alcohol
mycology needle
culture to be tested

Reagents

10% Yeast extract

Yeast extract	10 g
Distilled water	100 ml

Mix the yeast extract and distilled water in a flask and swirl to dissolve. Filter sterilize the solution and store it in a sterile flask in the refrigerator until it is needed.

Sterile hair

Select light-colored hair from a young child, preferably cut into lengths of approximately 1 cm to make it easier to handle. Place it in a glass Petri dish or screw-cap tube and autoclave it at 121°C (15 pounds pressure) for 15 minutes.

Cool the tube or dish completely so that moisture does not accumulate inside it, then seal the container and store it at room temperature.

Procedure

1. Put a piece of sterile filter paper into the sterile Petri dish; this helps contain the liquid you are adding and makes a spill less likely.
2. Use the Pasteur pipette to aseptically add 1 or 2 drops of yeast extract to the tube of distilled water, then cover the bottom of the dish with 2–3 ml of the dilute yeast extract. Don't drown the culture; more fluid can be added during incubation if the paper becomes dry.
3. Dip the tips of the forceps into the alcohol and flame them briefly to sterilize them. Transfer approximately 10–12 strands of hair onto the filter paper in the Petri dish.
4. Sterilize the mycology needle and transfer conidia from the original culture directly onto the hairs. Tape the two halves of the Petri dish together loosely—you don't want to seal it and cut off the oxygen supply, but you do want to prevent a spill if you can.
5. Incubate the hair perforation test at room temperature for up to 4 weeks. Check the test periodically (every 3–4 days) to ensure that it has not dried out. Obviously, if it has, you add more dilute yeast extract.
6. To read the test, remove a single hair from the dish and place it in a drop of LPCB on a microscope slide. Coverslip the preparation and examine it microscopically (see Fig. 5.6).

   Positive: wedge-shaped or conical perforations into the hair shaft
   Negative: no wedge-shaped or conical perforations

7. A positive test suggests that the mould is *Trichophyton mentagrophytes*; *Trichophyton rubrum* is unable to penetrate hair under these conditions *in vitro*. Controls

should be done to aid in reading and interpreting the results. Use known cultures of *Trichophyton mentagrophytes* and *Trichophyton rubrum* as the positive and negative controls, respectively.

HAY INFUSION AGAR

Hay infusion agar is used to stimulate the production of conidia or spores in fungi that have become genetically unstable, i.e., produce few reproductive structures or produce reproductive structures that are atypical. Colony morphology may also be atypical. This genetic change may occur in cultures that have lived too long in stock culture and been transferred many times. Sometimes the instability is seen in specimens from patients because of some therapy the patient is receiving. Of course the fungus may have been exposed to a mutagenic agent in nature—even something as simple as the ultraviolet rays in sunshine.

This medium is not chemically defined. The specific components contributed by the decomposing hay are not identified or quantitated. The medium must be prepared "from scratch," probably beginning with an expedition to get the hay. Then wet the hay thoroughly and let it hang around in a warm spot for 4–5 days, or a week, until it begins to decompose and turn brown. To prepare the medium from scratch follow the instructions for "Preparation of Media" in the "General Methods" section of this appendix. In preparing the medium note that the first round of autoclaving is not done to sterilize the hay. The purpose is to further break down the hay and "steep" it in the water to release the contents of the cells into solution—a process not unlike making a cup of tea from a tea bag. Soil extract agar can also be used to recover cultures that are genetically unstable.

Media Composition (desired pH 6.2)

Hay, decomposing	50 g
Dipotassium phosphate	2 g
Agar	15 g
Tap water	1000 ml

Media Preparation

Mix the hay and the tap water and autoclave the mixture at 121°C (15 pounds pressure) for 30 minutes. When the mixture has cooled enough to be handled safely, filter it through cheesecloth. Discard the hay with the cheesecloth.

Add dipotassium phosphate and agar to the infusion of hay and stir to mix. Cool the mixture and adjust the pH to 6.2. Then bring the mixture to a boil again and boil for 1 minute to get the agar into solution. *Before sterilization* dispense approximately 8 ml per 16 × 125 mm screw-cap tube for slants. Sterilize the medium by autoclaving it at 121°C (15 pounds pressure) for 15 minutes.

Slant it; when cooled, store it in the refrigerator (4–6°C) with the usual precautions to prevent drying.

Use and Interpretation

1. Subculture from the unknown colony to a slant of hay infusion agar. You may wish to inoculate several tubes, given that the fungus may be badly damaged or fastidious, to increase the likelihood of growth of the organism.[18]
2. Cap the tube loosely and incubate it at room temperature. Examine the tube regularly until growth appears. Hold the tube for a minimum of 21 days before discarding it as "no growth"; a longer incubation period may be appropriate, depending on the suspected identity of the fungus.
3. When good growth appears, do a tease mount (refer to "Preparation of Tease Mounts") of the colony for clues about the identity of the organism and to determine what to do next. NOTE that the fungus may have to go through several generations on the hay infusion agar before it is stable enough to respond typically on standard media and produce its identifiable gross and microscopic morphologies.

INDIA INK PREPARATION

India ink is a negative staining method that uses carbon particles as the background for the colorless transparent cells of fungi. The method was used initially to examine cerebrospinal fluid for the presence of *Cryptococcus neoformans*. India ink preparations are not very sensitive, so the method has been supplanted in many laboratories by immunologic methods such as the latex antigen test for detecting *Cryptococcus*. The results of India ink preparations are, on the other hand, obtained quickly, which makes it a good screening procedure. India ink preps are also done to examine colonies of suspected cryptococci.

Reagent

Pelikan brand India ink is available from art supply stores. Other brands can be used, but Pelikan is least likely to be contaminated with bacteria, and it can be purchased in a handy tube that can deliver exactly the desired number of drops of ink exactly where they should be placed. Formalinized nigrosin can also be used as the negative stain.

Procedure

1. Dilute the ink, using 1 part ink to 1 or 2 parts water. You can mix this on the slide, or in a small test tube if

---

[18]Let's get serious. You might as well use the slants; most of that batch of agar is likely to sit in the refrigerator and have to be discarded eventually anyhow.

more than one India ink prep is being done. Follow the "Procedure for Wet Mounts," described in the "General Methods" section of this appendix and in the text.

2. After streaming has stopped, examine the slide with the low- and high-power objectives of the microscope.

Positive: *Cryptococcus neoformans* is suggested by large transparent spheres, with little or no internal definition, against a dark background. The spheres may be surrounded by a bright "halo" created by the polysaccharide capsule (see Fig. 7.16)

Negative: no large transparent structures

Artifacts: lymphocytes are distinguished from *C. neoformans* by their more granular texture and the presence of a nucleus. Erythrocytes are smaller and less clear than *C. neoformans;* talc crystals from somebody's gloves are more refractile than the yeast, and irregular in shape

IN VITRO[19] CONVERSION OF DIMORPHIC FUNGI

Dimorphic fungi live in tissue as spherules or yeast. Most of them also assume the yeast form when they are cultured on artificial media at 37°C. When they are grown in culture at room temperature, all dimorphic fungi of medical importance develop mould-form colonies. One method for proving that a fungus is a dimorphic pathogen is to show that it can be converted from the mould form to the yeast (tissue) form. Conversion is effected by simulating life in tissue, i.e., simply subculturing the mould colony to rich media and using warmer (37°C) temperatures. To convert the yeast form or spherule to the mould subculture it to standard mycologic media and incubate at room temperature.

Converse medium and increased temperature and carbon dioxide levels must be used to convert *Coccidioides immitis* moulds to spherules. *Histoplasma capsulatum, Paracoccidioides brasiliensis,* and *Sporothrix schenckii* can be induced to convert on rich media such as BHIA, preferably BHIA with 5% to 10% blood added. Cottonseed conversion medium may be needed for *Blastomyces dermatitidis* moulds, although BHIA with blood works well for most isolates of this fungus.[20]

Under most circumstances cultural conversions of dimorphic fungi other than *Sporothrix schenckii* should

perhaps be considered something of a laboratory trick. Exoantigen tests and DNA probes can identify the dimorphic pathogens more rapidly with less risk. The only justification we recognize for conversion of the systemic pathogens—if there is a justification—may be for experienced mycologists working in optimum safety conditions to produce demonstration materials for teaching.

Materials

mycology needles
sterile distilled water or BHIB
fresh tubes of agar (BHIA with blood, cottonseed medium, Converse medium)
culture to be converted

Procedure

NOTE that every step of the conversion should be done within a biologic safety cabinet.

1. *If you are testing a mould colony,* cover the yeast or mould culture to be converted with sterile distilled water to reduce the release of aerosols containing conidia from the surface of the mould.
2. Aseptically transfer a portion of the yeast *or* mould colony to the surface of a fresh tube of the chosen medium. If the surface of the medium seems dry, dribble several drops of sterile distilled water or BHIB over it to provide moisture.
3. Cap the tube loosely and incubate it at the appropriate temperature for 2–3 days before examining it for growth. When growth appears, make a slide preparation and examine it microscopically. If you know that the initial growth was a pure culture, then a mixture of hyphal elements, conidia, and yeast forms in the subculture strongly suggests that the fungus is dimorphic. Several transfers may be needed to convert the fungus completely to its other form.

LACTOPHENOL–COTTON BLUE (LPCB) STAIN AND LPCB WITH POLYVINYL ALCOHOL (PVA)[21]

LPCB is perhaps the original staining method for the study of fungi. It is the preferred stain for the microscopic examination of mould-form colonies. The lactic acid enhances penetration of the solution into the hyphae, the phenol inactivates the living cells, the cotton blue does the staining, and the glycerol creates a semiper-

[19]*In vivo* conversion of fungi, by inoculating laboratory animals, is not recommended. First, better culture methods, DNA probes and the exoantigen tests make it unnecessary, even for *Coccidioides immitis.* Second, creating artificial infections in animals is potentially extremely hazardous for all personnel who have contact with the animals.
[20]The use of Converse medium and cottonseed conversion medium is described elsewhere in this appendix.

[21]Polyvinyl alcohol (PVA) is a potential carcinogen. The reagent should be prepared in a chemical hood or biologic safety cabinet. Avoid getting it on your body now and when you use it to make slide preparations.

manent preparation and reduces the likelihood of precipitation of the stain.

LPCB with PVA is a refinement of the original LPCB stain for the microscopic examination of mould-form colonies. The solution is fluid initially, allowing a tease mount to be done. One effect of PVA is to reduce evaporation of the stain so that you can take more time teasing the fungus. The addition of PVA also creates a mounting fluid that will harden in 24–36 hours, creating permanent slides without the messy extra step of sealing the edge of the coverslip with Permount or nail polish.

Basic LPCB Reagent

Phenol	20 g
Lactic acid	20 ml
Glycerol	40 g
Cotton blue (Poirrier's blue)	0.05 g

Mix the phenol with the lactic acid and glycerol. Gently heat the mixture to dissolve the phenol crystals. While it is still warm add the cotton blue dye and mix thoroughly. If cotton blue dye precipitates from the solution, filter it through Whatman #1 filter paper.

Stock solution of polyvinyl alcohol

PVA granules	15 g
Distilled water	100 ml

Place an Erlenmeyer flask containing the water in an 80°C water bath. Slowly add the PVA to the water and stir until the PVA dissolves and the solution thickens and clears. When the solution has cooled transfer it to a brown screw-cap bottle for storage. NOTE that any PVA that gets on the threads of the cap should be wiped away with alcohol or, when the PVA hardens, the bottle of stock solution will be sealed permanently (unless you choose to knock off the top to get to the solution).

Working solution of LPCB with PVA mounting medium

Stock solution of PVA	56 ml
Lactic acid	22 ml
Phenol (liquid concentrate)	22 ml
Cotton blue (Poirrier's blue)	0.05 g

To avoid a gummy mess that is unusable, *always* add the lactic acid to the stock solution of PVA and mix well. Then mix in the liquid phenol. Finally, add the cotton blue stain and mix until the stain is evenly distributed; you may need to warm the PVA–phenol–lactic acid mixture to get the cotton blue into solution. Place the working solution in a brown screw-cap bottle for storage.

Procedure

See *tease mounts* and *Scotch tape preps* in the "General Methods" section of this appendix.

MITE CONTROL

Yes, mite control—managing tiny insects that get into your cultures and destroy them (and your nerves). This procedure is included because we both have taught mycology in buildings with inadequate air conditioning that were not initially designed as laboratories. The preferred method might be to simply autoclave the cultures and go on, but this is not always possible. Usually some attempt must be made to recover the fungus so that it can be identified. More information about mite control is given in Chapter 2.

Because of the chemicals used, the media and reagents should be prepared in a chemical hood. The mite control methods should be done in a biologic safety cabinet.

Method #1

The medium

Prepare 1 L of any standard nonselective mycology medium. Add 10 mg of hexachlorocyclohexane to the medium and dispense it into 16 × 125 ml screw-cap tubes. After the tubes are autoclaved allow them to cool in a slant position. Subculture the infested fungus to one or more tubes of the medium and incubate at room temperature. The mites die in approximately 1 week on this medium. Unfortunately, not all fungi survive.

Method #2

The reagent

95% ethyl alcohol	95 ml
mercuric chloride	0.5 g
glycerin	5 ml
methylene blue dye	3 drops

Replace the cap of the culture tube with a cotton plug saturated in the above mixture. Wrap the top with Parafilm or plastic wrap to reduce evaporation and incubate the culture for 4 days.

or

Place the Petri dish or the culture tube (with the cap loosened) in a plastic bag that can be sealed. Before you seal the bag add 2 or 3 cotton balls soaked in the reagent. Incubate for 4 days at room temperature. Subculture the organism to fresh medium and trust that it survived the treatment and the mites did not.

POTASSIUM HYDROXIDE (KOH) SOLUTIONS

KOH is used in two different concentrations to clear specimens that are cloudy or opaque so that the mycotic elements are visible. The stronger (20%) solution is recommended for use with scrapings from fingernails or toenails; 10% KOH is used for all other specimens. Adding glycerol to the KOH helps keep the KOH from precipitating and retards dissolution of the fungal elements; this is especially useful for the 20% solution. DMSO can be added to the KOH solution to enhance penetration of the KOH into the solution and speed up the process of clearing debris. Combining the KOH with Parker's blue-black ink makes it easier to see any fungal elements against the clear background.

Reagents

NOTE that the reaction of KOH with water produces heat. Placing the container in an ice bath controls this.

10% (20%) KOH

| KOH | 10 g (20 g for 20%) |
| Distilled water | 100 ml |

Slowly add KOH crystals to approximately half the distilled water. Stir until they are completely dissolved. Transfer to a volumetric flask and make up to 100 ml with distilled water.

KOH with glycerol

Slowly add KOH crystals to approximately 40 ml of distilled water with stirring until the KOH is completely dissolved, then add 20 ml of the glycerol. Transfer to a volumetric flask and make up to 100 ml with distilled water.

KOH with DMSO

Mix 40 ml of the DMSO and approximately 30 ml of distilled water in a fume hood.[22] Slowly add 10 g of KOH and mix until the crystals are completely dissolved. Transfer to a volumetric flask and make up to 100 ml with distilled water.

KOH with ink

Mix 1 volume of Parker's blue-black ink with 2 volumes of KOH (10% or 20%) with or without additives. For a single slide preparation the reagents can be mixed on the slide. If more than one preparation is to be done you may wish to use a test tube or dropper bottle to prepare the mixture.

Procedure

Follow the **Procedure for Wet Preps** that is given in the "General Methods" section of this appendix.

---

[22]DMSO smells like garlic and the odor gets into everything. Unless you are very careful in working with DMSO, everything you eat, drink, and smell will be overlaid with garlic for about 24 hours.

POTATO FLAKES AGAR (PFA)

PFA is a nutritious medium that can be used for primary cultures. PFA encourages production of conidia and spores; this makes it a favorite for slide cultures of fungi. Potato starch also enhances development of pigment, especially among the dermatophytes. "Homemade" potato dextrose agar (PDA) is generally preferred over commercially prepared medium or PDA prepared from commercial bases because both pigmentation and conidiation are better on the homemade variety. For most routine laboratory work the difference in the quality of the results may not be great enough to justify the hassle of making the medium from raw potatoes. Rinaldi developed and tested this formula for a potato-based medium using dried potato flakes as a way to get homemade goodness without the peeling, dicing, and filtering. To prepare the medium "from scratch," follow the instructions for "Preparation of Media" in the "General Methods" section of this appendix.

CMA and rice infusion agar can also be used to encourage pigment production. Commercially available PDA is useful for studying both pigmentation and conidiation.

Media Composition

Potato flakes (any brand)	20 g
Dextrose	10 g
Agar	15 g
Distilled water	1000 ml

Media Preparation

Add the dry ingredients to the distilled water in a flask. Swirl the flask to distribute the ingredients, then heat the mixture to boiling. Boil long enough to get the agar into solution.

In dispensing the medium NOTE that the flakes tend to settle to the bottom of the container. This means that the flask must be swirled frequently as plates are being poured. You may also wish to tilt tubes as they cool to 45–50°C to ensure somewhat even distribution of the potato flakes through the medium as the agar solidifies.

Sterilize the medium by autoclaving it at 121°C (15 pounds pressure) for 15 minutes. PFA can be used in plates or slant tubes; for slants dispense approximately 8 ml per 16 × 125 mm screw-cap tube. After the medium has cooled, store it in the refrigerator (4–6°C) with the usual precautions to prevent drying.

Use and Interpretation

NOTE that growth of the fungus on the PFA subculture should take no longer than it took for the initial colony to develop, and growth is usually faster because (1) PFA is richer than most general purpose media, and (2) the organism has already overcome the shock of leaving the host and making do with artificial media.

To study conidiation/sporulation

To use PFA for slide cultures, follow the "Procedure for Slide Cultures" in the "General Methods" section of this appendix. An alternate way to study conidiation is to subculture the isolated unknown to a plate of PFA (see "Subculture of Moulds"). Incubate the plate at room temperature, and check it periodically. The amount of time to incubate the plate before discarding it varies with the organism.

To study pigmentation

For determining pigment production, subculture a portion of the original colony to the center of the PFA plate. Incubate the plate at room temperature[23] and check it periodically. The amount of time to incubate the plate before discarding it varies with the organism.

SOIL EXTRACT AGAR

Soil infusion agar is used to stimulate the production of conidia or spores in fungi that have become genetically unstable, i.e., produce few reproductive structures or produce reproductive structures that are atypical. Colony morphology may also be atypical. This genetic change may occur in cultures that have lived too long in stock culture and been transferred many times. Sometimes the instability is seen in specimens from patients because of some therapy the patient is receiving. Of course the fungus may have been exposed to a mutagenic agent in nature—even something as simple as the ultraviolet rays in sunshine.

Soil extract agar can also be used as a maintenance medium for cultures of *Histoplasma capsulatum* and *Blastomyces dermatitidis*. To maintain a fungus consult the section on "Maintenance of Stock Cultures" in this appendix for better methods than growth on agar.

This medium is not chemically defined. The specific components contributed by the soil are not identified or quantitated. The medium must be prepared from scratch, probably beginning with a trip to somebody's garden for the soil. To prepare the medium from scratch follow the instructions for "Preparation of Media" in the "General Methods" section of this appendix.

In preparing the medium note that the first round of autoclaving is not done to sterilize the soil. The purpose is to break down the soil and release the contents into solution by "steeping" it in the water, a process not unlike making a cup of tea from a tea bag.

Hay infusion agar can also be used to revitalize cultures that are genetically unstable. Malt extract agar has also been suggested as a maintenance medium for fungi, as noted earlier, although a number of other, better, methods exist (see "Maintenance of Stock Cultures" in this appendix).

Media Composition (desired pH 6.0–6.2)

Garden soil	500 g
Dextrose	2 g
Yeast extract	1 g
Potassium phosphate	0.5 g
Agar	15 g
Tap water	1000 ml

Media Preparation

Mix the soil and the tap water and autoclave the mixture at 121°C with 15 pounds pressure (121°C) for 10 minutes. When the mixture has cooled enough to be handled safely, filter it through Whatman's #2 filter paper. Discard the filter paper and its contents. Add the remaining ingredients to the filtrate and swirl the flask to mix the contents. Add enough tap water to bring the volume back to 1 L. Adjust the final pH to 6.0–6.2. Then bring the mixture to a boil and boil for 1 minute to get the agar into solution.

It can be used in plates or slant tubes; for slants dispense approximately 8 ml per 16 × 125 mm screw-cap tube. Sterilize the medium by autoclaving it at 121°C (15 pounds pressure) for 15 minutes. Slant the tubes. After the medium has cooled, store it in the refrigerator (4–6°C) with the usual precautions to prevent drying.

Use and Interpretation

Follow the usual procedure for subculture of a mould. You may wish to inoculate several tubes, given that the fungus may be badly damaged or fastidious, to increase the likelihood of growth of the organism.[24]

Cap the tube loosely and incubate it at room temperature. Examine the tube regularly until growth appears. Hold the tube for a minimum of 21 days before discarding it as "no growth"; a longer incubation period may be appropriate, depending on the likely identity of the fungus.

When good growth appears, do a tease mount (refer to "Preparation of Tease Mounts") of the colony for clues about the identity of the organism and to determine what to do next. NOTE that the fungus may have to go through several generations on the soil extract agar be-

---

[23]Pigment production is always better at room temperature than at 37°C, for bacteria as well as fungi.

[24]The reality is that you might as well use the slants; most of that batch of agar is likely to sit in the refrigerator and has to be discarded eventually anyhow.

fore it is stable enough to respond typically on standard media and produce its characteristic gross and microscopic morphologies.

STERILE RICE GRAINS

Sterile rice grains are used to distinguish *Microsporum audouinii* from *Microsporum canis*. *M. canis* produces conidia and usually produces a yellow pigment on the rice grains, while *Microsporum audouinii* just lies there, exerting itself very little. At best *M. audouinii* produces a light brown discoloration of the rice. Do not confuse sterile rice grains with the rice infusion/rice extract agar used for the study of yeast and yeastlike fungi.

This test is useful, especially for the inexperienced mycologist, for distinguishing these two species of *Microsporum*. Most isolates of *M. canis* (and many other fungi) readily produce typical macroconidia and other structures, but "lazy" atypical variants closely resemble *M. audouinii*, which is identified by its reluctance to grow and produce reproductive structures.

This medium is not commercially available but must be prepared from scratch.

Media Composition

White rice (*not* fortified with vitamins)	8 g
Distilled water	25 ml

Media Preparation

Dispense 8 g of rice into a 50 ml screw-cap bottle or flask with a wide mouth. Add 25 ml of distilled water and cap the container loosely. Mixing is unnecessary. Autoclave at 121°C (15 pounds pressure) for 15 minutes. After cooling, store it in the refrigerator (4–6°C) with the usual precautions to prevent drying.

Use and Interpretation

1. Bring the sterile rice grains to room temperature and label the container. Inoculate the top of the sterile rice grains heavily with the unknown culture. Transfer only mycelium and spores *without* including any medium from the initial culture; carryover of nutrients from the isolation plate can cause confusion by allowing *M. audouinii* to grow better than it ought to on the unfortified rice alone.

2. Incubate at room temperature (25–30°C) for 6–10 days.

   Positive: white woolly mycelium followed in several days (perhaps) by yellow pigment in the colony

   Negative: little or no growth, with (perhaps) brownish discoloration of the medium

3. Control cultures may also be inoculated:

   Positive: *M. canis*
   Negative: *M. audouinii*

4. When growth appears a wet mount should be done to differentiate between variants of *M. canis* that do not produce the characteristic pigment and other dermatophytes able to grow on sterile rice grains. Consult Chapter 5 of this text for the characteristic microscopic features of *M. canis* and other dermatophytes.

TEMPERATURE TESTS

The temperature at which a fungus can grow is sometimes an important part of differentiating it from similar organisms. Two factors must be considered in testing this. First (logically enough), select a medium on which the fungus is expected to grow well. Usually this is Emmon's modification of SDA or the medium used for the initial culture. Second, use the same medium for all of the temperatures being tested.

Incubate the tests for an interval at least as long as the fungus took for its initial growth in culture. The temperatures usually used are room temperature (25–30°C), 37°C, and 45°C, but temperatures as high as 54°C may sometimes be needed.

V-8 JUICE AGAR

V-8 juice agar is used to detect the production of ascospores and asci as one component of the identification of ascosporogenous ("perfect") yeast such as *Saccharomyces* and *Hansenula*. This medium may be prepared from the components or it may be available commercially. To prepare the medium from scratch, follow the instructions for "Preparation of Media" in the "General Methods" section of this appendix. If commercially prepared base is used, determine the amount of basal medium to use from the manufacturer's directions for preparation.

Acetate agar can also be used to detect ascospore production.

Media Composition (desired pH 6.8)

V-8 vegetable juice	350 ml
Dry yeast	5 g
Agar	14 g
Distilled water	340 ml

Media Preparation

Add agar to water in one flask and bring the mixture to a boil. In a second flask, mix the V-8 juice and dry yeast. Adjust the pH of the juice-yeast mixture to 6.8, then heat it in flowing steam in the autoclave for 10 minutes. Readjust the pH to 6.8 after the mixture has cooled.

Combine the agar solution with the juice-yeast mixture and mix well. To sterilize, autoclave at 121°C (15 pounds pressure) for 15 minutes. Approximately 8 ml can be dispensed per 16 × 125 mm screw-cap tube for slants or dispense approximately 25 ml per large screw-cap tube or bottle for later use as plates. Store it in the refrigerator (4–6°C) with the usual precautions to prevent drying.

Use and Interpretation

1. If multiple tests are to be done, prepare a *light* suspension of the colony to be tested in sterile saline or water. If this is the only differential test to be done, touch the colony lightly with a sterile inoculating loop. In either case, streak the surface of the agar plate as you would for bacterial isolation.

2. Incubate at room temperature (25–30°C). Examine the culture for growth after 48 hours and then at 72-hour intervals. The plate should be held for 3 weeks before the test is discarded as "negative," i.e., no ascospores or asci are produced.

3. To examine the culture for asci and ascospores, make a wet mount in a drop of saline on a microscope slide. Coverslip the suspension and examine it with a bright-field microscope, using both low- and high-power objectives.

4. Asci will be larger than the asexual yeast cells. NOTE the shape of the asci (round, hat shaped, kidney shaped, and so forth), because this characteristic is important in the identification of the yeast. If asci are seen, determine whether they contain ascospores and the average number of ascospores per ascus.

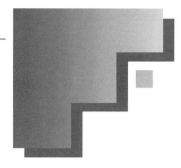

Bibliography: References and Suggested Readings

1. Campbell MC, Stewart JL: The Medical Mycology Handbook. New York, John Wiley & Sons, 1980.
2. Cook NB: Serodiagnosis of fungal infections. *In* Stevens CD (ed): Clinical Immunology and Serology—A Laboratory Perspective. Philadelphia, FA Davis, 1996, pp 299–306.
3. Cooper BH (section ed): Section VI: Taxonomy, Classification, and Nomenclature of Fungi. *In* Lennette EH, Balows A, Hausler WJ, et al (eds): Manual of Clinical Microbiology, 4th ed. Washington DC, American Society for Microbiology, 1985, pp 495–584.
4. Emmons CW, Binford CH, Utz JP, Kwon-Chung KJ: Medical Mycology, 3rd ed. Philadelphia, Lea & Febiger, 1977.
5. Fromtling RA (section ed): Section V: Fungi. *In* Balows A, Hausler WJ, Hermann KL, et al (eds): Manual of Clinical Microbiology, 5th ed. Washington, DC, American Society for Microbiology, 1991, pp 579–693.
6. Howard BJ, Keiser MD, Smith TF, et al: Fundamental Mycology. Clinical and Pathogenic Microbiology, 2nd ed. St. Louis, CV Mosby, 1994, pp 543–639.
7. Kaplan W, Bragg SL, Crane S, Ahearn DG: Serotyping *Cryptococcus neoformans* by immunofluorescence. J Clin Microbiol 1981; 14:313–317.
8. Kaufman L, Reiss E: Serodiagnosis of fungal diseases. *In* Rose NR, de Macario EC, Fahey JL, et al: Manual of Clinical Laboratory Immunology, 4th ed. Washington, DC, American Society for Microbiology, 1992, pp 506–527.
9. Kaufman L, Standard PG: Specific and rapid identification of medically important fungi by exoantigen detection. Annu Rev Microbiol 1987; 41:209–225.
10. Koneman EW, Allen SD, Janda WM, et al: Mycology. *In* Color Atlas and Textbook of Diagnostic Microbiology, 4th ed. Philadelphia, JB Lippincott, 1992, pp 791–877.
11. Koneman EW, Roberts GD (eds): Mycotic diseases. *In* Henry JB: Clinical Diagnosis and Management by Laboratory Methods, 19th ed. Philadelphia, WB Saunders, 1996, pp 1099–1157.
12. Koneman EW, Roberts GD: Practical Laboratory Mycology, 3rd ed. Baltimore, Williams & Wilkins, 1985.
13. Kwon-Chung KJ, Bennett JE: Medical Mycology. Philadelphia, Lea & Febiger, 1992.
14. Larone DH: Medically Important Fungi: A Guide to Identification, 2nd ed. New York, Elsevier, 1987.
15. McGinnis MR: Laboratory Handbook of Medical Mycology. New York, Academic Press, 1980.
16. McGinnis MR, Tilton RC: Immunologic diagnosis of fungal infection. *In* Howard BJ, Keiser JF, Smith TF, et al (eds): Clinical and Pathogenic Microbiology, 2nd ed. St. Louis, CV Mosby, 1994, pp 541–545.
17. Miller LE, et al: Manual of Laboratory Immunology, Infectious Disease Serology, (C) Fungal infections, 2nd ed. Philadelphia, Lea & Febiger, 1991, pp 291–306.
18. Murphy N, Buchanan CR, Damjanovic V, et al: Infection and colonization of neonates by *Hansenula anomala*. Lancet 1986; 1:291–293.
19. Pappaglanis D, Zimmer BI: Serology of coccidioidomycosis. Clin Microbiol Rev 1990; 3(3):247–268.
20. Rinaldi MG: Use of potato flake agar in medical mycology. J Clin Microbiol 1982; 15(6):1159–1160.
21. Rippon JW: Medical Mycology: The Pathogenic Fungi and Pathogenic Actinomycetes, 3rd ed. Philadelphia, WB Saunders, 1988.
22. Roberts G: Laboratory methods in basic mycology. *In* Baron EJ, Lance RP, Finegold SM (eds): Bailey and Scott's Diagnostic Microbiology, 9th ed. St. Louis, CV Mosby, 1994.
23. Rogers AL, Cole GT, Rippon JW, McGinnis MR: Identification of Saprophytic Fungi Commonly Encountered in a Clinical Environment Workshop Publication sponsored by the American Society for Microbiology. Washington, DC, 1988.
24. Sekhonm AS, Standard PG: Reliability of exoantigens for differentiation of blastomycosis, histoplasmosis, and coccidiomycosis. Diagn Microbiol Infect Dis 1986; 4:221–232.
25. Wheat LJ: Diagnosis and management of histoplasmosis. Eur J Clin Microbiol Infect Dis 1989; 8(5):480–490.

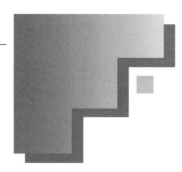

Index

Note: Page numbers in *italics* refer to illustrations.
Page numbers followed by (t) refer to tables.
Page numbers followed by (d) refer to definitions of glossary terms.

A

Abscesses, cutaneous, due to blastomycosis, 235
  exudate from, 14
Absidia species, 90-91
  differentiation of, from other members of Zygomycetes class, *89*, 92(t)
  macroscopic (colony) morphology of, 90
  microscopic morphology of, *89*, 90, *91*, Color Plate 12
Accidents, precautions against. See *Laboratory, safety precautions in.*
Acremonium species, 43-44
  differentiation of, from fungi of similar appearance, 45(t), *46, 185*
    from other fungi with multiple arrangements of conidia, 176(t)
  infection by, 43
  macroscopic (colony) morphology of, 43
  microscopic morphology of, *43*, 43-44, *44, 46*
Acropetal conidiogeny, 267(d)
Acrotheca-type conidiation (rhinocladiella-type conidiation), 161-162, *162*, 267(d), 284(d)
Actidione (cycloheximide), 23-24, 267(d)
Actinomycotic, 267(d)
Actinomycotic mycetoma, 158
Adiaspore, 267(d)
Adiaspormycosis, 59, 267(d)
Aerial hyphae, 4, *4*, 267(d)
Agar. See also particular media, e.g., *Cornmeal–Tween 80 agar.*
  preparation of, 322-323
  use of wetting agents in, 323
Aleuric release, 267(d)
  of conidia, from conidiophores of *Nigrospora* species, 75
Alopecia, 121, 267(d)
Alternaria species, 44, 47
  distinctiveness of, 47, *47*
  infection by, 44
  macroscopic (colony) morphology of, 47
  microscopic morphology of, 47, *47*, Color Plate 1
Anamorph(s), 2, 6, 7(t), 267(d). See also *Synanamorph(s).*

Anamorph(s) *(Continued)*
  of *Aureobasidium pullulans, Syctalidium* as, *57, 57*
  of *Exophiala jeanselmei, Phaeoannellomyces* as, 169, 177
  of *Pseudallescheria boydii, Graphium* as, 179, 180, 181, 242(t)
    Scedosporium apiospermum as, 160, 179, 180, 181, *181*, 242(t), *243*
  of *Wangiella (Exophiala) dermatitidis, Phaeococcomyces* as, 177, 186
Anergic patient, 28-29
Anergy, 267(d)
Annellation, 38, 163, 267(d)
Annellides (indeterminate conidiogenous cells), 37-38, *38*, 267(d), 278(d)
  of *Exophiala werneckii*, 106, *107*
  vs. phialides, *162*, 163
Annellidic conidiation, *162*
Annelloconidia, 38, 267(d)
Annellophores, 267(d)
  of *Exophiala werneckii*, 106, *107*
  of *Scopulariopsis* species, 82
Annular frills, on conidia, 267(d)
  of *Chrysosporium* species, 62, *62*
Antibiotic, 23, 268(d)
Antibodies, detection of. See *Immunologic testing.*
Antigenemia, 268(d)
  Aspergillus fumigatus and, 49
Antimicrobial agent, 23, 268(d)
Antimycotic agent, 23, 28, 268(d)
Apex (apices), 268(d)
Apiculate, 268(d)
Apiculate conidiogenous cells, surrounding ascospores of *Hansenula anomala*, 217
Apophysis, 88, 268(d)
Apothecium, 7, 8, 268(d)
Arthralgia, coccidioidomycosis and, 238
Arthroconidia, 111, 268(d)
  of *Coccidioides immitis*, 245, *245*
    disjuncture cells between, 246
Ascocarp, 7, 8, 268(d)
Ascomycetes, 8
  infection of hair by. See *Piedraia hortae.*
Ascomycetous yeasts and yeastlike organisms, 217-218, 220

Ascospores, *9*, 268(d)
  of *Hansenula anomala*, 217
Ascostroma, 8, 268(d)
Ascus (asci), 268(d)
  of *Hansenula anomala*, 217
Aseptate, 268(d)
Aseptate hyphae, 4, *4*
  saprobes with, 92(t)
Asexual reproduction, 6, 268(d)
Aspergilloma, 36, 268(d)
Aspergillosis, 36-37, 48, 268(d)
  immunologic testing for, 48(t), 48-49, 235(t)
Aspergillus flavus, 50, 53-54
  differentiation of, from other *Aspergillus* species, 51(t), *52*
    from *Scopulariopsis* species, 51(t)
  infection by, 50
  macroscopic (colony) morphology of, 53
  microscopic morphology of, *52*, 53, *53*
Aspergillus fumigatus, 47-50
  differentiation of, from other *Aspergillus* species, 51(t), *52*
    from *Scopulariopsis* species, 51(t)
    from *Syncephalastrum* species, *98*
  infection by, 36-37, 48
    immunologic testing for, 48(t), 48-49, 235(t)
  macroscopic (colony) morphology of, 49
  microscopic morphology of, *49*, 49-50, *50, 52*, Color Plate 2
Aspergillus niger, 54-55
  differentiation of, from other *Aspergillus* species, 51(t), *52*
    from *Scopulariopsis* species, 51(t)
  infection by, 54
  macroscopic (colony) morphology of, 54
  microscopic morphology of, *52*, 54, *54, 55*, Color Plate 3
Aspergillus species, 48, *48*
  biseriate, 48, *48*, 269(d)
  differentiation among, 51(t), *52*
  uniseriate, 48, *48*
Aspergillus terreus, 55-56
  differentiation of, from other *Aspergillus* species, 51(t), *52*
    from *Scopulariopsis* species, 51(t)

352   Index

Trichosporon beigelii, 112, 114
  biochemical reactions aiding identification of, 206(t)-207(t)
  differentiation of, from other superficial fungi, 105, 113(t)
  infection of hair by, 104, *104,* 104(t), 112, 122(t)
  macroscopic (colony) morphology of, 112, 209(t)
  microscopic morphology of, 112, *114,* 209(t), Color Plate 16
Trichosporon species. See also *Trichosporon beigelii.*
  differentiation of, from *Coccidioides immitis,* 216
    from *Geotrichum candidum,* 216
Trophozoites, 289(d)
  of *Pneumocystis carinii,* 218
"True" pathogens, fungi acting as. See *Pathogenic fungi.*
Truncate, 289(d)
Truncate microconidia, of *Trichophyton tonsurans,* 148
Tuberculariaceae, contaminant/opportunistic, 66-70
Tuberculate, 290(d)
Tuberculate conidia, 62
Tuberculate macroconidia, of *Histoplasma capsulatum,* 249
Tumefaction, 290(d)
  boggy, 121

U

Ulocladium species, vs. other dematiaceous saprobes with globose conidia, 69(t)
Unguium, 290(d). See also *Nail(s).*
Uniseriate, 290(d)
Uniseriate species, of *Aspergillus,* 48, *48*
Urinary tract, specimen collection from, 15(t)

V

V-8 vegetable juice agar, as culture medium, 340-341
Vagina, specimen collection from, 15(t)
Vaginitis, candidal, 198
Valley fever, 238, 290(d). See also *Coccidioidomycosis.*
Vegetative hyphae, *4,* 290(d)
Velvety texture (suede texture), of fungal colonies, 25, *26,* 287(d), 290(d)
Vermiform, 290(d)
Vermiform appearance, of granules, 44
Verrucoid, 290(d)

Verrucoid nodules, chromoblastomycosis and, 159
Verrucose topography, of fungal colonies, 26, *27,* 290(d)
Verticillium species, vs. other fungi resembling *Acremonium,* 45(t), *46*
Vesicle(s), 290(d)
  denticulated, at apices of conidiophores, of *Sporothrix schenckii,* 183
  fluid in, 120
  globose, of conidiophores of *Aspergillus species,* 53

W

Wangiella (Exophiala) dermatitidis, 186-187
  biologic tests for, 165(t)
  differentiation of, from other dematiaceous fungi with conidia in clusters, 172(t)
    from superficial fungi, 109(t)
  infection by, 186
    cyst due to, findings in specimen from, *160*
  macroscopic (colony) morphology of, 186
  microscopic morphology of, *186,* 186-187, *187*
Phaeococcomyces anamorph of, 177, 186
Water, addition of agar to, 323
  sterile, storage of cultures in, 328-329
Wet preparations (wet mounts), 19, 290(d), 330-331
  from specimens using KOH (potassium hydroxide), 331-332
  from yeast colonies, 331
White piedra, 104, *104,* 104(t), 112, 122(t), 290(d). See also *Trichosporon beigelii.*
Wood's lamp, 105, 290(d)
Woolly (cottony, floccose) texture, of fungal colonies, 25, *26,* 272(d), 275(d), 290(d)
Work sheets, for assessment of dimorphic fungi, *296, 304*
  for evaluation of monomorphic moulds, *295, 300*
  for identification of monomorphic yeasts, *297, 307*
Wright-Giemsa stain, 20, 290(d)

X

Xylohypha bantiana, 188-189
  biochemical tests for, 165(t)
  differentiation of, from other dematiaceous fungi with chains of conidia, *167,* 168(t)
  infection by, 188

Xylohypha bantiana (Continued)
  macroscopic (colony) morphology of, 188
  microscopic morphology of, *188,* 188-189, *189,* Color Plate 22

Y

Yeastlike texture, of fungal colonies, 25, *26*
Yeasts/yeastlike organisms, 5, 196-225, 240(t)-241(t), 290(d)
  black, 109(t), 177
  chlamydospores produced by, 201, *201*
  differentiation among, 202, 206(t)-209(t), *223-225, 200,* 239, 240(t)-241(t)
  germ tubes in, 202, *202*
  laboratory identification of, 198-202, 206(t)-209(t)
    assimilation tests in, 200, 207(t)
    cornmeal–Tween 80 agar in, 200, 201, 202, 206(t), 208(t)-209(t), 240(t)-241(t)
    detection of *Candida albicans* in, 202, 206(t)-207(t)
    detection of *Cryptococcus neoformans* in, 200, *200,* 206(t)-207(t)
    fermentation tests in, 200, 207(t)
    morphology in, 200-201. See also *Yeasts/yeastlike organisms, differentiation among.*
      macroscopic vs. microscopic. See *microscopic* and *macroscopic* subentries under particular fungi.
  purification of culture in, 325
  subculture in, 330
  wet preparations for, 331
  worksheet for, *297, 307*
  pseudohyphae produced by, 197, *197,* 200, *200*

Z

Zygomycetes, contaminant/opportunistic, 37, 38, 86-98
  sporangia of, 88, *88, 89,* 92(t)
  sporangiophores of, 88, *88, 89*
    columellae on, 88, *88, 89,* 90, 92(t)
    internodal, 88, 278(d)
    length and arrangement of, 92(t)
    nodal, 88, 281(d)
  sporangiospores of, 38, 88, *88, 89,* 92(t)
Zygomycosis (mucormycosis), 37, 87, 280(d), 290(d)
Zygosporangium, 291(d)
Zygospore, 8, 291(d)